Handbook of Research on Health and Environmental Benefits of Camel Products

Omar Amin Alhaj
University of Petra, Jordan

Bernard Faye
Independent Researcher, France

Rajendra Prasad Agrawal
Independent Researcher, India

A volume in the Practice, Progress, and Proficiency in Sustainability (PPPS) Book Series

Published in the United States of America by
IGI Global
Medical Information Science Reference (an imprint of IGI Global)
701 E. Chocolate Avenue
Hershey PA, USA 17033
Tel: 717-533-8845
Fax: 717-533-8661
E-mail: cust@igi-global.com
Web site: http://www.igi-global.com

Library of Congress Cataloging-in-Publication Data

Names: Alhaj, Omar Amin, 1979- editor. | Faye, Bernard, editor. | Agrawal, Rajendra Prasad, 1957- editor.
Title: Handbook of research on health and environmental benefits of camel products / Omar Amin Alhaj, Bernard Faye, Rajendra Prasad Agrawal, editors.
Description: Hershey, PA : Medical Information Science Reference, [2020] | Includes bibliographical references and index. | Summary: "This book discusses the nutritional, physical, and chemical factors of camel milk in comparison to other animal and plant-based milks and introduces benefits attributed to camel meat. It explores the health benefits of fresh and fermented camel milk in vitro and in vivo as well as the link between functional constituents and the functional properties of milk"-- Provided by publisher.
Identifiers: LCCN 2019031888 (print) | LCCN 2019031889 (ebook) | ISBN 9781799816041 (hardcover) | ISBN 9781799816058 (ebook)
Subjects: MESH: Camelus | Milk | Meat
Classification: LCC SF401.C2 (print) | LCC SF401.C2 (ebook) | NLM WB 428 | DDC 338.1/76295--dc23
LC record available at https://lccn.loc.gov/2019031888
LC ebook record available at https://lccn.loc.gov/2019031889

This book is published in the IGI Global book series Practice, Progress, and Proficiency in Sustainability (PPPS) (ISSN: 2330-3271; eISSN: 2330-328X)

British Cataloguing in Publication Data
A Cataloguing in Publication record for this book is available from the British Library.

Practice, Progress, and Proficiency in Sustainability (PPPS) Book Series

Ayman Batisha
International Sustainability Institute, Egypt

ISSN:2330-3271
EISSN:2330-328X

Mission

In a world where traditional business practices are reconsidered and economic activity is performed in a global context, new areas of economic developments are recognized as the key enablers of wealth and income production. This knowledge of information technologies provides infrastructures, systems, and services towards sustainable development.

The **Practices, Progress, and Proficiency in Sustainability (PPPS) Book Series** focuses on the local and global challenges, business opportunities, and societal needs surrounding international collaboration and sustainable development of technology. This series brings together academics, researchers, entrepreneurs, policy makers and government officers aiming to contribute to the progress and proficiency in sustainability.

Coverage

- Green Technology
- Outsourcing
- Sustainable Development
- Global Business
- Eco-Innovation
- Strategic Management of IT
- E-Development
- ICT and knowledge for development
- Innovation Networks
- Environmental informatics

IGI Global is currently accepting manuscripts for publication within this series. To submit a proposal for a volume in this series, please contact our Acquisition Editors at Acquisitions@igi-global.com or visit: http://www.igi-global.com/publish/.

The Practice, Progress, and Proficiency in Sustainability (PPPS) Book Series (ISSN 2330-3271) is published by IGI Global, 701 E. Chocolate Avenue, Hershey, PA 17033-1240, USA, www.igi-global.com. This series is composed of titles available for purchase individually; each title is edited to be contextually exclusive from any other title within the series. For pricing and ordering information please visit http://www.igi-global.com/book-series/practice-progress-proficiency-sustainability/73810. Postmaster: Send all address changes to above address.

Titles in this Series

For a list of additional titles in this series, please visit: www.igi-global.com/book-series

Implications of Mobility as a Service (MaaS) in Urban and Rural Environments
António Manuel Amaral (University of Minho, Portugal) Luís Barreto (ESCE-IPVC, Portugal) Sara Baltazar (ESCE-IPVC, Portugal) João Pedro Silva (IPLeiria, Portugal) and Luísa Gonçalves (IPLeiria, ortugal)
Engineering Science Reference • ©2020 • 200pp • H/C (ISBN: 9781799816140) • US $150.00

Social, Economic, and Environmental Impacts Between Sustainable Financial Systems and Financial Markets
Magdalena Ziolo (University of Szczecin, Poland)
Business Science Reference • ©2020 • 383pp • H/C (ISBN: 9781799810339) • US $245.00

Developing and Designing Circular Cities Emerging Research and Opportunities
Elżbieta Ryńska (Warsaw University of Technology, Poland)
Engineering Science Reference • ©2020 • 150pp • H/C (ISBN: 9781799818861) • US $135.00

Technological Innovations for Sustainability and Business Growth
Geetika Jain (UP Technical University, Lucknow, India) Harjit Singh (Amity University, Noida, India) Shahriar Akter (University of Wollongong, Australia) Alka Munjal (Amity University, Noida, India) and Harpal S. Grewal (Claflin University, USA)
Business Science Reference • ©2020 • 338pp • H/C (ISBN: 9781522599401) • US $225.00

Handbook of Research on the Conservation and Restoration of Tropical Dry Forests
Rahul Bhadouria (University of Delhi, India) Sachchidanand Tripathi (University of Delhi, India) Pratap Srivastava (University of Allahabad, India) and Pardeep Singh (University of Delhi, India)
Engineering Science Reference • ©2020 • 465pp • H/C (ISBN: 9781799800149) • US $295.00

Innovative Waste Management Technologies for Sustainable Development
Rouf Ahmad Bhat (Sri Pratap College, India) Humaira Qadri (Sri Pratap College, India & Cluster University Srinagar, India) Khursheed Ahmad Wani (Government Degree College Bijbehara, India) Gowhar Hamid Dar (Sri Pratap College, India & Cluster University Srinagar, India) and Mohammad Aneesul Mehmood (Sri Pratap College, India & Cluster University Srinagar, India)
Engineering Science Reference • ©2020 • 373pp • H/C (ISBN: 9781799800316) • US $195.00

Global Approaches to Sustainability Through Learning and Education
Abdalmuttaleb M.A. Musleh Al-Sartawi (Ahlia University, Bahrain) Khaled Hussainey (University of Portsmouth, UK) Azzam Hannoon (American University in the Emirates, UAE) and Allam Hamdan (Ahlia University, Bahrain)
Information Science Reference • ©2020 • 350pp • H/C (ISBN: 9781799800620) • US $195.00

IGI Global
DISSEMINATOR OF KNOWLEDGE

701 East Chocolate Avenue, Hershey, PA 17033, USA
Tel: 717-533-8845 x100 • Fax: 717-533-8661
E-Mail: cust@igi-global.com • www.igi-global.com

This book is dedicated to:

My mother, the first school of life, who taught me the life, your lessons live on;

My father who planted the seeds of knowledge and innovation within me;

My endless love "wife" for her patience, combination and kind support throughout writing and editing of this book, I love you today and forever, I am proud of you;

My family and joy of life: Aya, Abdullah, Dana, Ibrahim, and Talya, I am grateful you are in my life; your smile warms my heart and fill it with love;

Finally, to you, the passionate professional and readers of this book, whom have dedicated your time to read this book, my wish is that this book expand your knowledge in all topics related to Handbook of Research on Health and Environmental Benefits of Camel Products.

Omar Alhaj

List of Contributors

Table of Contents

Detailed Table of Contents

This chapter aimed to report the strategies and technologies for camel milk preservation. Raw camel milk is easily spoiled owing to its nutrient content, which provides an ideal substrate for the development of microorganisms. Several traditional methods have been conducted in order to increase the shelf life of camel milk including fumigation of milk containers, simple evaporative cooling, chilling, freezing, pasteurization, and milk processing into many products like fermented camel milk, butter, and ghee. Modern technologies are used nowadays to preserve camel milk including freeze-drying, spray drying, high hydrostatic pressure, and sterilization. Besides, many value-added products are produced like yoghurt, cheese, ice cream, snacks, and camel milk protein hydrolysates, which are used in the field of functional food and nutraceuticals. The non-marketed camel milk is sold at a lower price or consumed at the household level in tea or after processing it into naturally fermented milk.

Camel milk provides a common source of nutrition but also a potential rich source of beneficial, pathogenic, and potentially pathogenic microorganisms. This chapter reviews lactic acid and probiotic bacteria from camel milk, product innovation using such bacteria, and potential areas of improvement in technical as well as practical aspects of fermentation technologies. Lactic acid bacteria fermentation helps mitigate the impact of poor handling and storage conditions by enhancing shelf life and food safety. Traditionally-fermented sour milk products are culturally accepted and widely distributed worldwide with product-specific microbiota responsible for aroma, flavor, and texture. Knowledge of microbiota and predominant, technologically important microorganisms associated with camel milk is critical in developing products with enhanced quality and safety, as well as sustainable interventions for these products, including camel milk specific starter culture development. This chapter presents occurrence of LAB and probiotic bacteria in camel milk and technological aspects of camel dairy.

Camel milk is popular in the world as it has an excellent nutritive value and many health benefits. There are many dairy and non-dairy products that could be manufactured from camel milk such as milk powder, UHT-milk, yogurt and fermented products, cream, ghee, ice-cream, frozen products, sweets, and candy (such as chocolate bars and cookies). In general, camel milk processing encounters challenges. This chapter is aimed to cover the recent issues of the manufacturing and processing of the most popular above-mentioned camel milk products based on the recent studies and other available commercial resources. Camel milk seems to have many challenges during high temperature treatment as well as creaming to manufacture yogurt and other fermented dairy products, cream, and butter. On the other hand, ice cream and frozen yogurt and chocolate bar manufacturing from camel milk seems to be less challenging. Further research is recommended to solve the faced challenges and to develop different versions of these products such as skim, low fat, low sugar, and flavored products.

The difficulties in camel milk coagulation due to low concentration in κ-casein was the main obstacle for its processing into cheese. Thus, for 80 years, camel scientists concentrated their efforts on improving coagulation by different methods including use of plant or camel calf abomasum extracts. However, in all cases, poor cheese yield and organoleptic properties were obtained. The recent introduction of the CHY-Max – M1000®, on market solved the problem of clotting. Obtained by genetic engineering, this camel rennet allows high cheese yield. However, other challenges must be met: (1) investigation by fundamental studies of the "behavior" of camel milk during the different steps of cheese processing, (2) to set up final products corresponding to food preferences of local consumers, (3) to ensure transfer of camel cheese technology to camel dairy industry. Based on experiences in different camel countries, the chapter is taking stock of the challenges regarding technological development, cultural satisfaction, and commercialization of camel cheese.

This chapter highlights the potential health benefits of camel milk including antioxidant, anti-cancer activity, antihypertensive properties, antidiabetic activity, antimicrobial activity, hypoallergenicity activity, and anti-Crohn's disease. In addition to the most recent identified functional properties of camel milk. The bioactivity of conjugated linoleic acid (CLA), D and L amino acid, as well as oligosaccharide in camel milk will be also discussed. The proposed mechanisms behind these properties and potential health benefits are explained. This chapter also describes composition and nutritive value of camel milk and their association to functional properties. The current available information in the literature on camel milk is covered too.

Camel milk has been used as part of the human diet since ancient times. This chapter tries to elaborate the different aspects of nutraceutical functional properties of camel milk, focusing on the nutritional composition, presence of bioactive zoochemicals and peptides, antioxidant nutrients (vitamin C), and health rendering properties of this unique milk. Recent research has identified camel milk as a prophylactic and therapeutic functional food due to its noticeable content of essential macronutrients, namely bioactive functional proteins and peptides, along with its considerable content of essential micronutrients. Indeed, the presence of this unique mixture has shown to be promising contributors to the management and prevention of chronic diseases, such as cancer, diabetes, liver and kidney, metabolic syndrome, inflammatory bowel diseases in adults, and autism. In vivo, in vitro, and epidemiological and experimental studies were reviewed, and molecular mechanisms were highlighted for better understanding of the health-promoting, disease-preventing potential of camel milk.

Based on empirical observations regarding the low prevalence of diabetes mellitus in population drinking regularly camel milk, camel scientists have investigated and assessed the effect of regular camel milk consumption on glycaemic status of diabetic patients and animal models. All the experiments' results concluded to the reduction of blood glucose and glycosylated haemoglobin. The hypothesis of high quantity of natural insulin in camel milk was proposed, but the quantities reported in the literature could not explain by itself the beneficial effect of camel milk consumption. It is stated that the lack of coagulum formation of camel milk the stomach was supposed to act as an effective vehicle (under internal nanoparticles) to take the milk insulin unchanged throughout the digestive tract and absorbed in the intestine. Other proteins in higher concentrations in camel milk than in other milk could interact with insulin receptor and contribute by their antioxidant and inti-inflammatory effect to regeneration of beta-cells in pancreas.

Camel milk has a comparable gross composition with other milk sources including bovine milk with some minor differences in the molecular properties of proteins and fat. The limited amount of β-Lg and κ-Casein(CN) are involved in heat denaturation via formation of disulfide bridges in cow milk; their absence in camel milk result in different responses for heat treatment at different scale. Furthermore, differences between camel milk proteins compared to other milk resulted poor coagulation and reduce stability during processing of dairy products such as yogurt and cheese. The effect of different thermal processing methods on camel milk were discussed; however, high pressure processing (HPP) study on processing effect on camel milk is an area of research for more confirmation in-depth study. The industrial processing methods were found to effect important camel milk properties, nutritional values, and health properties compared to other animals including limiting bioactive proteins such as immunoglobulin, lactoferrin, lysozyme, and vitamins. This effect depends on the type of heat treatment applied.

generally contains less fat and ash, more moisture, and similar protein content. Camel meat products are receiving worldwide interest owing to its unique healthy features and the ability of camels to thrive in climatic regions of the world that may be a challenge to many other meat-producing species. Camel meat products contain many essential nutrients and some components with potential bioactive properties that could be beneficial for human health and wellbeing. Continued improvements in the understanding and optimization of the production processes of camel meat are required for successful industrial implementation and marketing. Advances in ingredient systems may be used to manufacture new meat products from camel meat where higher levels of nutrition are required to enhance consumer health and wellbeing. Camel meat as a functional food is one area that can be exploited.

Irwandi Jaswir, International Islamic University Malaysia, Malaysia
Hassan Abdullah Al-Kahtani, King Saud University, Saudi Arabia
Fitri Octavianti, Avicenna Dental Clinic, Malaysia
Widya Lestari, International Islamic University Malaysia, Malaysia
Nurlina Yusof, International Islamic University Malaysia, Malaysia

Gelatin is an important protein produced through partial hydrolysis of collagen from animal parts and byproducts such as cartilage, bones, tendons, and hides. The ability of gelatin to form a thermo-reversible gel at normal body temperature and high water content make it an exceptional food ingredient. A good quality gelatin is translucent, brittle, colorless (sometimes slightly yellow), bland in taste, and odorless. Gelatin has been found useful as stabilizer and filler in dairy products and other food industries. Recently, the global gelatin production net over 300,000 metric tons: 46% were from pigskin, 29.4% from bovine hides, 23.1% from bones, and 1.5% from other parts. Although camels have been recognized as source of meat and milk, utilization of camel bones and skins for gelatin production has not been fully explored. This chapter will discuss the processing of camel gelatin extraction.

Surong Hasi, Inner Mongolia Agricultural University, China
Guleng Amu, Inner Mongolia Agricultural University, China
Wenbin Zhang, Bactrian Camel Institute of Alxa, China

The camel coat can be divided into upper and lower layers based on the external shape. The upper layer is sparse and upright coarse wool; the lower layer is thick wool, which is mainly composed of camel cashmere mixed with small amount of coarse hair. This chapter introduces the basic characteristics of camel hair, such as morphological structure, microstructure, fiber type, and density. Then it introduces the process characteristics of camel wool, the net wool rate, camel hair grades, the photometric and thermodynamic properties of camel cashmere. Finally it gives some camel cashmere and hair products. All contents try to give detailed experimental data and images and insist on giving a more comprehensive and scientific explanation for camel hair.

This chapter conveys the untapped property of camel milk as cosmeceutical. The camel milk ingredients (i.e., water, ascorbic acid, alpha hydroxy acid, polyunsaturated fatty acid, peptides, and micronutrients) make it a cost-effective cosmeceutical with no adverse cutaneous or systemic reactions. It may be used as a photoprotective, moisturizing, anti-wrinkle, anti-aging skin softener. The bioactive ingredients may begin the new class of natural cosmeceutical when consumed orally or applied topically.

The close adaptation of camel to its desert environment could explain its weak expansion out of the arid lands of the world. This adaptation can contribute to the desertification combat, attesting to its small ecological footprint with traditional extensive farming. The camel population in the world, despite its active growth, remains marginal, and its contribution to the greenhouse gas emission is negligible. However, the current trends to the intensification of camel productions could change the impact of the species on the environment and on animal metabolism. The necessity to expect a better productivity face to the growing demand could lead to a "specialization" of the camel farms and a specific selection of the camel. Such trends require care with a possible erosion of the camel biodiversity and the consequences on the interactions between the emerging camel production system and the environment.

Foreword

For several thousands of years, camels have been domesticated and used for their fresh and fermented milk, their meat and other by-products as textile materials. In the last few decades, the importance of camel milk and the emphasis on its economic and therapeutic properties have been a focal point for much of the research worldwide. This book with its title "Health and Environmental Benefits of Camel Products" is an excellent reflection to the importance of this subject. It covers a wide range of topics of interest to those involved in the economic, social, scientific and technological aspect of camel husbandry, the derived products and the environment. Its comprehensive reporting includes milk production, processing, its chemical and microbiological properties, meat production and other uses. This stimulating book adds to the already existing knowledge but with more comprehensive reporting backed with relevant research findings by imminent scientist in their field across many countries.

Consumers' interest in camel milk in the last few decades, especially in more economically developed countries, has been mainly due to its perceived, and to some degree, experienced health benefits which have been well addressed. The health benefits cover the recent research about its role in ameliorating certain health concerns such as diabetes, cardiovascular diseases by reducing blood pressure through its ACE inhibitory action, antioxidant, anti-inflammatory and many other functions, with yet to be clinically proven its role in reducing the symptoms of autism. Its immune modulating and hypoallergenic property makes camel milk a good alternative source to cow milk based on their chemical composition regarding certain casein and whey protein fractions.

This is an interesting multi-authored textbook which has been written and edited by academics and research scientists. The editors and the contributors of the 17 chapters covered the subjects very well, complimenting each other, filling some research gaps in the nature and the functionality of the milk with some suggestion for future research. There are good range and up to date references for each chapter that are of importance to readers interested to investigate further research in this field. This book is a vital additional source and is highly recommended as a good basis of information for those already working in the field, for academics, university students, industrialist and business minded people to enhance their knowledge about this subject.

Ara Kanekanian
Independent Researcher, UK

Foreword

***Ara Kanekanian** has been in academia for 30 years with main interest in protein chemistry, bioactive compounds and probiotics. He is a member of editorial boards of several International journals and published several scientific as well as technical papers. He participated as keynote speaker to many international biotechnology conferences in the US, Europe and the Middle East. He worked in the food industry and undertook several consultancy and turnkey projects for food and dairy processing within Europe and the Middle East. He has run several training programmes for industrialists and large retail managers. Recently, worked in the development of dairy technology in collaboration with "Dairy Solutions Training" in the UK. He worked as consultant for USDA for developing new food technology curriculum for Caucus Countries.*

Preface

The increasing number of existing textbooks, monographs and scientific journals suggest that the field of camel history, behaviour, and products have huge scientific output. These different aspects of the subject to date have received little or no interest as these are relatively unexplained sciences but this is no longer the case. The large scientific knowledge in these fields coupled with impressive social interest is stimulating a new and fascinating challenge for scientists. However, we are sure that this textbook shall provide researchers worldwide with a platform of recent research and great interest for scientists, academicians, students and specialists alike.

This issue of *Handbook of Research on Health and Environmental Benefits of Camel Products* provides a collection of articles that describe our current understanding on the camel habitat and products. It contributes also efficiently to response to the growing interest of camel stakeholders and large public for camel milk, meat and wool.

There has been an important growth of convenient information on this subject over the past few years that offers many exciting opportunities for investigator, scientist and the people at large. We would therefore, like to thank all the contributing authors for their exclusive and scholarly reviews and for sharing their wisdom. I hope you will enjoy their perspective and incorporate the information into your practice and research. At the end of the chapter, our contributors have provided carefully selected references.

The enormous responsibility of preparing and publishing a textbook on educative and scientific knowledge of camel products is nothing but a monumental task. The consistent and persistent persuasion of our editorial team shall make this book very useful in the pursuit of longer motive and movement.

The chapters in this book have been written by a number of reputed international experts on the field. All these chapters are thoroughly revised with updated information. We also have earned much in the process of editing and hope that you shall find this book uniquely valuable as an educational resource. The textbook is only a beginning in the process of covering the incredible work that is going on around the world on the subject. It is the most befitting time to share our respective experiences, so that other providers may also get benefit in pursuit of their knowledge on the subject.

The editors and authors have been able to present this highly readable, informative and comprehensive book through rigorously curating and synthesizing the vast amount of updated information available on the subject. Editors really privileged to have the opportunity of compiling such a valuable book named *Health and Environmental Benefits of Camel Products.*

The first chapter, "Historical Background, and Population of Camels," provides us with some introductory remarks on the historical background, and population of camels. In this chapter, the origin of camels based on the most recent mitochondrial genome analyses and incisor fossils have been reviewed.

Different genus and species of camels are also presented. Additionally, the distribution of camel population worldwide as well as its uses are reported. This chapter also introduces some essential figures on economic value of camels based on the most recent statistics of the "Food and Agricultural Organization (FAO)". Though the camels have a long history and recent findings based on genomic research give new light on the origin of camels Organizations, whether local or international, are encouraged to estimate the data related to this animal, especially, the production, yield, and manufacture of different camel-based food products.

In the chapter "Camel Milk Composition and Nutritional Value," comprehensive composition and variation factors of camel milk composition have been explored along with comparison other animal milks. The latest knowledge regarding composition of camel milk has created with an interest in the scientists, the world over. The belief regarding the true or supposed "Medicinal Virtues" of camel milk is obviously an important motivation to deepen our knowledge on the finer composition of this remarkable product of the nature.

In the chapter "Strategies and Technologies for Camel Milk Preservation," the different strategies and technologies for camel milk preservation are detailed. The author stated that camel milk is an important source of essential nutrients. Consequently, there is a big need to preserve this worthily called "The White Gold of the Desert". The traditional methods include cooling, pasteurization and processing of camel milk. Numerous modern processes like freeze-drying, spray drying, high hydrostatic pressure and sterilization are being applied to preserve camel milk.

But, strategies and technologies for camel milk preservation are still limited and warrant further investigations. It is necessary to optimize and design a spray drying operation, which will result in desired physicochemical and functional properties of camel milk powder. The shelf life of camel milk that undergoes high hydrostatic pressure procedure should be determined. The effect of the addition of various plant extracts or their essential oils as preservatives to camel milk and its derived products should be well investigated. Besides, new value-added products from camel milk with long shelf life have to be made by the dairy industry to increase its availability.

The chapter "Microbial Aspect of Lactic Acid Bacteria Isolated From Camel Milk" reveals wide diversity of dairy products depending on agricultural practices, animal husbandry, seasonality, agro-ecological zones, animal species, stage of commercialization or industrialization, food preferences and cultural practices. These factors also influence the camel dairy microbiota. This chapter presents the occurrence of lactic acid bacteria and probiotic bacteria in camel milk; developments in typing and characterization; a high technological potential provided by a rich diversity of organisms. The traditional and modern practices for camel milk fermentation as well as constraints and opportunities are furnished for further innovation.

Knowledge of microbiome predominance, and technologically important microorganisms associated with camel milk is critical in developing products with enhanced quality and safety, as well as for its importance in development of sustainable interventions for these products, including development of novel camel milk specific starter cultures. The chapter concludes that the scale and technology of production, as well as marketing and distribution systems need have to be applied at industrial level. Demand for fermented food products is rising due to the health benefits associated with these products, as also due to migration, and urbanization. The increased demand by consumers calls for improvement in the safety and quality of fermented food products.

The chapter "Manufacturer of Dairy and Non-Dairy Camel Milk Products" presents better understanding, opportunities and tools in dairy manufacturing and production. Dairy products manufactured from camel milk are known to represent a source of energy and nutrients and probably replace fruits and vegetables for people who live in the harsh conditions of deserts. Several dairy and non-dairy camel milk products have been developed and standardized using different methods of preparation or production. This chapter covers the recent processing methods, and views on the most popular camel milk products as on the recent studies and other available commercial resources.

Dairy products and non-dairy products are successfully manufactured from camel milk at the experimental or commercial levels but other products are still facing processing challenges and encountering many difficulties compared with cow and sheep milk. The difficulties are the sensitivity of camel milk to high temperature treatment, hygienic conditions, poor stability, and short shelf life.

The physio-chemical properties of camel milk make it difficult to coagulate. Recent advances have been obtained in camel cheese processing in different parts of the world. These recent and significant advances are presented in chapter "Manufacture and Challenges of Camel Milk Cheese". In this chapter, the author has gone through the challenges like getting firm coagulum and camel cheese processing at a large scale. The author remarks that if the cheese made from cow or sheep's milk can claim of an experience of several millennia, the camel cheese is only at the beginning of its history and its development. Producers, developers, dairy plant managers, and scientists must work together to put camel cheese out of its present marginality. One point is regarding the high cost of camel cheese but the valorization of the lactoserum, which contains more valuable components than cow milk, could be a highly convenient way.

"Exploring Potential Therapeutic Properties of Camel Milk" highlights that camel milk has great potential medicinal value including antioxidant properties, anti-cancer activity, angiotensin converting enzyme (ACE) inhibitory, antidiabetic activity, antimicrobial activity, hypo-allergenicity property, and anti-Crohn's disease effect. In addition, the bioactivity of conjugated linoleic acid (CLA), D and L amino acid as well as oligosaccharide in camel milk can be mentioned. It shall help patients, doctors, nutritionists, research scholars, particularly, pharmaceutical houses to make nutriceutical products out of camel milk.

The chapter "Health-Improving and Disease-Preventing of Camel Milk Against Chronic Diseases and Autism" focuses on cumulative evidence has shown that camel milk is helpful in suppressing the carcinogenesis process, in halting initiated carcinogens, and in stopping metastasis for different neoplasms. Further, camel milk has shown to help in normalizing blood sugar and blood lipids and normalizing metabolic syndrome components. Finally, recent reports indicated that camel milk could be an effective adjuvant therapy for inflammatory bowel diseases and cancers, with a plausible beneficial effect for patients with autism.

In chapter "Potential Anti-Diabetic Effect of Camel Milk," the author opines on the basis of his researches that camel is going to benefit the society, specially, the diabetic patients. Medical professionals and pharma houses can produce useful medicines from camel milk for a better regulation of glycaemia in diabetic patients.

The chapter "Effects of Industrial Processing Methods on Camel Milk Composition, Nutritional Value, and Health Properties" deals with effects of industrial processing methods on camel milk composition, nutritional value and health properties. The author stated that heat treatment of milk is an essential step to render milk safe for human consumption and extend its shelf life. Heat treatment methods include low temperature long time pasteurization (LTLT), high temperature short time pasteurization (HTST), and sterilization at Ultra High Temperature (UHT). Among these, HTST pasteurization and UHT are the most commonly used methods in the dairy industry. Such treatment is mainly aimed at killing microorganisms and inactivating spoilage-induced enzymes, or at achieving some other changes, mainly chemical.

The chapter "Camel Colostrum Composition, Nutritional Value, and Nutraceuticals" provides in-depth information on the physico-chemical properties of camel colostrum of both camel species (dromedary and Bactrian) and also in detail the composition of camel colostrum, one by one (c.a. fat fraction, lactose, oligosaccharides, minerals, enzymes and whey proteins) as well as its role in human nutrition, compared to those of other animal colostrum including human, cow, goat, sheep, and buffalo. The chapter also emphasizes on the biological and therapeutic values of camel colostrum.

The chapter also reveals high nutritional value of camel colostrum compared with other studied species. It contains almost all the beneficial compounds found in other colostra, e.g., proteins, peptides, fatty acids, vitamins, and other bioactive compounds. Camel colostrum has higher levels of total protein, IgG, LF, long chain poly-unsaturated fatty acids, conjugated linoleic acid, vitamin C and oligosaccharides compared to those of cow, goat and buffalo colostra. Camel colostrum also contribute to human health care, both as part of a health promoting diet and as an alternative or supplement to the medical treatment of specified human diseases

The nutritional value of camel meat has been described in chapter "Camel Meat Production, Structure and Quality". Camels are a good source of high nutritional meat especially in areas where the climate adversely affects the survival of other livestock. The camel has unique physiological characteristics, including a great tolerance to high and low temperatures, solar radiation, water scarcity, rough topography and poor vegetation. Camels are mostly reared under traditional systems on poor levels of nutrition and are mostly slaughtered at old ages after completion of a career in work, racing or milk production. According to the quality parameters of camel meat, it can be successfully marketed alongside that of cattle, dear, sheep and goat. Pre and post-mortem factors should be carefully considered to improve meat quality characteristics. Future research is required for exploiting the potential of the camel as a source of meat through multi-disciplinary research into efficient production systems, and improved meat technology and marketing.

The perception of meat consumers has changed over recent decades from considering meat simply as a source of required nutrients and energy to seeing meat as a health-promoting component. Efforts in the meat industry have led towards improving and characterizing the quality and healthiness of meat and meat products. The chapter "Camel Meat Nutrient Content and Potential Health Benefits" aims to characterize the important nutrient components of camel meat and to consider future developments of camel meat and camel meat products.

The camel meat has high nutritional values compared to other red meats. It has higher amino acid and mineral contents than other animal meats while intramuscular fat level is lower. Knowing the composition and quality parameters of camel meat, it could be successfully launched to market alongside with cattle, deer, sheep and goat. With the increasing demand for high-protein and low-fat shelf stable products for recreational activities, the potential of some traditional products being marketed internationally is very high.

The chapter "Camel Gelatin Composition, Properties, Production, and Applications" reveals that Gelatin is an ingredient used widely in various industries, such as food, cosmetics, pharmaceuticals, and photography. It may be produced from the skins or bones of animals. In order to extract gelatin from camel bone, camel bone needs to be demineralised. Camel bone is suitable for production of gelatin with good potentials in food and non-food applications. Author also obtained gelatin from camel skin and bone. The extracted gelatins were categorized successfully.

The quality of wool fibre of camel and its use is described in chapter "Camel Hair Structure, Properties, and Commercial Products". The camel wool fibre have fineness, softness and curliness. The flakes made from camel cashmere have the advantages of being light, thin, fluffy, windproof, mildew proof, breathable and warm. The finished garment is comfortable to wear and not as bloated as a down jacket.

"Camel Milk Disguised Cosmeceutical" highlights the topical value of camel milk in certain diseases. Natural production having cosmeceutical value is a concern for dermatologist and public sufferers. This is a new concept of research.

The interactions of the camel with its environment is somewhat complex compared to other animal species domesticated by human. Author summarized these interactions at three main levels in the chapter "Interaction Between Camel Farming and Environment". First, by the proper characteristics of the camel who have an anatomy, physiology and metabolism entirely to its surviving in the harsh conditions of the desert. Second, the camel can valorize the remote areas of the world thanks to its wide production and services to human. The arid lands occupy more than 35% of terrestrial surface, and in such areas, camel farming is a blessing for rural activities. Third, the camel contributes to the global economy by its progressive integration to regional or international market. Beyond this contribution to the world economy, camel production and products can support the participation of the stakeholders living in desert or desert margins. However, intensification of camel production could modify this fragile balance between the meagre resources of the desert and the pressure of camel rearing. Camel scientists and developers must take in account this new equation in the development plan of camel farming.

This book provides the reader with a comprehensive review on camel milk composition, physical, chemical, nutritional, dairy preservation and therapeutic properties; in addition to the industrial methods affecting camel milk composition and up-to-date potential health properties compared to other animal milks. This publication also provides insight and supports executives concerned with the camel meat production, nutritional value, and potential health. The commercial camel products such as dairy, gelatin, cosmetics, as well as camel hair products are also presented. This book furthermore gives better understanding to the researchers in information related to interaction between camel farming and environment.

Acknowledgment

We have many people to thank for their efforts in producing this book. First, the authors have done a super job of producing authoritative chapters that synthesize vast amounts of recent scientific and clinical data to create informative and practical approaches to managing patients. In today's information-rich, rapidly evolving environment, they have ensured that this information is current. We are most grateful to our colleagues who worked closely with each other to facilitate communication with the authors and help us. We would like to acknowledge the expert support of IGI Publishing Group. It has inspired the creative and dynamic evolution in new formats.

Chapter 1
Historical Background and Population of Camels

Hiba Fathi Al-Sayyed
University of Petra, Jordan

ABSTRACT

Camels were designated as the ships of the desert. This chapter includes some introductory remarks on the historical background and population of camels. In this chapter, the origin of camels based on the most recent mitochondrial genome analysis and incisor fossils was reviewed. Based on the results of these studies, camels were found in different parts of the world such as North America, Africa, Russia, China, Magnolia, Iran, and Middle Eastern region. Different genus and species of camels were also reviewed in the chapter. Additionally, the distribution of camel population worldwide as well as the uses of camels were reviewed. This chapter introduces some essential figures on the economic value of camels based on the most recent statistics of the Food and Agricultural Organization (FAO).

INTRODUCTION

Camels have a long history, but even if recent discovers were available in the literature on the origin of the camels' ancestors (Rybczynski, Gosse, Harington, Wogelius, Hidy & Buckley, 2013) and on the domestication of modern camel (Almathen et al., 2016), some data are still lacking.

This chapter aims at introducing some introductory remarks on the historical background and present population of camels. The origin of camels based on the most recent mitochondrial genome analysis and incisor fossils are reviewed. Different genus and species of camels are also reviewed. Additionally, the present distribution of camel population worldwide as well as the uses of camels are reported here. This chapter introduces also some essential figures on the economic value of camels which based on the most recent statistics of the Food and Agricultural Organization (FAO), the only available data at world level.

DOI: 10.4018/978-1-7998-1604-1.ch001

Historical Background of Camels' Ancestors

Many people believe in the myth that camels have originated from rabbits because camels have grooved upper lip-like structures similar to those of rabbits. Nonetheless, many researchers showed that the origin of camel can be traced to *Protylopus;* a rabbit-sized animal with four-toed feet, low-crowned teeth, which lived in America during Eocene period 40-45 million years ago (Indra, Magash, & Biichee, 1998). Several genera of camelids developed and disappeared over the following million years (Rybczynski et al., 2013). After *Protolypus* (Eocene), paleontologists described the *Poebrotherium* (Oligocene), the *Procamelus* (Miocene), the *Paracamelus* (Pliocene) and others. The *Camelus* genus appeared at early or middle Pleistocene (Monchot, 2015). The ancestors of camelids are originated from North America. Fossil was found in Ellesmere Island at 97th parallel north or 1200 kilometers away from the Yukon early camel fossil remains place and it represents the most northerly record for early camels. The size of Ellesmere camel tibia was larger than that of the modern camels by 30% and lived at 20°C-30°C warmer than nowadays temperature (Yam & Khomeiri, 2015).

The *camelus'* ancestors reached Eurasia via the Bering strait around 6.5-7.5 Million years and fossils of direct ancestors of the modern *Camelus* (*Paracamelus, Camelus thomasi*), appearing as "giant camels" were recorded in Asia (Kozhamkulova, 1986), Spain (Pickford, Morales & Soria, 1995), Northern Africa (Peters 1998) and Syria (Martini, Costeur, Le Tonsorer & Schmid, 2015). In another hand, the ancestors of New-World camelids entered South America around 3 Million years ago (Rybczynski et al., 2013). So, according to the recent complete analysis of camel mitochondrial genome by Burger (2016), world camelids belong nowadays to either of the domestic New-World camelids (*Lamini*) or Old-World Camelids (*Camilini*) (Figure 1). Those two genera probably diverged more than 16 million years ago (Burger, Ciani, & Faye, 2019).

Figure 1. Classification of the camelidae family
(Adapted with permission from Burger, 2016)

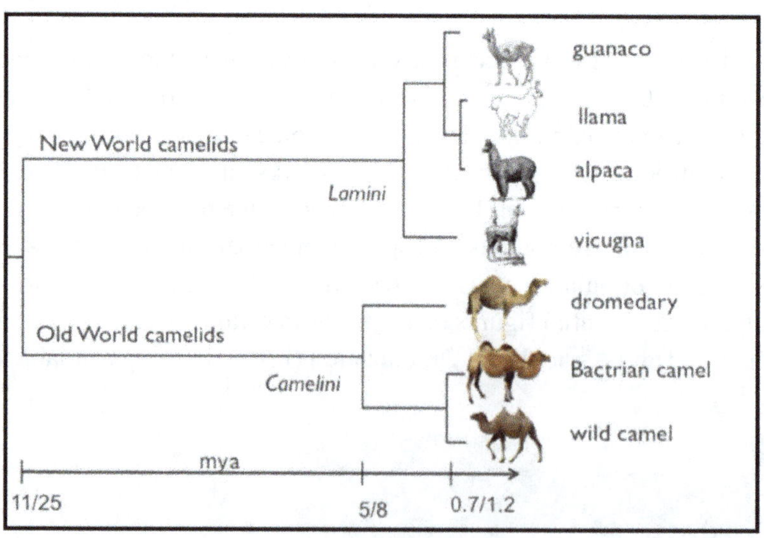

DOMESTICATION AND INTRODUCTION

According to Uerpman and Uerpman (2002) and Von den Driesch & Obermaier (2007), a wild form of dromedary was hunted 5000 years BC in the actual Arab Emirates concluding that the domestication was not achieved at this time. Domestication is a long and slow process probably achieved in the Iron Age between 2000- and 1000-years BC in the south of Arabian Peninsula, presently Yemen and Oman (Fowler, 1998). The first historic sources speaking on domestic camel were written 1100 years BC during the battle between the northern Arab tribes against those on the Mediterranean coasts.

Purpose of domestication was probably mainly for riding and packing in connection with the trade of spices, incense and possibly salt. Indeed, the caravan trade was flourishing between Arabia and the Near East and some prestigious civilizations took form on this activity as Nabatean who founded Petra. From this domestication focus, the spread of the dromedary camel followed the aridification of the milieu. From 3500 BP on, the camel was present in Socotra Island from where it occupied the Horn of Africa, and then, migrated through Sahelian zones. Around 3000 BP, the camel was used in the whole near and Middle East for pack and milk production. However, the spread of the domestic camel was also linked to the military uses (troops and materials transport) as attested by various documents in Palestine. The introduction of the camel into Egypt occurred later as no representation was depicted on any temple or palace wall in ancient Egypt (Epstein, 1971). This introduction dated from around 2200-2100 BP through Sinai Peninsula or by way of the Red Sea, in connection with the incense trade with Upper Egypt. The spread of the dromedary camel in the North Africa was contemporary to the Roman Empire including camels in the rural economy and trade as camel skeletons are observed along the roman ways up to Europe (Tomczyk, 2016). After Hegira, with the Arab conquest, the camel becomes present in Spain in 1020 and Sicily in 1059. In 1405, it was introduced in Canary Islands by a French landowner to help in agriculture (Bulliet, 1975) during European colonization (Wilson & Gutierrez, 2015). To the Easter direction, camel went to Mesopotamia, Assyria and up to India probably following the invasion of Alexander the Great at about 2300 B.P. (Faye, 2013).

Less information was available regarding domestication of Bactrian. It occurred probably in the same time in Central Asia, between actual Mongolia and Kazakhstan. In Iran empire, Near East, and Syrian, cylinders mentioned to domesticate Bactrian camel 1800 B.C. (Indra et al., 1998).

Present Taxonomy

Camels belong to the order of Artiodactyla (even-toed ungulates); sub-order Tylopoda (pad-footed), family of Camelidae. Three main genus of camelids are mentioned nowadays i,e. *Camelus, Lama* and *Vicugna* (Yam & Khomeiri, 2015). From the genus *Camelus*, two domesticated species exist including the one-humped (*Dromedarius;* the name of the dromedary derived from the Greek, *dromeus* which means runner or *dromos*- running (Jassim & Naji, 2002) and the two-humped (*Bactrianus;* the word Bactrian come from the word Bactriana in Asia, the old name of a Kingdom close to actual Iran (Bakhtar or Bactar) (Yam & Khomeiri, 2015)). As the name indicates, the one-humped camels are single-humped with spindled legs. The *Bactrianus* are double-humped, stockier, and covered by thicker wool (Chapman, 1991; Yam & Khomeiri, 2015).

On the other hand, Burger (2016) mentioned that the two humped camels of the Mongolian Gobi, the Chinese Taklimakan, and Lop Nor desert, discovered by Nikolaj Przewalski in 1878, were a unique evolutionary unit. Its mitogenome sequencing performed by Ji et al. (2009) and more recently by Mohandesan et al. (2017) as well as Ming et al., (2019) showed divergence between the domestic and wild Bactrian camels between 0.58-1.8 million years ago which necessitates the opportunities for conserving the *Camelus ferus* type of camels. Nonetheless, Ming et al. (2019) mentioned that the limited molecular markers as wells as archaeological findings of Bactrian camels provide inconclusive evidence on the camel domestication history.

Among the New World camels, two genera are described: genus *Lamini* with the species *L. glama, L. guanicoe, L. pacos*) and genus *Vicugna* (with the species *V. vicugna*) (Wilson & Reeder, 2005; Faye, 2013).

On the other hand, it has been thought that the Southern American camelids, at the tribe level, are divided into *Camelus peruvianus Glama dictus* or *Llamas* (*Lamas*) and *Camelus pacos* (*Camelus peruvianus laniger Pacos dictus*) or *Alpacas*. *Llamas* and *Alpacas* are camel-like loading animals that are found in the cold dry deserts of South America and lived 10,000 years ago. Nonetheless, López Aranguren, (1930), Webb (1974), Harrison (1985), and Menegaz, Goin, & Jaureguizar (1989) suggested that *Lamas* have originated from Argentina plains for about two million years ago (Larson, 2009). *Alpacas* share some features with *Lamas* such as color but more important than *Lamas* for meat production (see Chapter 12).

The genus *Vicugna* has been cited as an independent species in 1924 by Miller based on hypsodont incisors (Wheeler, 2012). At present, *Vicugna* genus resides between 9° 30' and 29° S latitude in the Andes. *Vicugna* animals grow in the high altitudes of more than 14,000 feet of Chile and Northern Peru. *Vicugna* animals do not have chest hair, covered with white-light beige mixed wool in most of their body surface area (Wheeler, 2012), and have finer wool than that of *Lama*. These animals weigh about 100 lbs. *Lamas* weigh 200 lbs. *Lamas* and *Alpacas* are known to be domestic animals (Larson, 2009) while *Vicugna* occur in a wild state (Nova, 1970).

Present Distribution

On the contrary to one-humped camels which live in hot deserts, the two-humped camels live in cold deserts and dry steppes of Asia (Yam & Khomeiri, 2015). Thus, the two-humped (*Bactrianus*) camels were found mainly in China, Mongolia and Kazakhstan, but it is present also in the borders of Iran and Turkmenistan and spread in the areas of Crimea, southern Siberia, north of Afghanistan, Pakistan and India. The dromedary is found in Northern part of Africa from Mauritania to the Horn of Africa, and in Asia from Arabian Peninsula to India (Rajasthan). Globally, 48 countries in the world declare a camel population in the FAO database (Figure 2).

Regarding later introductions, it includes Australia, USA, Europe and Namibia. In USA, President Jefferson Davis introduced camels for US Army in 1856. Nowadays, camel dairy farms are developing for providing camel milk based on the belief that it could have beneficial effect on diabetes and autism. Camel was recently also introduced in Kalahari Desert (Namibia), in arid zones from South America (Brazil, Peru) and in some parts of European countries (France, Italy, Spain, Netherland, Austria, Cyprus)

Figure 2. The worldwide production of camels by country (measured as heads; average values between the years 2006 and 2017)
(Source: Food and Agriculture Organization of the United Nations, [2019], [FAOSTAT], [http://www.fao.org/faostat/en/#data/QV/visualize]

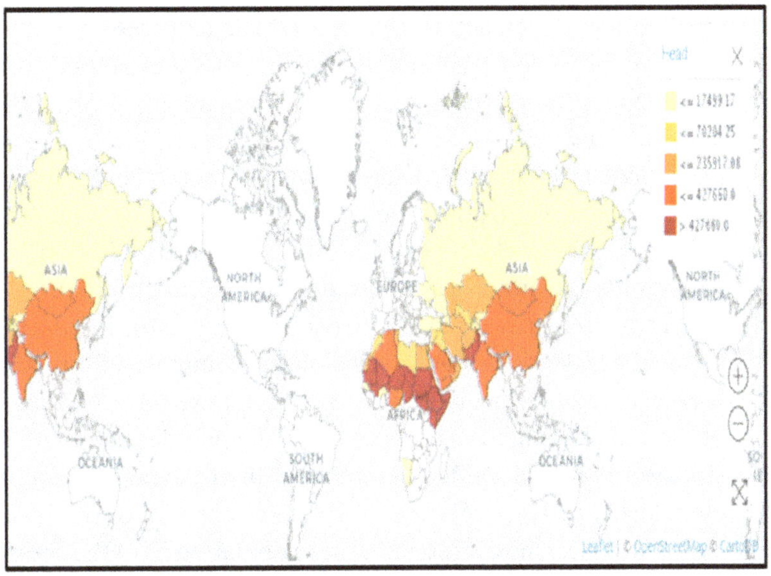

were used for tourism (Koç & Atasever, 2016). However, it was in Australia that camel introduction was perennial: Six camels were imported from Afghanistan and Pakistan in 1849, 121 in 1866; in 1895, the number of dromedary camels were 6000 (Saalfeld & Edwards, 2010). They were widely used for riding, ploughing and for the exploration of arid areas in Central Australia (Jones & Kenny, 2010). In 1920, farmers, postmen and policemen used 12000 domestic camels. However, the number of domestic animals decreased with the motorization and, 2000 domestic camels only were accounted for in the sixties of the 20th century while in the same time, many camels became "feral". In 1960, the population of wild camels was estimated at 90000 heads. In 1996, this number varied between 100000 and 500000 heads (Gee, 1996). At present, the population was more than one million feral camels which started to cause some environmental problems due to their high density and a Camel Destruction Act was published to limit the pressure of the wild population on the Australian desert environment (Edwards, Zeng, Saalfeld, Vaarzon-Morel, & McGregor, 2008). In the present book, the interaction between camel farming and environment will be discussed in details in Chapter 17.

Moreover, in the past thirty years, the expansion of the camel distribution area has been observed in several African countries (Faye, Chaibou & Vias, 2012). The "desert belt" of Sahara corresponded roughly to the location of camel farming. Today, the expansion of the camel is still intimately linked to the aridification of the milieu. Indeed, camel farms are nowadays present in the north of Nigeria, Cameroon, the Central African Republic (RCA), the north of Uganda and even Tanzania (Swai, Moshy, Mshanga, Lutatina, & Bwanga, 2011). For example, in Chad, camel herds usually reared under long transhumance patterns go today up to the RCA border or even beyond (Marty, Eberschweiler, & Dangbet, 2009). In Kenya, the camel population is occupied a wide part of the country, even areas inhabited by Massaï, yet traditionally cattle breeders (Cecchi, Shaw, Marletta, Mattioli, & Robinson, 2010).

Economic Value of Camels

Historically, camels played an essential role in the cultural heritage of residents in the arid and semi-arid regions of the world. For instance, camel ownership started after a boy delivery where camel (with the boy umbilical cord tied around the camel neck) and a female calf were presented (Hartley, 1979). In other cultures, the ownership of camels has been used to attract wives and pay off criminal offences (Dickson, 1951). But, beyond the cultural aspect, as multipurpose animals (Hjort af Örnas, 1993), camel play an important economic role. Indeed, it is used to obtain milk, meat, hide, transportation (Al-Juboori, Mohammed, Rashid, Kurian, & El Refaey, 2013), and wool (Sharma & Pant, 2013).

The first available statistics on the world population of camel herds, camels and Bactrian camels combined, date from 1961 on the FAOSTAT website (www.faostat.org). In 2017, the year of the latest available statistics, the world's population was estimated at 34.8 million heads. Such a figure is underestimated for several reasons: the lack of a comprehensive census in most breeding countries, the lack of identification of animals (largely related to the lack of mandatory vaccination campaigns for this species), the lack of declarations in Western countries and especially in Australia. These uncertainties explain, moreover, the sudden resurgence of the camel population observed over the past decade, more related to statistical adjustments following censuses than to a sudden natural growth of the population. For example, Chad, which reported 1.55 million head in 2014, declared, following a census of the national herd, more than 7 million in 2017 (7.85 million heads). However, comparing population growth for domestic herbivorous species gives a definite advantage to large camelids. Indeed, based on an index 100 in 1961 for all species, this index reaches 269 among camels in 2017, more than equines (97) whose numbers have rather declined, sheep (121), cattle (158), small Andean camelids (170), and buffalo (227), only goats (297) having higher growth. However, camels being concentrated in arid environments, unlike cattle and small ruminants with more ubiquitous distribution, the percentage of camels in the Domestic Herbivorous Biomass (DHB) can be locally important reaching 12% in the Horn of Africa, and even exceed 30% for example in Mauritania (37%), the Emirates and Qatar (47%), Chad (50%), Somalia (52%) or Western Sahara/Morocco's Saharan provinces (84%). The top ten countries of camels are Chad, Somalia, Sudan, Kenya, Niger, Mauritania, Ethiopia, Mali, Pakistan, and Saudi Arabia (Figure 3). Nonetheless, the United Arab Emirates and Qatar are estimated to contain the highest density of livestock density per agricultural land area (Figure 4). Camel population is increasing in all the countries except in India.

Regarding milk production, the added value is difficult to estimate for many reasons. The part of self-consumption, which is beyond any control of the market, is indeed largely predominant, although difficult to quantify. Even in Saudi Arabia where the sector is apparently well structured the part of milk produced in the Bedouin system not integrated into market could represent 62% of camel milk produced in the country (Faye, Madani & El-Rouili, 2014). FAO statistics show a global production of 2.8 million tons of camel milk in 2017, probably widely underestimated. Based on this reference, camel milk would account for only 0.37% of the milk consumed worldwide, but this part has doubled since 1961 (0.18%). Moreover, with a proportion of 23% of the camel herds devoted to dairy production (see Chapter 5), camels seem to be more widely used for milk production than cows (only 18% are used for milk production).

Despite this marginal place in world dairy economy, a real enthusiasm for camel milk is observed for three main reasons: (i) climate change resulting in an expansion of camel breeding areas especially in Africa as mentioned above, (ii) the "merchandising" of milk, i.e. its ability to integrate local, regional and even international markets (Faye, 2016), and (iii) the supposed or true medicinal "virtues" of camel

Figure 3. Distribution of the camel in the world countries in 2017
(Source: Food and Agriculture Organization of the United Nations, [2019], [FAOSTAT], [http://www.fao.org/faostat/en/#data/QV/visualize]

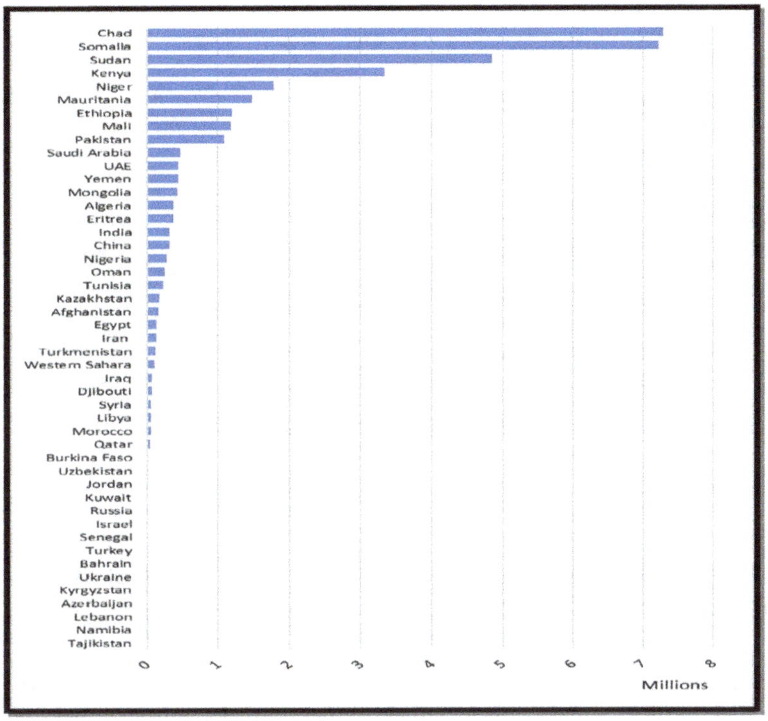

Figure 4. Density of camel in the different countries of the world
(Source: Food and Agriculture Organization of the United Nations, [2019], [FAOSTAT], [http://www.fao.org/faostat/en/#data/QV/visualize]

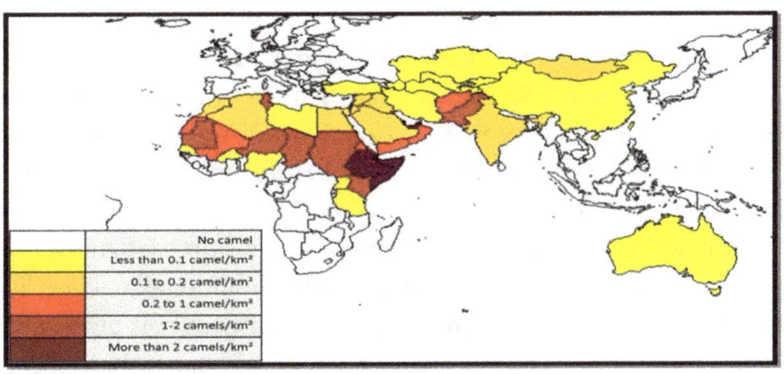

milk that make it a calling product in the current context of "welfare" product research (Yadav, Kumar, Priyadarshini, & Singh, 2015). Such growing interest for camel milk could explain its increase in higher proportion than the camel population (Figure 5).

Figure 5. Changes in camel population, milk and meat for the period 1961-2017 (calculated from FAOSTAT, 2019).

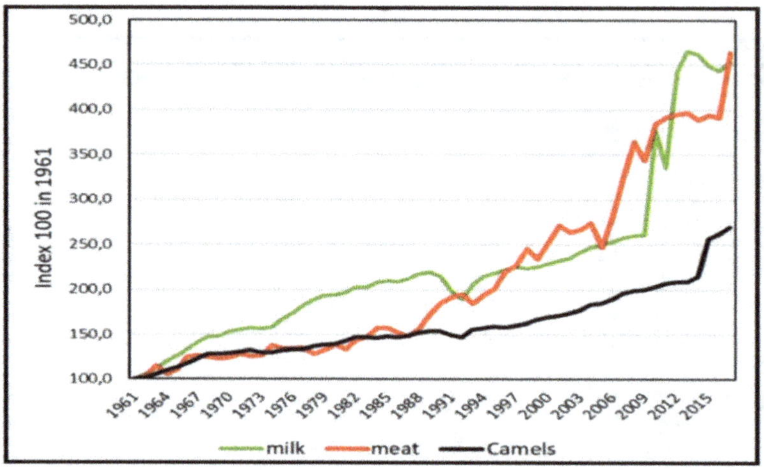

To satisfy the growing demand in camel milk, dairy intensification in the camel industry is occurring especially in Gulf countries, mobilizing modern management practices as the use of reproductive biotechnology (artificial insemination, embryo transfer), machine milking, health prevention, supplement feeding, settlement and genetic selection (Nagy, Faigl, Reiczigel & Juhasz, 2015). Despite a lower productivity of camel, the price of camel milk being 2 to 10 times higher than that of cow milk, the rentability of dairy camel farm could be interesting.

Unlike camel milk, which has only recently contributed to the global economy (see Chapter 12), camel meat is the subject of a very old cross-border trade, although poorly documented (Alary & Faye, 2016). Camel meat production at world level was reaching 312,000 tons in 2017 (FAOSTAT, 2019), i.e. 0.45% of the red meat consumed worldwide. This percentage ranges from 0.01% (Senegal, Turkey) to more than 60% (Western Sahara/South Morocco). However, while the mean slaughtering rate (number of animals slaughtered each year relative to the world's population) is 8.3%, the inter-country variability is considerable, between less than 10% (mostly Sahelian countries) to more than 20% in importing countries. Among them, two countries, Egypt (82.4%) and Saudi Arabia (96.4%) have slaughtering rates that are incompatible with livestock survival; such rate is possible thanks to the high number of imported camels for slaughterhouses.

While the camel meat sector remains largely traditional (pastoral fattening, live export, informal slaughtering, lack of carcass classification and cutting system, traditional butcher distribution network), the modernization is at work in countries where the demand for quality is emerging among urban consumers. Such modernization can be achieved both in the development of feed-lots for fattening, for example in Tunisia (Khorchani, Hammadi & Moslah, 2005) or in the Gulf countries (Faye, Abdelhadi, Raiymbek, Kadim & Hocquette, 2013) as well as in the establishment of a carcass classification system (Herrman & Fisher, 2004) or the distribution of camel meat in supermarkets. Moreover, as for camel milk, camel meat is introduced in market under more diversified forms than before (sausage, jam, camel burger, etc…) (Farouk & Bekhit, 2012).

Other major productions include wool and leather (see Chapter 15). There are no international statistics regarding camel wool, but an estimate, based on the average wool productivity of the camel and especially that of Bactrian, makes it possible to consider that large camelids have an annual production potential of 40,000 tons, to be compared to the 2.1 million tons of wool supplied by sheep worldwide.

Bactrian camel is providing the best part of camel wool. The fineness of Bactrian's wool is much higher than that of sheep (Saipolda, 2005). In this niche, Mongolia and recently China are carving out the largest part of the international market with exports to luxury boutiques in Western capitals. This development has been made possible by some technical innovations such as the technique of combing rather than shearing, the processing of wool after collection, the industrialization of weaving and the modernization of cuttings. Traditional use is reserved for the manufacture of local traditional clothes such as *burnous* in North Africa.

Camel has heavy skin (22 to 47 kg) large in size, but its economic valorization is generally poor for several reasons: (i) the high frequency of skin diseases (Driot et al., 2014), (ii) the presence of the hump on the back, (iii) the poor collection and storage conditions, (iv) the cost of preparing the skins in relation to the possible valorization. Finally, camel's skin is of low commercial value, and in many contexts, producers and slaughterers destroyed this product. However, recent technical innovations (particularly implemented in North Africa), based on better prevention of skin diseases, improved collection and storage as well as preparation techniques (scrubbing, thinning, trimming and tanning) have enabled a certain development of the leather sector in the tourism industry for the manufacture of artisanal products (handicrafts), including in luxury sectors (handbag, shoes). In the present book, the camel hair and disguised cosmeceutical products will be discussed in Chapter 15 and 16, respectively.

Other productions remain anecdotal, except for the use of camel in agricultural work, transport or leisure (Faye & Bonnet, 2012). In the Gulf countries, the use of camels as a racing animal is part of a true industry involving biotechnology of reproduction, rational feeding, training, anti-doping control and rigorous management. The price of the progenitors of animals renowned for their velocity can reach high prices up to millions USD.

FUTURE RESEARCH DIRECTIONS

Scientists are encouraged to continue genomic research in order to know the exact origin of camels. Organizations whether local or international are encouraged to estimate the data related to this animal specially the production, yield, and manufacturing of different camel-based food products. National censuses could help also to have a clear idea of the camel population in the world.

CONCLUSION

Camels has a long history, better known since recent research results. Camels are used for many purposes and its production is increasing worldwide. Based on its demographic place at world level, the economic potential of camel appears marginal, but it can become significant locally. The amount of direct production can be estimated at around 9 billion USD, as indirect productions are more difficult to quantify.

However, camel production is expanding for three main reasons: (i) climate change that seems to benefit the species due to its adaptive capacity, (ii) the increasing economic integration of camel producers in various parts of the world, and (iii) the increasing demand for camel products, milk, meat and leisure in the first places.

ACKNOWLEDGMENT

I would like to thank the Food and Agricultural Organization [FAO] for their permission of adopting the Figures.

Additionally I would like to thank Prof.Bernard Faye for his convenient remarks in this chapter.

REFERENCES

Al-Juboori, A. T., Mohammed, M., Rashid, J., Kurian, J., & El Refaey, S. (2013). Nutritional and medicinal value of camel (*Camelus dromedarius*) milk. *WIT Transactions on Ecology and the Environment, 170*, 221–232. doi:10.2495/FENV130201

Alary, V., & Faye, B. (2016). The camel chains in East Africa- Importance of gaps between the data and the apparent reality. *Journal of Camelid Science, 9*, 1–2.

Almathen, F., Charruau, P., Mohandesan, E., Mwacharo, J. M., Orozco-ter Wengel, P., Pitt, D., & ... Burger, P.A. (2016) Ancient and modern DNA reveal dynamics of domestication and cross-continental dispersal of the dromedary. *Proceedings of the National Academy of Sciences* USA, *113*, 6707-12. 10.1073/pnas.1519508113

Bulliet, R. W. (1975). *The camel and the wheel.* Cambridge, MA: Harvard University Press.

Burger, P. (2016). The history of old world camelids in the light of molecular genetics. *Tropical Animal Production, 48*(5), 905–913. doi:10.100711250-016-1032-7 PMID:27048619

Burger, P., Ciani, E., & Faye, B. (2019). Old World camels in a modern world – a balancing act between conservation and genetic improvement. *Animal Genetics, 50*(6), 598–612. doi:10.1111/age.12858 PMID:31532019

Cecchi, G. W., Shaw, W., Marletta, A., Mattioli, A., & Robinson, T. (2010). Geographic distribution and environmental characterization of livestock production systems in Eastern Africa. *Agriculture, Ecosystems & Environment, 135*(1-2), 98–110. doi:10.1016/j.agee.2009.08.011

Chapman, M. J. (1991). Camels. *Biologist, 38*, 41-44.

Dickson, H. R. (1951). *The Arab of the desert.* London: George Allen & Unwin Ltd.

Driot, C., Kamili, A., Bengoumi, M., Faye, B., Delverdier, M., & Taleban, Y. (2011). Study on the epidemiology and of sarcoptic mange and ringworm in the one-humped camel in South of Morocco. *Journal of Camel Practice and Research, 18*(1), 107–114.

Edwards, G. P., Zeng, B., Saalfeld, W. K., Vaarzon-Morel, P., & McGregor, M. (Eds.). (2008). *Managing the impacts of feral camels in Australia: a new way of doing business. DKCRC Report 47*. Alice Springs: Desert Knowledge Cooperative Research Centre. Available at http://www.desertknowledgecrc.com.au/publications/contractresearch.html

Epstein, H. (1971). History and origin of the African camel. In *The origin of the domestic animals in Africa* (pp. 558–564). New York: African Publishing Corporation.

Farouk, M. M., & Bekhit, A. E. (2012). Processed camel meats. CAB International publ.

Faye, B. (2013). Classification, history and distribution of the camel. In I. Kadim, O. Maghoub, B. Faye, & M. Farouk (Eds.), *Camel meat and meat products* (pp. 1–7). Oxfordshire, UK: CAB International. doi:10.1079/9781780641010.0001

Faye, B. (2016). The camel, new challenges for a sustainable development. *Tropical Animal Health and Production*, *48*(4), 689–692. doi:10.100711250-016-0995-8 PMID:26922737

Faye, B., Abdelhadi, O., Raiymbek, G., Kadim, I., & Hocquette, J. F. (2013). La production de viande de chameau: État des connaissances, situation actuelle et perspectives. *Productions Animales*, *26*(3), 247–258.

Faye, B., & Bonnet, P. (2012). Camel sciences and economy in the world: Current situation and perspectives. In *Proceedings of the 3rd ISOCARD Conference. Keynote presentations* (pp. 2-15). Muscat, Oman: Sultan Qaboos University.

Faye, B., Chaibou, M., & Vias, G. F. (2012). Integrated impact of climate change and socioeconomic development on the evolution of camel farming systems. *British Journal of Environment & Climate Change*, *2*(3), 227–244. doi:10.9734/BJECC/2012/1548

Faye, B., Madani, H., & El-Rouili, A. H. (2014). Camel milk value chain in Northern Saudi Arabia. *Emirates Journal of Food and Agriculture*, *26*(4), 359–365. doi:10.9755/ejfa.v26i4.17278

Food and Agriculture Organization. FAOSTAT. (2019). *Food and Agricultural Organization of the United Nations/Statistics*. Retrieved May 4, 2019 from: http://www.fao.org/faostat/en/#data/QV/visualize

Fowler, M. E. (1998). *Medicine and surgery of south American camelids*. Iowa State Press Blackwell.

Gee, P. (1996). The camel in Australia. *Journal of Camel Practice and Research*, *3*(2), 139–140.

Harrison, J. A. (1985). Giant Camels from the Cenozoic of North America. *Smithsonian Contributions to Paleobiology*, *57*(57), 1–29. doi:10.5479i.00810266.57.1

Hartley, J. B. (1979). *Camels in the Horn of Africa*. Paper presented in IFS Symposium Camels.

Herrman, K., & Fischer, A. (2004). Method for hygienic slaughter of camels. In Z. Farah, & A. Fisher (Eds.), Milk and meat from the camel. Handbook on products and processing. Zuric: vdf Hochschulverlag AG an der ETH Zurich.

Hjort af Ornäs, A. (1993). *The Multi-Purpose Camel: Interdisciplinary Studies on Pastoral Production in Somalia*. Uppsala, Sweden: EPOS, MO Print.

Indra, R., Magash, A., & Biichee, N. (1998). *Studies of Bactrian camel*. Washington, DC: Institution Press.

Jassim, S. A., & Naji, M. A. (2002). The desert ship: Heritage and science - unique camel antibodies. *Middle East Laboratory*, *5*, 6–11.

Ji, R., Cui, P., Ding, F., Geng, J., Gao, H., Zhang, H., ... Meng, H. (2009). Monophyletic origin of domestic bactrian camel (*Camelus bactrianus*) and its evolutionary relationship with the extant wild camel (*Camelus bactrianus ferus*). *Animal Genetics*, *40*(4), 377–382. doi:10.1111/j.1365-2052.2008.01848.x PMID:19292708

Jones, P., & Kenny, A. (2010). *Australia's Muslim Cameleers: Pioneers of the Inland, 1860s-1930s*. Wakefield press Publishers.

Khorchani, T., Hammadi, M., & Moslah, M. (2005). Artificial nursing of camel calves: an effective technique for calves' safeguard and improving herd productivity. In *Proceedings of the International Workshop Desertification Combat and Food Safety: The Added Value of Camel Producers, Ashkabad (Turkmenistan)*, (Vol. 362, pp. 177-182). Amsterdam, The Netherlands: IOS press Publishers.

Koç, A., & Atasever, S. (2016). *Production and characteristics of camel milk*. Paper presented in International Selçuk-Ephesus Symposium on Culture of Camel-Dealing and Camel Wrestling, Turkey.

Kozhamkulova, B. S. (1986). The Late Cenozoic two-humped (Bactrian) camels of Asia. *Quartärpläontolgie*, *6*, 93–97.

Larson, J. A. (2009). *Information Resources on the South American Camelids: Llamas, Alpacas, Guanacos, and Vicunas 2004-2008*. AWIC Resource Series No. 12. Retrieved from: https://pubs.nal.usda.gov/sites/pubs.nal.usda.gov/files/Camelids2009.pdf

López Aranguren, D. J. (1930). Camélidos fósiles argentinos. *Anales de la Sociedad Científica Argentina (Buenos Aires)*, *109*, 97–126.

Martini, P., Costeur, L., Le Tonsorer, J.-M., & Schmid, P. (2015). Pleistocene camelids from the Syrian Desert: The diversity in El Kowm. *L'Anthropologie*, *119*(5), 687–693. doi:10.1016/j.anthro.2015.10.005

Marty, A., Eberschweiler, A., & Dangbet, Z. (2009). *Au Cœur De La Transhumance. Un Campement Chamelier Au Tchad Central*. Paris, France: Khartala.

Menegaz, A. N., Goin, F. J., & Jaureguizar, E. O. (1989). Análisis morfológico y morfométrico multivariado de los representantes fósiles y vivientes del género *Lama* (*Artiodactyla, Camelidae*). *Sus implicancias sistemáticas biogeográficas, ecológicas y biocronológicas. Ameghiniana*, *26*, 153–172.

Ming, L., Yuan, L., Yi, L., Ding, G., Hasi, S., Chen, G., Jambl, T., … Jirimutu. (2019). *Whole-genome sequencing of 128 camels across Asia provides insights into origin and migration of domestic Bactrian camels*. Retrieved from https://www.biorxiv.org/content/biorxiv/early/2019/06/03/656231.full.pdf

Mohandesan, E., Fitak, R., Corander, J., Yadamsuren, A., Chuluunbat, B., Abdelhadi, O., ... Burger, P. A. (2017). Mitogenome sequencing in the genus camelus reveals evidence for purifying selection and long-term divergence between wild and domestic Bactrian camels. *Scientific Reports*, *7*(1), 9970–9982. doi:10.103841598-017-08995-8 PMID:28855525

Monchot, H. (2015). From paleontology to zooarchaeology, importance of camels through time and history. *Proceedings of 4th Conference of ISOCARD, "Silk Road Camel: The Camelids, main stakes for sustainable development"*.

Nagy, P., Faigl, V., Reiczigel, J., & Juhasz, J. (2015). Effect of pregnancy and embryonic mortality on milk production in dromedary camels (*Camelus dromedarius*). *Journal of Dairy Science*, *98*(2), 975–986. doi:10.3168/jds.2014-8546 PMID:25434338

Nova, C. L. (1970). Reproduction in *Camelidae. Journal of Reproduction and Fertility*, *22*(1), 3–20. doi:10.1530/jrf.0.0220003 PMID:4911974

Peters, J. (1998). *Camelus thomasi Pomel*, 1893, a possible ancestor of the one-humped camel? *Mammalian Biology*, *63*, 372–376.

Pickford, M., Morales, J., & Soria, D. (1995). Fossil camels from the Upper Miocene of Europe: Implications for biogeography and faunal change. *Geobios-Lyon*, *28*(5), 641–650. doi:10.1016/S0016-6995(95)80217-7

Rybczynski, N., Gosse, J. C., Harington, R., Wogelius, R. A., Hidy, A. J., & Buckley, M. (2013). Mid-Pliocene warm-period deposits in the High Arctic yield insight into camel evolution. *Nature Communications*, *4*(1550), 1–9. PMID:23462993

Saalfeld, W. K., & Edwards, G. P. (2010). Distribution and abundance of the feral camel (*Camelus dromedarius*) in Australia. *The Rangeland Journal*, *32*(1), 1–9. doi:10.1071/RJ09058

Saipolda, T. (2005). Mongolian camels: current status of genetic resources, recording and production system in African, Asian and American Camelids. *Proceedings of the 34th meeting FAO/ICAR (International Committee for Animal Recording)* (pp. 73-80). Academic Press.

Sharma, A., & Pant, S. (2013). Studies on camel hair merino-wool blended knitted fabrics. *Indian Journal of Fibre and Textile Research*, *38*, 317–319.

Swai, E. S., Moshy, W., Mshanga, D., Lutatina, J., & Bwanga, S. (2011). Intestinal parasitic infections of camels in the agro and pastoral areas of northern Tanzania. *Veterinary Research*, *4*, 4–38.

Tomczyk, W. (2016). Camels on the Northeastern Frontier of the Roman Empire. *Papers from the Institute of Archaeology*, *26*(1), 1–13. doi:10.5334/pia-485

Uerpmann, H., & Uerpmann, M. (2002). The appearance of the domestic camel in south-east Arabia. *Journal of Oman Studies*, *12*, 235–260.

Von den Driesch, A., & Obermaier, H. (2007). The hunt for wild dromedaries during the 3rd and 2nd millennia BC on the United Arab Emirates coast. Camel bone finds from the excavations at Al Sufouh 2 Dubai, UAE. In Documenta Archaeobiologiae Bd. 5 – Skeletal series and their socio-economic context (pp. 133-167). Rahden, Germany: Verlag Marie Leidorf GmbH.

Webb, S. D. (Ed.). (1974). *Pleistocene mammals of Florida.* The University Press of Florida.

Wheeler, J. C. (2012). South American camelids - past, present and future. *Wheeler. Journal of Camelid Science*, *5*, 1–24.

Wilson, D. E., & Reeder, D. M. (2005). *Mammal species of the world*. Smithsonian.

Wilson, R. T., & Gutierrez, C. (2015). The one-humped camel in the Canary Islands: History and present status. *Tropicultura*, *33*(4), 288–298.

Yadav, A. K., Kumar, R., Priyadarshini, L., & Singh, J. (2015). Composition and medicinal properties of camel milk: A Review. *Asian Journal of Dairy & Food Research*, *34*(2), 83–91. doi:10.5958/0976-0563.2015.00018.4

Yam, B. A., & Khomeiri, M. (2015). Introduction to Camel origin, history, raising, characteristics, and wool, hair and skin: A review. *Research Journal of Agriculture and Environmental Management*, *4*, 496–508.

Chapter 2
Camel Milk Composition and Nutritional Value

Gaukhar S. Konuspayeva
Al-Farabi Kazakh National University, Kazakhstan

ABSTRACT

If gross composition of camel milk is roughly comparable to cow milk, fine composition shows significant differences explaining potential health benefit for regular consumers. The main particularities of camel milk are (1) better atherogenicity index thanks to its higher proportion of mono-unsaturated and polyunsaturated fatty acids compared to other milks, (2) different proportion of caseins than cow milk leading to difficult clotting, (3) lack of β-lactoglobulin, often responsible for cow milk allergy, (4) slightly higher concentration in antibacterial and immunity support proteins with higher bio-activity than in other milk, (5) presence of WAP (whey acidic protein) and PGRP (peptidoglycan-recognition protein) not available in cow milk, (6) probable efficient insulin for supporting better glycemia regulation, (7) better metabolization of lactose leading to lower intolerance in consumers, (8) richness in sodium and iron compared to other milks, and (9) contrasted values of vitamins (less vitamins B, high quantity of vitamins C and D). This chapter explores camel milk composition and nutritional value.

INTRODUCTION

The gross composition of camel milk has been investigated for more than one century. Indeed, the first available reference in the literature regarding this milk is that of Barthe in 1905 (Barthe, 1905). However, the number of references remains modest compared to that regarding cow milk. In a meta-analysis of the camel milk composition published in 2009 (Konuspayeva, Faye & Loiseau, 2009a), an almost comprehensive list of 82 references only was explored. For the last 10 years, the number of references increased significantly, in relation to the growing interest for camel milk in the world (Faye, 2018). Such growing interest is partly associated with the dietetic or medicinal values attributed to this milk. This

DOI: 10.4018/978-1-7998-1604-1.ch002

aspect discussed in other chapters of the present book. In the present chapter, the comprehensive list published in 2009 completed with some recent publications regarding the gross composition, while a second part is discussing the variation factors of this milk composition. In a last part, the particularities of camel milk in its fine composition is explored and compared with other milk of dairy species.

THE GROSS COMPOSITION OF CAMEL MILK

The compilation of 121 references published between 1905 and 2019 gives a mean and standard deviation of 3.68±1.00 for percentage of fat matter, 3.28±0.59 for total protein, 4.47±0.66 for lactose and 0.81±0.19 for ash with dry matter varying between 8.25 and 16.70% (mean=12.2±1.62%). To assess the average changes in this gross composition throughout the century, the references were gathered into 6 periods: per1 (1905-1960, 6 references), per2 (1961-1980, 12 references), per3 (1981-1990, 23 references), per4 (1991-2000, 32 references), per5 (2001-2010, 18 references), and per6 (2011-2019, 30 references). If lactose and mineral content doesn't change significantly across periods, there is a significant difference in fat matter and total protein (and consequently in dry matter percentage) according to the time of analysis, with a regular decrease of protein content and a maximum of fat in the period 1991-2000 (figure 1).

Such variation could be explained by the changes in the analytical methods used (Konuspayeva et al., 2009a), but could be also linked to the increasing references based on data from intensive camel farm where a certain degradation of fat and protein concentration in milk is observed (Benmohamed, Siboukeur & Ehoud, 2018). However, the variability is also observed according to origin of the camel milk samples. In the compilation of our 121 references, 15 were issued from Central Asia, 20 from South Asia, 24 from Middle East, 27 from East Africa, 27 from North Africa, 1 from West Africa and 1 from Europe,

Figure 1. Changes (mean ± SD) in fat matter (□) and total protein (○) in camel milk at different periods between 1905 and 2019 based on the compilation of 121 references

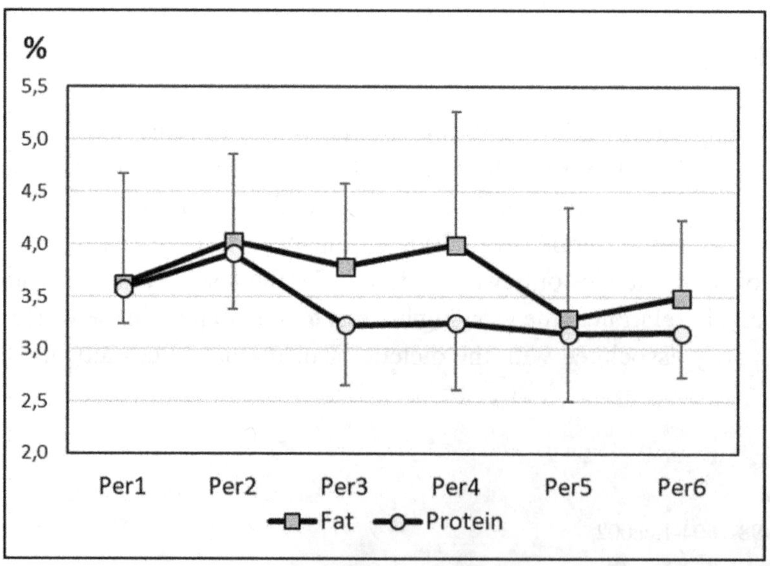

6 being undetermined. The samples from Central Asia were significantly richer in fat (4,87±0,77%) and in total protein (3,86±0,57%) than in other regions while the lower concentrations in fat is observed in North and West Africa, and for protein in Middle East and West Africa (Figures 2a and b).

The samples from Central Asia are issued mainly from Bactrian camel known for their lower milk productivity and their relative richness in fat matter and protein. Indeed, Bactrian camel produced around 1.5 to 2kg/day only while dromedary milk yield can reach more than 10 liters/day (Faye, 2004). In their comparative study based on the analysis of 57 Bactrian, 70 dromedaries and 20 hybrids reared in the same farms from Kazakhstan, Faye, Konuspayeva, Messad & Loiseau (2008a) observed significant higher concentration in fat matter, vitamin C and minerals in Bactrian compared to dromedary milk, the concentrations in hybrid milk being intermediary (Table 1). No significant difference was reported for lactose content.

As for milk from other dairy species, fat matter and protein concentrations are highly correlated. The investigation of our 121 references shows linear equation:

Protein=0.261Fat+2.32 ($P<0.0001$; $r=0.44$) (Figure 3).

Figure 2. Mean and SD of fat matter (a) and total protein (b) concentrations in camel milk from different regions of the world based on the compilation of 121 references (in %)

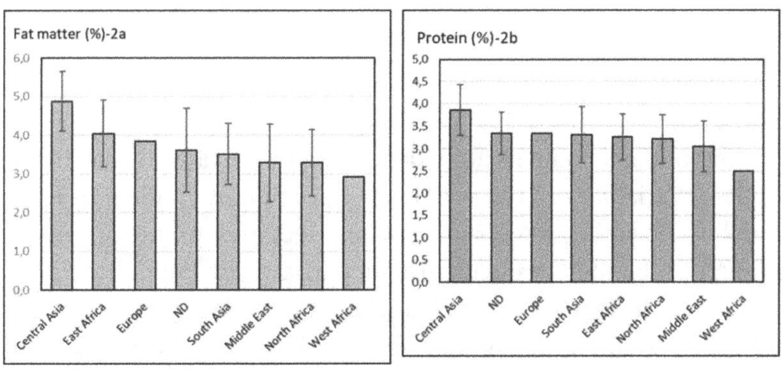

Table 1. Differences in the gross composition of Bactrian, dromedary and hybrid milk in animals reared in the same farms from Kazakhstan (from after Faye et al., 2008a)

Parameters	Bactrian	Dromedary	Hybrid	*P* value
Fat	6.67 ± 2.93	5.94 ± 2.26	6.09 ± 1.81	0.04
Lactose	2.77 ± 0.96	3.12 ± 0.92	3.04 ± 0.60	0.45
Vit C (mg/l)	177 ± 109	152 ± 91	133 ± 133	<0.001
TP	5.23 ± 1.17	4.76 ± 1.13	5.15 ± 1.59	0.11
Ca (g/L)	1.303 ± 0.287	1.163 ± 0.273	1.257 ± 0.268	0.003
P (g/L)	1.075 ± 0.177	0.915 ± 0.190	1.067 ± 0.273	<0.001
Fe (mg/L)	2.11 ± 1.63	1.93 ± 1.06	2.01 ± 0.78	0.55

Figure 3. Correlation between fat matter and total protein in camel milk reported in 121 references from the literature between 1905 and 2019

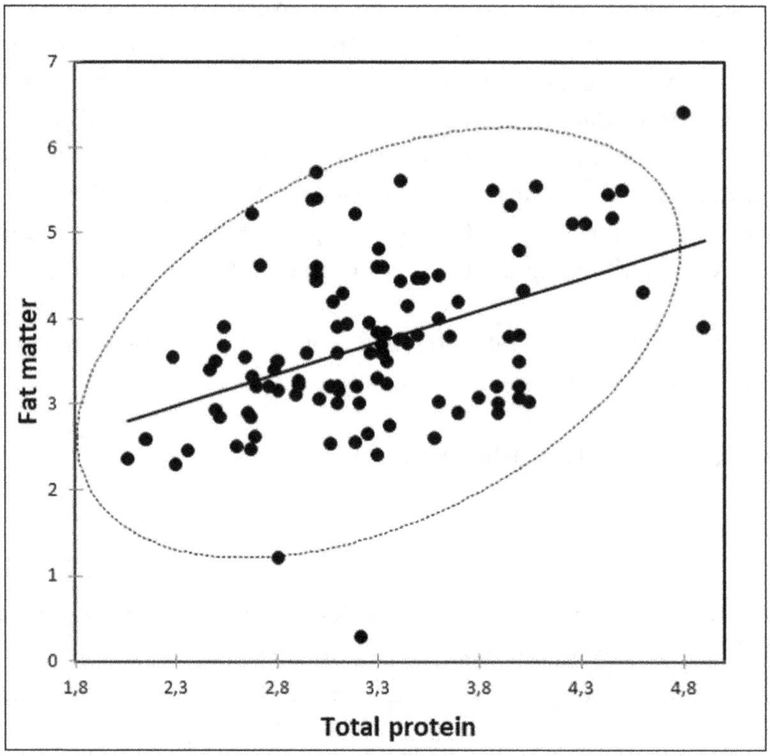

At reverse, lactose and mineral contents are independent of the fat and protein concentrations. However, due to the high daily variability in the composition, both in individual or bulk milk, and because the conditions of sampling (lactation stage, parity, breed, feeding) are not always recorded in the publications, the compilation of the literature data gives a partial view only of the proper values of camel milk composition. For example, in a 2-years monitoring in intensive camel dairy farm in Saudi Arabia (Al-Gedan, Al-Aguili, Alomayri, Konuspayeva & Faye, 2015), fat percentage in bulk milk varied between 0.8 and 5.7% while protein concentrations were in the range 2.16-3.99% and lactose 3.69-5.13%.

The daily variability is especially high for fat content while lactose and protein appear to be more stable (Figure 4). Similar variations at individual level occur, partly due to the milking practice. Indeed, when the milking is complete (including alveolar milk), fat concentration in milk is significantly higher: 3.59±0.18 vs 2.98±0.17% in cisternal milk, while there was no difference for protein and lactose (Ayadi et al., 2013).

However, the variability can be linked also to the animal itself even within the same farm environment. In an intensive camel dairy farm in Saudi Arabia, the gross composition of milk was monitored weekly in 46 camels over their entire lactation (Faye, 2015). The range of mean fat concentration values was between 1.19±1.01 and 4.84±1.61% while it was between 2.09±0.28 and 3.58±0.28% for protein and between 3.27±0.36 and 5.26±0.43% for lactose with respective coefficient of variation 0.48, 0.18 and 0.16 underlining the highest variability of fat concentration.

Figure 4. Daily chronicles of fat, protein and lactose content in camel bulk milk in intensive dairy farm from Saudi Arabia (from after Al-Gedan et al., 2015)

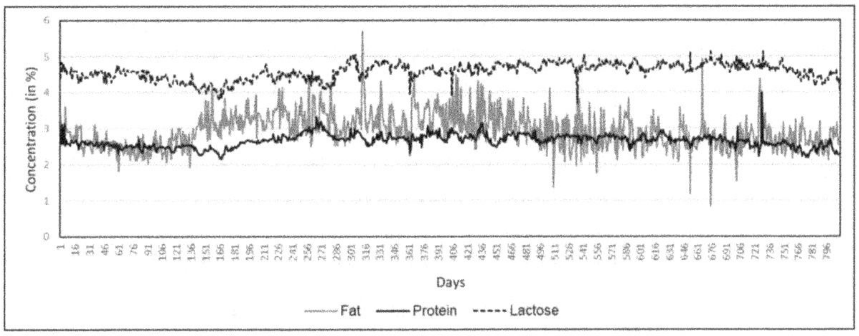

MAIN VARIATION FACTORS OF GROSS COMPOSITION

The variation in camel milk composition as in other species is under control of genetic (breed) and non-genetic (physiological stage, feeding management practices, health status) factors. In camel, those factors were relatively poorly investigated.

Genetic Factors of Variation

The difference between Bactrian and dromedary milk composition was investigated, showing the possibility to predict the species origin with 75.4% well-classed after quadratic discriminant analysis (Faye et al., 2008a). The between-breed within species variability was sometimes reported. Some authors explored differences between 3 Kenyan camel breeds (Wangoh, Farah & Puhan, 1998), 3 other breeds also in Sudan (Dowelmadina, El Zubeir, Salim & Arabi, 2014; Elobied et al., 2015) or in 3 camel breeds from India (Mal & Sena, 2007). Most of the references were reported in Saudi Arabia. For example, Mehaia, Hablas, Abdel-Rahman & El-Mougy (1995) reported values for 3 main camel breeds in the country with higher fat and protein concentrations in Majaheem (3.22 and 2.91% respectively), than in Wadah (2.46 and 2.36%) and Hamra breed (2.85 and 2.52%) while no significant difference occurred for lactose and ash. Later, Gaili, Al-Eknah & Sadek (2000) found also richer content (fat and protein) in Majaheem compared to Wadah and Awarik milk throughout the lactation. From their side, Aljumaah et al., (2012) reported higher mean fat content in Shoal breed milk (3.26%) than in Majaheem (2.84%), Wadah (2.79%) and Sofor (2.96%) while protein and lactose were in higher concentration in Sofor (3.7 and 5.44% respectively) than in the other breeds (3.25-3.48 and 5.07-5.12% respectively).

More complete comparison was published recently by Nagy et al. (2017). Comparing 2332 milk samples from 7 camel breeds or ecotypes (namely Emirati, crossbreed-Emirati, Majaheem (black), Pakistani, Saudi, Saudi-crossbreed and Sudanese) belonging to the same intensive dairy farm in Emirates, high fat content was observed in Pakistani breed (2.81%) and low-fat milk in Saudi-crossbreed (2.3%) while protein was in higher concentration in Emirati-crossbreed (3.05%) and lower in Saudi and Saudi-crossbreed (2.85 and 2.87% respectively). Conversely, lactose was higher in Saudi-crossbreed (4.27%) while Pakistani breed was poor in lactose (3.7%).

Such results show the relative inconsistence between studies leading to difficult conclusions. First, a large variability in the mean values is observed in literature for a specific breed (for example Majaheem);second, several factors of confusion (as lactation stage, milk productivity or parity) could occur in the different published studies. Moreover, despite the phenotype variability observed in camel breeds and ecotypes (Abdallah & Faye, 2012), there is no high genotypes distances (Almathen et al., 2016).

Physiological Stage

The components of milk are varying throughout the lactation in all dairy species. This factor of variation was investigated in Bactrian camel (Zhang et al., 2005; Konuspayeva et al., 2009b) and dromedary (El-Mougy, 1995; Zeleke et al., 2007; Ahmad et al., 2012; Musaad, Faye & Al-Mutairi, 2013a; Babiker & Elzubeir, 2014). In most of the cases, data are available on monthly reported data or even quarterly, except in the observations of Musaad et al., (2013a) achieved on weekly basis showing lower fat content between week12 and week32 while other parameters show a slight regular decrease throughout the lactation period (figure 5).

All references agree with the higher impact of physiological stage on fat content than on protein while lactose and ash content appear relatively stable although some authors observed a seasonal effect on lactose content (Bakheit, Majid & Nikhala 2008). Globally, in the studies on seasonal variability of camel milk composition, there is a confusion with the lactation stage as the calving season in camel is generally grouped within 3-4 months. For example, in the study of Musaad et al., (2013a), the fat content dropped to a lower level during the hot months (April to September), corresponding to the maximum of milk production which occurs usually at the 3rd and 4th months of lactation both in Bactrian (Zhao, Bai, & Niu, 2015) and dromedary camel (Musaad, Faye & Abu-Nikhela, 2013b). Thus, the fat component is

Figure 5. Weekly chronicles of fat, protein, lactose and ash content in camel milk throughout the lactation period (from after Musaad et al., 2013a)

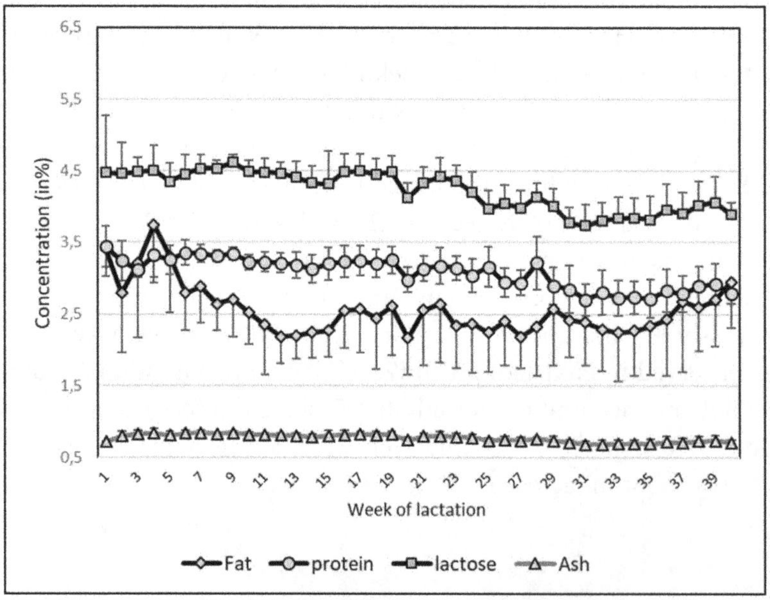

the most sensitive parameter to the dilution effect linked to the production increase. Shuiep & Elzubeir (2008) and Haddadin, Gammoh & Robinson (2008) reported similar results with lower fat at the hot season. However, the total quantity of the different components excreted in milk is following the lactation curve, with a maximum of excretion at lactation peak (Musaad et al., 2013a).

Feeding and Management Effect

The investigation of camel milk composition according to farming system effect has been undertaken only recently. Some authors compared extensive to intensive system but with contradictory results. For example, in Sudan, fat content was significantly higher in intensive system compared to "grazing" system (4.05±1.5 *vs* 3.29±1.06%) while protein and lactose content were significantly higher in "semi-intensive" system (Babiker & Elzubeir, 2014). At reverse, in Algeria, no significant difference was observed between extensive and semi-intensive breeding farms except for vitamin C concentration which was higher in extensive system (Benmohamed et al., 2018). In Morocco, Bouhaddaoui et al., (2019) compared 3 highly contrasted locations in the country, covering in fact different farming and feeding systems. They reported higher quantity of fat and lactose in milk sampled at Dakhla in the south of the country where farming system is more extensive while there was no difference in protein and ash. In Tunisia, Fguiri et al., (2018) reported higher fat (3.47%) and protein (4.36%) in extensive system compared to intensive one (2.14 and 3.17% respectively) while Aljumaah et al., (2012) in Saudi-Arabia found higher fat content (3.16%) in settled system compared to semi-nomadic one (2.86%) and higher protein (3.6%) and lactose (5,25%) in semi-nomadic system compared to nomadic herd (3.11 and 4.59% respectively). It appears however, that on average, milk collected in camel grazing in the desert is richer in useful matter and the effect is more noticeable on fat content, but the inconsistent observations could be linked to the feed provided to the camel and other parameters.

Few references explored the impact of different diet on camel milk gross composition (Musaad et al., 2013a; Benmohamed et al., 2018). In the experiment of Faye et al., (2013a) regarding the introduction of olive cake in the diet, no difference was observed in fat content (3.42 ±0.8 in group receiving olive cake *vs* 3.35±0.81% in control group) and protein concentration (3.20±0.19 *vs* 3.16±0.20%, respectively).

Other variation factors were investigated as milking interval (Alshaikh & Salah, 1994; Abdalla et al., 2016), parity (Ahmad et al., 2012; Musaad at al., 2013a; Dowelmadina et al., 2014; Elobied et al., 2015), sex of the camel calf (Nagy et al., 2017), machine milking effect (Hammadi et al., 2010) or even the quarter of udder (Eisa & Hassabo, 2009). Thus, the concentration of fat and protein in milk decreased linearly with increase in milking interval, but for most of the variation factors, the observed effect on the main components does not appear constant.

Comparison with Milk from Other Dairy Animals

In several references, comparison with milk from other species is reported. For example, Sabahelkhier, Faten & Omer (2012) compared camel to cow, goat, sheep and human. Yoganandi, Mehta, Wadhwani, Darji & Aparnathi (2014) compared camel milk composition to cow and buffalo milk. Globally, camel milk gross composition is close to that of cow and goat (Figure 6). Camel milk gross composition appears close to that of cow and goat milk for fat and protein content and to all other common domestic ruminants for lactose and minerals. However, there is a lack of comparative studies in similar feeding and management context throughout the lactation.

Figure 6. Normal ranges of fat (a), protein (b), lactose (c) and minerals (d) in different dairy animals (in g/l)

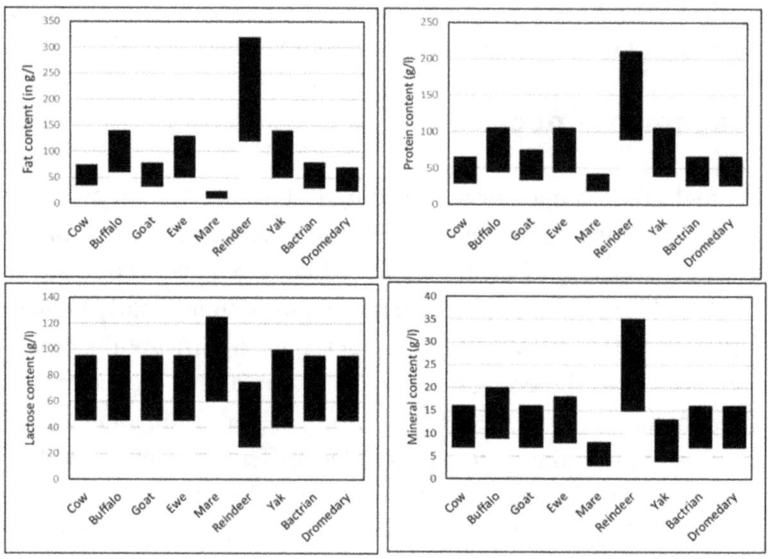

Some differences between camel milk and other milk from dairy species were reported also regarding physical parameters as foaming, emulsion, buffering capacity, acidity and pH. The foaming and emulsion capabilities are considered of the important functional properties (Mati et al., 2017). The foam is the fine continuous dispersion of gas bubbles in an aqueous solution. Foaming is essential in the structure of many food products (Stave & Törner, 2007) such as whipped toppings, ice cream, mousse, espresso coffee (Sharma, Jana, & Chavan, 2012), and cookies (Ikechukwu et al., (2017). The proteins from bovine or camel milk exhibited similar surface-active properties, which lead to similar foaming capacity (Maqsood et al., 2019). Furthermore, foaming capacity of bovine and camel milk proteins at specific pH values did not show any significant difference. This makes camel milk proteins or protein hydrolysates (Al-Shamsi, Mudgil, Hassan, & Maqsood, 2017) good substitutes for other mammalian milk proteins (Al-Ghsyar, Salem, & Ahmad, 2018).

Foaming ability and stability are related to pH and emulsion droplet diameter. At pH 5, 88% of camel whey droplets are sized > 2µm, while 80% and 1.5% of the bovine whey particles are sized < 2µm and >3µm respectively. The addition of HCl improved the foaming ability of camel milk (Laleye, Jobe, & Wasesa, 2008). In another study, proteins from camel and bovine milk at different pH possessed high foaming capacity, emulsifying activity index, and protein solubility at acidic and alkaline pH, while these functional properties were low at isoelectric point of pH 4 (Maqsood et al., 2019). In contrast, emulsifying activity index of camel milk proteins is higher compared to those of bovine milk at isoelectric points of pH 4 and pH 2. This might be due to the lack of β-lactoglobulin and amino acid content of camel milk proteins. On the other hand, it can be attributed to the structural variation between camel and bovine milk proteins as well as conformity (Maqsood et al., 2019).

Similar to the acidity of sheep milk (Yagil, Saran, & Etzion, 1984), the pH of camel milk range between 4 and 6.7 (Abu-Taraboush, Al-Dagal, & Al-Royli, 1998; Khaskheli, Arain, Chaudhry, Soomro, & Qureshi, 2005). Camel milk was reported to have buffering capacity at pH 4.95, which is lower than that of bovine milk (Sawaya, Khalil, Al-Shalhat, & Al-Mohammad, 1984) while skimmed camel milk has higher buffering capacity at the pH 5.65.

SOME SPECIFIC CHARACTERISTICS OF THE FINE COMPOSITION

If the gross composition of camel milk is relatively close to that of cow milk, some components of the fine composition (fatty acids, caseins and other proteins, vitamins, main and trace minerals) can be specific in terms of concentration or even qualitatively (Al haj & Al Kanhal, 2010). The exhaustivity in the presentation of the fine composition should require a full book. So, in the present chapter, only some specific characteristics of the camel milk were chosen.

FAT MATTER COMPONENTS

Fatty Acids

Compared to cow milk, the content of unsaturated fatty acids in camel milk is in higher proportion in both dromedary (Cardak, Yetismeyen & Brückner, 2003; Dreiucker & Vetter, 2011; Ereifej Alu'datt, Al-Khalidy, Alli & Rababah, 2011) and Bactrian camel (Narmuratova et al., 2006; Konuspayeva, Lemarie, Faye, Loiseau & Montet, 2008). At reverse, camel milk is poor in short-chain fatty acids. For example, cow milk contains more than 3% of the shortest one (butyric acid-C4:0) while camel milk contains 0.37% only (Abu-Lehia, 1989; Attia, Kherouatou, Fakhfakh, Khorchani & Trigui, 2000). The sum of short-chain fatty acids C4:0 to C8:0 was only 1.15% in camel's milk, and 8.99% in the milk of cows fed with a nutritionally balanced diet. The medium-chain fatty acids (C4:0 to C14:0) were 16.38% in camel's milk and 21.44% in cow's milk. The long-chain fatty acids C15:0 to C20:1 were much higher (82.43%) in camel's milk than in cow's milk (66.1%) but less than in mare milk (Faye, Konuspayeva, Narmuratova, & Loiseau, 2008b). If the ratio saturated/unsaturated FA was closed for the two dairy species: 67.7 for camel's milk and 69.9 for cow's milk, the proportion of unsaturated fatty acid content is in favor of camel milk (Figure 7). For example, content of C18:3 was about 10 times higher in camel's milk (0.6) than in cow's milk (0.07).

In consequence, camel milk has a better atherogenicity index (AI) than cow milk. This index is highly associated with the onset of coronary heart diseases in consumers. AI was estimated to 2.7 in camel milk (Konuspayeva et al., 2008) while it was between 3.3 and 3.5 in cow milk with standard feeding (Chilliard, Ferlay & Doreau, 2001).

Few differences in FA profiles were observed between dromedary and Bactrian camel (Konuspayeva et al., 2008): C14:0 (myristic acid) was in higher proportion in Bactrian milk while C17:0iso (iso-heptadecanoic) and C18:1 (oleic acid) were in higher percentage in dromedary milk. However, no significant variation was observed for the total of short-chain FA, medium-chain FA and long-chain FA (Table 2).

Figure 7. Proportions of saturated (SAT), mono-unsaturated (MUSAT) and poly-unsaturated (PUSAT) fatty acids in milk of different dairy species (from after Faye et al., 2008b)

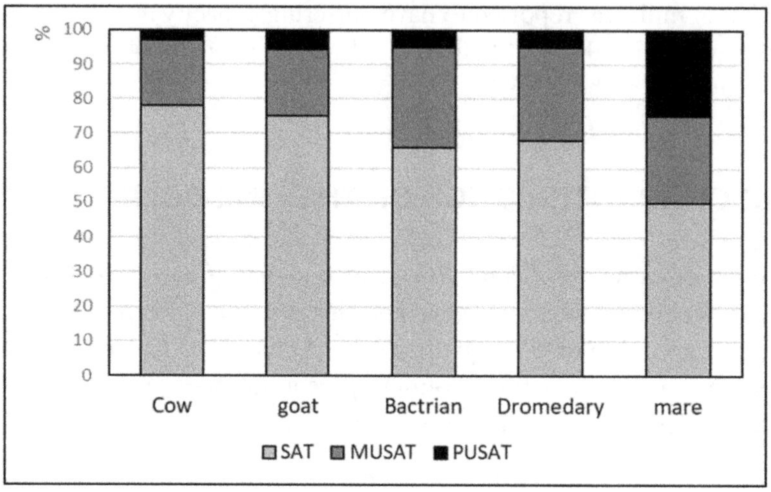

The dietetic interest of camel milk is reinforced by its relative richness in conjugated linoleic acid (CLA) compared to human and cow milk, respectively 1.23, 0.42 and 0.65 g/100g fat (Dreiucker & Vetter, 2011).

Cholesterol

Despite the general agreement on the low cholesterol content in camel meat (see Chapter 13), the situation is controversial for camel milk (Faye, Bengoumi, Al-Masaud & Konuspayeva, 2015a). Many consumers and scientists argue that camel milk contains less cholesterol than cow milk (Kamal & Salama, 2009; Raziq, Younas & Kakar, 2008) while others reported opposite results (Gorban & Izzeldin, 1999; Konuspayeva et al., 2008). In their comparative study, Gorban & Izzeldin (1999) reported total cholesterol in camel colostrum of 27.6 mg/100 ml and 31.3 mg/100 ml in mature camel milk *vs* 25.6 mg/100 ml in mature cow milk. Moreover, the proportion of total cholesterol to total fat was reported to 0.93% in camel milk compared to 0.69% in cow milk (Gorban & Izzeldin, 1999). In dromedary and Bactrian camels from Kazakhstan, the mean value of cholesterol in camel milk was reported as 37.1 mg/100 ml (Konuspayeva et al., 2008), but the animals had a high level of fat in milk (5.9%). Indeed, the level of cholesterol in the milk is closely dependent on the quantity of fat matter. Therefore, it is not possible to ascertain that camel milk contains less or more cholesterol than cow milk, the ratio cholesterol/fat being quite comparable between the two species (Faye Bengoumi, Al-Masaud & Konuspayeva, 2015b).

Phospholipids

In a comparative study, phospholipids were identified and quantified by ^{31}P NMR spectroscopy procedure showing higher concentrations in total phospholipids in camel milk (0.503 mM) than in cow (0.265 mM) and mare milk (0.101 mM) and a more abundant sphingomyelin (117.5 µg/ml) and plasmalogens (24 µg/ml) than in other dairy species (Garcia, Lutz, Confort-Gouny, Cozzone, Armand & Bernard, 2012).

Table 2. Fatty acid composition of camel milk fat by species (IA: index of atherogenicity; SCFA: short chain fatty acid; MCFA: medium chain fatty acid; LCFA: long chain fatty acid; ns: insignificant) (from after Konuspayeva et al., 2008)

Acids	Bactrian (n=7)	Dromedary (n=10)	Hybrids (n=3)	*P* value
C4:0	0.54 ± 0.63	0.34 ± 0.29	0.20 ± 0.20	ns
C6:0	0.46 ± 0.39	0.29 ± 0.16	0.35 ± 0.34	ns
C8:0	0.53 ± 0.41 [b]	0.27 ± 0.19 [a]	0.41 ± 0.44 [a]	0.02
C10:0	0.46 ± 0.51	0.27 ± 0.39	0.30 ± 0.34	ns
C10:1	1.15 ± 1.44	0.81 ± 1.22	0.54 ± 0.60	ns
C12:0	1.24 ± 0.58 [b]	0.80 ± 0.20 [a]	1.00 ± 0.69 [a]	0.03
C13:0	0.17 ± 0.38	0.03 ± 0.06	0.01 ± 0.01	ns
C14:0iso	0.20 ± 0.19	0.17 ± 0.17	0.06 ± 0.02	ns
C14:0	15.43 ± 4.09 [a]	10.10 ± 1.32 [b]	12.95 ± 5.71 [a]	0.001
C14:1	0.80 ± 0.42 [a]	0.57 ± 0.15 [b]	0.86 ± 0.52 [a]	0.04
C14:0 dm	0.32 ± 0.17	0.50 ± 0.33	0.28 ± 0.21	ns
C15:0iso	0.77 ± 0.21	0.88 ± 0.20	0.60 ± 0.13	ns
C15:0	1.41 ± 0.50	1.24 ± 0.18	1.07 ± 0.16	ns
C16:0iso	0.22 ± 0.14	0.34 ± 0.21	0.21 ± 0.05	ns
C16:0	32.05 ± 3.83	29.74 ± 4.62	32.56 ± 2.66	ns
C16:1	7.01 ± 2.01	6.60 ± 1.31	6.74 ± 1.01	ns
C16:0dm	0.38 ± 0.20	0.44 ± 0.30	0.34 ± 0.21	ns
C17:0iso	0.55 ± 0.27 [a]	0.82 ± 0.24 [b]	0.49 ± 0.21 [a]	0.003
C17:0	0.65 ± 0.32	0.76 ± 0.17	0.61 ± 0.12	ns
C17:1	0.33 ± 0.25	0.38 ± 0.13	0.33 ± 0.17	ns
C18:0	14.75 ± 5.55	17.82 ± 3.70	17.69 ± 5.35	ns
C18:1	18.78 ± 4.68 [a]	24.66 ± 4.63 [b]	20.64 ± 5.38 [b]	0.002
C18:2	1.19 ± 0.45	1.61 ± 0.51	1.10 ± 0.41	ns
C18:3	0.60 ± 0.41	0.51 ± 0.71	0.67 ± 0.36	ns
C20:0	0.01 ± 0.02	0.05 ± 0.09	0.00	ns
C20:1	0.00 [a]	0.01 ± 0.03 [a]	0.00 [a]	0.05
IA	2.30 ± 0.71	2.75 ± 0.91	2.85 ± 1.12	ns
SCFA	1.52 ± 1.25	0.89 ± 0.55	0.95 ± 0.79	ns
MCFA	21.95 ± 5.70	15.38 ± 2.42	17.67 ± 6.32	ns
LCFA	76.51 ± 6.76	83.73 ± 2.80	81.37 ± 7.10	ns

Some Proteins Components

The protein composition of milk is complex. It includes four groups of proteins: caseins, whey protein (lactoglobulin, lactalbumin, immunoglobulins, serum albumin, and lactoferrin), proteins of the fat globule membranes and secretory components (enzymes). According to Omar, Harbourne & Oruna-Concha

(2016), camel milk has high concentration in α-lactalbumin (2.01 ± 0.02 mg/ml), lactoferrin (1.74 ± 0.06 mg/ml) and serum albumin (0.46 ± 0.01 mg/ml).

The proteomic investigation of camel milk from Bactrian, dromedary and hybrids allowed detecting 1010 functional groups of proteins including 893 common proteins between these three camel species. Thirty-one proteins were unique to Bactrian, five to dromedary and twelve to hybrids (Ryskalieva et al., 2018).

The caseins represent 76% of the proteins in camel milk (82% in cow and buffalo milk, 78% in sheep and goat milk, 52% in mare milk and 33% only in human milk). Moreover, the distribution of the types of caseins and whey proteins differed between species (Figure 8).

The concentration of β-casein is 12.78 ± 0.92 mg/ml) followed by α-casein (2.89 ± 0.29 mg/ml) while κ-casein is in minor amount (1.67 ± 0.01 mg/ml) (Omar et al., 2016). The particularities of camel milk proteins are the low proportion of κ-casein, the lack of β-lactoglobulin, the higher proportion of α-lactalbumin and the presence of WAP (Whey Acidic Protein) and PGRP (Peptidoglycan-recognition protein) not available in cow milk. Recently, a new variant of α-S2-casein was detected in camel from Kazakhstan (Ryskalieva et al., 2019a). The low proportion of κ-casein should be the main cause of the clotting difficulties during cheese processing (Chapter 6) as shown by Kappeler, Farah & Puhan (2003). The lack of β-lactoglobulin could contribute to the low induction of allergy with camel milk consumption (Shabo et al., 2005). WAP could play an important role in regulating the proliferation of mammary epithelial cells and in bacteriostatic activity (Ryskalieva et al., 2019b). PGRP is a pathogen recognition protein having antimicrobial and immunostimulant properties (Chapter 7) that could contribute to the health effect of camel milk (Kappeler, Heuberger, Farah & Puhan, 2004).

Regarding the essential amino-acid composition, camel milk compared to cow milk contains significantly less lysine, phenylalanine and histidine in α-casein, but more lysine, threonine, methionine and isoleucine in β-casein (Salmen, Abu-Tarboush Al-Saleh & Metwalli, 2012).

Lactoferrin (Lf) is a glycoprotein having affinity to iron playing different biological roles, beneficial for health (Chapter 7). From the first quantification of camel lactoferrin published in 1996 (El-Gawad, El-Sayed, Mahfouz & Abd El-Salam, 1996), it was reported that Lf concentration in raw camel milk was more than 10 times higher (2.48 mg/mL) than in cow's milk (0.07-0.28 mg/mL). Later, Zhang et al., (2005) reported that Lf values were between 2.35 and 7.28% of the total protein in the Bactrian milk, i.e around 0.7 to 2.1 mg/mL representing again 10 times the cow's values. In fact, the analytical methods used by these authors induced bias. By using gel radial immunodiffusion, Lf in camel milk

Figure 8. Distribution in % of the caseins (a) and whey protein in camel and cow (from after Kappeler, Farah & Puhan, 1998)

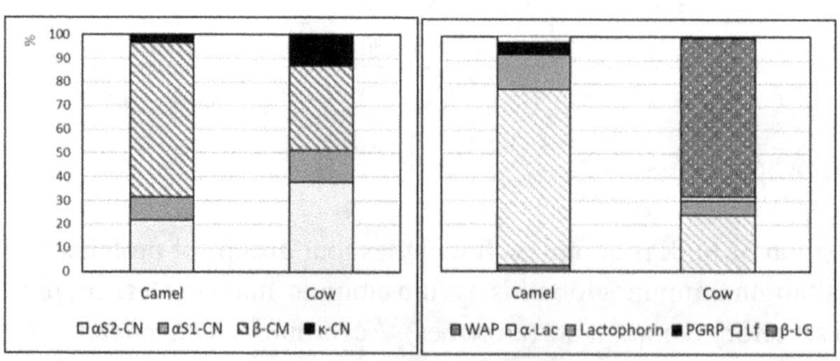

was estimated to 0.229±0.135 mg/ml in dromedary and Bactrian camels (Konuspayeva, Faye, Loiseau & Levieux, 2007). Using similar analytical methods, El Hatmi, Levieux & Levieux, (2006) and Kappeler, Manfred, Farah & Puhan, (1999) found in dromedary camel 0.14 and 0.22 mg/mL respectively, i.e. values only slightly higher than in cow. However, a comparative study showed that camel Lf has the highest antimicrobial activity (Conesa et al., 2008) compared to other mammals.

The concentration in immunoglobulins, proteins playing a considerable role in the immune protection of the new-born, vary according to the lactation stage, with especially a quite higher quantity in colostrum (see chapter 11).

Insulin is not a common protein in milk, but the traditional belief that regular consumption of camel milk could contribute to the prevention and control of diabetes due to its high insulin concentration is a common report in scientific literature (see Chapter 9), although few references are available. Moreover, the values are highly variable because the differences in analytical methods. The total quantity should be around 50 μU/ml, comparable to sheep milk, but higher than cow milk (30 μU/ml) (Zagorski et al., 1998). In measurement over one lactation, Wernery, Johnson & Tawfig Ishmail (2006) observed variation between 25 and 75 μU/ml with an average of 40.5 ±10.7 μU/ml, comparable to the 52 μU/ml cited by Agrawal et al. (2003). Diaz-Medina (2017) reported insulin concentration in camel milk as 57.3 ±3.46 at early lactation, then 25.3 ±10.7 at the middle and 47.26 ±9.8 μU/l at late lactation.

The enzymes are not commonly investigated in camel milk (Yadav, Kumar, Priyadarshini & Singh, 2015). Among the enzymes useful for dairy industry, Alkaline phosphatases (ALP) are determined to control the pasteurization because it disappears after heat treatment (Chapter 10). However, camel ALP being thermoresistant, its use as marker of milk pasteurization is not convenient (Loiseau, Faye, Serikbaeva & Montet, 2001; Wernery, Fischbach, Johnson, & Jose, 2008). In fresh camel milk, the average ALP activity was lower (21.31 μg/ ml) than in cow and buffalo milk samples: 575 μg/ ml and 253.75 μg/ml respectively (Yoganandi, Jain, Mehta, Wadhwani & Aparnathi, 2014). However, after pasteurization, ALP activities are disappearing in pasteurized cow milk but remain between 5.8 to 10.2 U/l in pasteurized camel milk (Lorenzen, Wernery, Johnson, Jose & Wernery, 2011).

Reverse to ALP, Gamma Glutamyl Transferase (GGT) being destroyed at 72°C, it has been proposed as indicator for the pasteurization of camel milk (Loiseau et al., 2001). Lorenzen et al., (2011) reported values at 342 ± 37.5 U/l and 329 ± 22.4 U/l in two different pools of raw milk while the remain activity after heat treatment at 2.2 ± 4.0 and 0.1 ±0.3 U/l respectively.

Lactose

As reported above, the concentration of lactose in camel milk is comparable to that of cow milk (Al-Haj & Kanhal, 2010), i.e. 4.47±0.66 g/100ml according to the compilation of published references cited above whereas it was 4.5 to 5.0 g/100ml in cow milk (Gaucheron, 2011). Yet, camel milk is known to have less effect on lactose intolerance than cow milk, and seems more easily metabolized by consumers, even those having no lactase (Cardoso, Santos, Cardoso & Carvalho, 2010). The explanation advanced by these authors is that camel milk produces less casomorphin, leading to lower intestinal motility and consequently a longer exposition of lactose to the action of lactase. Another hypothesis could be linked to the type of lactate as final product of lactose fermentation in the digestive tract of milk consumers. Indeed, two stereoisomers of lactate are described according to the position of hydroxyl radical on the molecule: D-Lactate (for dextrogyre) and L-Lactate (for levogyre). D-lactate has negative effect on the health of the new-born up to one year old due to the lack of the enzyme responsible of its degradation.

The consecutive accumulation of lactate could provoke acidosis. In contrast, L-lactate is well supported by the consumers as they possess the oxidative enzyme Lactate dehydrogenase (LDH) which recognizes only the L(+) form of lactate. Thus, if the content of total lactate in camel milk was comparable to cow milk (1.82 – 2.49 g/l), the quantity of L-Lactate was 100 times more in camel milk (2.21% of the total lactate) than in cow milk (0.02%) (Konuspayeva, Baubekova, Akhmetsadykova, Akhmetsadykov & Faye., 2019). The appearance of these products of lactose metabolism mainly depends of microflora of camel milk. L- and D-lactate production are linked to lactic microflora and the difference with the microflora of cow milk could explain some dietetic properties of camel milk.

In addition of lactose, camel milk as for other milk contains oligosaccharides. In mature Bactrian milk, the total concentration of oligosaccharides was 0.12 g/100 ml vs 0.04 g/100ml only for cow milk while the ratio was reverse in colostrum (0.20 and 0.29 g/100 ml in camel and cow respectively). The composition and nutraceuticals properties of oligosaccharides in camel colostrum will be discussed in Chapter 11. Three main oligosaccharides were described in mature camel milk (3′-galactosyllactose, lacto-N-novopentaose I and 3′-sialyllactose) and 10 in Bactrian colostrum: 3-fucosyllactose, 3’-galactosyllactose, 6’-galactosyllactose, 3’-sialyllactose, 6’-sialyllactose, sialyl-3’-galactosyllactose, sialyllacto-N-tetraose, sialyllacto-N-novopentaose sialyllacto-N-novopentaose and monosialyllacto-N-neohexaose (Fukuda et al., 2010). A more complex structure of oligosaccharides was described in a comparative study reporting 48 structures in dromedary camel milk compared to 41 in goat milk, 40 in pig and horse milk, 38 in sheep and 35 only in bovine milk (Albrecht et al., 2014). The potential health properties of oligosaccharides in camel milk will be discussed in Chapter 7.

Minerals

The richness of camel milk in minerals is regularly stated by different authors for promoting its supposed dietetic virtues. Yet, compared to other species, this trait is contrasted.

On average in the literature, **calcium** concentrations in camel milk are in a wide range between 30 and 257 mg/100ml (Faye & Bengoumi, 2018) with variations linked to breed, lactation stage and management systems but with contradictory observations. However, in most of the studies, the means varied between 100 and 150 mg/100ml. For example, in Morocco, Bengoumi, Faye & Tressol (1998) reported a mean value of 146 ± 24 mg/100ml. Comparing cow, goat, sheep and camel milk, Al-Wabel (2008) found similar concentration of calcium: 69.9 ± 9.6 (camel) *vs* 66.1 ± 4.2 (cow), 75.1 ± 7.27 (goat) and 82.2 ± 11.3 mg/100ml (sheep) although higher concentration was reported in domestic Bactrian camel (Jirimutu et al., 2010) with a range 122.9 ± 0.8 to 183.4 ± 1.87 mg/100ml.High regional variations were also observed for example in 25 Iranian camels with extreme values between 78.2 ± 3.1 and 151 ± 9.1 mg/100ml (Mostafidi, Moslehishad, Piravivanak, & Pouretedal, 2016).

Phosphorus varies in camel milk between 34 and 100 mg/100ml (Faye & Bengoumi, 2018) and is on average in a lower concentration than in buffalo, cow and goat milk (Soliman, 2005). For **magnesium,** contradictory observations were reported, some authors considering comparable concentrations than in cow milk while other found significantly lower. On average, the values varied between 6.7 and 14 mg/100ml (Soliman, 2005; Shamsia, 2009).

Among the main minerals, **sodium** has a special status as it appeared in quite higher quantity in camel milk than in cow or goat milk (Al-Wabel, 2008; Wang, Shao & Wen., 2011). Globally, the range of sodium in camel milk is 220-990 mg/l (Faye & Bengoumi, 2018). The grazing of desert halophytes containing high quantity of salt could explain the differences with milk from other species, giving notably a saltier taste to camel milk. The range for **potassium** in camel milk in literature is between 520 and 1800 mg/l (Faye & Bengoumi, 2018), i.e. in similar quantity than in other species except human milk (Shamsia, 2009).

Data regarding trace elements in camel milk are scattered and important gap is observed between the reported values and in the differences with the milk from other species. For example, globally, reported **copper** contents in camel milk are highly variable, between 30 to 800 µg/100ml (Faye & Bengoumi, 2018). In the study of Omer & Eltinay (2008) including 350 milk samples, the range was 1-118 µg/100ml with an average of 40 µg/100ml. In Bactrian milk, values around 5-7µg/100ml were observed (Konuspayeva et al., 2011a). Such values are sometimes comparable and sometimes higher or lower to that of other milk according to the comparative studies (Faye & Bengoumi, 2018).

Similar observations can be done for **zinc** concentration in milk. With a range of 0.06 to 0.50 mg/100ml according to different authors, the values in camel milk appear sometimes higher, comparable or lower than cow or goat milk. Zinc content in milk is sensitive to zinc supplementation in the diet (Dell'Orto, Cattaneo, Beretta, Baldi & Savoini, 2000).

Except for Elhardallou & El-Naggar (2016), it seems that with concentration varying between 0.20 and 350 mg/100ml according to different references, camel milk contains more **iron** than in cow and goat milk (Faye & Bengoumi, 2018). Iron is also a discriminating component between Bactrian and dromedary camel milk, the first one being slightly richer than dromedary milk (Faye et al., 2008a).

Manganese in milk does not reflect nutritional status in this element. Moreover, the results of the literature appear not to be homogeneous and the comparisons with other species are contradictory (Faye & Bengoumi, 2018). Reverse to manganese, **selenium** status of milk is sensitive to the oral supplementation of the camel. In their experiment, Seboussi, Faye, Askar, Hassan & Alhadrami, (2009) observed an average of 86.4 ± 39.1 ng/mL in the control group and 167.1 ± 97.3 ng/mL in the orally supplemented group. Similar figure is reported after organic and inorganic supplementation (Faye et al, 2013b) or selenium injection (Faye, Althamma, Musaad, Bengoumi & Seboussi, 2014). It seems that the maternal transfer of selenium to camel milk is more efficient than in cow (Faye, Seboussi & Alhadrami, 2011).

Vitamins

Many authors claim that vitamin composition of camel milk is partly at the origin of certain number of its health benefits for consumers (Al haj & Al Kanhal, 2010). Potential therapeutic and disease preventing properties of camel milk will be discussed in details in Chapter 7 and 8. Yet, except for vitamin C, relatively few references are available regarding the concentrations in camel milk.

With a range of 50 to 390 µg/l according to different authors, camel milk is relatively poor in **vitamin A** as confirmed in few comparative references. For example, Wernery (2003) found 100-150 µg/l *vs* 170-380 µg/l in milk of camels and cows respectively, living in the same environment. In their comparative study, Claeys et al., (2014) reported lower vitamin A concentration in camel milk (50-970) than in sheep (410-500), goat (500-680), cow (170-500) or buffalo milk (690 µg/l). Bactrian camel seems to contain higher concentration, up to 970 µg/l (Zhang, et al., 2005). The camel milk concentration in pro-vitamin A (β-carotene) is also low compared to cow milk as could be noticed from its white color while cow milk presents a creamey color.

At reverse, it is well established that camel milk contains higher quantity of **vitamin D** than does cow milk. For example, Sboui, Djegham, Belhadj & Khorchani, (2016) found 8 times more vitamin D in fresh camel milk (15.6 ± 2.01 ng/ml) than in cow milk (1.78 ± 0.99 ng/ml). According to other authors, the values vary between 1 and 6 ng/ml in camel milk (Faye & Bengoumi, 2018) while in cow milk, the concentrations are expressed in pg/ml (Kunz, Niesem, Lilienfeld Toal & Burmeister, 1984).

Some authors stated that there is no **vitamin E** in camel milk (Ronald de Almeida, 2011; Alavi, Salami, Emam-Djomeh & Mohammadian, 2017) which is not confirmed by many other authors. Farah, Rettenmaier & Atkins (1992) found similar concentrations than in cow milk, respectively 56 and 60 µg/100ml. Unfortunately, important gaps are observed between reported values in the literature, from 1.78 ± 0.58 µg/100ml (Stahl, Sallmann, Duehlmeier & Wernery, 2006) to 12.8 mg/100ml (Wang et al., 2011). Nonetheless, in almost all comparative studies, vitamin E appears in normal ranges compared to cow milk (Faye & Bengoumi, 2018).

To our knowledge, there is a lack of data regarding vitamin K content in camel milk. In their comparative study, Sboui et al., (2016) found 3 times more vitamin K in cow milk than in camel milk but without mentioning the units.

Thiamine (**vitamin B1**) concentration in camel milk was first determined by Sawaya, Khalil, Al-Shalahat & Al-Mohammed (1984) with a range of 28-90 µg/100ml that is lower than in cow milk as confirmed by Sboui et al., (2016). **Vitamin B2** (riboflavin) varies between 6.4 (Nahar, Khan & Shoeb, 2016) and 124 µg/100ml (Zhang et al., 2005) with slightly lower values than in cow milk (range 80-250 µg/100ml). Regarding niacin (**vitamin B3**), high differences occurred according to the references, between 11.6 and 520 µg/100ml with higher values than in cow milk (Faye & Bengoumi, 2018). For the **vitamin B5** (panthotenic acid), the references agree to consider that the values (88 ± 22 µg/100ml for Sawaya et al., 1984; 81.3 ± 8 µg/100ml for Ibrahim & Khalifa, 2015) are quite lower than in cow milk although higher concentration was reported by Haddadin et al., (2008). With values around 50 µg/100ml, camel milk contains similar values of **vitamin B6** (piridoxin) than cow milk (Sawaya et al., 1984, Haddadin et al., 2008, Zhang et al., 2005). While there is no data on biotin (vitamin B7), camel milk appears to be poor in folic acid (**vitamin B9**). Its concentration should be 10 times lower than in cow milk, with 0.41 ± 0.06 and 3.8 to 4.3 µg/100ml respectively (Sawaya et al., 1984), a ratio that was confirmed by Sboui et al., (2016). **Vitamin B12** (cyancobalamin) is also in low quantity in camel milk (0.15 µg/100ml) compared to cow (0.44) or sheep milk (0.71 µg/100ml) as stated by Sawaya et al., (1984). Thus, on average, camel milk is not rich in vitamins of group B with the exception of niacin.

Contrary to vitamins B, camel milk is renowned for its richness in **vitamin C** since the publication of Sawaya et al., (1984) who reported a value of 23.7 ± 2.65 mg/l. Farah et al., (1992) confirmed later such high concentration (range of 26-61 mg/l) as well as Saini, Bhati, Singh & Tuteja, in 2007 (32.3 ± 9 mg/l) and many other authors (Faye & Bengoumi, 2018).

On average, the quantity of vitamin C would be 3-5 times higher than in cow as confirmed by the comparative study of Claeys et al., 2014) or Ahmed, Alhassan & Elobeid, (2017). In Bactrian camel, Konuspayeva, Faye & Loiseau (2011b) observed higher values (range 48-256 mg/l) than in dromedary. Besides, vitamin C content is an important parameter to discriminate Bactrian from dromedary milk (Faye et al., 2008a)

Thus, except for vitamin C and to a lesser extent for niacin (vitamin B3) and vitamin D, camel milk is not exceptional in term of vitamins concentrations. Finally, the statement that camel milk is "rich in vitamins" is based on a limited number of references.

CONCLUSION

The knowledge regarding the composition of camel milk is being increasingly accurate due to the higher interest of scientists through the world for this product. The beliefs regarding the true or supposed "medicinal virtues" of camel milk is obviously an important motivation to further explore the fine composition of this remarkable product of the nature. However, it is the responsibility of the camel scientific community to sort between the beliefs, the empirical observations and the scientific findings. Obviously, further research works are required because despite the noticeable advances obtained for the last decades in the knowledge of its composition, camel milk has still many secrets to reveal. Especially, data regarding oligosaccharides, vitamins, trace elements, and bioactive proteins could be more widely investigated.

ACKNOWLEDGMENT

I would like to thank Dr. Bernard Faye for his convenient remarks on this chapter.

REFERENCES

Abdalla, E. B., Ashmawya, A. E. A., Salama, O. A. E., Farouk, M. H., Khalila, F. A., Seioudy, A. E., & Caja, G. (2016). Effect of milking interval on milk partitioning between udder compartments, milk yield and milk composition in Maghrebi camels. *Small Ruminant Research*, *136*, 214–220. doi:10.1016/j.smallrumres.2016.02.001

Abdallah, H. R., & Faye, B. (2012). Phenotypic classification of Saudi Arabian camel (Camelus dromedarius) by their body measurements. *Emirates Journal of Food and Agriculture*, *24*(3), 272–280.

Abu-Lehia, I. H. (1989). Physical and chemical characteristics of camel milk fat and its fractions. *Food Chemistry*, *34*(4), 267–271. doi:10.1016/0308-8146(89)90103-9

Abu-Taraboush, H. M., Al-Dagal, M. M., & Al-Royli, M. A. (1998). Growth, viability, and proteolytic activity of Bifidobacteria in whole camel milk. *Journal of Dairy Science*, *81*(2), 354–361. doi:10.3168/jds.S0022-0302(98)75584-5 PMID:9532489

Agrawal, R. P., Swami, S. C., Beniwal, R., Kochar, D. K., Sahani, M., Tuteja, F. C., & Ghouri, S. K. (2003). Effect of camel milk on glycemic control, risk factors and diabetes quality of life in type-1 diabetes: A randomized prospective controlled study. *Journal of Camel Practice and Research*, *10*(1), 45–50.

Ahmad, S., Yaqoob, M., Bilal, M. Q., Khan, M. K., Muhammad, G., Yang, L.-G., & Tariq, M. (2012). Factors affecting yield and composition of camel milk kept under desert conditions of central Punjab, Pakistan. *Tropical Animal Health and Production*, *44*(7), 1403–1410. doi:10.100711250-012-0079-3 PMID:22270241

Ahmed, M., Alhassan, A., & Elobeid, E. (2017). Comparison of chemical composition, major metals and vitamin C of camel. *International Journal of Advanced Research*, *5*(3), 712–717. doi:10.21474/IJAR01/3562

Al-Gedan, M. M., Al-Aguili, H., Alomayri, A., Konuspayeva, G., & Faye, B. (2015). Monitoring of camel milk production and composition in intensive dairy farm. *Scientific and Practical Journal Veterinariya*, *2*(42), 164-166.

Al-Ghsyar, M. A., Salem, S. A., & Ahmad, S. H. (2018). Studies on Physiochemical and functional properties of Protein Co-Precipitates from Camel's and Goat's Milk. *Health Science Journal*, *12*(5), 587–594.

Al haj, O. A. & Al Kanhal, H. A. (2010). Compositional, technological and nutritional aspects of dromedary camel milk. *International Dairy Journal, 20*, 811-821.

Al-Shamsi, K. A., Mudgil, P., Hassan, H. M., & Maqsood, S. (2017). Camel milk protein hydrolysates with improved technofunctional properties and enhanced antioxidant potential in in vitro and in food model systems. *Journal of Dairy Science*, *101*(1), 47–60. doi:10.3168/jds.2017-13194 PMID:29128226

Al-Wabel, N. A. (2008). Mineral contents of milk of cattle, camels, goats and sheep in the central region of Saudi Arabia. *Asian Journal of Biochemistry*, *3*(6), 373–375. doi:10.3923/ajb.2008.373.375

Alavi, F., Salami, M., Emam-Djomeh, Z., & Mohammadian, M. (2017). Neutraceutical properties of camel milk. In R. Watson, R. Collier, & V. Preedy (Eds.), *Nutrients in dairy and their implications for health and disease* (pp. 451–468). New York: Academic Press. doi:10.1016/B978-0-12-809762-5.00036-X

Albrecht, S., Lane, J. A., Marin, K., Al Busadah, K. A., Carrington, S. D., Hickey, R. M., & Rudd, P. M. (2014). A comparative study of free oligosaccharides in the milk of domestic animals. *British Journal of Nutrition*, *111*(7), 1313–1328. doi:10.1017/S0007114513003772 PMID:24635885

Aljumaah, R. S., Almutairi, F. F., Ismail, E., Alshaik, M. A., Sami, A., & Ayadi, M. (2012). Effects of production system, breed, parity and stage of lactation on milk composition of dromedary camels in Saudi Arabia. *Journal of Animal and Veterinary Advances*, *11*(1), 141–147. doi:10.3923/javaa.2012.141.147

Almathen, F., Charruau, P., Mohandesan, E., Mwaharo, J. M., Orozco-Terwengel, P., Pitt, D., ... Burger, P. (2016). Ancient and modern DNA reveal dynamics of domestication and cross-continental dispersal of the dromedary. *Proceedings of the National Academy of Sciences of the United States of America*, *113*(24), 6707–6712. doi:10.1073/pnas.1519508113 PMID:27162355

Alshaikh, M. A., & Salah, M. S. (1994). Effect of milking interval on secretion rate and composition of camel milk in late lactation. *The Journal of Dairy Research*, *61*(4), 451–456. doi:10.1017/S0022029900028375 PMID:7829750

Attia, H., Kherouatou, N., Fakhfakh, N., Khorchani, T., & Trigui, N. (2000). Dromedary milk fat: Biochemical, microscopic and rheological characterics. *Journal of Food Lipids*, *7*(2), 95–112. doi:10.1111/j.1745-4522.2000.tb00164.x

Ayadi, M., Musaad, A., Aljumaah, R. S., Samara, E. M., Abelrahman, M. M., Alshaikh, M. A., ... Faye, B. (2013). Relationship between udder morphology traits, alveolar and cisternal milk compartments and machine milking performances of dairy camels (Camelus dromedarius). *Spanish Journal of Agricultural Research*, *11*(3), 790–797. doi:10.5424jar/2013113-4060

Babiker, W. I. A., & El-Zubeir, I. E. M. (2014). Impact of husbandry, stages of lactation and parity number on milk yield and chemical composition of dromedary camel milk. *Emirates Journal of Food and Agriculture*, *26*(4), 333–341. doi:10.9755/ejfa.v26i4.17664

Bakheit, S. A., Majid, A. A., & Nikhala, A. M. (2008). Camels (Camelus dromedarius) under pastoral systems in North Kordofan, Sudan: Seasonal and parity effects on milk composition. *Journal of Camelid Science*, *1*, 32–36.

Barthe, L. (1905). La composition du lait de chamelle. *Journal de Pharmacie et de Chimie*, *21*, 386–388.

Bengoumi, M., Faye, B., & Tressol, J. C. (1998). Composition minérale du lait de chamelle du Sud marocain. In Actes de l'atelier « Chameaux et dromadaires, animaux laitiers », 24-26 Oct. 1994, Nouakchott. CIRAD (coll. Colloques).

Benmohamed, C., Siboukeur, O., & Edoud, A. (2018). Influence of feeding on some physicochemical and biochemical characteristics of camel milk (*Camelus dromadarius*). *Emirates Journal of Food and Agriculture*, *30*(4), 251–255. doi:10.9755/ejfa.2018.v30.i4.1658

Bouhaddaoui, S., Chabir, R., Errachidi, F., El Ghadraoui, L., El Khalfi, B., Benjelloun, M., & Soukri, A. (2019). Study of the Biochemical Biodiversity of Camel Milk. The Scientific World Journal.

Cardak, A. D., Yetismeyen, A., & Brückner, H. (2003). Quantitative comparison of free fatty acids in camel, goat and cow milk. *Milchwissenschaft. Milk Science International*, *58*, 127–130.

Cardoso, R. R. A., Santos, R., Cardoso, C., & Carvalho, M. (2010). Consumption of camel's milk by patients intolerant to lactose: A preliminary study. *Revista Alergia Mexico*, *57*, 3–26. PMID:20857626

Chilliard, Y., Ferlay, A., & Doreau, M. (2001). Contrôle de la qualité nutritionnelle des matières grasses du lait par l'alimentation des vaches laitières: Acides gras trans, polyinsaturés, acide linoléique conjugué. *Productions Animales*, *14*, 323–335.

Claeys, W. L., Verraes, C., Cardoen, S., De Block, J., Huyghebaert, A., Raes, K., & Herman, L. (2014). Consumption of raw or heated milk from different species: An evaluation of the nutritional and potential health benefits. *Food Control*, *42*, 188–201. doi:10.1016/j.foodcont.2014.01.045

Conesa, C., Sanchez, L., Rota, C., Pérez, M. D., Calvo, M., Farnaud, S., & Ewans, R. W. (2008). Isolation of lactoferrin from milk of different species: Calorimetric and antimicrobial studies. *Comparative Biochemistry & Physiology, Part B.*, *150*(1), 131–139. doi:10.1016/j.cbpb.2008.02.005 PMID:18387837

Dell'Orto, V., Cattaneo, D., Beretta, E., Baldi, A., & Savoini, G. (2000). Effect of trace element supplementation on milk yield and composition in camels. *International Dairy Journal*, *10*(12), 873–879. doi:10.1016/S0958-6946(01)00023-1

Diaz-Medina, E. (2017) *Studies on identification, lactation and rearing of dromedaries in the Island of Fuerteventura (Canary Islands)* (PhD thesis). University Autonomous of Barcelona, Spain. Available: http://camelides.cirad.fr/fr/science/these_diaz_medina.html

Dowelmadina, M. M., El Zubeir, I. E. M., Salim, A. D. A., & Arabi, O. H. M. H. (2014). Influence of Some Factors on Composition of Dromedary Camel Milk in Sudan. *Global Journal of Animal Scientific Research*, *2*(2), 120–129.

Dreiucker, J., & Vetter, W. (2011). Fatty acids patterns in camel, moose, cow and human milk as determined with GC/MS after silver ion solid phase extraction. *Food Chemistry*, *126*(2), 762–771. doi:10.1016/j.foodchem.2010.11.061

Eisa, M. O., & Hassabo, A. A. (2009). Variations in milk yield and composition between fore and rear udder-halves in she-camel (*Camelus dromedarius*). *Pakistan Journal of Nutrition*, *8*(12), 1868–1872. doi:10.3923/pjn.2009.1868.1872

El-Gawad, I. A., El-Sayed, E. M., Mahfouz, M. B., & Abd El-Salam, A. M. (1996). Changes of lactoferrin concentration in colostrum and milk from different species. *Egyptian Journal of Dairy Science*, *24*, 297–308.

El-Hatmi, H., Levieux, A., & Levieux, D. (2006). Camel (*Camelus dromedarius*) immunoglobulin G, α-lactalbumin, serum albumin and lactoferrin in colostrum and milk during the early *post-partum* period. *The Journal of Dairy Research*, *73*(3), 288–293. doi:10.1017/S0022029906001713 PMID:16566855

Elhardallou, S. B., & El-Naggar, A. Y. (2016). Determination of Micro Minerals in Milk from Farm and Pasture-Reared Cow, Goat and Camel using Inductively Coupled Plasma-Optical Emission Spectrometry. *Oriental Journal of Chemistry*, *32*(1), 341–347. doi:10.13005/ojc/320138

Elobied, A. A., Osman, A. M., Abu Kashwa, S. M., Ali, A. S., Ibrahim, M. T., & Salih, M. M. (2015). Effect of parity and breed on some physico-chemical components of Sudanese camel milk. *Research Opinions in Animal & Veterinary Sciences*, *5*(1), 20–24.

Ereifej, K. I., Alu'datt, M. H., Al-Khalidy, A., Alli, I., & Rabab, T. (2011). Comparison and characterization of fat and protein composition for camel milk from eight Jordanian locations. *Food Chemistry*, *127*(1), 282–289. doi:10.1016/j.foodchem.2010.12.112

Farah, Z., Rettenmaier, R., & Atkins, D. (1992). Vitamin Content of Camel Milk. *International Journal for Vitamin and Nutrition Research*, *62*, 30–33. PMID:1587705

Faye, B. (2004). Dairy productivity potential of camels. *Proc. of the 34th meeting FAO/ICAR (International Committee for Animal Recording)*, 93-105.

Faye, B. (2015). *Activity report UTF/SAU/044/SAU Improvement of research for sustainable development of camel production in the Kingdom of Saudi Arabia*. FAO.

Faye, B. (2018). The enthusiasm for camel production [Editorial]. *Emirates Journal of Food and Agriculture*, *30*(4), 249–250.

Faye, B., Althamma, O. M., Musaad, A., Konuspayeva, G., & Bengoumi, M. (2014). Effect of selenium injection in pregnant camels on selenium status of their new-born and milk. *Emirates Journal of Food and Agriculture*, *26*(4), 342–348. doi:10.9755/ejfa.v26i4.17272

Faye, B., & Bengoumi, M. (2018). *Camel clinical biochemistry and hematology*. Springer Publ. doi:10.1007/978-3-319-95562-9

Faye, B., Bengoumi, M., Al-Masaud, A., & Konuspayeva, G. (2015a). Low milk cholesterol in camel milk: true or not? *Scientific and Practical Journal Veterinariya*, *2*(42), 189-191.

Faye, B., Bengoumi, M., Al-Masaud, A. & Konuspayeva, G. (2015b). Comparative milk and serum cholesterol content in dairy cow and camel. *Journal of King Saud University-Science*, *27*, 168-175.

Faye, B., Konuspayeva, G., Messad, S., & Loiseau, G. (2008a). Discriminant milk components of Bactrian camel (*Camelus bactrianus*), dromedary (*Camelus dromedarius*) and hybrids. *Dairy Science & Technology*, *88*(6), 607–617. doi:10.1051/dst:2008008

Faye, B., Konuspayeva, G., Narmuratova, M., & Loiseau, G. (2008b). The comparative fatty acid composition of milk in Bactrian camel, dromedary, mare, cow and goat. *Journal of Camelid Science*, *1*, 49–54.

Faye, B., Konuspayeva, G., Narmuratova, M., Serikbaeva, A., Musaad, A. M., & Mehri, H. (2013a). Effect of crude olive cake supplementation on camel milk production and fatty acid composition. *Dairy Science & Technology*, *93*(3), 225–239. doi:10.100713594-013-0117-6

Faye, B., Saleh, S., Konuspayeva, G., Musaad, A., Bengoumi, M., & Seboussi, R. (2013b). Comparative effect of organic and inorganic selenium supplementation on selenium status in camel. *Journal of King Saud University-Science*, *26*(2), 149–158. doi:10.1016/j.jksus.2013.10.003

Faye, B., Seboussi, R., & Alhadrami, G. (2011). Maternal transfer of selenium by blood and milk in camels. *Journal of Camelid Science*, *4*, 30–39.

Fguiri, I., Ziadi, M., Sboui, A., Ayeb, N., Atigui, M., Arroum, S., & Khorchani, T. (2018). Effect of the production system and stage of lactation on the microbiological and biochemical characteristics of camel milk. *Journal of Camelid Science*, *11*, 57–63.

Fukuda, K., Yamamoto, A., Ganzorig, K., Khuukhenbaatar, J., Senda, A., Saito, T., & Urashima, T. (2010). Chemical characterization of the oligosaccharides in Bactrian camel (*Camelus bactrianus)* milk and colostrum. *Journal of Dairy Science*, *93*(12), 5572–5587. doi:10.3168/jds.2010-3151 PMID:21094729

Gaili, E. S. E., Al-Eknah, M. M., & Sadek, M. H. (2000). Comparative milking performance of three types of Saudi camels (*Camelus dromedarius*). *Journal of Camel Practice and Research*, *7*(1), 73–76.

Garcia, C., Lutz, N. W., Confort-Gouny, S., Cozzone, P., Armand, M., & Bernard, M. (2012). Phospholipid fingerprints of milk from different mammalians determined by 31P NMR: Towards specific interest in human health. *Food Chemistry*, *135*(3), 1777–1783. doi:10.1016/j.foodchem.2012.05.111 PMID:22953921

Gaucheron, F. (2011). Diversité des laits et des produits laitiers dans le monde. In *Culture des laits du monde*. Paris, France: Les cahiers de l'OCHA.

Gorban, A. M., & Izzeldin, O. M. (1999). Study on cholesteryl ester fatty acids in camel and cow milk lipid. *International Journal of Food Science & Technology*, *34*(3), 229–234. doi:10.1046/j.1365-2621.1999.00254.x

Haddadin, M. S. Y., Gammoh, S. I., & Robinson, R. K. (2008). Seasonal variations in the chemical composition of camel milk in Jordan. *The Journal of Dairy Research*, *75*(1), 8–12. doi:10.1017/S0022029907002750 PMID:17971263

Hammadi, M., Atigui, M., Ayadi, M., Barmat, A., Belgacem, A., Khaldi, G., & Khorchani, T. (2010). Training period and short time effects of machine milking on milk yield and milk composition in Tunisian Maghrebi camels (*Camelus dromedarius*). *Journal of Camel Research and Practice*, *17*(1), 1–7.

Ibrahim, A., & Khalifa, S. (2015). Effect of freeze-drying on camel's milk nutritional properties. *International Food Research Journal*, *22*(4), 1438–1445.

Ikechukwu, P., Okafor, D., Kabuo, N., Ibeabuchi, J., Odimegwu, O., Alagbaoso, E., ... Mbah, N. (2017). Production and evaluation of cookies from whole wheat and date palm fruit pulp as sugar substitute. *International Journal of Advancement in Engineering Technology Management and Applied Science*, *4*(4), 1–31.

Jirimutu, B., Li, J., Alam, M. S., Li, H., Guo, M., & Zhang, H. (2010). Fatty acid and protein profiles, and mineral content of milk from the wild Bactrian camel (*Camelus bactrianus ferus*) in Mongolia. *Milchwissenschaft. Milk Science International*, *65*, 21–25.

Kamal, A. M., & Salama, O. A. (2009). Lipid fractions and fatty acid composition of colostrums, transitional and mature she-camel milk during the first month of lactation. *Asian Journal of Clinical Nutrition*, *1*, 23–30. doi:10.3923/ajcn.2009.23.30

Kappeler, S., Farah, Z., & Puhan, Z. (1998). Sequence analysis of *Camelus dromedarius* milk caseins. *The Journal of Dairy Research*, *65*(2), 209–222. doi:10.1017/S0022029997002847 PMID:9627840

Kappeler, S., Farah, Z., & Puhan, Z. (2003). 5′-Flanking regions of camel milk genes are highly similar to homologue regions of other species and can be divided into two distinct groups. *Journal of Dairy Science*, *86*(2), 498–508. doi:10.3168/jds.S0022-0302(03)73628-5 PMID:12647956

Kappeler, S., Heuberger, C., Farah, Z., & Puhan, Z. (2004). Expression of the Peptidoglycan Recognition Protein, PGRP, in the Lactating Mammary Gland. *Journal of Dairy Science*, *87*(8), 2660–2668. doi:10.3168/jds.S0022-0302(04)73392-5 PMID:15328291

Kappeler, S., Manfred, A., Farah, Z., & Puhan, Z. (1999). Sequence analysis of camel milk (*Camelus dromedarius*) lactoferrin. *International Dairy Journal*, *9*(7), 481–486. doi:10.1016/S0958-6946(99)00117-X

Khaskheli, M., Arain, M. A., Chaudhry, S., Soomro, A. H., & Qureshi, T. A. (2005). Physico-chemical quality of camel milk. *Journal of Agriculture and Social Sciences*, *2*, 164–166.

Konuspayeva, G., Baubekova, A., Akhmetsadykova, Sh., Akhmetsadykov, N., & Faye, B. (2019). Concentrations in D- and L-lactate in rawx cow and camel milk. *Journal of Camel Practice and Research*, *26*(1), 111–113. doi:10.5958/2277-8934.2019.00016.X

Konuspayeva, G., Faye, B., & Loiseau, G. (2009a). The composition of camel milk: A meta-analysis of the literature data. *Journal of Food Composition and Analysis*, *22*(2), 95–101. doi:10.1016/j.jfca.2008.09.008

Konuspayeva, G., Faye, B., & Loiseau, G. (2011b). Variability of vitamin C content in camel milk from Kazakhstan. *Journal of Camelid Science*, *4*, 63–69.

Konuspayeva, G., Faye, B., Loiseau, G., Ivashchenko, A., Meldebekova, A., & Davletov, S. (2009b). Physiological change in camel milk composition 1- Effect of lactation stage. *Tropical Animal Health and Production*, *42*, 495–499. doi:10.100711250-009-9449-x PMID:19757134

Konuspayeva, G., Faye, B., Loiseau, G., & Levieux, D. (2007). Lactoferrin and Immunoglobin content in camel milk from Kazakhstan. *Journal of Dairy Science*, *90*, 38–46. doi:10.3168/jds.S0022-0302(07)72606-1 PMID:17183073

Konuspayeva, G., Jurjanz, S., Loiseau, G., Barci, V., Akhmetsadykova, Sh., Meldebekova, A., & Faye, B. (2011a). Contamination of Camel milk (heavy metals, organic pollutants and radionuclides) in Kazakhstan. *Journal of Environmental Protection*, *2*(01), 90–96. doi:10.4236/jep.2011.21010

Konuspayeva, G., Lemarie, E., Faye, B., Loiseau, G., & Montet, D. (2008). Fatty acid and cholesterol composition of camel's (*Camelus bactrianus, Camelus dromedarius* and hybrids) milk in Kazakhstan. *Dairy Science & Technology*, *88*(3), 327–340. doi:10.1051/dst:2008005

Kunz, C., Niesem, M., Lilienfeld Toal, H., & Burmeister, W. (1984). Vitamin D, 25-hydroxyvitamin D and 1,25-dihydroxyvitamin D in cow milk, infant formulas and breast milk during different stages of lactation. *International Journal for Vitamin and Nutrition Research*, *54*, 141–148. PMID:6548730

Laleye, L. C., Jobe, B., & Wasesa, A. A. (2008). Comparative study on heat stability and functionality of camel and bovine whey proteins. *Journal of Dairy Science*, *91*(12), 4527–4534. doi:10.3168/jds.2008-1446 PMID:19038927

Loiseau, G., Faye, B., Serikbaeva, A., & Montet, D. (2001). Enzymes ability to serve as markers of pasteurized camel milk. *Int. Conf. On new horizons in biotechnology.*

Lorenzen, P. C., Wernery, R., Johnson, B., Jose, S., & Wernery, U. (2011). Evaluation of indigenous enzyme activities in raw and pasteurised camel milk. *Small Ruminant Research*, *97*(1-3), 79–82. doi:10.1016/j.smallrumres.2011.01.014

Mal, G. D., & Sena, S. (2007). Milk composition among different breeds of camel. *The Indian Veterinary Journal*, *84*(10), 1064–1065.

Maqsood, S., Al-Dowaila, A., Mudgil, P., Kamal, H., Jobe, B., & Hassan, H. M. (2019). Comparative characterization of protein and lipid fractions from camel and cow milk, their functionality, antioxidant and antihypertensive properties upon simulated gastro-intestinal digestion. *Food Chemistry*, *279*, 328–338. doi:10.1016/j.foodchem.2018.12.011 PMID:30611498

Mati, A., Senoussi-Ghezali, C., Zennia, S., Almi-Sebbane, D., Elhatmi, H., & Giradet, J.-M. (2017). Dromedary camel milk proteins, a source of peptides having biological activities: A review. *International Dairy Journal*, *73*, 25–37. doi:10.1016/j.idairyj.2016.12.001

Mehaia, M. A., Hablas, M. A., Abdel-Rahman, K. M., & El-Mougy, S. A. (1995). Milk composition of Majaheim, Wadah and Hamra camels in Saudi Arabia. *Food Chemistry*, *52*(2), 115–122. doi:10.1016/0308-8146(94)P4189-M

Mostafidi, M., Moslehishad, M., Piravivanak, Z., & Pouretedal, Z. (2016). Evaluation of mineral content and heavy metals of dromedary camel milk in Iran. *Food Science and Technology (Campinas), 36*(4), 717–723. doi:10.1590/1678-457x.16116

Musaad, A., Faye, B., & Abu-Nikhela, A. (2013b). Lactation curves of dairy camels in an intensive system. *Tropical Animal Health and Production, 4*(4), 1039–1046. doi:10.100711250-012-0331-x PMID:23212839

Musaad, A., Faye, B., & Al-Mutairi, S. (2013a). Seasonal and physiological variation of gross composition of camel milk in Saudi Arabia. *Emirates Journal of Food and Agriculture, 25*(8), 618–624. doi:10.9755/ejfa.v25i8.16095

Nagy, P., Fábri, Zs. N., Varga, L., Reiczigel, J., & Juhász, J. (2017). Effect of genetic and nongenetic factors on chemical composition of individual milk samples from dromedary camels (*Camelus dromedarius*) under intensive management. *Journal of Dairy Science, 100*(11), 8680–8693. doi:10.3168/jds.2017-12814 PMID:28843681

Nahar, N., Khan, W., & Shoeb, M. (2016). Physico-Chemical analysis and composition of camel milk of Bangladesh. *Journal of Basic and Applied Sciences*, 231–235.

Narmuratova, M., Konuspayeva, G., Loiseau, G., Serikbaeva, A., Barouh, N., Montet, D., & Faye, B. (2006). Fatty acids composition of dromedary and Bactrian camel milk in Kazakhstan. *Journal of Camel Practice and Research, 13*(1), 45–50.

Omar, A., Harbourne, N., & Oruna-Concha, M. J. (2016). Quantification of major camel milk proteins by capillary electrophoresis. *International Dairy Journal, 58*, 31–35. doi:10.1016/j.idairyj.2016.01.015

Omer, R. H., & Eltinay, A. H. (2008). Chemical composition of camel's colostrum and milk in United Arab Emirates. *Arab University Journal of Agricultural Science, 16*(1), 127–134. doi:10.21608/ajs.2008.14620

Raziq, K., Younas, M., & Kakar, M. A. (2008). Camel – a potential dairy animal in difficult environments. *Pakistan Journal of Agricultural Sciences, 45*(2), 263–267.

Ronald de Almeida, C. (2011). Camel milk: Characteristics and perspectives for use in clinical practice. *Revista Chilena de Nutrición, 38*(2), 211–218.

Ryskaliyeva, A., Henry, C., Miranda, G., Faye, B., Konuspayeva, G., & Martin, P. (2018). Complex milk protein fractions' in Bactrian camel milk. In *The 5th Conference ISOCARD "Recent advances in camelids biology, health and Production"*, 275-277.

Ryskaliyeva, A., Henry, C., Miranda, G., Faye, B., Konuspayeva, G., & Martin, P. (2019a). Alternative splicing events expand molecular diversity of camel CSN1S2 increasing its ability to generate potentially bioactive peptides. *Scientific Reports, 9*(1), 5243. doi:10.103841598-019-41649-5 PMID:30918277

Ryskaliyeva, A., Henry, C., Miranda, G., Faye, B., Konuspayeva, G., & Martin, P. (2019b). The main WAP isoform usually found in camel milk arises from the usage of an improbable intron cryptic splice site in the precursor to mRNA in which a GC-AG intron occurs. BMC Genetics, 20, 14. doi:10.118612863-018-0704-x

Sabahelkhier, M. K., Faten, M. M., & Omer, F. I. (2012). Comparative determination of biochemical constituents between animals (goat, sheep, cow and camel) milk with human milk. *Research Journal of Recent Sciences*, *1*(5), 69–71.

Saini, N., Bhati, A., Singh, N., & Tuteja, F. (2007). Trace mineral and vitamin C content of camel milk: A comparative study. *Veterinary Practitioner*, *8*(1), 20–21.

Salmen, S. H., Abu-Tarboush, H. M., Al-Saleh, A. A., & Metwalli, A. A. (2012). Amino acids content and electrophoretic profile of camel milk casein from different camel breeds in Saudi Arabia. *Saudi Journal of Biological Sciences*, *19*(2), 177–183. doi:10.1016/j.sjbs.2011.12.002 PMID:23961177

Sawaya, W. N., Khalil, J. K., Al-Shalahat, A., & Al-Mohammed, H. (1984). Chemical composition and nutritional quality of camel milk. *Journal of Food Science*, *49*(3), 744–747. doi:10.1111/j.1365-2621.1984.tb13200.x

Sboui, A., Djegham, M., Belhadj, O. & Khorchani, T. (2016). Le lait de chamelle: qualités nutritives et effet sur les variations de la glycémie. *Options Méditerranéennes, A, 115*, 487-492.

Seboussi, R., Faye, B., Askar, M., Hassan, K., & Alhadrami, G. (2009). Effect of selenium supplementation on blood status and milk, urine and fecal excretion in pregnant and lactating camel. *Biological Trace Element Research*, *128*(1), 45–57. doi:10.100712011-008-8251-3 PMID:18972072

Shabo, Y., Barzel, R., Margoulis, M., & Yagil, R. (2005). Camel Milk for Food Allergies in Children. *Immunology and Allergies*, *7*, 796–798. PMID:16382703

Shamsia, S. M. (2009). Nutritional and therapeutic properties of camel and human milks. *International Journal of Genetics and Molecular Biology*, *1*(2), 52–58.

Sharma, A., Jana, A., & Chavan, R. (2012). Functionality of milk powders and milk-based powders for end use applications—A review. *Comprehensive Reviews in Food Science and Food Safety*, *11*(5), 518–528. doi:10.1111/j.1541-4337.2012.00199.x

Shuiep, E. S., Zubeir, I. E. M., El Owni, O. A. O., & Musa, H. H. (2008). Raw camel (*Camelus dromedarius*) milk in Khartoum state, Sudan. *Tropical and Subtropical Agroecosystems*, *8*, 101–106.

Soliman, G. Z. A. (2005). Comparison of chemical and mineral content of milk from human, cow, buffalo, camel and goat in Egypt. *Egyptian Journal of Hospital Medicine*, *21*, 116–130.

Stahl, T., Sallmann, H. P., Duehlmeier, R., & Wernery, U. (2006). Selected vitamins and fatty acid patterns in dromedary milk and colostrum. *Journal of Camel Practice and Research*, *13*(1), 53–57.

Stave, C., & Törner, M. (2007). Exploring the organisational preconditions for occupational accidents in food industry: A qualitative approach. *Safety Science*, *45*(3), 355–371. doi:10.1016/j.ssci.2006.07.001

Wang, S. Y., Liang, J. P., Shao, W. J., & Wen, H. (2011). Mineral, vitamin and fatty acid contents in the camel milk of dromedaries in the Anxi Gansu China. *Journal of Camel Practice and Research*, *18*(2), 273–276.

Wangoh, J., Farah, Z., & Puhan, Z. (1998). Composition of milk from three camel (*Camelus dromedarius*) breeds in Kenya during lactation. *Milchwissenschaft. Milk Science International*, *53*(3), 136–139.

Wernery, U. (2003). Novel observations on camel milk. *Proc. 9th Kenya camel forum.*

Wernery, U., Fischbach, S., Johnson, B., & Jose, S. (2008). Evaluation of alkaline phosphatase (ALP), γ-glutamyl transferase (GGT) and lactoperoxidase (LPO) activities for their suitability as markers of camel milk heat inactivation. *Milchwissenschaft. Milk Science International, 63*(3), 265–267.

Wernery, U., Johnson, B., & Tawfig Ishmail, W. (2006). Insulin content in raw dromedary milk and serum measured over one lactation period. *Journal of Camel Practice and Research, 13*(2), 89–90.

Yadav, A. K., Kumar, R., Priyadarshini, L., & Singh, J. (2015). Composition and medicinal properties of camel milk: A Review. *Asian Journal of Dairy & Food Research, 34*(2), 83–91. doi:10.5958/0976-0563.2015.00018.4

Yagil, R., Saran, A., & Etzion, Z. (1984). *Camels milk: for drinking only?* Academic Press.

Yoganandi, J., Mehta, M. B., Wadhwani, K. N., Darji, V. B., & Aparnathi, K. D. (2014). Comparison of physico-chemical properties of camel milk with cow milk and buffalo milk. *Journal of Camel Practice and Research, 21*(2), 253–258. doi:10.5958/2277-8934.2014.00045.9

Zagorski, O., Maman, A., Yafee, A., Meisles, A., Van Creveld, C., & Yagil, R. (1998). Insulin in milk – a comparative study. *International Journal of Animal Science, 13*, 241–244.

Zeleke, Z. M. (2007). Non-genetic factors affecting milk yield and milk composition of traditionally managed camels (*Camelus dromedarius*) in Eastern Ethiopia. *Livestock Research for Rural Development, 19*(6), 85. Retrieved from http://www.lrrd.org/lrrd19/6/zele19085.htm

Zhang, H., Yao, J., Zhao, D., Liu, H., Li, M., & Guo, M. (2005). Change in chemical composition of Alxa Bactrian camel milk during lactation. *Journal of Dairy Science, 88*(10), 3402–3410. doi:10.3168/jds.S0022-0302(05)73024-1 PMID:16162513

Zhao, D. B., Bai, Y. H., & Niu, Y. B. (2015). Composition and characteristics of Chinese Bactrian camel milk. *Small Ruminant Research, 127*, 58–67. doi:10.1016/j.smallrumres.2015.04.008

Chapter 3
Strategies and Technologies for Camel Milk Preservation

Olfa Oussaief
https://orcid.org/0000-0003-3785-6083
Arid Lands Institute of Medenine, Tunisia

Zeineb Jrad
https://orcid.org/0000-0003-0463-4353
Arid Lands Institute of Medenine, Tunisia

Touhami Khorchani
Arid Lands Institute of Medenine, Tunisia

Halima El-Hatmi
Arid Lands Institute of Medenine, Tunisia

ABSTRACT

This chapter aimed to report the strategies and technologies for camel milk preservation. Raw camel milk is easily spoiled owing to its nutrient content, which provides an ideal substrate for the development of microorganisms. Several traditional methods have been conducted in order to increase the shelf life of camel milk including fumigation of milk containers, simple evaporative cooling, chilling, freezing, pasteurization, and milk processing into many products like fermented camel milk, butter, and ghee. Modern technologies are used nowadays to preserve camel milk including freeze-drying, spray drying, high hydrostatic pressure, and sterilization. Besides, many value-added products are produced like yoghurt, cheese, ice cream, snacks, and camel milk protein hydrolysates, which are used in the field of functional food and nutraceuticals. The non-marketed camel milk is sold at a lower price or consumed at the household level in tea or after processing it into naturally fermented milk.

DOI: 10.4018/978-1-7998-1604-1.ch003

INTRODUCTION

Camel milk is often consumed raw or naturally fermented. The sale of camel milk was considered as a taboo in pastoral communities. However, in recent years, camel milk utilization has been shifted from subsistence to commercialization all over the world (Konuspayeva & Faye, 2004). Hence, there has been a great interest in increasing the amount of milk marketed. Camel milk has longer shelf compared to the milk of other animals due to its high content in antimicrobial factors (Rahmeh, Alomirah, Akbar, & Sidhu, 2019). Yet, camel milk is easily spoiled owing to its nutrient content, which provides an ideal substrate for the development of microorganisms, especially at high temperatures. Thus, camel milk preservation is a must. Subsequently, different preservation strategies and technologies that increase its shelf life have been conducted to limit microbial contamination (Ogolla, Dede, Okoth, Hensel, & Sturm, 2017). The processing of camel milk into value-added products is among the most adequate methods to increase its shelf life. However, the manufacturing of camel dairy products using the same technology as for dairy products from cow milk results in processing difficulties and products with inferior quality (Berhe, Seifu, Ipsen, Kurtu, & Hansen, 2017). This data has prompted several researchers around the world to conduct studies to overcome these difficulties and allow populations to consume these products during all the year thanks to their longer shelf life compared to raw camel milk (Mati et al., 2017). In this chapter, the different strategies and technologies for camel milk preservation are detailed.

Strategies and Technologies for Camel Milk Preservation

Since long time ago, pastoralists used traditional preservation procedures, which are adapted to their lifestyle but don't necessarily offer the quality and safety standards required by ever changing modern lifestyles and growing population. Thereby, this has led to the search for new modern technologies to preserve camel milk aiming to satisfy the demand for quantity, quality, and safety (Ogolla et al., 2017). The main strategies and technologies used for the preservation of camel milk are summarized in Table 1.

Table 1. Main strategies and technologies for camel milk preservation

Camel milk preservation	
Traditional methods	**Modern methods**
Heat Treatment	
Simple evaporative cooling, pasteurization, refrigeration, freezing	Sterilization, UHT, high hydrostatic pressure treatment
Value added products	
Spontaneously fermented camel milk, butter, ghee	Fermented milk with probiotic starters, cheese, yogurt, ice cream, snacks, protein hydrolysates…
Others	
Fumigation of milk containers, special milk containers: Qoodha, condensation	Drying technologies: Freeze-drying, Spray drying

TRADITIONAL PRESERVATION METHODS

Fumigation of Milk Containers

Fumigation of milk containers is commonly referred to as smoking of camel milk. It is a common traditional practice performed by the pastoralists to preserve camel milk for 12–24 hours without refrigeration (Ogolla et al., 2017; Wayua, Okoth, & Wangoh, 2012). The milk containers are fumigated by smoke from burned wood of special trees like *Olea africana*, *Acacia nilotica*, *Cardia quercifolia*, *Balanities aegyptica,* and *Combretum* spp as a means of disinfection after cleaning (Seifu, 2007; Wayua et al., 2012; Ogolla et al., 2017). The usage is dependent on the effectiveness of the tree variety and its availability in the area of use (Odongo, Lamuka, Matofari, & Abong, 2016). During smoking, the containers are inverted over hot smoking chips until the smoke stops coming out of the container. Fresh camel milk to be stored is then poured into these containers (Wayua et al., 2012). Farmers report that the smoke prolongs the shelf life of the milk and imparts a distinct and desirable flavour to the milk for the consumers (Muloi et al., 2018). Smoke treatment decreases the microbial load inside milk containers resulting in the preservation of camel milk. Indeed, smoke compounds including acids, alcohols, carbonyls, esters, furans, lactones, and phenols are natural antimicrobials and are responsible for the preservation of milk and milk products and the enhancement of organoleptic properties of smoke-treated products (Wanjala, Matofari, & Nduko, 2016; Odongo et al., 2016). Nigussie and Seifu (2007) reported also that the use of smoked containers improves the microbial quality and extends the shelf life of cows' milk up to 7 hours during storage at an ambient temperature. However, the inhalation of the smoke from the incomplete combustion of charcoal and firewood, can be harmful to the health of pastoralists since it is associated with respiratory diseases (Ogolla et al., 2017) as well as esophageal cancer (Patel, Wakhisi, Mining, Mwangi, & Patel, 2013).

Cooling

Use of Qoodha

Milk could be stored for up to 72 hours in a traditional container named Qoodha (Ogolla et al., 2017). The Qoodha is specially woven from the roots of the *Ergemis sp* tree and decorated with cowrie shells. The top part of the Qoodha is made by fibres obtained from the stem of *Adansonia digitata* L. The fibres are woven into a pot like a basket using a metal needle. Camel milk is put in the Qoodha readably smoked with branches from *Cordia monoica*. Camel milk could be conserved in the smoked Qoodha due to its cooling and antimicrobial properties (Ogolla et al., 2017). This technique, mainly used in Kenya, was reported to be becoming extinct, but it is still optimally used in isolated rural communities away from commercial centers (Ogolla et al., 2017).

Evaporative Cooling

Simple evaporative cooling is another traditional method to preserve camel milk (Adongo, Coppock, & Wayua, 2013; Ogolla et al., 2017). Evaporative cooling technique requires the use of containers soaked in water. Adongo et al. (2013) reported that simple evaporative cooling could improve the chemical and bacteriological quality of camel milk that is marketed in challenging environments since it reduces camel milk temperature and therefore retards bacterial growth. Furthermore, chilling and freezing are low-temperature treatments that prevent quality deterioration through inhibiting biochemical and microbial activities (Ogolla et al., 2017). Milk storage at low-temperature does not destroy microorganisms but it delays their development. Hence, it is necessary to cool milk within four hours of milking to prevent the growth of microorganisms (Ogolla et al., 2017).

Refrigeration and Freezing

Sboui, Khorchani, Djegham and Belhadj (2009) reported that refrigeration and freezing are commonly used as a means of preservation of camel milk. The nutritional value of camel milk can be maintained almost intact during 7 days versus 5 days for cow milk at 4 °C and several weeks under freezing, making it accessible far from its place of production. According to Omer and Eltinay (2009), the storage duration of raw camel milk was 42 days at 4 °C, 15 days at 7 °C and 3 days at room temperature while the keeping quality of the raw cow milk samples was 7 days, 70 h and 2 days at the same temperatures mentioned above, respectively. However, chilling and freezing of camel milk are highly energy intensive and costly (Ogolla et al., 2017).

Pasteurization

Pasteurization of camel milk is carried out by primary milk traders at collection points to preserve milk during times when transport to the market is unavailable and access to cooling facilities is limited. Milk is boiled to a temperature of approximately 60 °C and then cooled to preserve it for sale the following day (Wayua et al., 2012; Ogolla et al., 2017). Pasteurization was conducted to rid camel milk of harmful pathogens, especially tuberculosis (Yagil, Zagorski, Van Creveld, & Saran, 1994). Pasteurized camel milk could be conserved for 10 days at cold (Al haj & Al Kanhal, 2010). Mohamed and El Zubeir (2012) reported that pasteurized camel milk at (63 °C, 30 min) and (72 °C, 15 s) could be conserved for 7 and 20 days, respectively. Heat treatment caused a decrease of pH, protein and lactose content of full-fat camel milk with an increase of its acidity, while solid non-fat (SNF), fat and density of milk remained stable (Elhasan et al., 2017). According to Elagamy (2000), pasteurization of camel, cow and buffalo milk at 65 °C for 30 min had no significant effect on lactoferrin and lysozyme while IgGs were significantly affected in the three kinds of milk. Camel milk IgGs lose 68.7% of their activity after pasteurization at 75°C for 30 min whereas the whole activity of IgGs in cow and buffalo milk was completely lost (see Chapter 10). Pasteurization of camel, cow and buffalo milk at 85 °C for 30 min resulted in a loss of the activity of lysozyme (56, 74 and 81.7%, respectively) whereas the activity of lactoferrin was completely lost for these three kinds of milk at this level of temperature. Interestingly, camel milk antimicrobial factors including lysozyme, lactoferrin, and IgGs were significantly more heat resistant than cow and buffalo milk proteins (see Chapter 7 and 10). However, the heat treatment of camel milk at 100 °C for 30 min results in a total loss of the activity of the antimicrobial factors. Similarly, bovine α-lactalbumin was not detected and only 26% of β-lactoglobulin remained in bovine milk after heating at 80 °C for 60 min (Felfoul, Jardin, Gaucheron, Attia, & Ayadi, 2017).

Camel Milk Condensation

Condensation of camel milk is being practiced in Samburu, Kenya. The process involves mixing one part by volume of sugar to four parts by volume of camel milk and then heating in an open metal pan to evaporate the majority of water (Kinoti, 1997). The main process is the reduction of water to minimize growth of microorganisms (Robinson, 1990). The condensed milk is then filled into tin cans, fitted with lids. This product is then stored and thereafter drank either directly, spread on bread, mixed with porridge or used in preparing tea (Kinoti, 1997).

The keeping quality of sweetened condensed milk is largely the result of the increase in osmotic pressure (reduction in water activity) due to the binding of the water by the added sugar. The increased concentration of the milk solids brought about by the removal of water by evaporation also contributes to the increase in osmotic pressure, but this is relatively minor compared to the effect of the added sugar (Robinson, 1990).

The shelf life of condensed camel milk depends on several factors such as the water content, the amount of air with the closed can, the level of hygiene and handling of the milk. When these factors are controlled, condensed milk may be kept for up to 6 months at room temperature. Once the container is opened, further contamination may be introduced, and therefore it is advisable, once the tin is opened, to finish the contents without undue delay (Kinoti, 1997). Author reported, significant losses of vitamins A and lactose during the storage of condensed camel milk whereas the amount of protein, fat and vitamin C remain stable (Kinoti, 1997).

Fermentation

Fermentation is one of the oldest forms of food preservation in the world (Leroy & De Vuyst, 2004). Lactic acid fermentation corresponds to the transformation of lactose of milk into lactic acid under the action of specific, natural or added microorganisms called lactic acid bacteria (lactic leavens) (Leroy & De Vuyst, 2004). The microbial aspect of lactic acid bacteria isolated from camel milk will be discussed in detail in Chapter 4. Different kinds of traditional fermented camel milk are produced by the pastoralist worldwide, for instance, *Suusac* (Kenya), *Gariss* (Sudan), *shubat* (Kazakhstan) or yogurt etc (see Chapter 5). It increases the stability of the product through the inhibition of possible microbial and enzymatic deteriorations and consequently lengthen its shelf life (Ramet, 1993; Leroy & De Vuyst, 2004). Konuspayeva (2007) indicated that the manufacturing processes of fermented camel milk are globally quite similar with some differences regarding the method of treatment, regions and seasons. Due to spontaneous nature of the fermentation, this traditional method results in products with varying taste and flavor and often of poor hygienic quality (Attia, Kherouatou, & Dhouib, 2001).

RECENT TRENDS IN PRESERVATION TECHNOLOGIES

Freeze Drying

Freeze-drying or lyophilization of camel milk is a process in which water is removed from frozen milk through sublimation. Lyophilization is an excellent drying process for heat sensitive products. The nutritional characteristics of camel milk as well as cow milk remain basically unchanged after lyophilization compared with fresh milk (Ibrahim & Khalifa, 2015; Sulieman, Elamin, Elkhalifa, & Laleye, 2018). Camel milk powder obtained after lyophilization possess stable physicochemical and biological properties during long term storage at ambient temperature as well as good appearance and flavor. Interestingly, freeze-dried camel milk powder is easy to transport and does not require special conditions for prolonged storage (Ibrahim & Khalifa, 2015). When stored under adequate dry and cool conditions, whole milk powder has a shelf life of twelve months and skim milk powder over two years (Sulieman, Elamin, Elkhalifa, & Laleye, 2014). However, it is notable that freeze-drying has been considered as the costliest process (Sulieman et al., 2018).

Spray Drying

Spray drying is a method of producing a dry powder from a liquid by rapidly drying with a hot gas. This process is among the most used techniques for drying milk (See Chapter 5) owing to the very short time of heat contact and the high rate of evaporation that give a high-quality product at a relatively low cost (Sulieman et al., 2014). The spray drying operating conditions like inlet temperature, drying air flow rate, outlet temperature, atomization pressure and even the composition of camel milk itself play a key role in the drying rate and the functional properties of the final product. Therefore, it is necessary to optimize spray-drying operation conditions to obtain the desired surface and physicochemical properties of camel milk powder. Generally, spray-drying of camel milk does not damage its physicochemical characteristics if the operating conditions are well designed (Smits., et al, Huppertz, Alting, & Kiers, 2011; Sulieman et al., 2014; Habtegebriel, Edward, Wawire, Sila, & Seifu, 2018). Ho et al. (2019) indicated that the changes in lactose, fat, and proteins did not induce significant alterations in true density, powder appearance (e.g. colour and morphology) and solubility of spray-dried camel milk powders kept at 37 °C and low relative humidity levels (< 32%) up to 18 weeks. The water activity of spray dried camel milk was less than that of spray dried cow milk, indicating the possibility of its longer shelf life (Sulieman et al., 2014). As compared to freeze-drying process, it is elucidated that spray drying retains a lesser amount of proteins, fat-soluble vitamins, minerals, and water. Since freeze-drying is a cold process, it is advantageous in that it does not destroy the fatty acid and amino acid profiles of camel milk (Ibrahim & Khalifa, 2015; Habtegebriel et al., 2018).

High Hydrostatic Pressure

High hydrostatic pressure is a non-thermal technique used to inactivate microorganisms including food-borne pathogens without altering the nutritional and sensorial quality of the products and therefore enhance their shelf life (see Chapter 10). Interestingly, this process provides the potential to reduce energy requirements in food processing industries (Chawla, Patil, & Singh, 2011). Hamad et al. (2013) reported that the high-pressure treatment of camel milk above 200 MPa for 5 minutes at 40 °C could reduce microbial contamination of camel milk. Moreover, color, aroma, and taste of treated milk are not affected. However, camel milk clots at pressures up to 300 MPa thereby reducing the effect of pressure on bacteria lethality. Omar, Harbourne, and Oruna-Concha (2018) indicated that high-pressure treatments at 200–800 MPa do not alter the composition of camel milk. However, high-pressure treatment of camel milk at 200 MPa causes a lower level of denaturation of camel whey proteins compared with

UHT (Ultra High Treatment) treatment (Omar et al., 2018). However, increasing the pressure from 400 to 800 MPa results in a significant increase in denaturation of α-lactalbumin up to 32.5%, which is still significantly lower than in the UHT, treated camel milk. Serum albumin and lactoferrin are more resistant to pressure with lower denaturation levels of 3.94% and 2.93%, respectively. Interestingly, the stability of camel whey proteins is higher than that of their counterparts in bovine milk during high-pressure processing (Omar et al., 2018).

Sterilization

Pasteurized camel milk appears straightforward and is used at industrial scale (Alhaj, Metwalli, & Ismail, 2011). UHT process together with refrigeration could achieve five weeks of shelf life while sterilization treatment of camel milk cause protein sedimentation, a phenomena not observed in cow milk (Alhaj et al., 2011). The authors reported that casein micelle size or deficiency of β-lactoglobulin and κ-casein in camel milk could be the reason beyond its heat instability. Nevertheless, increase in pH of camel milk was beneficial for heat stability. However, very small change in pH could result in large effect on protein heat stability. Camel milk was shown to be sterilized if its pH is increased to 7.0 - 7.2 or certain additives are added like κ-casein or EDTA. Besides, some additives such as phosphate could be used to improve heat stability of camel milk (Alhaj et al., 2011).

Microfiltration

To maintain the highest possible proportion of heat-sensitive and valuable components of camel milk, the use of microfiltration method as the most gentle shelf life extending procedure could be recommended. By pasteurization, average shelf life of fresh cow milk can be increased to 5-7 days. By the combined use of germ-count reducing microfiltration (MF) and pasteurization the shelf life of cow's milk can be extended to 21-30 days. For camel milk, only experimental trial was achieved (Bukovics, Hucker & Szafner, 2015) with the following procedure: after heating up to 50°C, the raw camel milk was skimmed (fat content 0.05%). For microfiltration, α-alumina ultrafiltration membrane was used (pore size 1.4 µm - CMF), with a total area of 1.68 m2. Operating temperature of microfiltration was 50 °C. The microfiltration was carried out with permeate re-circulation (UTP), maintaining uniform trans-membrane pressure drop (0.8-1.0 bar). The low germ-count permeate emerging from microfiltration was heat-treated at 72°C, the cream at 85°C with 5 minutes holding time. Then the two materials were mixed and cold stored (5°C). The mesophilic bacteria were present in raw milk at $3x10^3$ cfu/g while the concentration was 30 cfu/g only in permeate. For thermophilic micro-organisms, the concentrations decreased from <100 to 1 cfu/g, respectively in raw milk and permeate, while mesophilic bacterial spores decreased from 20 to <1 cfu/g. Reversely, bacteria retained by the membrane are concentrating in the retentate up to $3x10^5$ for mesophilic bacteria. On average, the germ-count was decreasing by 99%.

The microbiological status of micro-filtrated milk was stable throughout the entire (60 days) storage period with the maintain of organoleptic properties. By combining microfiltration and pasteurization, shelf life can be substantially extended. Low filtration temperature does not damage the heat-sensitive milk components. Moreover, the process besides live bacteria cells also removes the dead bacteria with their enzymes which could provoke an alteration of the organoleptic quality.

Modern Value-Added Products

Nowadays, fermented camel milk is manufactured using selected starter culture with technological and probiotic properties instead of being fermented traditionally, aiming to obtain products with high nutritional hygienic quality and extended shelf life (Mati et al., 2017). Interestingly, the biological activities of fermented camel milk were preserved during the storage for 21 days at 4°C (El-Hatmi et al., 2018; Ayyash et al., 2018b). In the present book, manufacturing of fermented camel milk products will be discussed in detail in Chapter 5.

Camel milk yogurt is manufactured using hydrocolloids and stabilizers (Al-Zoreky & Al-Otaibi, 2015; Chen, Wang, Zhang, Zhang, & Ren, 2019). Jrad et al. (2019) reported that camel milk yogurt obtained after milk ultrafiltration and supplementation with date powder was stable for 28 days during storage at 4 °C. In addition, camel milk cheese with high yield and good acceptability is successfully manufactured thanks to the ultrafiltration process as well as the use of camel chymosin (Mehaia et al., 2006; Konuspayeva et al., 2017). Soft cheese made from camel milk can be stored up to 22 days at lower temperature (4±1 °C) and for 6 days at 18±1 °C (Mohammed, Eshetu, Tadesse, & Hailu, 2019).

Moreover, adding essential oils of plants with medicinal properties like spearmint (*Mentha spicata*) and wild thyme (*Zataria multiflora*) to camel milk result in higher organoleptic properties and extend shelf life while keeping its nutritional properties, which can enhance the consumption rate of camel milk (Maaroufi, Rezaei, Raftaniamiri, & Mirzaei, 2015).

Camel milk protein hydrolysis is another way to produce high value-added products as well as to preserve camel milk. Protein hydrolysates are mixtures of polypeptides and amino acids, which are manufactured from protein sources using partial hydrolysis via food-grade proteolytic enzymes. Several reasons are behind the enzymatic hydrolysis of proteins since protein hydrolysates could find applications in food, cosmetic and pharmaceutical industries due to their great biological activities (Abd El-Salam & El-Shibiny, 2017). Several authors reported higher antioxidant, antimicrobial and hypertensive activities of camel milk protein hydrolysates compared to the protein source (see Chapter 7), via the hydrolysis of this latter by pepsin, chymotrypsin, papain, bromelaine and alaclase (Kumar, Chatli, Singh, Mehta, & Kumar, 2016; Al-Shamsi, Mudgil, Hassan, & Maqsood, 2018; Jrad et al., 2019). Potential therapeutic and disease preventing properties of camel milk will be discussed later in this book.

Overall, the modern preservation methods of camel milk present many advantages compared to traditional ones. Modern preservation methods results in products with higher shelf life. For instance, milk powder produced through freeze-drying can be preserved for more than one year. Besides, modern techniques of camel milk preservation result in more various products with great hygienic quality. However, traditional methods are cheaper than modern methods (spray drying, freeze drying, high-pressure treatment...).

Utilization of Non-Marketed Camel Milk

Physicochemical and organoleptic quality of camel milk was controlled before its acceptability from the producers for further processing. Milk was rejected when it is naturally fermented and returned to the producers. Therefore, sugar was added to the returned milk, which is thereafter sold at a lower price or consumed at the household level in tea or after processing it into naturally fermented milk (Ogolla et al, 2017).

CONCLUSION

There is a big need to preserve this worth called the white gold of the desert. Several traditional methods were used erstwhile by the pastoralists to preserve camel milk including fumigation of milk containers, condensation, cooling, pasteurization and processing it into value-added products. These traditional preservation procedures are adapted to their lifestyle. However, the negative effects of some preservation procedures on human health (fumigation), the ineffectiveness of certain processes to preserve camel milk for long periods as well as changing lifestyles and growing populations require process modifications to satisfy the demand for quantity, quality and safety. Numerous modern processes were used to preserve milk like freeze-drying, spray drying, high hydrostatic pressure and sterilization. Many value-added camel milk products are now available in the market all-over the year because the difficulties of camel milk processing, related to its unique structural and functional properties, were encountered.

FUTURE RESEARCH DIRECTIONS

Strategies and technologies for camel milk preservation are still limited and need further investigations. It is necessary to optimize and design a spray drying operation that will result in desired physicochemical and functional properties of camel milk powder. Condensed camel milk should be investigated deeply since informations are very limited concerning this type of milk conservation. The shelf life of camel milk that undergone high hydrostatic pressure procedure should be determined. New probiotic starter cultures should be isolated from camel milk to apply them in camel milk-controlled fermentation, in cheese making as well as in milk-derived products. The stability of the bioactive peptides during the storage of camel milk protein hydrolysates should be explored. The effect of the addition of various plant extract or their essential oils as preservatives to camel milk and its derived products should be well investigated. Besides, new value-added products from camel milk with long shelf life have to be made by the dairy industry to increase its availability in time and space. The effect of the different treatments used for camel milk preservation on its therapeutic potential should be studied deeply.

ACKNOWLEDGMENT

This research received no specific grant from any funding agency in the public, commercial, or not-for-profit sectors.

REFERENCES

Abd El-Salam, M. H., & El-Shibiny, S. (2017). Preparation, properties, and uses of enzymatic milk protein hydrolysates. *Critical Reviews in Food Science and Nutrition*, *57*(6), 1119–1132. doi:10.1080/10408398.2014.899200 PMID:25880259

Adongo, A. O., Coppock, D. L., & Wayua, F. O. (2013). Simple evaporative cooling method reduces bacterial content of traditionally marketed camel milk in Isiolo County, Kenya. *African Journal of Food, Agriculture, Nutrition and Development*, *13*(01), 7213–7224. doi:10.18697/ajfand.56.12460

Al Haj, O. A., & Al Kanhal, H. A. (2010). Compositional, technological and nutritional aspects of dromedary camel milk. A review. *International Dairy Journal*, *20*, 811–821.

Al-Shamsi, K. A., Mudgil, P., Hassan, H. M., & Maqsood, S. (2018). Camel milk protein hydrolysates with improved technofunctional properties and enhanced antioxidant potential in in vitro and in food model systems. *Journal of Dairy Science*, *101*(1), 47–60. doi:10.3168/jds.2017-13194 PMID:29128226

Al-Zoreky, N. S., & Al-Otaibi, M. M. (2015). Suitability of camel milk for making yogurt. *Food Science and Biotechnology*, *24*(2), 601–606. doi:10.100710068-015-0078-z

Alhaj, O. A., Metwalli, A. A., & Ismail, E. A. (2011). Heat stability of camel milk proteins after sterilization process. *Journal of Camel Practice and Research*, *18*, 277–282.

Attia, H., Kherouatou, N., & Dhouib, A. (2001). Dromedary milk lactic acid fermentation: Microbiological and rheological characteristics. *Journal of Industrial Microbiology & Biotechnology*, *26*(5), 263–270. doi:10.1038j.jim.7000111 PMID:11494100

Ayyash, M., Abushelaibi, A., Al-Mahadin, S., Enan, M., El-Tarabily, K., & Shah, N. (2018a). *In-vitro* investigation into probiotic characterisation of *Streptococcus* and *Enterococcus* isolated from camel milk. *Lebensmittel-Wissenschaft + Technologie*, *87*, 478–487. doi:10.1016/j.lwt.2017.09.019

Ayyash, M., Al-Nuaimi, A. K., Al-Mahadin, S., & Liu, S. Q. (2018b). *In vitro* investigation of anticancer and ACE-inhibiting activity, α-amylase and α-glucosidase inhibition, and antioxidant activity of camel milk fermented with camel milk probiotic: A comparative study with fermented bovine milk. *Food Chemistry*, *239*, 588–597. doi:10.1016/j.foodchem.2017.06.149 PMID:28873609

Benabdelkamel, H., Masood, A., Alanazi, I., Alzahrani, D., Alrabiah, D., AlYahya, S., & Alfadda, A. (2017). Proteomic profiling comparing the effects of different heat treatments on camel (*Camelus dromedarius*) milk whey proteins. *International Journal of Molecular Sciences*, *18*(4), 721. doi:10.3390/ijms18040721 PMID:28350354

Berhe, T., Seifu, E., Ipsen, R., Kurtu, M. Y., & Hansen, E. B. (2017). Processing challenges and opportunities of camel dairy products. *International Journal of Food Sciences*, *2017*, 9061757. doi:10.1155/2017/9061757 PMID:29109953

Bukovics, S., Hucker, A., & Szafner, G. (2015). Impact of microfiltration on camel milk's microbiological and organoleptic characteristics. *Scientific and Practical Journal Veterinariya, 2*(42), 168-170.

Chawla, R., Patil, G. R., & Singh, A. K. (2011). High hydrostatic pressure technology in dairy processing: A review. *Journal of Food Science and Technology*, *48*(3), 260–268. doi:10.100713197-010-0180-4 PMID:23572744

Chen, C., Wang, P., Zhang, N., Zhang, W., & Ren, F. (2019). Improving the textural properties of camel milk acid gel by treatment with trisodium citrate and transglutaminase. *Lebensmittel-Wissenschaft + Technologie*, *103*, 53–59. doi:10.1016/j.lwt.2018.12.063

El Hatmi, H., Jrad, Z., Oussaief, O., Nasri, W., Sbissi, I., Khorchani, T., & Canabady-Rochelle, L. L. (2018). Fermentation of dromedary camel (*Camelus dromedarius*) milk by *Enterococcus faecium, Streptococcus macedonicus* as a potential alternative of fermented cow milk. *Lebensmittel-Wissenschaft + Technologie*, *90*, 373–380. doi:10.1016/j.lwt.2017.12.040

Elagamy, E. I. (2000). Effect of heat treatment on camel milk proteins with respect to antimicrobial factors: A comparison with cows' and buffalo milk proteins. *Food Chemistry*, *68*(2), 227–232. doi:10.1016/S0308-8146(99)00199-5

Elhasan, S. M., Bushara, A. M., Abdelhakam, K. E., Elfaki, H. A., Eibaid, A. I., Farahat, F. H., ... Sukrab, A. M. (2017). Effect of heat treatments on physico-chemical properties of milk samples. *Journal of Academia and Industrial Research*, *6*, 40–46.

Felfoul, I., Jardin, J., Gaucheron, F., Attia, H., & Ayadi, M. A. (2017). Proteomic profiling of camel and cow milk proteins under heat treatment. *Food Chemistry*, *216*, 161–169. doi:10.1016/j.foodchem.2016.08.007 PMID:27596405

Habtegebriel, H., Edward, D., Wawire, M., Sila, D., & Seifu, E. (2018). Effect of operating parameters on the surface and physico-chemical properties of spray-dried camel milk powders. *Food and Bioproducts Processing*, *112*, 137–149. doi:10.1016/j.fbp.2018.09.010

Hamad, S.H., Al Eid, S.M., Al Jassas, F.M., & Abu Tarboush, H. (2013). Use of high hydrostatic pressure for the preservation of camel's milk. *Journal of Veterinary Science and Technology, 4*.

Ho, T. M., Chan, S., Yago, A. J., Shravya, R., Bhandari, B. R., & Bansal, N. (2019). Changes in physicochemical properties of spray-dried camel milk powder over accelerated storage. *Food Chemistry*, *295*, 224–233. doi:10.1016/j.foodchem.2019.05.122 PMID:31174753

Ibrahim, A. H., & Khalifa, S. A. (2015). Effect of freeze-drying on camel's milk nutritional properties. *International Food Research Journal*, *22*, 1438.

Jrad, Z., El-Hatmi, H., Adt, I., Gouin, S., Jardin, J., Oussaief, O., ... Oulahal, N. (2019). Antilisterial activity of dromedary lactoferrin peptic hydrolysates. *Journal of Dairy Science*, *102*(6), 4844–4856. doi:10.3168/jds.2018-15548 PMID:31005319

Jrad, Z., Oussaief, O., Bouhemda, T., Khorchani, T., & EL-Hatmi, H. (2019). Potential effects of ultrafiltration process and date powder on textural, sensory, bacterial viability, antioxidant properties and phenolic profile of dromedary Greek yogurt. *International Journal of Food Science & Technology*, *54*(3), 854–861. doi:10.1111/ijfs.14005

Kinoti, M. F. (1996). *The potential of condensed camel milk in contributing to food security in greater Baragoi, Samburu district* (Doctoral dissertation). University of Nairobi.

Konuspayeva, G. (2007). *Variabilité physico-chimique et biochimique du lait des grands camélidés (Camelus bactrianus, Camelus dromedarius et hybrides) au Kazakhstan* (Doctoral dissertation). Université Montpellier II, France.

Konuspayeva, G., Camier, B., Aleilawi, N., Al-Shumeimyri, M., Al-Hammad, K., Algruin, K., & Faye, B. (2017). Manufacture of dry-and brine-salted soft camel cheeses for the camel dairy industry. *International Journal of Dairy Technology, 70*(1), 92–101. doi:10.1111/1471-0307.12319

Konuspayeva, G., & Faye, B. (2004, November). A better knowledge of milk quality parameters: A preliminary step for improving the camel milk market opportunity in a transition economy–The case of Kazakhstan. In *Saving the Camel and Peoples' Livelihoods Building a Multi-Stakeholder Platform for the Conservation of the Camel in Rajasthan. International Conference* (pp. 28-36). Academic Press.

Kumar, D., Chatli, M. K., Singh, R., Mehta, N., & Kumar, P. (2016). Enzymatic hydrolysis of camel milk casein and its antioxidant properties. *Dairy Science & Technology, 96*(3), 391–404. doi:10.100713594-015-0275-9

Leroy, F., & De Vuyst, L. (2004). Lactic acid bacteria as functional starter cultures for the food fermentation industry. *Trends in Food Science & Technology, 15*(2), 67–78. doi:10.1016/j.tifs.2003.09.004

Maaroufi, S. H., Rezaei, K., Raftaniamiri, Z., & Mirzaei, F. (2015). Evaluating the effects of herbal essences from spearmint and wild thyme on the quality of camel's milk. *International Journal of Food Science & Technology, 50*(10), 2168–2174. doi:10.1111/ijfs.12855

Mati, A., Senoussi-Ghezali, C., Zennia, S. S. A., Almi-Sebbane, D., El-Hatmi, H., & Girardet, J. M. (2017). Dromedary camel milk proteins, a source of peptides having biological activities–A review. *International Dairy Journal, 73*, 25–37. doi:10.1016/j.idairyj.2016.12.001

Mehaia, M. A. (2006). Manufacture of fresh soft white cheese (Domiati type) from dromedary camel's milk using ultrafiltration process. *Journal of Food Technology, 4*, 206–212.

Mohamed, I. M. A., & El Zubeir, E. M. I. (2012). Effect of pasteurization on the keeping quality of camel milk. In *ISOCARD International Conference Sultanate of Oman 29thJanuary–1th February* (Vol. *3*, pp. 232-233). Academic Press.

Mohammed, S., Eshetu, M., Tadesse, Y., & Hailu, Y. (2019). Rheological Properties and Shelf Life of Soft Cheese Made from Camel Milk Using Camel Chymosin. *Journal ofDairy & Veterinary Sciences, 10*.

Muloi, D., Alarcon, P., Ombui, J., Ngeiywa, K. J., Abdullahi, B., Muinde, P., ... Fèvre, E. M. (2018). Value chain analysis and sanitary risks of the camel milk system supplying Nairobi city, Kenya. *Preventive Veterinary Medicine, 159*, 203–210. doi:10.1016/j.prevetmed.2018.09.010 PMID:30314783

Nigussie, H., & Seifu, E. (2007). Effect of the lactoperoxidase system and container smoking on the microbial quality of cows' milk produced in Kombolcha woreda, eastern Ethiopia. *Livestock Research for Rural Development, 19*, 157.

Odongo, N. O., Lamuka, P. O., Matofari, J. W., & Abong, G. O. (2016). Risk factors associated with the post-harvest loss of milk along camel milk value chain in Isiolo County, Kenya. *African Journal of Agricultural Research, 11*(8), 674–682. doi:10.5897/AJAR2015.9988

Ogolla, J. A., Dede, C., Okoth, M. W., Hensel, O., & Sturm, B. (2017). Strategies and technologies for camel milk preservation and utilization of non-marketed milk in arid and semi-arid areas. *East African Agricultural and Forestry Journal, 82*(2-4), 144–167. doi:10.1080/00128325.2017.1363686

Omar, A., Harbourne, N., & Oruna-Concha, M. J. (2018). Effects of industrial processing methods on camel skimmed milk properties. *International Dairy Journal*, *84*, 15–22. doi:10.1016/j.idairyj.2018.03.011

Omer, R. H., & Eltinay, A. H. (2009). Changes in chemical composition of camel's raw milk during storage. *Pakistan Journal of Nutrition*, *8*(5), 607–610. doi:10.3923/pjn.2009.607.610

Patel, K., Wakhisi, J., Mining, S., Mwangi, A., & Patel, R. (2013). Esophageal cancer, the topmost cancer at MTRH in the Rift Valley, Kenya, and its potential risk factors. *ISRN Oncology*. PMID:24490085

Rahmeh, R., Alomirah, H., Akbar, A., & Sidhu, J. (2019). Composition and properties of camel milk. In Milk Production, Processing and Marketing. IntechOpen. doi:10.5772/intechopen.82592

Ramet, J. P. (1993). *La technologie des fromages au lait de dromadaire (Camelus dromedarius)* (Vol. 113). Food & Agriculture Org.

Robinson, R. K. (1990). Dairy microbiology: Volume 1-The microbiology of milk. Elsevier Applied Science Publishers Ltd.

Sboui, A., Khorchani, T., Djegham, M., & Belhadj, O. (2009). Comparaison de la composition physicochimique du lait camelin et bovin du Sud tunisien; variation du pH et de l'acidité à différentes températures. *Afrique Science: revue internationale des sciences et technologie, 5.*

Seifu, E. (2007). Handling, preservation and utilization of camel milk and camel milk products in Shinile and Jijiga Zones, eastern Ethiopia. *Marketing, 10.*

Smits, M. G., Huppertz, T., Alting, A. C., & Kiers, J. (2011). Composition, constituents and properties of Dutch camel milk. *Journal of Camel Practice and Research*, *18*, 1–6.

Sulieman, A. E., Elamin, O. M., Elkhalifa, E. A., & Laleye, L. (2018). A comparative study of physicochemical properties of freeze-dried camel's milk and cow's milk powder. *Discourse Journal of Agriculture & Food Science*, *6*, 11–16.

Sulieman, A. M. E., Elamin, O. M., Elkhalifa, E. A., & Laleye, L. (2014). Comparison of physicochemical properties of spray-dried camel's milk and cow's milk powder. *International Journal of Food Science and Nutrition Engineering*, *4*(1), 15–19.

Wanjala, N. W., Matofari, J. W., & Nduko, J. M. (2016). Antimicrobial effect of smoking milk handling containers' inner surfaces as a preservation method in pastoral systems in Kenya. *Pastoralism*, *6*(1), 17. doi:10.118613570-016-0064-y

Wayua, F. O., Okoth, M. W., & Wangoh, J. (2012). Survey of postharvest handling, preservation and processing practices along the camel milk chain in Isiolo district, Kenya. *African Journal of Food, Agriculture, Nutrition and Development*, 12.

Yagil, R., Zagorski, O., Van Creveld, C., & Saran, A. (1994, October). Science and camel's milk production. In *Actes du Colloque: Dromadaires et chameaux animaux laitier*. Academic Press.

Chapter 4
Microbial Aspect of Lactic Acid Bacteria Isolated From Camel Milk

Dasel Wambua Mulwa Kaindi
https://orcid.org/0000-0003-1561-2408
University of Nairobi, Kenya

Patrick Murigu Kamau Njage
https://orcid.org/0000-0002-4364-5314
Technical University of Denmark, Denmark

ABSTRACT

Camel milk provides a common source of nutrition but also a potential rich source of beneficial, pathogenic, and potentially pathogenic microorganisms. This chapter reviews lactic acid and probiotic bacteria from camel milk, product innovation using such bacteria, and potential areas of improvement in technical as well as practical aspects of fermentation technologies. Lactic acid bacteria fermentation helps mitigate the impact of poor handling and storage conditions by enhancing shelf life and food safety. Traditionally-fermented sour milk products are culturally accepted and widely distributed worldwide with product-specific microbiota responsible for aroma, flavor, and texture. Knowledge of microbiota and predominant, technologically important microorganisms associated with camel milk is critical in developing products with enhanced quality and safety, as well as sustainable interventions for these products, including camel milk specific starter culture development. This chapter presents occurrence of LAB and probiotic bacteria in camel milk and technological aspects of camel dairy.

DOI: 10.4018/978-1-7998-1604-1.ch004

INTRODUCTION

The preparation of most traditional fermented dairy products was reviewed in detail by Food and Agricultural Organization (FAO, 1990) and will be discussed in details in Chapter 5. There is a wide diversity in the products depending on agricultural practices, animal husbandry, seasonality, agroecological zones, animal species, stage of commercialization or industrialization, food preferences and cultural practices. Same factors also influence the camel dairy microbiota. Fermented foods and beverages serve as a major component of diets in the world (Savadogo et al., 2004). This chapter presents the occurrence of LAB and probiotic bacteria in camel milk; developments in typing and characterization; a high technological potential provided by a rich diversity of organisms; traditional and modern camel milk fermentation practices as well as constraints and opportunities for further innovation. Knowledge of microbiome predominant, and technologically important microorganisms associated with camel milk is critical in developing products with enhanced quality and safety, as well as its importance in development of sustainable interventions for these products, including development of novel camel milk specific starter cultures.

LACTIC ACID FERMENTATION

Milk fermentation is a preservation process and occurs through the conversion of lactose into lactic acid with the use of lactic acid bacteria (LAB) and other microorganisms. The application of lactic acid fermentation to prolong the shelf life of food has existed for many generations (Djadouni & Kihal, 2012). LAB is the main microorganism involved in the fermentation of various products. They are a collection of functionally related organisms that are all fermentative, gram-positive, non-motile bacteria and generally have no functional catalase. LABs convert lactose and other sugars in milk to lactic acid (Rhee, Lee, & Lee, 2011). The process also leads to the development of aromatic substances, improved digestibility of proteins, development of sugar polymers, vitamins and useful enzymes (Shori & Baba, 2012). Some LABs produce antimicrobial substances and bacteriocins that inhibit the growth of pathogenic and spoilage microorganisms (Hernåndez et al., 2005). Lactic acid development leads to an acidic environment that suppresses the growth of undesirable pathogenic and spoilage bacteria (Ross, Desmond, Fitzgerald, & Stanton, 2005). This also plays an important role in food preservation and is considered an effective tool for food safety applications (Cotelo et al., 2013; Christoph, Gerber, et al., 2012; Christoph et al., 2017). During the early stages of fermentation, the growth of certain groups of microorganisms is high compared to others when the levels of lactic acid are still low. Some microorganisms can adapt to acidic conditions and therefore, continue to survive in the food. Some pathogens, for instance, *Escherichia coli* O157:H7, can survive the low acid condition of fermented products (Tamime & McNulty, 1999), leading to health risk towards the consumers.

Bacteria present in camel milk products are shown in Table 1. Most of the microorganisms involved in fermentations belong to LAB. In many occasions, fermentations of camel milk results in a wide variety of LAB populations in fermented foods such as *Streptococcus lactis, Lactobacillus casei, Streptococcus diacetylactis, Lactobacillus lactis, Leuconostoc cremoris, Lactobacillus bulgaricus* and *Lactobacillus acidophilus* (Lore, Mbugua, & Wangoh, 2005). The microflora plays a vital role in producing acid, texture, taste, and aroma of dairy and other fermented products (Leroy & De Vuyst, 2004).

Table 1. Bacteria and yeast present in camel milk products in Africa

Country	Type of milk	Organisms present	References
Algeria	Raw camel milk	*E. durans, E. faecalis, E. faecium, Lc. lactis* subsp. *lactis, Lb. paracasei* subsp. *paracasei, Lb. plantarum, Lb. rhamnosus.* No predominance recorded.	(Hassaïne, Zadi-Karam, & Karam, 2007)
Morocco	Raw camel milk	Predominant: *E. casseliflavus, Lc. lactis* subsp. *lactis, Lb. delbrueckii, Lb. casei* subsp. *casei, Lb. helveticus, Lb. plantarum, S. thermophilus* Others: *E. faecalis, Lb. amylophilus, Lb. brevis, Lb. rhamnosus, Lc. lactis* subsp. *cremoris, Lc. lactis* biovar *diacetylactis, Lc. garvieae, Lc. raffinolactis, Leuc. mesenteroides* subsp. *mesenteroides, Leuc. mesenteroides* subsp. *cremoris, Leuc. lactis, P. acidilactici, P. damnosus, P. pentosaceus*	(Khedid, Faid, Mokhtari, Soulaymani, & Zinedine, 2009)
Morocco	Raw camel milk	*S. cameli, S. tangierensis.* No predominance reported	(Khedid et al., 2009)
Kenya	Raw camel milk	Predominant: *E. faecalis, S. agalactiae, W. confusa; Rhodotorula mucilanginosa, Cryptococcus albidus, Candida lusitaniae* Others: *E. faecium, Lc. lactis, S. salivarius/thermophilus, Vagococcus* spp.; *Candida famata, Candida inconspicua, Candida krusei, Cryptococcus laurentii, Trichosporon mucoides*	(C Jans, 2011; P. M. K. Njage, 2011)
Kenya/Somalia	Fermented camel milk	Predominant: *E. faecium, Lb. helveticus,* Sii, *S. salivarius/thermophilus, W. confusa; Candida famata, Candida inconspicua* *Others: E. faecalis, Lb. fermentum, Lc. lactis* subsp. *lactis, Leuc. lactis, Leuc. mesenteroides, Sgm; Candida lusitaniae, Cryptococcus laurentii, Rhodotorula mucilaginosa, Saccharomyces cerevisiae, Trichosporon mucoides, Trichosporon cutaneum*	(C Jans, 2011; P. M. K. Njage, 2011)
Kazakhstan	Fermented Bactrian milk	Predominant: *E. durans ; E. faecalis; E. faecium; Lb casei; Lb casei subsp. casei; Lb curvatus; Lb kefiri; Lbs paracasei; Lbs sakei; Lc lactis subsp. lactis; Leuconostoc mesenteroides. Kazakhstania unispora, Saccharomyces cerevisiae; Kluyveromyces marxianus*	(Akhmetsadykova, Baubekova, Konuspayeva, Akhmetsadykov & Loiseau, 2014)

This table has been partly reprinted from Christoph Jans et al., (2017) with permission from Elsevier

PROCESSING OF FERMENTED MILK

In most parts of the world, especially, camel keeping regions, both traditional and modern camel milk processing techniques are equally available. Traditional fermentation practices vary from community to community and involve either the use of raw or pasteurized camel milk for fermentation (Cissé et al., 2019; Christoph et al., 2017; Mwangi, Matofari, Muliro, & Bebe, 2016). Manufacturing of camel milk dairy products will be discussed in detail in Chapter 5 of the present book. Consumption of unpasteurized raw milk has been shown to have safety concerns as demonstrated by presence of unwanted microorganisms in the fermented dairy products (Abera, Legesse, Mummed, & Urga, 2016; Alaoui Ismaili, Saidi, Zahar, Hamama, & Ezzaier, 2019; Maitha, Kaindi, Wangoh, & Mbugua, 2019), while many pastoralists prefer it due to therapeutic or medicinal value (Khatoon & Najam, 2017; Zibaee et al., 2015). On the other hand, informally traded fermented camel milk products in many occasions are a result of spontaneous fermentation process of milk stored in containers such as traditional gourds although quite rare these days or in plastic vessels used to hold fresh un-boiled camel milk during trade. In this case, mixtures of cultures/microorganisms originating from a natural flora of the raw materials or handling containers are involved in the food fermentation process (Holzapfel, 2002).

The modern techniques of milk fermentation involve the use of starter cultures leading to consistent and safe products with increased shelf-life as opposed to those of natural or spontaneous fermentation (Nduko, Matofari, Nandi, & Sichangi, 2017). The use of specifically defined starter cultures under controlled conditions in the production of fermented foods gives high-quality final products in terms of texture, taste, and aroma (Panesar, 2011). Additionally, this renders the process tenable to standardization leading to products that are consistent in uniformity and quality (Faye & Konuspayeva, 2016).

DIVERSITY OF LACTIC ACID BACTERIA AND YEASTS IN CAMEL MILK

Many species of LAB and other species are present in milk including *Lactococcus* spp., *Lactobacillus* spp., *Streptococcus* spp., *Enterococcus* spp., Bifidobacteria, fungi (Christoph et al., 2017) and *Leuconostoc* (Heller, 2001; Panesar, 2011; Rhee et al., 2011). Most of these are accepted for use in foods because they are considered safe (GRAS) for human consumption (Panesar, 2011).

Lactococcus

Lactococcus lactis, a mesophilic LAB has been isolated in *Suusac* in Kenya and other African countries or in *Shubat* in Kazakhstan and China (Akhmetsadykova et al., 2015). *Lactococcus lactis* is involved in the fermentation of lactose leading to the formation of diacetyl which is important for food preservation and flavor development (Teuber, 2009).

Lactobacillus

Lactobacillus species have also been isolated in fermented products. The most identified subspecies are *Lactobacillus plantarum*, *Lactobacillus fermentum* and *Lactobacillus delbrueckii* (Christoph et al., 2017).

Enterococcus

Enterococcus species have also been isolated and mainly represent milk contaminants. Most *Enterococci species* represent part of the intestinal microbiota of birds and mammals, but are also found in water and plants (Ludwig, Schleifer, & Whitman, 2009). *Enterococci faecalis* and *Enterococci faecium* are the most identified species in camel milk products and their presence in milk is an indicator of fecal contamination from either animal or human sources (Quigley et al., 2013). *Enterococcus* has been associated with human infections and this renders the genus unsafe for the production of safe products although some strains have been incorporated in the production of cheese since they contribute to the development of aroma and flavor (Ogier & Serror, 2008).

Streptococcus in Camel Milk

Members of the *Streptococcus* species are always identified in milk and milk products across the world. Those that are commonly identified in Africa include; *Streptococcus thermophilus*, *Streptococcus salivarius*, *Streptococcus infantarius* subsp *infantarius* (Sii), and *Streptococcus macedonicus* (Christoph et al., 2017). Of these, only *S. thermophilus* is approved for use in dairy processes. However, most of the African spontaneously fermented camel milk products are dominated by Sii rather than *S. thermophilus*. Sii is a member of the SBSEC (*Streptococcus bovis/Streptococcus equinus* complex) which is mainly associated with pathogenic microorganisms and the predominant LAB in fermented dairy products. The role of Sii in milk fermentation was not well known until it was isolated as the predominant LAB in camel fermented milk in Kenya, and Somalia (Christoph, Gerber, et al., 2012; Christoph, Kaindi, et al., 2013; Christoph Jans, Meile, Lacroix, & Stevens, 2015; Wullschleger et al., 2012). The first discovery of Sii was in Sudan, in the year 2008 (Abdelgadir, Nielsen, Hamad, Jakobsen, & Leo Meile, 2008).

Genomic analyses on Sii isolates have revealed an adaptation to lactose metabolism that is parallel to that of *S. thermophilus*. The common ancestor of *S. thermophilus* strains is believed to have lived between 3,000 - 30,000 years ago based on genome decay and this is approximately when human dairy activity started (Bolotin et al., 2004; Fox, 1993). In East Africa, Camels were introduced around 2,500 years ago (Epstein, 1971; Mikesell, 1955) and the less genome decay in Sii strain CJ 18 may be attributed to the start of fermentation of camel milk which came later (Christoph, Kaindi, et al., 2013). The analysis of the African strain of Sii, CJ18 has also revealed more dairy adaptations and events involving loss of function that is still parallel to the adaptation of *S. thermophillus* to the dairy niche. Sii has therefore been found to carry a partial additional gal-lac operon consisting of genes lac*S* and lac*Z* and exhibiting same phenotypic lactose/galactose exchange as *S. thermophilus* (Christoph, Gerber, et al., 2012). The Sii has not been classified as GRAS (generally recognized as safe). Its occurrence in intestinal tracts of humans and animals, together with its presence in fermented dairy products (FDPs) requires research to identify its phylogeny and host associations and the ability to survive in different ecological niches and hosts (Christoph et al., 2015). Further research on the functional analysis of Sii is required to ensure that innovations such as the developing of starter cultures for optimization of the manufacturing processes are implemented taking into account their ecological, safety and functional properties.

TAXONOMY AND PREVALENCE OF STREPTOCOCCUS BOVIS/ STREPTOCOCCUS EQUINUS COMPLEX MEMBERS

The *Streptococcus bovis/Streptococcus equinus complex* (SBSEC) consists of an extensive group of species categorized as *Streptococcus bovis* including several biotype subclasses (Christoph et al., 2015). The members of SBSEC are commensal inhabitants of human and animal gastrointestinal tracts where they establish a constant population in the rumen of the sheep, cattle, goats between 10^5 and 10^7 cells mL^{-1} (Christoph, Kaindi, et al., 2013). Despite its close relationship to pathogens (Alexander Bolotin et al., 2004), *S. thermophilus* was accepted for use in dairy products based on its long history of use in dairy fermentations and inactivation of virulence factors (Alexander Bolotin et al., 2004). Other members of SBSEC show similar gene decay and evolution in similar pattern to that of *S. thermophilus* e.g. *S.*

macedonicus ACA-DC 198, isolated from Greek cheese. Other members of the SBSEC, therefore, may have been similarly adapted to the dairy environment (Christoph et al., 2015). This could also suggest that certain members of the SBSEC could have vital contributions to dairy fermentations (Christoph, Gerber, et al., 2012). The predominance of African variant Sii in dairy environment indicates that it is highly adapted. Gal-lac operon in Sii is responsible for predominance of bacteriocin producers in the African variant Sii a feature that is absent in other members of SBSEC (Rusniok et al., 2010; Tettelin et al., 2002).

Sii is a member of SBSEC is a predominant bacterium in spontaneously fermented milk products in Africa (Abdelgadir et al., 2008; Christoph, Kaindi, et al., 2013; Christoph et al., 2015). It plays an important role in spontaneous dairy fermentation where it occurs at counts of up to 10^8 CFU/mL in the final product (Christoph, Gerber, et al., 2012). A study carried out by Jans et al., (2013a) indicated that CJ18, a strain of Sii contains several unique genetic regions when compared to Sii ATCC BAA-102^T (isolated from human stool) associated with several human infections such as bacteremia, endocarditis and colorectal cancer. Their functional and genomic analysis revealed adapted lactose uptake metabolism that is identical to that of GRAS approved *S. thermophilus* (Christoph, Follador, Lacroix, Meile, & Stevens, 2012). It also displayed loss of functional events paralleling the evolutionary adaptation of *S. thermophilus* to dairy environment (Christoph, Gerber, et al., 2012). Hence, the role of Sii CJ18 in dairy fermentations for possible adaptations in dairy environment needs to be investigated. This will also shed light on the strain's predominance in fermented African milk and milk products. Lactic acid bacteria like African dairy Sii has been reported to produce inhibitory substances against other pathogenic bacteria such as *Listeria* spp., *S. aureus* or *E. coli*. Despite other members of SBSEC being pathogenic, virulence factors have not been reported in African Sii isolates (Christoph, Follador, et al., 2013). Lack of reports on virulence factors of Sii and its ability to ferment lactose in a similar way to *S. thermophilus* suggests a possible application of this strain in developing novel camel dairy products applying *Streptococcus infantarius* subsp. *infantarius* as starter culture (Christoph, Follador, et al., 2013).

Yeasts

The occurrence and potential of yeast in both raw and fermented dairy products, remains underestimated. Various studies involving the presence of microorganisms in African fermented dairy products have reported the presence of yeast (Beukes, Bester, & Mostert, 2001) as well as *Shubat* from Kazakhstan (Baubekova et al., 2015). Yeasts play significant roles in product development during fermentation of dairy products mainly through the metabolism of lactose, lipolysis and proteolysis which altogether lead to flavor development (L. Quigley et al., 2013). The yeast species mostly identified in raw milk that are important in dairy product development include *Saccharomyces cerevisiae*, *Debaryomyces*, *Issatchenkia*, *Geotrichum*, *Kluyveromyces* and *Candida* (Quigley et al., 2013).

Njage (2011) studied the occurrence of yeast species in the raw and *suusac* value chain using a combination of phenotypic and molecular methods. The study identified 21 yeast species with most prevalent including *Saccharomyces cerevisiae* (19%), *Candida inconspicua* (12%), *Trichosporon mucoides* (11%), *Candida famata* (11%), *Rhodotorula mucilaginosa* (8%), *Candida lusitaniae* (6%), *Cryptococcus laurentii* (5%), *Cryptococcus albidus* (5%), *Candida guilliermondii* (5%) and *Trichosporon cutaneum* (5%). These yeast species belonged to the genera *Rhodotorula*, *Cryptococcus*, *Candida*, *Saccharomyces*,

Trichosporon, *Geotrichum* and *Issatchenkia.* There were high yeast counts (log cfu mL^{-1}) ranging from 2.4 log cfu mL^{-1} for *C. tropicalis* to highest counts of 7.6 log cfu mL^{-1} (range; 2.4-8.5) for *C. famata* and 8.0 log cfu mL^{-1} (range; 2.6-8.5) for *C. guilliermondii*. This high diversity and numbers of yeasts suggests they may play an important role in the spontaneously fermented camel milk. Further studies are recommended to support the exploitation of useful yeasts and the prevention of contamination by detrimental yeasts.

LIMITATIONS OF SPONTANEOUS FERMENTATION

Natural or traditional fermentation occurs because of inherent microflora in milk, normally through a spontaneous process and in many occasions back-slopping inoculating method is used (Holzapfel, 2002). Back-slopping is the use of samples from the previously fermented batch to inoculate subsequent products. Although back-slopping produces products with consistency in quality, meanwhile, the safety of the products is not assured (Nduko et al., 2017). In spontaneous fermentation, the pathogens are likely to dominate because the initial pH is too high to suppress their growth. The use of starter culture results in fast pH drop hence controlling the level of pathogenic microorganisms often to below infectious doses (Holzapfel, 1997). The traditional natural fermentation process leads to variation in the pH of the fermented product, hence undesirable quality attributes. For instance, Njage et al. (2012) studied the prevalence and distribution of *Escherichia coli* O157 and non-O157 Shiga toxin-producing *Escherichia coli* (STEC) in raw camel milk and *suusac* collected along the marketing chain from farm to the final market. They reported a high prevalence of both O157 and non-O157 STEC from serotypes O157, O111, and O113. The higher prevalence of STEC in camel milk than reported in other species indicated that the milk could be an important vehicle for transmission of STEC to humans. Both coagulase positive and negative staphylococci have also been reported in camel milk including *Staphylococcus aureus*, *S. epidermidis*, *S. simulans*, *S. saprophyticus*, *S. haemolyticus*, *S. hyicus*, *S. xylosus*, *S. lentus*, *S. carnosus* and *S. microti*. This diversity of Staphylococci was also accompanied by a high prevalence of enterotoxin genes indicating that these staphylococci may be of potential public health significance. The pathogens were inhibited when the milk was fermented under controlled conditions using a starter culture due to a rapid decrease in pH (Njage et al. 2012).

IMPROVEMENT OF MICROBIAL AND PROBIOTIC QUALITY OF FERMENTED CAMEL MILK PRODUCTS USING STARTER CULTURES

LABs are like small machines that manufacture fermented products. Each group of LAB has its own health-promoting, functional and technological capacities (See Chapter 7 and 8). Therefore, the microbial diversity of fermented camel dairy products must be studied for either product improvement or conservation.

Starter cultures are preparations containing high numbers of live microbial strains inoculated in food either as single, multiple or mixed species to overcome and dominate the existing flora by fermenting lactose to lactic acid. The cultures give good sensorial properties to the food by contributing to flavor, texture, and taste. They also enhance preservation, digestibility, nutrition and detoxification of the final product (Ray & Mishra, 2017). Starter cultures also help improve and accelerate predictable fermentation processes, which leads to improved product safety and reduced hygienic risks (Kimaryo, Massawe, Olasupo, & Holzapfel, 2000). Moreover, the addition of starter culture ensures that processing is done properly in a timed and repeatable schedule, in the same time maintaining the quality and consistency of the final product.

In high and upper-middle-income countries, the technology on starter culture design has been used to produce products like enzymes and microbial cultures which in most cases are imported to low and lower-middle income countries (Marshall & Mejia, 2011). This included starter cultures applied in the development of products such as yogurt. There is a growing need to incorporate probiotic bacteria in the fermentation of dairy products. The traditionally fermented dairy products are a source of these microorganisms, but the opportunities are yet to be exploited (see Chapter 5). There exists a huge diversity of fermented products due to traditional methods of fermentation such as back-slopping or natural fermentation in both high- and low-income economies. In the present book, the recent processing methods, and issues of the most popular camel milk dairy products will be discussed in details in Chapter 5.

The safety of fermented food is improved when starter cultures are used because they produce enough lactic acid from lactose that inhibits the growth of pathogenic microorganisms. An effective starter culture is one that produces sufficient acid in early stages of fermentation where rapid drop in pH inhibits pathogenic and spoilage microorganisms and maintains low pH level during storage (Cenci-Goga et al., 2015). The efficacy of a starter culture is influenced by among other things, the initial level of contamination of product, sanitation, overall hygiene conditions and the activity of the starter culture itself (Motarjemi, Käferstein, Moy, & Quevedo, 1993). It also depends on the type of tested microorganism, the ability of food to maintain appropriate conditions for growth and the amount of undissociated acid produced. The undissociated acid is the active form of lactic acid. The undissociated acid interferes with the metabolism of bacterial pathogens by diffusing and reducing the intracellular pH. During lactic acid fermentation, it is desired that the pH decreases to around 4.6. At this pH, growth of most undesirable microorganisms is suppressed (El-Ziney, De Mayer, & Debeyera, 1997).

In industrial dairy fermentations, starter cultures are deliberately added, and the process is controlled. The natural flora in the milk must first be destroyed by heat treatment process. High throughput technologies involving the use of starter cultures can lead to products with improved flavor and aroma. The use of a specified starter culture leads to products with enhanced safety and consistency of quality parameters (Faye & Konuspayeva, 2016).

CHARACTERISTICS OF LACTIC ACID BACTERIA IN CAMEL MILK

Antimicrobial Activity

Improved technologies have resulted to development of lactic acid bacteria (LAB) starter cultures (Leroy & De Vuyst, 2004). Use of starter cultures results for fermentation under controlled conditions yields a product of desired quality such texture, taste, flavour, aroma and improved microbial quality (Platteeuw, Alen-Boerrigter, Schalkwijk, & Vos, 1996). Fermented foods are usually considered safe as starter cultures are able to produce weak organic acids, diacetyl, ethanol, hydrogen peroxide, reuterin and antimicrobial-peptides such as bacteriocins that inhibit food-borne pathogens and spoilage bacteria (Savadogo et al., 2004). This result to improved storage period by producing antimicrobial substances such as bacteriocins (García, Rodríguez, Rodríguez, & Martínez, 2010). The most commonly used bacteriocin as bio-preservative in food is nisin (Hernández et al., 2005). It is produced by *Lactococcus lactis* and it the only bacteriocin recognized as safe for use in dairy products (Delves-Broughton, Blackburn, Evans, & Hugenholtz, 1996; Siboukeur & Siboukeur, 2013). Because of changing lifestyle and eating habits, food is often contaminated with a variety of food-pathogens especially, *L. monocytogenes*, *S. typhimurium*, Methicillin-resistant *Staphylococcus aureus* (MRSA) (Lynch, Tauxe, & Hedberg, 2009). This has led to an increase in the use of antibiotics resulting in evolution of antibiotic-resistant microorganisms (Saikia, 2008). Therefore, there has been continued interest in development of probiotics with the ability to produce bacteriocins that act as natural agents to inhibit food-borne pathogens in order to enhance the quality and safety of fermented milk products (Buyong, Kok, & Luchansky, 1998).

The ability of fermented foods to inhibit undesirable microorganisms is determined by assessing the antimicrobial activity against selected test microorganism and/ or their ability to improve the microbial quality of that particular food (García et al., 2010; Ross, Morgan, & Hill, 2002). The total viable counts of *C. botulinum* and *L. monocytogenes* reduces with time during fermentation process (Ross et al., 2002). Pathogenic *E. coli* survive under low pH for longer period compared other common food-borne pathogens (Gadaga, Nyanga, & Mutukumira, 2004). *Enterococcus faecalis*, *S. aureus* and *B. cereus* are susceptible to bacteriocins extracted from fermented milk products (Savadogo et al., 2004). Wambui et al., (2017) characterized the potential of LAB from camel milk as potential protective cultures against ten members of Enterobacteriaceae from *suusac*. *Citrobacter* spp., S*higella* spp. *E. coli* isolates were inhibited though *Salmonella* spp. was not inhibited by the LAB isolates. LABs were reported as potential protective cultures in improving safety and quality of camel products including milk and meat (Wambui et al., 2017). The antimicrobial effect of camel milk will be discussed in detail in Chapter 7.

Acidification

Camel milk takes longer time to ferment compared to cow milk, which is good for prolonging milk shelf life (Berhe et al., 2017). However, this represents a disadvantage point in view of fermentation process. Delays in fermentation have been previously been linked to ultra-composition of camel milk, especially high antimicrobial factors, functional and structural properties of camel milk proteins (Berhe, Seifu, Ipsen, Kurtu, & Hansen, 2017; FAO, 1982).

Some researchers have isolated starter cultures from the raw and traditional fermented camel milk products (see Chapter 5). To date, there is no suitable starter cultures from camel milk have been released into the industries except in Kazakhstan (Faye & Konuspayeva, 2016). Recently, the ability of various strains to ferment camel and cow milk were tested (Berhe et al. 2018). The results confirmed the difficulty experienced in fermenting camel milk by mesophilic, thermophilic commercial starter cultures and their combinations. In view of mesophilic group, culture R-704 (*Lactococcus lactis* subsp. *lactis* and *Lactococcus lactis* subsp. *cremoris*; Chr. Hansen A/S, Denmark) showed to be the fastest acidifier strain of camel milk with a rate of 33% slower than in cow milk at 37°C (Table 2). It is recommended to use culture R-704 at 30°C to ferment camel milk compared to R-707 and CHN-22 as it took 8:10 (hr:min) to reach pH 4.6.

Thermophilic cultures followed by a mixture of mesophilic and thermophilic cultures yielded acidification rates which were 48% to 81% slower than in camel milk. The use of yoghurt cultures led to acidification rates between 45 and 55% slower at 42°C (Berhe et al. 2018).

Table 2. The percent difference between camel's and cow's milk acidification rate by different Lactic Acid Bacteria cultures

		Temperature of incubation		
Cultures	**Strains**	**30°C**	**37°C**	**42°C**
Mesophilic	R 704	-62%	-33%	
	R 707	-81%	-51%	
	CHN – 22	-75%	-79%	
Mixture of mesophilic and thermophilic	RST-743	-81%	-51%	-48%
	XPL-2	-53%	-53%	-59%
Thermophilic	Yoflex mild 1.0		-58%	-45%
	YF-L904		-49%	-50%
	STI-12		-52%	-54%

Modified from (Berhe et al., 2018)

These results indicated that camel milk needs more time to reach a desirable pH of 4.6, compared to cow milk. But the thermophilic cultures (STI-12) were the best, since, at 37 and 42°C the difference is reduced to 1:14 and 1:35 hours: mins, respectively using culture ST-12 (Table 3). Camel milk needs a minimum of 5:10 hours: mins to reach a complete fermentation using ST-12 at 42°C. Mesophilic cultures take between 12 to 21 hours to achieve final required pH in camel milk. However, combination of mesophilic and thermophilic cultures gained the shortest fermentation time, as it was found with mixture of cultures RST-743. Also, authors suggested different mixtures between camel's and cow's milk or by supplementation of camel milk with casein hydrolysate to enhance the fermentation process and reduce the fermentation time of camel milk to a level comparable to that of cow milk (Berhe et al., 2018).

In Kenya, most of tested LABs isolated from camel milk belonged to the *Streptococcus infantarius* subsp *infantarius* in comparison to *Streptococcus thermophilus*. The *S. infantarius* strains were described in detail by Jans et al., (2015, 2013a). Most of the work on fermentation properties of the *S. infantarius*

Table 3. Required Fermentation Time of camel milk to reach pH 4.6 by different Lactic Acid Bacteria cultures

		Temperature of Incubation					
Cultures	**Strains**	**30°C**		**37°C**		**42°C**	
	R 704	12:40	(-4:15)	16:48	(-7:13)		
Mesophilic	R 707	8:10	(-2:15)	16:05	(-8:30)		
	CHN - 22	12:35	(-3:25)	21:15	(-1:30)		
Mixture of mesophilic and thermophilic	RST-743	7:55	(-0:15)	7:52	(-2:47)	7:23	(-2:33)
	XPL-2	13:40	(-2:20)	15:08	(-6:14)	9:58	(-2:28)
	Yoflex mild 1.0			8:30	(-4:00)	8:27	(-4:42)
Thermophilic	YF-L904			8:42	(-4:03)	8:37	(-4:34)
	STI-12			5:32	(-1:14)	5:10	(-1:35)

Modified from (Berhe et al., 2018) (- difference between cow and camel milk)

have not been published yet (Maitha, 2019; P. Njage, 2010; Nyagoya, 2016). Both thesis by Nyangoya (2015) and Maitha (2019) tried to compare the fermentation ability of *S. infantarius* to that by western cultures – *Streptococcus thermophilus*. Key findings were that camel milk still needed more time to ferment up to 6 to 9 hours at 37 ° C to reach a pH of less than 4.6. The effect of the *S. infantarious* was tested on pathogens and was found able to inhibit *E. coli* and *L. monocytogenes* but was not effective against *Salmonella* spp, and *Staphylococcus aureus (Nyagoya 2015)*. Maitha (2019) also tested fermentation ability of an African *Streptococcus thermophilus* strain isolated from *Susaac*, and the results were comparable to those of *S. infantarius*. Njage (2010) studied the acidification and metabolic properties of 95 lactic acid bacterial cultures (LAB) which were mainly belong to *Lb. helveticus, Lb. fermentum, Lc. Lactis* subsp. *lactis, S. infantarius* and *S. thermophilus*. The cultures were isolated from various camel milks and their associated production points in Kenya and Somalia. The LABs were ranked in the decreasing order of acidification capability as *S. infantarius, Lb. helveticus, Lc. Lactis* subsp. *lactis, Lb. fermentum* and *S. thermophilus*. Even though *S. infantarius* reached a lower pH at final experimental time and acidified for a longer time when compared with other strains (Njage 2010).

a. Bacteriocins Production

The inhibitory substances produced during lactic acid fermentation act differently depend on pathogenic reference indicators. Gram-positive bacteria are more sensitive to bacteriocin than gram-negative bacteria (Savadogo et al., 2004). The particular nature of gram-negative bacteria makes them resistance to bacteriocin compared to gram-positive bacteria (Savadogo, Ouattara, Bassole, & Traore, 2006). Lactic acid bacteria which are gram-positive bacteria produce bacteriocins that have a broad spectrum of activity (Leroy & De Vuyst, 2004). The efficacy of the bacteriocin against a given bacteria also depends on the strain of the microorganism (Vuyst & Leroy, 2007). This is due to the fact, some strains have to receive sites of immunoproteins and are thus easily hurt by inhibitory factors while other strains lack such sites and are therefore more resistant to such bacteriocins (Savadogo et al., 2006).

The potential of bacteriocin-producing starters is widely studied especially on Lactococci, Enterococci, and Lactobacilli (Vuyst & Leroy, 2007). Bacteriocins have been used successfully in milk products such as Cheddar cheese using *Lactococcus* as a starter culture (produces nisin) to control *Listeria (L.) monocytogenes*, *Clostridium sporogenes,* and *Staphylococcus aureus* (Zottola, Yezzi, Ajao, & Roberts, 1994). Sulzer and Busse, (1991) carried out research on the ability of *Lactococcus* spp., *Enterococcus* spp. and *Lactobacillus* spp. alone and in combination with other commercial starters to produce inhibitory substances against *L. monocytogenes* in Camembert cheese. They found out that the strains were more effective when they were used alone than when they were used in combination with other commercial cultures. *L. monocytogenes* was also suppressed more if contamination took place in the early stages of ripening of Camembert cheese.

Exopolysaccharide Production

Exopolysaccharide (EPS) plays an important role in milk thickness or viscosity. Some EPS produced by LABs have showed potential for application as food viscosifiers, thickeners, emulsifiers or stabilizers (Bajpai et al., 2016). EPS are of potential importance in fermented camel milk manufacture since camel milk does not form a thick coagulum upon fermentation (Ruas-Madiedo, Hugenholtz, & Zoon,

2002). The EPS concentration was between 41.3 and 269.3 mg/kg in the yoghurt made with non-EPS and EPS-producing starter cultures, respectively (Ibrahim, 2015). This gives dairy products viscosity or thickness, texture, more enhanced mouth feel and reduces syneresis. However, many additives are proposed to increase firmness and avoid syneresis of fermented camel milk (Ibrahim & Khalifa, 2015). Conventional yoghurt cultures composed of *S. thermophilus* and *Lactobacillus delbrueckii* are known for producing low amounts of EPS (De Vuyst et al., 2003). The role of additives in improving the functional properties of camel milk dairy products will be discussed in detail in Chapter 5.

Characteristics of Probiotics in FTA

The LAB found in camel milk consists of probiotics such as *Bifidobacterium*, *Streptococcus*, *Lactococcus*, *Lactobacillus*, *Leuconostoc,* and *Enterococcus* which are GRAS (Fernández, Hudson, Korpela, & de los Reyes-Gavilán, 2015; Lisa Quigley et al., 2011). *Streptococcus macedonicus (S. macedonicus)* is used as a starter culture in industrial dairy fermentations due to its ability to quickly acidify milk and to prevent the growth of spoilage bacteria (Samet-Bali, Bellila, Ayadi, Marzouk, & Attia, 2010). The proteolytic activity of *S. macedonicus* in fermented dromedary milk generates potential bioactive peptides from casein such as the glycosylation-dependent cell adhesion molecule-1 (GlyCAM-1) and peptidoglycan recognition protein-1 (PGRP-1). According to El Hatmi et al. (2018), all these biomolecules produced by milk fermentation can improve the health benefits of dromedary's dairy products (Chapter 7).

Strains of *Enterococcus faecium (E. faecium)* have demonstrated probiotic characteristics including several health effects and are safe for human consumption (Cavallini, Bedani, Bomdespacho, Vendramini, & Rossi, 2009). Witzler et al. (2017), developed a diet micro-capsule containing *E. faecium* probiotic strain for which a bacteriocinogenic anti-listeria activity was observed in thermized milk (Lianou, Kakouri, Pappa, & Samelis, 2017). Combination of *E. faecium* with *S. macedonicus* also enhances the viscosity of both dromedary and cow milk as compared to milk fermented by a single strain (El Hatmi et al., 2018).

Lactococcus lactis is one of the most frequent used bacteria in probiotic preparations in fermented dairy products (Odamaki, Xiao, Yonezawa, Yaeshima, & Iwatsuki, 2011). According to a previous study, *Lactococcus lactis* subsp *cremoris* exhibits a good inhibition of angiotensin converting enzyme (ACE) in vitro (Rodríguez-Figueroa et al., 2010). ACE showed a capacity to improve heart fibrosis (Chiang, Chen, Wang, Hsieh, & Chen, 2011).

Fermented camel milk by *Lactococcus lactis subsp cremoris* has demonstrated the preventive effect against carbon tetrachloride induced cardiotoxicity lesions with heart oxidative damage and histopathological changes (Hamed et al., 2018). The results from the study suggested that pretreatment with fermented camel milk by *Lactococcus lactis subsp cremoris* is beneficial for reduce heart injury induced by carbon tetrachloride (Hamed et al., 2018).

Indigenous strains of *Lactobacillus spp* (*Lb. reuteri* KX881777, *Lb. plantarum* KX881772 and *Lb. planturum* KX881779) isolated from camel milk have demonstrated robust probiotic characteristics (Abushelaibi, Al-Mahadin, El-Tarabily, Shah, & Ayyash, 2017). A study by Ayyash et al. (2018), found that the water soluble extracts from camel milk fermented by indigenous *Lactobacillus spp* Lr .K777, Lp .K779, and Lp. K772 exhibited greater health benefits than non-indigenous strains. These strains are promising starter cultures for the dairy food industries.

Abushelaibi et al. (2017) isolated several probiotic bacteria and examined their effect after testing their survival in camel and cow milk. The three probiotic strains *Lb. reuteri* KX881777 (Lp.K777), *Lb. plantarum* KX881772 (Lp.K772), *Lb. plantarum* KX881779 (Lp.K779). All the strains grew well in camel and cow milk but the change in pH of camel milk was lower than that of cow milk. Microbial counts were all higher than 10^8 cfumL^{-1}, giving an indication that they can be suitable as probiotic cultures. The *in vitro* probiotic characteristics of these strains were tested by Ayyash et al., (2018). The proteolytic and antioxidant activity was higher in camel milk compared to cow milk. LrK772 strain showed the highest angiotensin-converting-enzyme (ACE)-inhibition of over 80%. The study also indicated that the anticancer activity was higher when water- soluble extracts were from camel milk rather than cow milk. This implies that peptides emanating from camel milk as a result of fermentation possess bioactivity (Ayyash et al., 2018; Park, 2009). A possible explanation for the role of the peptides is their ability to outcompete other cancer-promoting factors for the cancer cell membrane receptors. The second explanation is that peptides from camel milk fermentation could have anticancer toxicity specific enough to target and induce death of the cancer cells (Park, 2009; Pessione & Cirrincione, 2016; Picot et al., 2006). In the present book, the potential therapeutic and disease prevention properties of camel milk will be discussed in details in Chapter 7 and 8.

CONCLUSION

There is a great consensus that traditional fermented dairy products play a pivotal role all over the world. However, the scale and technology of production, as well as marketing and distribution systems, need to be scaled to industrial level (FAO, 1990). Demand for fermented food products is rising due to the health benefits associated with these products, migration, and urbanization. The increased demand by consumers calls for improvement in the safety and quality of fermented food products. Several limitations have been accrued to spontaneous fermentation of food products, which include; low yields, inefficiency, and production of products with varying quality standards. In addition, there are concerns regarding the safety of products of spontaneous fermentation due to the presence of pathogenic bacteria and chemical toxins produced by the bacteria.

FUTURE RESEARCH DIRECTIONS

In comparison with current fermentation technologies used in developing countries, there is a need to develop and describe bacteria and their ecological characteristics. This process will enable the development of novel starter cultures for the fermentation of camel milk under controlled conditions. This will give high-quality camel milk products with desirable thick viscosity and probiotic potential. In addition, there is a need for investment towards research, since most of the studies have used culture-dependent techniques in the identification of microorganisms. However, the use of synthetic media has been shown to be inaccurate and inconclusive. Therefore, it is proposed to use culture-independent techniques to further determine the population diversity of fermented camel milk in the various camel keeping regions.

REFERENCES

Abdelgadir, W., Nielsen, D. S., Hamad, S., & Jakobsen, M. (2008). A traditional Sudanese fermented camel's milk product, Gariss, as a habitat of Streptococcus infantarius subsp. Infantarius. *International Journal of Food Microbiology*, *127*(3), 215–219. doi:10.1016/j.ijfoodmicro.2008.07.008

Abera, T., Legesse, Y., Mummed, B., & Urga, B. (2016). Bacteriological quality of raw camel milk along the market value chain in Fafen zone, Ethiopian Somali regional state. *BMC Research Notes*, *9*(1), 285–285. doi:10.118613104-016-2088-1

Abushelaibi, A., Al-Mahadin, S., El-Tarabily, K., Shah, N. P., & Ayyash, M. (2017). Characterization of potential probiotic lactic acid bacteria isolated from camel milk. *Lebensmittel-Wissenschaft + Technologie*, *79*, 316–325. doi:10.1016/j.lwt.2017.01.041

Akhmetsadykova, Sh., Baubekova, A., Konuspayeva, G., Akhmetsadykov, N., Faye, B., & Loiseau, G. (2015). Lactic acid bacteria biodiversity in raw and fermented camel milk. *African Journal of Food Science and Technology*, *6*(3), 84–88.

Akhmetsadykova, Sh., Baubekova, A., Konuspayeva, G., Akhmetsadykov, N., & Loiseau, G. (2014). Microflora identification of fresh and fermented camel milk from Kazakhstan. *Emirates Journal of Food and Agriculture*, *26*(4), 327–332. doi:10.9755/ejfa.v26i4.17641

Alaoui Ismaili, M., Saidi, B., Zahar, M., Hamama, A., & Ezzaier, R. (2019). Composition and microbial quality of raw camel milk produced in Morocco. *Journal of the Saudi Society of Agricultural Sciences*, *18*(1), 17–21. doi:10.1016/j.jssas.2016.12.001

Ayyash, M., Al-Nuaimi, A. K., Al-Mahadin, S., & Liu, S.-Q. (2018). In vitro investigation of anticancer and ACE-inhibiting activity, alpha-amylase and alpha-glucosidase inhibition, and antioxidant activity of camel milk fermented with camel milk probiotic: A comparative study with fermented bovine milk. *Food Chemistry*, *239*, 588–597. doi:10.1016/j.foodchem.2017.06.149

Baubekova, A., Akhmetsadykova, S., Konuspayeva, G., Akhmetsadykov, N., Faye, B., & Loiseau, G. (2015). Biodiversity study of the yeast in fresh and fermented camel and mare's milk by denaturing gradient gel electrophoresis. *Journal of Camel Practice and Research*, *22*(1), 91–95. doi:10.5958/2277-8934.2015.00014.4

Berhe, T., Ipsen, R., Seifu, E., Kurtu, M. Y., Eshetu, M., & Hansen, E. B. (2018). Comparison of the acidification activities of commercial starter cultures in camel and bovine milk. *LWT*, *89*, 123–127. doi:10.1016/j.lwt.2017.10.041

Berhe, T., Seifu, E., Ipsen, R., Kurtu, M. Y., & Hansen, E. B. (2017). Processing Challenges and Opportunities of Camel Dairy Products. *International Journal of Food Sciences*, *2017*, 9061757–9061757. doi:10.1155/2017/9061757

Beukes, E. M., Bester, B. H., & Mostert, J. F. (2001). The microbiology of South African traditional fermented milks. *International Journal of Food Microbiology*, *63*(3), 189–197. doi:10.1016/S0168-1605(00)00417-7

Bolotin, A., Quinquis, B., Renault, P., Sorokin, A., Ehrlich, S. D., Kulakauskas, S., ... Hols, P. (2004). Complete sequence and comparative genome analysis of the dairy bacterium Streptococcus thermophilus. *Nature Biotechnology*, *22*(12), 1554–1558. doi:10.1038/nbt1034

Bolotin, A., Quinquis, B., Renault, P., Sorokin, A., Ehrlich, S. D., Kulakauskas, S., ... Hols, P. (2004). Complete sequence and comparative genome analysis of the dairy bacterium Streptococcus thermophilus. *Nature Biotechnology*, *22*(12), 1554–1558. doi:10.1038/nbt1034

Buyong, N., Kok, J., & Luchansky, J. B. (1998). Use of a Genetically Enhanced, Pediocin-Producing Starter Culture, Lactococcus lactis subsp. Lactis MM217, To Control Listeria monocytogenes in Cheddar Cheese. *Applied and Environmental Microbiology*, *64*(12), 4842–4845.

Cavallini, D. C., Bedani, R., Bomdespacho, L. Q., Vendramini, R. C., & Rossi, E. A. (2009). Effects of probiotic bacteria, isoflavones and simvastatin on lipid profile and atherosclerosis in cholesterol-fed rabbits: A randomized double-blind study. *Lipids in Health and Disease*, *8*(1), 1. doi:10.1186/1476-511X-8-1

Cenci-Goga, B. T., Karama, M., Sechi, P., Iulietto, M. F., Novelli, S., Selvaggini, R., & Mattei, S. (2015). Growth Inhibition of Selected Microorganisms by an Association of Dairy Starter Cultures and Probiotics. *Italian Journal of Animal Science*, *14*(2), 3745. doi:10.4081/ijas.2015.3745

Chiang, M.-L., Chen, H.-C., Wang, S.-Y., Hsieh, Y.-L., & Chen, M.-J. (2011). Use of Taiwanese Ropy Fermented Milk (TRFM) and Lactococcus lactis subsp. Cremoris Isolated from TRFM in Manufacturing of Functional Low-Fat Cheeses. *Journal of Food Science*, *76*(7), M504–M510. doi:10.1111/j.1750-3841.2011.02320.x

Cissé, H., Muandze-Nzambe, J. U., Somda, N. S., Sawadogo, A., Drabo, S. M., Tapsoba, F., ... Savadogo, A. (2019). Assessment of safety and quality of fermented milk of camels, cows, and goats sold and consumed in five localities of Burkina Faso. *Veterinary World*, *12*(2), 295–304. doi:10.14202/vetworld.2019.295-304

De Vuyst, L., Zamfir, M., Mozzi, F., Adriany, T., Marshall, V., Degeest, B., & Vaningelgem, F. (2003). Exopolysaccharide-producing Streptococcus thermophilus strains as functional starter cultures in the production of fermented milks. *3rd NIZO Dairy Conference - Dynamics of Texture, Process and Perception (Part 1)*, *13*(8), 707–717. 10.1016/S0958-6946(03)00105-5

Delves-Broughton, J., Blackburn, P., Evans, R. J., & Hugenholtz, J. (1996). Applications of the bacteriocin, nisin. *Antonie van Leeuwenhoek*, *69*(2), 193–202. doi:10.1007/BF00399424

Djadouni, F., & Kihal, M. (2012). Antimicrobial activity of lactic acid bacteria and the spectrum of their biopeptides against spoiling germs in foods. *Brazilian Archives of Biology and Technology*, *55*(3), 435–444. doi:10.1590/S1516-89132012000300015

El Hatmi, H., Jrad, Z., Oussaief, O., Nasri, W., Sbissi, I., Khorchani, T., & Canabady-Rochelle, L. L. S. (2018). Fermentation of dromedary camel (Camelus dromedarius) milk by Enterococcus faecium, Streptococcus macedonicus as a potential alternative of fermented cow milk. *LWT*, *90*, 373–380. doi:10.1016/j.lwt.2017.12.040

El-Ziney, M., De Mayer, H., & Debeyera, J. (1997). Growth and survival kinetics of Yersinia enterocolitica IP 383 0:9 as affected by equimolar concentrations of undissociated short-chain organic acids. *International Journal of Food Microbiology, 34*(3), 233–247. doi:10.1016/S0168-1605(96)01194-4

Epstein, H. (1971). *The origin of domestic animals of Africa*. New York: Africana Publ. Corp.

FAO. (1982). *Camels and camel milk*. Retrieved from http://www.fao.org/3/X6528E/X6528E03.htm#chIII

FAO. (1990). *The technology of traditional milk products in developing countries*. Rome, Italy: FAO.

Faye, B., & Konuspayeva, G. (2016). Innovations in camel milk processing: The new challenges for marketing camel dairy products and the consequences on genetic selection. In: *Regional conf. for animal genetic resources conservation. Towards Sustainable Utilization.* Available on: https://oapgrc.gov.om/Documents/The new challenges for marketing camel dairy products and the consequences on genetic selection_Bernard Fye.pdf

Fernández, M., Hudson, J. A., Korpela, R., & de los Reyes-Gavilán, C. G. (2015). Impact on human health of microorganisms present in fermented dairy products: An overview. *BioMed Research International, 2015*, 412714–412714. doi:10.1155/2015/412714

Fox, P. F. (1993). *Cheese: Chemistry, physics and microbiology*. London, UK: Chapman & Hall.

Fraga Cotelo, M., Perelmuter Schein, K., Salvo, G., Solange, S., Abirad, Z., Miguel, P., ... Beatriz, S. (2013). Antimicrobial properties of lactic acid bacteria isolated from uruguayan artisan cheese. *Food Science and Technology (Campinas), 33*(4), 801–804. doi:10.1590/S0101-20612013000400029

Gadaga, T. H., Nyanga, L. K., & Mutukumira, A. N. (2004). The occurrence, growth and control of pathogens in African fermented foods. *African Journal of Food, Agriculture, Nutrition and Development, 4*(1). doi:10.4314/ajfand.v4i1.19155

García, P., Rodríguez, L., Rodríguez, A., & Martínez, B. (2010). Food biopreservation: Promising strategies using bacteriocins, bacteriophages and endolysins. *Trends in Food Science & Technology, 21*(8), 373–382. doi:10.1016/j.tifs.2010.04.010

Hamed, H., Chaari, F., Ghannoudi, Z., ElFeki, A., Ellouz, S. C., & Gargouri, A. (2018). Beneficial effects of fermented camel milk by lactococcus lactis subsp cremoris on cardiotoxicity induced by carbon tetrachloride in mice. *Biomedicine & Pharmacotherapy = Biomedecine & Pharmacotherapie, 97*, 107–114. doi:10.1016/j.biopha.2017.10.057

Hassaïne, O., & Zadi-Karam, H., & Karam. (2007). Technologically important properties of lactic acid bacteria isolated from raw milk of three breeds of Algerian dromedary (Camelus dromedarius). *African Journal of Biotechnology, 6*(14), 1720–1727.

Heller, K. J. (2001). Probiotic bacteria in fermented foods: Product characteristics and starter organisms. *The American Journal of Clinical Nutrition, 73*(2), 374s–379s. doi:10.1093/ajcn/73.2.374s

Hernández, D., Cardell, E., & Zárate, V. (2005). Antimicrobial activity of lactic acid bacteria isolated from Tenerife cheese: Initial characterization of plantaricin TF711, a bacteriocin-like substance produced by Lactobacillus plantarum TF711. *Journal of Applied Microbiology, 99*(1), 77–84. doi:10.1111/j.1365-2672.2005.02576.x

Holzapfel, W. (1997). Use of starter cultures in fermentation on a household scale. *Food Control, 8*(5), 241–258. doi:10.1016/S0956-7135(97)00017-0

Holzapfel, W. H. (2002). Appropriate starter culture technologies for small-scale fermentation in developing countries. *International Journal of Food Microbiology, 75*(3), 197–212. doi:10.1016/S0168-1605(01)00707-3

Ibrahim, A. (2015). *Effects of exopolysaccharide-producing starter cultures on physicochemical, rheological and sensory properties of fermented camel's milk* (Vol. 27). doi:10.9755/ejfa.v27i4.19911

Ibrahim, A., & Khalifa, S. (2015). *The effects of various stabilizers on physiochemical properties of camel milk yoghurt* (Vol. 11).

Jans, C. (2011). *Biodiversity of lactic acid bacteria in raw camel milk products of East Africa including genomic and functional characterization of predominant lactose-adapted Streptococcus infantarius subsp. Infantarius.* (PhD Thesis No. 19835). ETH Zurich, Zurich, Switzerland.

Jans, C., Follador, R., Hochstrasser, M., Lacroix, C., Meile, L., & Stevens, M. J. A. (2013). Comparative genome analysis of Streptococcus infantarius subsp. InfantariusCJ18, an African fermented camel milk isolate with adaptations to dairy environment. *BMC Genomics, 14*(1), 200. doi:10.1186/1471-2164-14-200

Jans, C., Follador, R., Lacroix, C., Meile, L., & Stevens, M. J. A. (2012). Complete Genome Sequence of the African Dairy Isolate Streptococcus infantarius subsp. Infantarius Strain CJ18. *Journal of Bacteriology, 194*(8), 2105–2106. doi:10.1128/JB.00160-12

Jans, C., Gerber, A., Bugnard, J., Njage, P. M. K., Lacroix, C., & Meile, L. (2012). Novel Streptococcus infantarius subsp. Infantarius variants harboring lactose metabolism genes homologous to Streptococcus thermophilus. *Food Microbiology, 31*(1), 33–42. doi:10.1016/j.fm.2012.02.001

Jans, C., Kaindi, D. W. M., Böck, D., Njage, P. M. K., Kouamé-Sina, S. M., Bonfoh, B., ... Meile, L. (2013). Prevalence and comparison of Streptococcus infantarius subsp. Infantarius and Streptococcus gallolyticus subsp. Macedonicus in raw and fermented dairy products from East and West Africa. *International Journal of Food Microbiology, 167*(2), 186–195. doi:10.1016/j.ijfoodmicro.2013.09.008

Jans, C., Meile, L., Kaindi, D. W. M., Kogi-Makau, W., Lamuka, P., Renault, P., ... Bonfoh, B. (2017). African fermented dairy products – Overview of predominant technologically important microorganisms focusing on African Streptococcus infantarius variants and potential future applications for enhanced food safety and security. *International Journal of Food Microbiology, 250*, 27–36. doi:10.1016/j.ijfoodmicro.2017.03.012

Jans, C., Meile, L., Lacroix, C., & Stevens, M. J. A. (2015). Genomics, evolution, and molecular epidemiology of the Streptococcus bovis/Streptococcus equinus complex (SBSEC). *Infection, Genetics and Evolution, 33*, 419–436. doi:10.1016/j.meegid.2014.09.017

Khatoon, H., & Najam, R. (2017). Bioactive Components in Camel Milk: Their Nutritive Value and Therapeutic Application. In R. R. Watson, R. J. Collier, & V. R. Preedy (Eds.), Nutrients in Dairy and their Implications on Health and Disease (pp. 377–387). Academic Press. doi:10.1016/B978-0-12-809762-5.00029-2

Khedid, K., Faid, M., Mokhtari, A., Soulaymani, A., & Zinedine, A. (2009). Characterization of lactic acid bacteria isolated from the one humped camel milk produced in Morocco. *Microbiological Research*, *164*(1), 81–91. doi:10.1016/j.micres.2006.10.008

Kimaryo, V. M., Massawe, G. A., Olasupo, N. A., & Holzapfel, W. H. (2000). The use of a starter culture in the fermentation of cassava for the production of "kivunde", a traditional Tanzanian food product. *International Journal of Food Microbiology*, *56*(2–3), 179–190. doi:10.1016/S0168-1605(00)00159-8

Leroy, F., & De Vuyst, L. (2004). Lactic acid bacteria as functional starter cultures for the food fermentation industry. *Trends in Food Science & Technology*, *15*(2), 67–78. doi:10.1016/j.tifs.2003.09.004

Lianou, A., Kakouri, A., Pappa, E. C., & Samelis, J. (2017). Growth interactions and antilisterial effects of the bacteriocinogenic Lactococcus lactis subsp. Cremoris M104 and Enterococcus faecium KE82 strains in thermized milk in the presence or absence of a commercial starter culture. *Food Microbiology*, *64*, 145–154. doi:10.1016/j.fm.2016.12.019

Lore, T. A., Mbugua, S. K., & Wangoh, J. (2005). Enumeration and identification of microflora in suusac, a Kenyan traditional fermented camel milk product. *Lebensmittel-Wissenschaft + Technologie*, *38*(2), 125–130. doi:10.1016/j.lwt.2004.05.008

Ludwig, W., Schleifer, K. H., & Whitman, W. B. (2009). Order II. Lactobacillales ord. Nov. In P. De Vos, G. M. Garrity, D. Jones, N. R. Krieg, W. Ludwig, F. A. Rainey, … W. B. Whitman (Eds.), Bergey's manual of systematic bacteriology. The firmicutes (2nd ed.; Vol. 3, pp. 464–735). New York, NY: Springer.

Lynch, M. F., Tauxe, R. V., & Hedberg, C. W. (2009). The growing burden of foodborne outbreaks due to contaminated fresh produce: Risks and opportunities. *Epidemiology and Infection*, *137*(03), 307–315. doi:10.1017/S0950268808001969

Maitha, I. (2019). *Microbial safety of traditional milk products From North Eastern Kenya and functional characterization of selected Lactic Acid Bacteria* (Thesis). University of Nairobi, Nairobi, Kenya.

Maitha, I., Kaindi, D. W. M., Wangoh, J., & Mbugua, S. K. (2019). Microbial Quality and Safety of Traditional Fermented Camel Milk Product Suusac Sampled from Different Regions in North Eastern, Kenya. *Asian Food Science Journal*, *8*(2), 1–9. doi:10.9734/afsj/2019/v8i229986

Marshall, E., & Mejia, D. (2011). *Traditional fermented food and beverage for improved livelihoods*. Rome, Italy: FAO.

Mikesell, M. W. (1955). Notes on the dispersal of the dromedary. *Southwestern Journal of Anthropology*, *11*(3), 231–245. doi:10.1086outjanth.11.3.3629022

Motarjemi, Y., Käferstein, F., Moy, G., & Quevedo, F. (1993). Contaminated weaning food: A major risk factor for diarrhoea and associated malnutrition. *Bulletin of the World Health Organization*, *71*(1), 79–92.

Mwangi, L. W., Matofari, J. W., Muliro, P. S., & Bebe, B. O. (2016). Hygienic assessment of spontaneously fermented raw camel milk (suusa) along the informal value chain in Kenya. *International Journal of Food Contamination*, *3*(1), 18. doi:10.118640550-016-0040-8

Nduko, J. M., Matofari, J. W., Nandi, Z. O., & Sichangi, M. B. (2017). Spontaneously fermented kenyan milk products: A review of the current state and future perspectives. *African Journal of Food Science, 11*(1), 1–11. doi:10.5897/AJFS2016.1516

Njage, P. (2010). *Microbial diversity, safety and role of predominant lactic acid bacteria in raw and spontaneously fermented camel milk from Kenya and Somalia* (PhD Thesis). University of Nairobi, Nairobi, Kenya.

Njage, P. M. K. (2011). *Microbial diversity, safety and role of predominant lactic acid bacteria in raw and spontaneously fermented camel milk in Kenya and Somalia* (PhD Thesis). University of Nairobi, Kenya.

Nyagoya, S. (2016). *Cow Milk Fermentation trials with Streptococcus infantarius subsp. Infantarius and its effect on the growth of selected pathogenic bacteria* (Thesis). University of Nairobi. Retrieved from https://foodtech.uonbi.ac.ke/sites/default/files/cavs/agriculture/foodtech/Final%20dissertation.pdf

Odamaki, T., Xiao, J. Z., Yonezawa, S., Yaeshima, T., & Iwatsuki, K. (2011). Improved viability of bifidobacteria in fermented milk by cocultivation with Lactococcus lactis subspecies lactis. *Journal of Dairy Science, 94*(3), 1112–1121. doi:10.3168/jds.2010-3286

Ogier, J., & Serror, P. (2008). Safety assessment of dairy microorganisms: The Enterococcus genus. *International Journal of Food Microbiology, 126*(3), 291–301. doi:10.1016/j.ijfoodmicro.2007.08.017

Panesar, P. S. (2011). Fermented Dairy Products: Starters Cultures and Potential Nutritional Benefits. *Food and Nutrition Sciences, 02*(01), 47–51. doi:10.4236/fns.2011.21006

Park, Y. (2009). Overview of bioactive components in milk and dairy products. In *Bioactive Components in Milk and Dairy Products* (p. 14). Ames, IA: Wiley-Blackwell Publishers. doi:10.1002/9780813821504.ch1

Pessione, E., & Cirrincione, S. (2016). Bioactive Molecules Released in Food by Lactic Acid Bacteria: Encrypted Peptides and Biogenic Amines. *Frontiers in Microbiology, 7*, 876. doi:10.3389/fmicb.2016.00876

Picot, L., Bordenave, S., Didelot, S., Fruitier-Arnaudin, I., Sannier, F., Thorkelsson, G., ... Piot, J. M. (2006). Antiproliferative activity of fish protein hydrolysates on human breast cancer cell lines. *Process Biochemistry, 41*(5), 1217–1222. doi:10.1016/j.procbio.2005.11.024

Platteeuw, C., van Alen-Boerrigter, I., van Schalkwijk, S., & de Vos, W. M. (1996). Food-grade cloning and expression system for Lactococcus lactis. *Applied and Environmental Microbiology, 62*(3), 1008–1013.

Quigley, L., McCarthy, R., O'Sullivan, O., Beresford, T. P., Fitzgerald, G. F., Ross, R. P., ... Cotter, P. D. (2013). The microbial content of raw and pasteurized cow milk as determined by molecular approaches. *Journal of Dairy Science, 96*(8), 4928–4937. doi:10.3168/jds.2013-6688

Quigley, L., O'Sullivan, O., Beresford, T. P., Ross, R. P., Fitzgerald, G. F., & Cotter, P. D. (2011). Molecular approaches to analysing the microbial composition of raw milk and raw milk cheese. *International Journal of Food Microbiology, 150*(2–3), 81–94. doi:10.1016/j.ijfoodmicro.2011.08.001

Ray, R., & Mishra, S. (2017). Technological Innovations in Processing of Fermented Foods An Overview. In *Fermented Foods, Part II Technological Interventions* (1st ed.; pp. 21–45). Boca Raton, FL: CRC Press.

Rhee, S. J., Lee, J.-E., & Lee, C.-H. (2011). Importance of lactic acid bacteria in Asian fermented foods. *Microbial Cell Factories*, *10*(1Suppl 1), S5. doi:10.1186/1475-2859-10-S1-S5

Rodríguez-Figueroa, J. C., Reyes-Díaz, R., González-Córdova, A. F., Troncoso-Rojas, R., Vargas-Arispuro, I., & Vallejo-Cordoba, B. (2010). Angiotensin-converting enzyme inhibitory activity of milk fermented by wild and industrial Lactococcus lactis strains. *Journal of Dairy Science*, *93*(11), 5032–5038. doi:10.3168/jds.2010-3103

Ross, P. R., Morgan, S., & Hill, C. (2002). Preservation and fermentation: Past, present and future. *International Journal of Food Microbiology*, *79*(1–2), 3–16. doi:10.1016/S0168-1605(02)00174-5

Ross, R., Desmond, C., Fitzgerald, G., & Stanton, C. (2005). Overcoming the technological hurdles in the development of probiotic foods. *Journal of Applied Microbiology*, *98*(6), 1410–1417. doi:10.1111/j.1365-2672.2005.02654.x

Ruas-Madiedo, P., Hugenholtz, J., & Zoon, P. (2002). An overview of the functionality of exopolysaccharides produced by lactic acid bacteria. *NIZO Dairy Conference on Food Microbes 2001*, *12*(2), 163–171. 10.1016/S0958-6946(01)00160-1

Rusniok, C., Couvé, E., Cunha, V. D., Gana, R. E., Zidane, N., Bouchier, C., ... Glaser, P. (2010). Genome Sequence of Streptococcus gallolyticus: Insights into Its Adaptation to the Bovine Rumen and Its Ability To Cause Endocarditis. *Journal of Bacteriology*, *192*(8), 2266–2276. doi:10.1128/JB.01659-09

Saikia, R. (2008). *Microbial Biotechnology*. New India Publishing.

Samet-Bali, O., Bellila, A., Ayadi, M.-A., Marzouk, B., & Attia, H. (2010). A comparison of the physicochemical, microbiological and aromatic composition of Traditional and Industrial Leben in Tunisia. *International Journal of Dairy Technology*, *63*(1), 98–104. doi:10.1111/j.1471-0307.2009.00546.x

Savadogo, A., Ouattara, C. A., Savadogo, P. W., Barro, N., Ouattara, A. S., & Traoré, A. S. (2004). Identification of exopolysaccharides-producing lactic acid bacteria from Burkina Faso fermented milk samples. *African Journal of Biotechnology*, *3*(3), 189–194. doi:10.5897/AJB2004.000-2034

Savadogo, A., Ouattara, A. C., Bassole, H. I., & Traore, S. A. (2006). Bacteriocins and lactic acid bacteria—A minireview. *African Journal of Biotechnology*, *5*(9). Retrieved from https://www.ajol.info/index.php/ajb/article/view/42771

Shori, A. B., & Baba, A. S. (2012). Viability of lactic acid bacteria and sensory evaluation in Cinnamomum verum and Allium sativum-bio-yogurts made from camel and cow milk. *Journal of the Association of Arab Universities for Basic and Applied Sciences*, *11*(1), 50–55. doi:10.1016/j.jaubas.2011.11.001

Siboukeur, A. (2013). Effect of cameline nisin isolated from Lactococcus lactis sub sp. lactis on Staphylococcus aureus sp. *Emirates Journal of Food and Agriculture*, *25*(5), 398–402. doi:10.9755/ejfa.v25i5.15511

Sulzer, G., & Busse, M. (1991). Growth inhibition of Listeria spp. On Camembert cheese by bacteria producing inhibitory substances. *International Journal of Food Microbiology*, *14*(3), 287–296. doi:10.1016/0168-1605(91)90120-E

Tamime, A. Y., & McNulty, D. (1999). Kishk—A dried fermented milk / cereal mixture. 4. Microbiological quality. *Le Lait*, *79*(4), 449–456. doi:10.1051/lait:1999437

Tettelin, H., Masignani, V., Cieslewicz, M. J., Eisen, J. A., Peterson, S., & Wessels, M. R., … Fraser, C. M. (2002). Complete genome sequence and comparative genomic analysis of an emerging human pathogen, serotype V Streptococcus agalactiae. *Proceedings of the National Academy of Sciences of the United States of America*, *99*(19), 12391–12396. 10.1073/pnas.182380799

Teuber, M. (2009). Genus II. Lactococcus. In P. De Vos, G. M. Garrity, D. Jones, N. R. Krieg, W. Ludwig, F. A. Rainey, … W. B. Whitman (Eds.), Bergey's manual of systematic bacteriology. The firmicutes (2nd ed.; Vol. 3, pp. 711–722). New York, NY: Springer.

Vuyst, L. D., & Leroy, F. (2007). Bacteriocins from Lactic Acid Bacteria: Production, Purification, and Food Applications. *Journal of Molecular Microbiology and Biotechnology*, *13*(4), 194–199. doi:10.1159/000104752

Wambui, J. M., Lamuka, P. O., & Njage, P. M. K. (2017). Lactic acid bacteria isolates from fermented camel milk (suusac) are potential protective cultures of raw camel meat. *International Journal of Agriculture and Environmental Research*, *3*, 2960–2975.

Witzler, J. J. P., Pinto, R. A., Font de Valdez, G., de Castro, A. D., & Cavallini, D. C. U. (2017). Development of a potential probiotic lozenge containing Enterococcus faecium CRL 183. *LWT*, *77*, 193–199. doi:10.1016/j.lwt.2016.11.011

Wullschleger, S., Lacroix, C., Bonfoh, B., Sissoko-Thiam, A., Hugenschmidt, S., & Romanens, E. … Meile, L. (2012). Analysis of lactic acid bacteria communities and their seasonal variations in a spontaneously fermented dairy product (Malian fènè) by applying a cultivation/genotype-based binary model. *International Dairy Journal*. doi:10.1016/j.idairyj.2012.08.001

Zibaee, S., Hosseini, S. M. A.-R., Yousefi, M., Taghipour, A., Kiani, M. A., & Noras, M. R. (2015). Nutritional and Therapeutic Characteristics of Camel Milk in Children: A Systematic Review. *Electronic Physician*, *7*(7), 1523–1528. doi:10.19082/1523

Zottola, E. A., Yezzi, T. L., Ajao, D. B., & Roberts, R. F. (1994). Utilization of cheddar cheese containing nisin as an antimicrobial agent in other foods. *International Journal of Food Microbiology*, *24*(1), 227–238. doi:10.1016/0168-1605(94)90121-X

Chapter 5
Manufacture of Dairy and Non-Dairy Camel Milk Products

Nour Amin Elsahoryi
University of Petra, Jordan

Hiba Fathi Al-Sayyed
University of Petra, Jordan

ABSTRACT

Camel milk is popular in the world as it has an excellent nutritive value and many health benefits. There are many dairy and non-dairy products that could be manufactured from camel milk such as milk powder, UHT-milk, yogurt and fermented products, cream, ghee, ice-cream, frozen products, sweets, and candy (such as chocolate bars and cookies). In general, camel milk processing encounters challenges. This chapter is aimed to cover the recent issues of the manufacturing and processing of the most popular above-mentioned camel milk products based on the recent studies and other available commercial resources. Camel milk seems to have many challenges during high temperature treatment as well as creaming to manufacture yogurt and other fermented dairy products, cream, and butter. On the other hand, ice cream and frozen yogurt and chocolate bar manufacturing from camel milk seems to be less challenging. Further research is recommended to solve the faced challenges and to develop different versions of these products such as skim, low fat, low sugar, and flavored products.

INTRODUCTION

Camel milk is popular in the world as it has an excellent nutritive value and many health benefits. Camel milk is known to be richer than bovine milk in vitamin C (Stahl, Sallmann, Duehlmeier, & Wernery, 2006). Dairy products manufactured from camel milk represent a source of energy and nutrients (Brezovecki et al., 2015) and probably replace fruits and vegetables for people who live in the harsh condition of deserts (Sawaya, Khalil, Al-Shalhat, & Al-Mohammad, 1984). It had been recognised that camel milk is only suitable for drinking as fresh or sour milk due to challenges associated with the production. Recently, several dairy and non-dairy camel milk products have been developed and standardized us-

DOI: 10.4018/978-1-7998-1604-1.ch005

ing different preparation or production method (Korlepara, Kalla, Manthani, & Keerthi, 2017). These products are available commercially in India, Mongolia, Kazakhstan, Sudan, and Turkmenistan (Solanki & Hati, 2018) as well as in Saudi Arabia, United Arab Emirates, and United states of America including milk powder, ultrahigh temperature (UHT) treated milk, yogurt and fermented products, cream, butter, ghee, ice-cream, frozen products, sweets and candy (such as chocolate bars and cookies). According to the latest FAO statistics, the demand on camel products has increased due to the increase in the camel population and slaughtering (Galeboe, Seifu, & Sekwati-Monang, 2018). A recent study showed that camel population has grown faster than cattle, sheep, horse, and lama populations but it is similar to buffalo population and lower than that of goat population (Faye& Bonnet, 2012). Moreover, camel dairy plants are developed in many countries market especially in the Horn of Africa and Arabian Peninsula, but the global economy still marginal except for camel meat (Faye, 2016). However, the new products such as cheese, yogurt, or ice cream, has led to significant changes in the added value chains of camel milk (Faye et al., 2014). This chapter is aimed to cover the recent processing methods, and issues of the most popular camel milk products based on the recent studies and other available commercial resources.

BACKGROUND

Camel milk is popular in the world specially in the Middle Eastern, Asian, and African cultures (Zibaee et al., 2015). Camel milk is receiving more recognition as a global product in optimizing human health as drinking milk (Nikkhah, 2011). Many studies indicated that camel milk has benefits and nutritional values and traditionally prescribed as a cure for disease recovery such as kidney, liver, cancer, and children diseases (Zibaee et al., 2015). In the present book, the potential therapeutic and disease prevention properties of camel milk will be discussed in details in Chapter 7 and 8. Yagil (1982) and the Food and Agriculture Organization of the United Nations (FAO, 2008) predicted that dairy products manufactured from camel milk will appear on European supermarket shelves. In addition, the demand on camel milk is increased from Sahara to Mongolia despite the production arrived approximately to 5.4 million tonnes annually, but it is still greatly inadequate. Therefore, many sectors and local investments in the Middle East and the Western world would made effort to meet demands and create gainful markets (Zibaee et al., 2015).

Camel milk composition was discussed in details in Chapter 2 of the present book. Only few physiochemical properties of camel milk compared with cow and buffalo milk is given here (table 1). The chemical composition of camel milk gives the milk and milk products higher nutritional values but, on the other hand, dairy products manufacturing from camel milk do not proceed as other milk types such as cow and goat milk. Camel milk dairy products production is challenging and encounters number of obstacles.

The popular consumption of camel milk occurs as fresh or fermented form, but there are many dairy products could be manufactured. Moreover, these products constitute a major part of the diet of the population in rural areas such as Africa and Asia, by virtue of the geographical nature of living, because they consider these products source of main nutrients and energy too (Brezovečki, Cagalj, Dermit, Mikulec, Ljoljić, & Antunac, 2015). Therefore, it is valuable to focus nutritionally and practically (manufacturing method) on the major products of camel milk.

Table 1. Some physiochemical properties of camel milk compared with cow and buffalo milk

Physiochemical property	Camel	Cow	Buffalo	Standard error of mean	Critical difference (0.05 significant level)	Coefficient of variance %
Acidity (% Lactic acid)	0.14±0.003	0.14±0.003	0.13±0.003	0.0030	0.0089	6.2841
Specific gravity	1.03±0.000	1.03±0.000	1.03±0.000	0.0003	0.0008	0.0785
Viscosity (cp)	1.77±0.016	1.54±0.021	1.79±0.023	0.0219	0.0640	3.6400
Surface tension (dyne/ cm)	58.39±0.421	51.77±0.184	50.78±0.259	0.3257	0.9579	1.7200
Refractive index	1.34±0.001	1.35±0.000	1.35±0.000	0.0056	0.0017	0.1195
Freezing point (°C)	-0.52±0.001	-0.53±0.003	-0.54±0.006	0.0044	0.0130	2.3900
Electrical conductivity (millimohs)	6.08±0.057	4.60±0.072	4.65±0.031	0.0596	0.1753	3.3000

Table was adapted with permission from Yoganandi, Mehta, Wadhwani, Darji, & Aparnathi (2014).

In general, camel milk processing has many challenges including incompatibility with the Ultra High Temperature (Nikkhah, 2011), poor firmness and consistency of camel milk yogurt and higher melting point which make the butter churning difficult (Berhe et al., 2017).

PRODUCTS OF CAMEL MILK

Ultra-High Temperature Heat-Treated Milk (UHT Milk)

Heat treatment of camel milk improves the microbial quality (Shewangizaw, 2016) and extends milk shelf life (Omar, Harbourne, & Oruna-Concha, 2018). One of the commonly used heat treatments for camel milk is ultrahigh temperature (UHT) treatment (Benabdelkamel et al., 2017). In the present book, the preservation strategies and technologies for camel milk was discussed in Chapter 3.

UHT milk is a pasteurized packaged milk that can stay on shelf without refrigeration up to 9 months. During UHT pasteurization treatment of camel milk, raw milk heated quickly to 135°C for a relatively short time (2-8 seconds). Then, milk cooled down to room temperature (Tay & Chua, 2015).

The most important concern of UHT camel milk is the heat stability. Heat stability is defined as the ability of milk to stay stable at high temperature treatment without gelatin, thickening, or coagulation (Augustin, 2000). In 2004, Farah et al., showed that UHT camel milk failed to attain physical stability without additive.

In terms of coagulation, UHT treatment denatures rennet and coagulation fails accordingly (Ham et al., 2008; Omar,et al. 2018). This is probably due to the association between casein and denatured whey protein micelles and the reduction in ionic Ca concentration (Vasbinder, Rollema, & Kruif, 2003). In terms of color, skimmed UHT milk was found (Omar et al. 2018) to have lower lightness compared with raw camel and bovine milk. The authors attributed this reduction to the disintegration of casein protein particles. In terms of flavor, UHT treatment known to develop off flavors of milk such as sulfur compounds (for example: methyl ketones and aldehydes). These compounds known to reduce milk acceptability and affect sensory properties (Contarini, Povolo, Leardi, & Toppino, 1997). In addition, upon UHT treatment, aldehyde (such as (E)-2- nonenal, nonanal, octanal, heptanal, and hexanal) concentration increases compared to raw camel milk and pasteurized camel milk (Vazquez-Landaverde, Velazquez, Torres, and Qian, 2005). Other aldehydes such as [E, E]-2, 4-nonadienal, (E, E)-2, 6-nonadienal, heptanal, and (E)-2- hexenal were detected in UHT camel milk. The formation of aldehydes can be induced by amino acid degradation during Maillard reaction as well as heat-induced breakdown of hydroperoxides. Aldehyde formation is responsible for the developed off-flavors (Vazquez-Landaverde, Torres, & Qian, 2006) and stale flavor (Perkins, D'Arcy, Lisle, & Deeth, 2005) of UHT camel milk.

Camel milk contains casein and whey protein. The casein fraction of camel milk contains Beta casein (β-CN) predominantly, Alpha casein (α-CN) and a small fraction of Kappa casein (κ-CN) (Omar, et al. 2018). The whey protein fractions of camel milk consist in Alpha lactalbumin (α-La), Beta lactoglobulin (β-Lg), serum albumin (SA), and lactoferrin (LF). Among different milk types including raw bovine, raw camel milk, high temperature short time (HTST) treated camel milk and bovine milk, UHT camel milk was shown to contain the lowest ($P<0.05$) amounts of these proteins. Within the same context, camel milk casein micelle size decreased by 19.55% upon UHT treatment due to the dissociation of ƙ-CN and/or calcium phosphates out of the casein micelles (Anema & Li, 2003).

UHT skimmed camel milk contains the same amino acid concentrations of raw camel milk except for glutamic acid (Newton, Fairbanks, Golding, Andrewes, & Gerrard, 2012), alanine, glycine, serine, and aspartic acid. Upon UHT treatment, the concentration of these amino acids increases. Glutamic acid and aspartic acid are responsible for the umami and sour taste of the UHT milk while serine is responsible for the sweet taste of milk. Other amino acids such as lysine, leucine, and phenylalanine are reduced upon UHT treatment (Omar et al. 2018).

On the other hand, lactose content in camel milk is 3.02 g/100 mL. This content was found to remain unchanged using UHT treatment. While, lactose content was found to have some losses after UHT treatment (Omar et al. 2018).

Milk Powder (MP)

Milk drying techniques have developed several centuries ago. In 1810, Nicholas Appert was the first scientist who dried milk to 1/3 of its initial volume in an opened vessel- by evaporation. In 1859, commercial dry milk production has started after a British patent granted to Grimwade (Hal & Hedrick, 1975). In 1872, spray drying has been developed while the first drum dryer was developed in 1902 (Anonymous, 1986). Milk powder (MP) industry become nowadays an integral part of dairy industry (Kalyankar et al., 2016).

MP is defined as a product which can be obtained by partial removal of water from milk in which the composition of fat and/or protein content(s) can be manipulated to comply with the Codex definition(s) without altering whey protein/casein ratio. MP has many advantages over fresh milk in terms of size and volume, cost, supply upon demand, and stability (Kalyankar et al., 2016).

Upon milking, camel milk faces microbial contamination necessitating heat treatment before manufacturing (Odongo, Lamuka, Matofari, & Abong, 2016). For instance, Hussen, Selamawit, Ashenafi, Fikre & Ashenafi (2016) detected *Salmonella*, *Staphylococcus aureus*, and *Escherichia coli* in Northeast Ethiopia fresh camel milk samples. Heat treatment of camel milk reduces microbial contamination and increases the shelf life (Shori & Baha, 2014; Zubeir, 2015). Heat treatment of camel milk, therefore, will improve the microbial quality upon manufacturing products from camel milk (Shewangizaw, 2016).

Differences between camel milk compositions and other mammalian milks (Chapter 2) obligate following different manufacturing process for camel milk production (Food and Agricultural Organization (FAO), 1982). For instance, heat treatment during manufacturing affects some physiochemical properties of camel milk. Generally, camel milk has longer shelf life than cow milk (Hassan, El Zubeir, & Babiker, 2006). Pasteurized camel milk has been found to stand at 4°C for 10 days (Wernery, 2008).

Conventional drying of milk affects milk proteins negatively (Desrosier, 2008). Camel milk proteins such as whey are stable at up to 150°C compared to bovine milk due to the absence or deficiency of β-lactoglobulin and κ-casein (Al-Saleh, 1996; Farah & Atkins, 1992). Similarly, sterilization at 135°C for 2-5 seconds denatures camel milk whey protein despite the fact that this denaturation is less occurring in cow milk. Camel milk whey proteins are therefore more heat stable at 80°C and 90°C than those of cow milk by about 2 folds (Farah, 1993; Shewangizaw, 2016). For instance, Wernery (2007) found that heat treatment at 72°C for 5 minutes revealed no denaturation of milk proteins. Moreover, the antimicrobial proteins of camel milk completely lose their functionality upon heat treatment at 100°C for 30 minutes (see Chapter 10). Nonetheless, camel milk lysozymes, lactoferrin, and immunoglobulins are more heat stable than those of cow milk (El-Agamy, 2000). On the other hand, heat stability of camel milk ingredients especially the functional ones represent a great challenge in camel MP manufacturing. For instance, vitamin C content of camel milk has been reduced by about 6-8% upon treatment at 72°C for 5 minutes (Wernery, 2007).

Taking into consideration the functional properties of camel milk, it has been thought that this milk will be probably the super food in the future (Desrosier, 2008); this opens many opportunities to keep camel milk for longer time probably by manufacturing MP.

Methods of Manufacturing Camel MP

Generally, there are four methods used for milk drying as follow: drum roll drying, spray drying, foam mat drying, and freeze-drying (Kalyankar et al., 2016). Currently, camel MP is being manufactured either by spray drying or freeze-drying only (AbdAlmageed, 2005; Zouari et al., 2018). This is due to the sensitivity of camel milk proteins to heat treatment which lead to the risk of whey protein denaturation. Accordingly, drying of camel milk by this method needs to be optimized in terms of temperature, pressure, and milk flow rate (Habtegebriel, Edwardb, Wawire, Silaa, & Seifu, 2018). Nowadays, camel MP has been manufactured by spray drying at the experimental level.

Recently, Zouari et al., (2018) showed that camel milk was not affected significantly (P>0.05) using spray-drying at the laboratory scale, moreover, neither the water activity nor the glass transition temperature (T_g). Fortunately, the treatment increased significantly the bulk density and without leading to whey protein denaturation. On the other hand, spray-drying increased the free fat eventually increase the risk of rancidity in whole MP. No data was shown regarding the crystallization of the final product. Similarly, Ho, Chan, Yago, & Shravya (2019) found that upon controlled storage at 37°C over 18 weeks and at low relative humidity (RH) (<32% RH), spray-dried camel milk crystals exhibited almost the same true density, morphology and colour (L* (lightness), a* (redness to greenness), and whiteness). On the other hand, the reduction in moisture content and water activity (a_w) caused glass transition of lactose crystals. With time, b* (yellowness to blueness) colour values associated with non-enzymatic browning and fat oxidation into volatile compounds increased steadily while crystal solubility declined. Moreover, the secondary protein structures tend to unfold from α-helices to β-sheets.

Moreover, AbdAlmageed (2005) showed that spray-dried camel MP showed acceptable chemical (in terms of moisture, fat, protein, and ash contents), physicochemical (in terms of total solids, lactose content, pH, titrable acidity, specific gravity, and boiling point), and sensible characteristics compared to cow and goat MP. Nonetheless, chemical, physical, and sensible properties of the final product need to be studied more extensively (AbdAlmageed, 2005; Zouari et al., 2018).

The quality of spray-dried camel milk greatly depends on the raw milk composition as well as the drying conditions (Habtegebriel et al., 2018). For example, fat globules of whole camel milk are exposed to the milk surface, hence influence the moisture passage between milk particles as a result increase the final product particle size (Birchal, Passos, Wildhagen, & Mujumdar, 2005). Furthermore, total solid content was shown to affect cyclon recovery and outlet temperature (Habtegebriel et al., 2018). Moreover, the physico-chemical properties of spray-dried camel milk greatly depends on the operating parameters such as drying flow rate by affecting the solubility of milk proteins (Habtegebriel et al., 2018).

Spray-dried MP is very sensitive to the storage conditions due to the presence of amorphous lactose particles leading to changes in milk properties including stickiness, caking, degradation, and non-enzymatic browning (Fitzpatrick et al., 2007; Jouppila & Roos, 1994). In the presence of very low concentrations of moisture, lactose can adsorb water leading to stickiness of the final product and bridge with other particles causing caking (Yazdanpanah & Langrish, 2011). Probably, this problem would be more obvious in cow milk than in camel milk because camel milk could contain less amount of lactose than cow milk at least in Middle-East (3.3 vs. 4.8-4.9 g/100g) (Al haj & Al Kanhal, 2010; Rafiq et al., 2016). Nonetheless, lactose crystallization can be prevented by simultaneous drying and crystallization (Nijdam, Ibach, & Kind, 2008; Saito, 1985; Yazdanpanah & Langrish, 2011). Additionally, Hynd (1980) suggested the presence of whey crystals within the MP manufactured by spray drying.

Freeze-dried camel milk product is now available at the industrial level (CamilkDairy®, 2019). Freeze-drying is a cold-process in which water is removed from a solution via sublimation process (Fonseca, Passot, Cunin, & Marin, 2004). Initially, the water is frozen slowly. Then, ice crystals are evaporated under vacuum leaving the final product dry without defrosting (Sulieman, Elamin, Elkhalifa, & Laleye, 2018). Freeze-drying is usually used for heat sensitive foods in which the final product keeps the high-quality chemical and nutritional sensitive properties of the initial product with a moisture content down to 2% (Ibrahim & Khalifa, 2015). Freeze-drying method of milk produces lighter final product than other dehydration methods beside no refrigeration is needed (Ibrahim & Khalifa, 2015). Hence, this process is a suitable method for camel milk drying to keep the functional properties of camel milk. Nonetheless, the effect of this process on the functional properties of camel milk is not documented yet (Ibrahim & Khalifa, 2015).

Ibrahim & Khalifa (2015) studied the effect of freeze-drying process on the nutritive value and reconstitution properties of whole and skimmed camel milk. Freezing was performed at -45°C, initial drying was performed at 30°C, using 0.10 mbar pressure for 48 h and secondary drying at 5°C for 3 h at the same pressure. As a result of freeze-drying, moisture content was reduced, while total protein, casein, whey protein, lactose, and ash were concentrated ($P<0.05$) as shown by Kumar & Mishra (2004). Moreover, upon reconstitution, the energy value of freeze-dried milk was similar to that of fresh camel milk (Ibrahim & Khalifa, 2015). In another study, freeze-dried camel milk yielded the same concentrations of trace minerals except for Ca, K, and Zn. The concentrations of these three minerals were significantly ($P<0.05$) higher than those of the original milk due to the concentration caused by evaporation. On the other hand, the process reduced vitamin C content of camel milk significantly (P<0.05) and tended to reduce the concentrations of the vitamins A, D, and E. This study confirmed the possibility of producing lyophilized camel MP. What is noteworthy to mention here is that these analyses were performed without any pre-heat treatment for the fresh milk and with the camel udder washing to improve the microbial quality.

Concluding, that freeze drying of camel milk might provide an excellent opportunity for keeping physicochemical as well as functional characteristics compared with cow milk with keeping in mind that camel milk should be kept under vacuum packaging (Sulieman et al., 2018). The preservation strategies of freeze drying and spry drying methods for camel milk were discussed in Chapter 3.

To date, foam-mat drying (mechanical-drying foam) and fluidized-bed drying technique have not been used in camel MP. Mechanical-drying foam is a method in which the raw material is converted into a stable foam initially (Mounir, 2017), then dried (Desrosier, 2008). This method of drying has the advantages of using lower temperature (50-80°C) for drying since foaming allows more water evaporation, lower cost, and most importantly, keeping of the physical and chemical properties, and easiness of application (Jagtiani, Chan, & Sakai, 1998). While, Fluidized-bed drying method use lower heat than drum drying and spray drying methods. Aforementioned drying methods seems to suit camel milk proteins which is resistant to heat temperature of up to 90°C. Back to mechanical-drying foam method, which used foaming agents such as proteins including egg albumin, whey protein, and casein; with their hydrocolloidal properties. These can stabilize foams even at low concentrations; perform well at different pH range even at the presence of foam inhibitors such as fat, alcohol, or flavouring substances (Zayas, 1997). On the other hand, whey protein isolate was shown to have an excellent foaming agent due to the absence of lysozyme, which reduces the electrostatic interactions, and the absence of β-lactoglobulin (Abirached et al., 2012). Fortunately, camel milk whey proteins is absent in β-lactoglobulin providing an opportunity for successful foaming when dried using this method. Thus, extensive research in this area is required to know the feasibility of drying camel milk by this technique.

Commercially Available Camel MP Products

Nowadays, camel MP manufactured commercially by the following companies:

1. Emirates industry for camel milk & products factory of BurDubai: where camel MP manufacturing started since 2006. This factory produces camel MP under the brand name of Camelicious®. Interestingly, this factory manufactures camel MP for infants aged 1-3 years with the claim of (growing up formula). The camel farms are located in the UAE also (AliBaba, 2019).
2. Camilk® Dairy: manufactures freeze-dried milk in Australia with the claim of the same health and nutritional benefits of fresh and dried camel MP. The camel farms are located in Australia (CamilkDairy®, 2019).
3. Aadvik®: the first camel MP manufacturer in India with the claim that camel MP is beneficial in lactose intolerance, gut healing, body and brain development, controlling blood sugar level, and in boosting immunity. Additionally, camel MP is claimed to have the same nutritional value of fresh camel milk (Aadvik®, 2019).
4. Desert farms® company of California: where the camel farms are located in many parts of the USA. The manufactured camel MP is claimed to be non-homogenized non-pasteurized to keep the natural colour, flavour, and consistency of milk (Deserfarms®, 2019).

5. Al-Ain Camilait® Company: the plant is located in Al-Ain city of UAE. The camel MP is manufactured by freeze-drying method with the claims to be beneficial for diabetic and autistic patients (Camelait®, 2019) based on the claim that camel milk is a natural pharmacy that protects human body from several ailments.
6. Camel milk South Africa ® Company: the plant as well as the farms are located in South Africa. Camel MP is manufactured and sold with the disclaimer that despite the scientifically cited health benefits of camel milk, South Africa camel milk® doesn't claim that camel milk heals or will help the health in any way (Camel milk South Africa®, 2019).

Yogurt and Fermented Dairy Products

Milk and milk products are the most valuable foods in terms of nutritive and biological quality, which represent the biggest share among the agricultural industrial sector (Temerbayeva et al., 2018a). Yogurt is the most popular sour milk produced by bacterial fermentation of milk. Yogurt is consumed within healthy meals worldwide due to its high digestibility and bioavailability of nutrients (Temerbayeva et al., 2018b). It can be made from cow, goat, mare and camel milk but the last two are less often used in manufacturing (Akanova et al., 2017). Numerous studies showed the positive association between milk yogurt consumption and many health benefits such as improving the lactose and gastrointestinal disorders such as inflammatory bowel disease and irritable bowel disease, and helping in immune function and weight control (Ahmed et al., 2014).

The nutritional value of yogurt could be determined by three main aspects; 1/ consequence of lactic acid production, which is important for lactose-intolerant people, by limiting the formation of organic acids, hydrogen, methane, and carbon dioxide in the human gut. 2/ calcium, phosphorus and potassium levels which are higher in yogurt than milk as a result of non-fat solid adjustment (Corrieu & Béal, 2016). 3/ folic acid content which present in higher amount in yogurt compared to milk (Corrieu & Béal, 2016). The higher the level of some elements in yogurt compared to milk could refer to the change of the casein micelles and their destabilization which lead to increase the acidity electrostatic and the casein–casein attractions increase due to enhanced hydrophobic interactions (Aswal et al., 2012; Corrieu & Béal, 2016). For example; during acidification, the net negative charge on casein micelles decreases, leading to reduce the electrostatic repulsion between charged groups and the size of the casein micelles which remains unchanged as the small amount of colloidal calcium phosphate is solubilized at pH > 6.0 (Corrieu & Béal, 2016).

Classification

Yogurt could be classified in to many type depending on milk source, fat content, texture, flavor, and storage temperature (Corrieu & Béal, 2016). The common milk types used in yogurt manufacturing include cow, sheep, and goat. Yogurt could contain free fat or low or full-fat milk. Furthermore, yogurt could be classified according to its texture (firm, stirred, concentrated, drinking, frozen and powder) or/and flavour (plain, sweetened and flavoured). On the other hand, yogurt could be stored on chilled temperature of 4 °C, dehydrated (Ambient) or frozen at -20 °C (Corrieu & Béal, 2016).

Traditional Yogurt Processing

The traditional method for manufacturing yogurt back to thousands of years (see Chapter 3). Briefly, milk is standardized, pasteurized, homogenized at 55-65 °C for 15- 20 s, then incubated at 43- 45°C, with yogurt starter culture. After these main steps, milk is either produced as set-yogurt or stirred yogurt (Weerathilake, Rasika, Ruwanmali, & Munasinghe, 2014). The fermentation process is the cornerstone step in the fermented dairy products production. In yogurt manufacturing, milk is subjected to fermentation using a mixture of bacterial cultures: *Lactobacillus bulgaricus* and *Streptococcus thermophilus.* They are the main (starter) cultures in yogurt that are responsible for the fermentation process with the lactose (milk sugar) to obtain lactic acid, which generates the texture and flavor of yogurt (Afolabi *et al*, 2013). The fermentation of lactose also produces the flavor compounds as a main characteristic of yogurt. If the lactic acid increase, the pH decreases and causes milk clotting, or form a soft gel that also affects yogurt characteristics (Gorelik et al., 2017; Temerbayeva et al., 2018b). However, the main ingredient in yogurt is milk but another ingredient could be added such as other bacterial cultures including *Lactobacillus acidophilus, Lactobacillus subsp. casei,* and *Bifido*-bacteria as probiotic cultures to improve lactose digestion, gastrointestinal function, and stimulate the immune system (Gorelik et al., 2017; Temerbayeva et al., 2018b). More details related to yogurt manufacturing was mentioned recently by Corrieu and Béal (Corrieu & Béal, 2016).

Processing Challenges of Camel Milk Yogurt

Recently, yogurt from camel milk has been developed and became one of the main products in Middle East and Africa. The composition of camel milk differ from other mammalian milks (see Chapter 2) including cows, sheep and goats (Galeboe et al., 2018). This is due to intrinsic factors, camel milk behaves differently from the bovine milk during the lactic fermentation process (Hassan, Zubei, & Babiker, 2007). The challenges associated with production of yogurt from camel milk include presence of small casein fragments at the surface, fragile and heterogeneous and consists of dispersed flakes are produced result unsuccessful coagulation curd (Berhe et al., 2017; Hassan et al., 2007). Some researchers referred this behavior to the presence of antibacterial factors in camel milk because the starter culture showed a longer lag phase and an earlier decline phase resulting in a fragile coagulum (Attia & Dhouib, 2001). These antibacterial factors are available in camel milk and not similar to cow and buffalo milks curd (Berhe et al., 2017; Hassan et al., 2007).

Moreover, the antibacterial properties effect on fermentation process reduce the acidification rate (most important parameter to assess yogurt appearance) compared to bovine milk (Berhe et al., 2017). This level of acidity effect the texture of yogurt, lower acidity lead to a very weak texture while the consistency is very thin (Berhe et al., 2017). This property affects mouth feel and the overall consumer acceptability (Berhe et al., 2017). In addition, the total solid content and fat content play a vital role in the final product texture and consequently consumer acceptability. This factor related to other factors such as seasonal variation, fermentation process and additive types as well as concentrations. For example, the texture of camel milk products varies depending on season; in summer the content of fat is lower while water content is higher (Galeboe et al., 2018).

Structure-forming agents such as pectin, starch, and alginate usually added to improve the consistency and texture of camel yogurt. Likewise, stabilizers such as carrageenan, starch and gelatin could be added to improve the body and texture by increasing firmness, preventing separation of the whey, and help keeping the fruit uniformly mixed in yogurt (Al-Zoreky & Al-Otaibi, 2015; Galeboe et al., 2018; Hashim et al., 2009; Ibrahem & El Zubeir, 2016; Ibrahim & Khalifa, 2015). Flavoured yogurt is another product derived from the original yogurt by adding different types of flavour and sweeteners such as fruits to provide more variety to the consumer (Corrieu & Béal, 2016).

Overall, the challenges in camel milk yogurt manufacturing could be referred as the unique structural and functional properties of the camel milk compositions (see Chapter 7 and 8), which make fermented camel product manufacturing different from bovine milk. Hence, the common and traditional method used to produce yogurt from bovine milk sources are not suitable for camel yogurt production.

Opportunities of Camel Milk Yogurt Production

There have been several attempts to produce yogurt from camel milk (Al-Zoreky & Al-Otaibi, 2015; Galeboe et al., 2018; Hashim et al., 2009; Ibrahem & El Zubeir, 2016; Ibrahim & Khalifa, 2015; Mohsin et al. 2019; Mudgil et al. 2018). Most of these trials have reported improvement in yogurt characteristics at laboratory scale but no industrial scale were established due to challenges in camel milk composition (see Chapter 2). Coagulum of camel milk yogurt is different from other mammalian milk. Whereas, yogurt from camel milk exhibits longer coagulation time compared with sheep milk and the properties of casein particles are different. While, coagulum of camel milk have larger casein micelles than bovine milk coagulum (Ibrahem & El Zubeir, 2016).

Most trails focused to improve yogurt's texture, consistency and overall quality. These includes using stabilizers such as gelatin or alginate and calcium together to yield acceptable sensory quality (Hashim et al., 2009; Mohsin et al. 2019; Mudgil et al. 2018).

Stabilizers were one of the choices to improve yogurt characteristics. To date, three studies used different types and concentrations of stabilizers but their trials yielded contradictory results (Al-Zoreky & Al-Otaibi, 2015; Hashim et al., 2009; Ibrahim & Khalifa, 2015).

Ibrahim and Khalifa (2015) reported using three different combination and ratios of stabilizers to produce yogurt from fresh camel milk. The combinations were A (gelatin E441, mono & diglyceride of fatty acids E471), B (guar gum E412, sodium carboxymethyl cellulose E466 and mono & diglyceride of fatty acids E471) and C (modified starch E1422, mono, and diglyceride of fatty acids E471). The results showed significant increase in yogurt acidity with all stabilizers combinations compared to the control sample. This could be due to the acidity of added stabilizers and continued fermentation by lactic acid bacteria (Ibrahim & Khalifa, 2015). Moreover, stabilizers added to camel milk to produce yogurt samples have increased the total solids, protein and fat contents compared to control yogurt. While, water holding capacity was significantly higher in yogurt from camel milk than fresh control samples due to the action stabilizers. The combinations of stabilizers have improved the texture by reducing water flow in the matrix space and increasing hydration behaviour leading to significant differences in viscosity depending on type and concentrations of stabilizers. For example, the highest viscosity in yogurt manufactured from camel milk was observed using gelatin E441, mono & diglyceride of fatty acids E471; in return exhibited greater effect on flavour of the final product. On the other hand, stabilizers combinations have significantly decreased syneresis. While viscosity, water holding capacity and sensory acceptability were increased ($p \leq 0.05$) in the final product (Ibrahim & Khalifa, 2015). Furthermore, the addition of all stabilizer types have a positive effect on the rate of acidity, moisture content and total solids. Similarly, the use of stabilizers improved the distribution of protein and casein network, which increased smoothness and decreased porosity in yogurt. While no significant differences were reported between different concentration of added stabilizers (Al-Zoreky & Al-Otaibi, 2015; Hashim et al., 2009; Ibrahim & Khalifa, 2015). The type and amount of stabilizers were found to enhance water holding capacity and susceptibility to syneresis of yogurt produced from camel milk. Concluding that the higher the concentration of stabilizers result in lower serum separation. The best results in this study were upon using stabilizers A, B and C compared to control sample. In particular, combination A (gelatin E441, mono & diglycerids of fatty acids E471) at a level of up to 1.5% was superior than other combinations in terms of improving texture without affecting the overall acceptability of the final product (Ibrahim & Khalifa, 2015). Overall, the study concluded that adding stabilizers to camel milk for yogurt production have a significant effect on taste, odour, consistency and overall acceptability (Ibrahim & Khalifa, 2015).

In another study, Hashim and researchers used 12 different treatments of stabilizers with camel milk at different levels including gelatin, alginate, and calcium (Hashim et al., 2009). The results showed that one of the formulas contains 0.75% sodium alginate + 0.075% calcium chloride has improved the texture of yogurt and provided similar sensory attributes and acceptability as cow milk. The researchers also reported the possibility of using this formula along with cherry, strawberry, peach + apricot + mandarin, and date paste + date syrup to produce flavoured yogurt (Hashim et al., 2009). In another study adding different types of stabilizers (CMC, pectin, gum acacia, or alginate) to camel milk did not improve consistency and angulation properties of camel milk yogurt (Al-Zoreky & Al-Otaibi, 2015).

Another approach was reported of mixing camel milk and other milk livestock species such as sheep, goat and bovine milk (Ibrahem & El Zubeir, 2016). Mixing camel milk and sheep milk exhibited 40–60% improvement in composition, nutrition value and acceptability, and offered better quality than making yogurt from camel milk alone (Ibrahem & El Zubeir, 2016). Likewise, mixing cow sheep and goat milk with camel milk yogurt was found to be an excellent choice to produce yogurt because due to their high total solid and physical characteristics (Park et al., 2007).

This approach was found to improve the weak texture of yogurt manufactured from camel milk. Mixing camel milk with other milk types might improve the weak texture and thin consistency of camel milk yogurt through replacing the lack of β-LG and k-CN in camel milk, as well as improving the high whey protein to casein ratio (Shamsia, 2009). Similarly, mixing camel milk with 5% bovine skim milk powder and adding 1.2% gelatin and 1.5 ml/L of calcium chloride before pasteurization along with flavour (strawberry syrup) yielded acceptable consistency yogurt (Galeboe et al., 2018). In another study, researchers compared the rheological, micro-structural and sensorial properties of camel milk yogurt influenced by addition of gelatin and bovine milk (Mudgil et al., 2018). In this study, gelatin was added to camel milk at different levels (0, 0.5%, 0.75%, 1.0% and 1.25%), while the bovine milk used as a control. The results indicated that high levels of gelatin improved the texture and appearance of yogurt from camel milk compared with low levels (0.75–1.0%), on the other hand, high levels of gelatin affected the taste and flavor of yogurt and resulted more rigid and solid consistency (Mudgil et al., 2018). Recently, (Mohsin et al. (2019) used xanthan from orange waste to improve the quality of camel milk date yogurt. The researchers added Biosynthesized xanthan at different levels (0.255, 0.505 and 0.75%), along with 1%gelatin as control. The addition of biosynthesized xanthan has adversely affected most quality parameters in yogurt such as rheology, viscosity, texture, syneresis and sensory parameters. Among all levels, 0.75% xanthan exhibited the best results (Mohsin et al., 2019).

In another approach, yogurt was manufactured from camel milk using either YC-X11 Thermophilic yogurt culture or CH-1 Thermophilic yogurt culture following the traditional method, however, the consistency of yogurt was fluidic and could be consumed as drinking yogurt (Ibrahem & El Zubeir, 2016).

In another study, Ibrahim & Khalifa (2015) added all aforementioned stabilizers to fresh camel milk and homogenised at 400 Kpa, then heated at 90°C for 10 min, finally cooled to 42°C and inoculated with 2% freeze-dried ABY-1 culture and Nu-TRISH yogurt cultures containing *Streptococcus thermophilus, Lactobacillus delbrueckii subsp. bulgaricus, L. acidophilus LA-5 and Bifidobacterium.* These samples incubated at 42 °C until a pH reach to 4.5– 4.6 and finally stored at 5± 2°C for 21 days. Hashim et al. (2009) added stabilizers to the fresh camel milk and heated without homogenization in a water bath at 85°C for 30 min, then cooled to 42°C, finally inoculated with commercial yogurt culture at 43°C for 4 h, and stored at 4°C. Concluding that all studies in the literature used similar procedures and approaches to produce yogurt from camel milk with minor differences by either adding stabilizers or mixing camel milk with other milk types; these trails reported improvement in overall characteristics of camel yogurt.

TRADITIONALLY FERMENTED CAMEL DAIRY PRODUCTS

Labneh

Labneh is the Middle Eastern name of the concentrated yogurt. It is the same of strained yogurt of Greece and Europe (Desouky, Shalaby, & Soryal, 2013) which can be manufactured by removing a part of yogurt whey to reach total solids of 23-25% of which 8-11% is fat (Konuspayeva, Faye, Loiseau, & Levieux, 2007). To date, the only attempt for manufacturing Labneh from camel milk processed by Desouky et al., (2013). These researchers used three different heating temperatures for milk at 63, 85, and 95°C for 30 minutes. The fermentation of yogurt performed using *Streptococcus thermophilus* and *Lactobacillus delbrueckii* ssp. *bulgaricus*.

The total solids especially protein content of Labneh increased significantly ($P<0.05$) throughout heat treatment at 85°C and 95°C. This treatment found to be crucial in Labneh production in terms of improving viscosity and fermentation (decrease in lactose content). Meanwhile, syneresis was found to decrease due to fermentation and increase with heat treatment. Furthermore, casein was shown (under electron microscopic examination) to form strong particle-particle chains rather than particle fusion. Best physicochemical, sensory and texture results of Labneh found to be at thermal treatment of 90°C for 30 minutes.

Kefir

Kefir is a drinkable foamy whitish (Hertzler & Clancy, 2017; Mistry, 2004; Yuksekdag, Beyatli, & Aslim, 2004) fermented milk product which contains 1.2% ethanol and 1% lactic acid (Nuñez, 2016). This product is traditionally consumed in Iran (Saljooghi, Mansouri-Najand, Ebrahimnejad, Doostan, & Askari, 2017), Turkey (Altay, Karbancıoglu-Güler, Daskaya-Dikmen, & Heperkan, 2013) and by Caucasian mountain residents (Irigoyen, Arana, Castiella, Torre, & Ibànez, 2005). The traditional Caucasian Kefir is prepared by subjecting milk to fermentation with Kefir grains. These grains have irregular shape, gelatinous 1-6 mm diameter and contains a mixed culture of lactic acid bacteria (*Lactobacilli, Lactococci, Leuconostocs*), acetic acid bacteria, lactose-fermenting yeast (*Kluyveromyces lactis*, *Kluyveromyces marxianus*, *Torula kefir*), and non-lactose fermenting yeast (*Kluyveromyces lactis*, *Kluyveromyces marxianus*, *Torula kefir*) as reported by Guzel-Seydim, Kök-Tas, & Greene, (2010); Irigoyen et al., (2005); Angulo, Lopez, & Lema, (1993). These grains also contain casein and polysaccharides (Irigoyen et al.,

2005; Toba, Arihara, & Adachi, 1987). The milk used for the manufacturing of Kefir could be whole or skim milk, or subjected to pasteurization, or unpasteurized, (Altay et al., 2013). After fermentation, Kefir contain a mixture of compounds including lactic acid, acetaldehyde, acetoin, carbon dioxide, ethanol, and diacetyle (Guzel-Seydim, Seydim, Grenee, & Bodine, 2000), vitamins K, B_1 and B_{12}, and folic acid, calcium, amino acids (Otles & Cadingi, 2003).

At the experimental scale, Kefir was prepared by heating camel milk at 95°C for15 minutes, then starter culture added at a level of 0.5g/100 ml. Thereafter, cooled down to the inoculation temperature of 45°C and incubated for 5 hours to reach the desirable acidity of 11g per Litre, later further cooled to 43°C for 12-18 hours to obtain the proper taste development (Saljooghi et al., 2017).

In 2015, Kavas studied the possibility of manufacturing grain-fermented Kefir from glucose-enriched fresh camel milk and compared the results with that from cow's milk. The enrichment of camel milk with 1% glucose and the use of 10% Kefir grains have significantly improved many physiochemical characteristics of Kefir such as: dry matter content, fat, titrable acidity, ash, and lactose contents; while, sensory characteristic of Kefir from camel milk was likely to be more sour. On the other hand, no significant differences were found between cow and camel milk Kefir in terms of fatty acid and cholesterol contents (Kavas, 2015).

Nowadays, frozen Kefir produced commercially from camel milk by Desert farms® company with the claim of being 100% natural and fermented traditionally in small batches with living Kefir cultures without added sugars. Interestingly, Kefir of Desert farms® is claimed to contain billions of *Bifidobacterium, Lactobacillus brevis, Lactobacillus paracasei, Lactococcus lactis* and *Saccharomyces cerevisiae* (Desert farms®, 2019).

Chal

Chal is a white sparkling fermented beverage manufactured from camel milk (Lakosa and Shokir, 1964) with sour taste (Brezovečki et al., 2015). This product is traditionally consumed in Iran, Turkman Sahra, and Golestan provinces, (Solanki & Hati, 2018) and in Turkmenistan (Konuspayeva, Faye & Serikbaeva, 2003). Chal is prepared by diluting camel milk with warm water in a 1:1 ratio, then incubated at 25-30°C for 2-8 hours (depends on desirable taste of final product) in goat skin bag or ceramic containers within a capacity of 30-kg (Yagil & Etzion, 1979). Ceramic containers are inoculated with previously fermented camel milk (1/4-1/3 weight/weigh) (Korlepara et al., 2017). The microbial strains used for Chal manufacturing contain *Lactobacilli lactic, Lactobacillus casei, Streptococcus thermophilus*, and yeast (Kieselev, 1956). The lactic acid bacterial strains of *Lactobacillus plantarum, L. paracasei, L. kefiri, L. gasseri, Enterococcus faecium* and *Weissella cibaria* are isolated from Chal by Soleymanzadeh, Mirdamadi, & Kianirad (2016). The microbial aspect of lactic acid bacteria isolated from camel milk was discussed in details in Chapter 4.

Yam, Khomeiri, Mahounak, & Jafari (2014) analyzed the hygienic characteristics of 18 samples of household as well as commercially produced Chal products compared to fresh and pasteurized camel milk. Researchers analyzed pH, total count, total yeast and mold counts, *Enterobacteriaceae*, lactic acid bacteria, and total *Staphylococcal* counts, anas well as presence of *Salmonella* and *Shigella*. The pH of camel milk was 6.4-6.7 compared to 3.8-4.5 of Chal. The total bacterial count was ranged between (4.11-3.90) and (3.77-1.95) log CFU/ml in milk and Chal, respectively. The counts of *Enterobacteriaceae,* Lactic acid bacteria and *Staphylococcal* were 2.60-1.90 and 2.04-1.77 log CFU/ml, 4.58-4.04 and 2.60-1.95 log CFU/ml, and 1.95-1.30 and 2.00-1.00 log cfu/ml for Chal and milk samples, respectively.

On the other hand, neither *Shigella* nor *Salmonella* present in Chal and camel milk samples. The results of this research concluded that fresh camel milk and Chal were produced under poor hygienic conditions compared to commercially available pasteurized milk.

In similar study, Zahedi, Salami, & Moslehishad (2016) studied the physiochemical, microbiological, and antioxidant properties of different Chal samples manufactured from camel milk. These samples collected from different household ranchers with different hygienic conditions. Chal contained 5.82±0.27%, 3.07±0.073%, and 12.24±0.16% of fat, protein, and total solids respectively. The acidity and pH values were 4.52±0.10 and 80±7 °D respectively. The Ca and P content in Chal were 103.29±3.87% and 10.25±0.1%, respectively. Furthermore, Chal found to have potential antioxidant activity. On the other hand, the total bacterial and coliform counts of Chal were 6.54±0.19 log CFU/mL and 2.34±0.23 log CFU/mL, respectively.

Soleymanzadeh et al. (2016) isolated and identified eight types of lactic acid bacteria from commercially available Chal products manufactured from camel and bovine milks. The lactic acid bacteria types are *Lactobacillus* (L.) *plantarum*, *L. paraplantarum*, *L. kefiri*, *L. gasseri*, *L. paracasei*, *Leuconostoc lactis*, *Weissella cibaria*, and *Enterococcus faecium*. Researchers also examined the antioxidant activity of Chal and were found to be high. In the present book, the antioxidant properties of camel milk will be discussed in details in Chapter 7 and 8.

Shubat

Shubat is a non-diluted fermented camel milk mainly made by Kazakh people from Kazakhstan, Uzbekistan, Russia, in Xinjiang region of China and Western part of Mongolia. Traditional *shubat* made by spontaneous fermentation yielding gas and foam, particularly white and very acid. Among the lactic bacteria, three genera were in majority: *Lactococcus*, *Lactobacillus* and *Enterococcus*. The following microorganisms were identified in Shubat of Kazakhstan: *Enterococcus durans; Enterococcus faecalis; Enterococcus faecium; Lactobacillus casei; Lactobacillus casei subsp. casei; Lactobacillus curvatus; Lactobacillus kefiri; Lactobacillus paracasei; Lactobacillus sakei; Lactococcus lactis subsp. lactis; Leuconostoc mesenteroides* (Akhmetsadykova, Baubekova, Konuspayeva, Akhmetsadykov, Faye & Loiseau, 2015). Such high microflora biodiversity is already reported in China (Wu, Huang, Zhang, Li, Xu, Wang & Shi, 2011). In addition, seven species of yeast were identified, *Kazakhstania unispora* and *Kluyveromyces marxianus* being predominant (Baubekova, Akhmetsadykova, Konuspayeva, Akhmetsadykov, Faye & Loiseau, 2015). The yeasts are generally responsible for the specific aroma of the fermented beverages (Koroleva, 1991). The production of specific starters after identification of the most convenient lactic bacteria strains (easy to cultivate in bio-fermenter, good aroma, few gas production) for making standardized *shubat* at industrial scale was implemented in local enterprises in Kazakhstan (Faye & Konuspayeva, 2016)

Gariss and Dhanaan

Gariss is an alcoholic fermented product (Mirghani, 1994) of acidic nature (pH 3.4-3.7) commonly consumed in Sudan (Abdel-Rahman, 2017), and in Jijiga and Shinile areas of Ethiopia (Omar, et al. 2018). The product known as Gariss in Sudan (Omar et al. 2018) and Dhanaan (Biratu & Seifu, 2016) in Ethiopia. Hassan et al., (2006) prepared Gariss using traditional method by placing raw camel milk in goat's skin bags along with black cumin (*Nigella sativa*) and onion bulb (Shori, 2012). These bags usually covered with moistened green or dry palm leaves then rapped with grass, thereafter hanged on camel saddle. The continuous movement during the camel journey causes the raw product stirring and allow air to mix with milk to aid in fermentation (Korlepara et al., 2017). The composition of gariss, especially its fatty acid composition, could vary according season, location and stage of fermentation (Ahmed, Mohamed, Elyousif, Faye, Loiseau & Montet, 2015). Fermentation in Gariss occurred due to the presence of lactic acid bacteria (such as *Lactobacillus paracasei* ssp. *paracasei*, *L. fermentum*, and *L. plantarum* (Sulieman et al., 2006), *Lactobacillus animalis*, *Lactobacillus brevis*, *Lactobacillus divergens*, *Lactobacillus rhamnosus*, *Lactobacillus gasseri*, *Lactobacillus paracasei*, *Lactobacillus fermentum*, and *Lactococcus alimentarium* (Ashmaig, Hasan, & El Gaali, 2009) as well as yeast (Mirghani, 1994). Moreover, Abdelgadir, Dennis, Nielsen, Hamad, & Jakobsen, (2008) also reported the presence of *Streptococcus infantarius* subsp. *infantarius* in camel milk as a potential human pathogen. Among the 19 lactic bacteria strains isolated in Gariss by Ahmed et al. (Ahmed, Mohamed, Yousif, Faye & Loiseau, 2012), none of them have shown antimicrobial effect (also see Chapter 7) on *staphylococcus aureus* and *escherichia coli*. The microbial aspect of lactic acid bacteria isolated from camel milk was discussed in Chapter 4.

Like, other fermented dairy products Gariss can stand for 10 days under refrigeration (Awad, El Zubeir, & Babiker, 2006). This shelf life can be extended to 234 hours if camel milk subjected to heat treatment of 63°C for 30 minutes and then stored at 25°C and 37°C (Awad et al., 2006).

Suusac

Suusac is a traditional fermented camel milk in Kenya (Solanki & Hati, 2018) and Ethiopia (Awad et al., 2006). Suusac contains 12.5% dry matter, 4% fat, 3% protein, and 1.1% alcohol (Farah, Streiff, & Bachmann, 1990). Suusac usually produced using raw camel milk incubated previously in pumpkin-smoked containers at 25-30 °C for 2 days (Lore, Mbugua, & Wangoh, 2005).

Hurunge

Hurunge is a traditional fermented product in China (Solanki & Hati, 2018) manufactured from camel milk and gourd (Shori, 2012) The fermentation of hurunge occurred using lactic acid bacteria strains such as *Lactococcus lactis* ssp. *lactis*, *Lactococcus raffinolactis*, *Lactococcus lactis* ssp. *cremoris*, *Leuconostoc mesenteroides* ssp. *cremoris*, *Lactobacillus casei*, *Lactobacillus homohiochii*, *Lactobacillus plantarum*, *Lactobacillus acetotolerans* and *Lactobacillus kefiranofaciens*. In addition to few strains of yeasts isolated from Hurunge such as Candida *kefyr*, *Candida valida*, *Candida krusei Kluyveromyces marxianus* var. *lactis* and *Saccharomyces cerevisiae* (Quan, Burentegusi, & Miyamoto, 2006).

Shmen (Semma)

Shmen or Semma is a popular fermented product consumed by Touareg communities of Sahar region made from camel milk butter (Mourad & Nour-Eddine, 2006; Asresie, Eyassu, Seifu, & Kurtu, 2013). Shmen is produced by melting butter at 100-120°C for 30 minutes to destroy bacteria, then clarified with a clarifying agent. Thereafter, stirred with a wooden spoon. Later, the clarifying agent is grated and collected, and then some grass or dates added to enhance color and aroma of the final product (Yagil & Etzion, 1979). Mourad and Nour-Eddine (2006) analyzed the total bacterial count of Shmen collected from four different areas of Algerian Sahara; researchers reported the presence of high bacterial counts which range between 2.76±0.19 - 3.88±0.23 log CFU/g.

OTHER FERMENTED DAIRY PRODUCTS

There are a number of fermented camel milk products reported in the literature, which have different names such as **Tarag** consumed as fermented camel milk similar to yogurt (Accolas et al., 1975), while **Unda** is a fermented product made by alcoholic fermentation of camel milk and other milks (Accolas et al., 1975). **Kheer** is a popular fermented dairy product known in the Raika's community of Rajasthan (Mal & Pathak, 2010). In Saudi Arabia, a fermented camel milk called **leben** was proposed. The making included 8 steps described as follow: (i) Preparation of mother solution with starter lambda 6 and 12 (Coquard©, France), (ii) acidification of the mother solution (pH=5.0) in stove 42°C for 7-8 hours, (iii) fresh camel milk heated at 70°C, then cooled down to 45°C, (iv) camel milk mixed with mother solution (60:1 V/V) for 20 min., then let at ambient temperature, (iv) put in bottle after 2 hours when pH=5.0, (v) stored in refrigerator, lifetime being 10 days (Algruin & Konuspayeva, 2015). Similar technology was used in Algeria.

Cream

Cream is classified according to the fat content and milk sources. For example, low cow cream contains 10 – 18% of fat, and high fat cow cream contains typically 35 – 40% of fat, the higher the fat content the thicker the cream will be. Cow cream is pasteurized at a high temperature of 95°C or higher without any holding time (Bylund, 1983).

Cream production from camel milk is different from cow cream due to deficiency of fat agglutinin in camel milk. This is why camel milk is not forming cream layer; however, protein is also responsible for rapid formation of a cream layer and promotes clustering of globules. Farah and Rüegg, (1991) reported that camel milk has a very slow creaming rate at all temperatures compared to cow milk and creaming layers of camel milk varied from 0.5 to 2 ml at 4 °C . Researchers also found that increasing the creaming time to 48 h did not produce any significant increase in creaming layer (Farah & Rüegg, 1991).

In another recent study, camel milk shows little tendency to cream up, compared to cow milk, this is because fat is distributed as small micelle-like globules in milk (Attia, Kherouatou, Fakhfakh, Khorchani & Trigui, 2000). Hence following the same churning method to produce cream and butter from cow milk is not successful to produce the same products from camel milk (Korlepara et al., 2017). The bonds between protein and fat in camel milk are firm, lead to higher melting point of camel milk fat (41- 42 °C) compared to cow milk. This could make churning of camel cream is more difficult for the same temperatures used for cow milk churning (8-12 °C)(Lore et al., 2005). Compared to butter from cow cream, butter from camel cream is richer in polyunsaturated fatty acids (oleic and linoleic acids C-18) and contain a normal amounts of palmitic acid (C-16) and only a small amount short chain of fatty acids of lower than C-12 lauric acid (Korlepara et al., 2017).

Several attempts were undertaken to churn camel milk cream into butter. Lore *et al.*, (2005) attempt to keep small amount of camel milk fat on the top of the milk after heating, then milk was cooled and churned to turn fat drops into butter grains. In another attempt, camel milk was hold in goat skin to produce butter (FAO, 1982). Recently, Korlepara et al., (2017) attempts to produce butter at industrial scale in the rural part of north-eastern Kenya, camel milk was heated to 65 °C then centrifuged. The resultant fat was standardized to 20-30%, thereafter churned at temperatures between 15 and 36°C to produce butter and cream. Overall conclusion from all attempts that the rate of camel milk creaming is very slow in raw, heated, refrigerated milk and even at room temperatures. This is attributed to the insufficient quantity of agglutinin in camel milk lead to slow creaming rate. Other factors could have effect the formation of creaming layer such as electrical charges on the globules, ionic distribution, and interfacial tension between milk sera and fat globules.

Ghee

Ghee is a pure clarified fat derived from milk and milk products (Kumar et al., 2017) or defined as an anhydrous milk fat (Hazra & Parmar, 2014). Ghee is an essential diet in some cultures such as Indian diet (Hazra & Parmar, 2014). Ghee is also known as "Samna" as in Egypt, "Samn" as in Middle East, "Rogan" as in Iran, "Samuli" as in Uganda and dhadha baksa/ Neter Kibe as in Ethiopia (Gemechu & Tola, 2017).The major criterion for accepting ghee is flavor and aroma (Hazra & Parmar, 2014; Gemechu & Tola, 2017). Ghee is a complex lipid of mixed glycerides together with a small amount of free fatty acids, phospholipids, sterols and their esters, fat soluble vitamins (A, D, E and K), carotenoids, carbonyl compounds, hydrocarbons, charred casein, moisture and trace elements such as copper and iron (Hazra & Parmar, 2014; Gemechu & Tola, 2017).

The most common industrial method to produce ghee is by chilling raw milk immediately below 5 °C, then warmed at 55- 60°C and subjected to separation. The resultant cream is warmed at 78- 84 °C for 16 s then cooled to 10- 12 °C. Pasteurized fresh cream is stored in insulated cream storage tanks to produce butter. Finally, resultant buttermilk added to melting butter vat at 40- 45 °C then transform to serum separator to separate the product into serum and ghee (Kumar et al., 2017). The main difference between butter and ghee in addition to the flavour, aroma and texture is the shelf. Ghee is a more stable product than butter due to its better shelf life even under warm conditions (Gemechu & Tola, 2017).

Many references in the literature reported that butter and ghee could not be produced from camel milk. This is due to the small diameter of fat globules but some local and foreign workers have successfully developed methods to make butter and ghee (Knoess et al., 1986). El-Bashir, (1997) reported that butter could be produced after shaking camel milk for 15-20 minutes or 3-4 hours at 24-25 °C; but it is difficult to keep butter fresh, unless heated at 100- 120 °C for 30 minutes to convert butter it into Ghee. In another study, Parmar (Parmar, 2013), attempted to produce ghee from camel milk and compared with that from cow milk and buffalo milk. The research produced all ghee samples using direct creaming method by heating cream to 115 °C with no holding time. The results revealed that camel milk yielded lower quantity of ghee than cow and buffalo. Moreover, all tested physical properties of camel ghee including solidification, melting points, refraction index and density were higher than cow and buffalo ghee. While, chemical tests such as cholesterol content and free fatty acid were lower but found to be more susceptible to oxidative deterioration. The sensory evaluation of this research (Parmar, 2013) showed that colour, appearance and flavour of camel ghee was preferable more than cow and buffalo ghee.

ICE CREAM AND FROZEN YOGURT

Ice Cream

There is a global increase in the demands of frozen dairy products (Salem, Fardous, Meead, & El-Rashody, 2017). Ice cream is defined as a smooth, sweet, cold dessert food prepared from a frozen mixture of milk ingredients including milk products, sweetening materials, stabilizers, colors, flavors, and egg products. Ice cream contains a minimum of 10% milk fat (Karaman et al., 2014) with ice crystals using continuous agitation (Deosarkar, Khedkar, Kalyankar, & Sarode, 2016).

The production of ice cream from camel milk has started since 1989 (Abu-Lehia, Al-Mohiezea, & El-Behry, 1989) at the laboratory scale and at industrial scale using a mixture of 12% fat, 11% milk solids nonfat (MSNF) and 37% total solids (Mehta, Jain, Patel, & Aparnathi, 2019).

It has been reported (Deosarkar et al., 2016) that successful ice cream manufacturing depends on several factors such as choosing the right ingredients and mixture processing (mixing, homogenizing, pasteurizing, aging, freezing, and packaging). The overall quality of ice cream assessed by studying viscosity, overrun, rheological and melting properties (Salem et al., 2017). Furthermore, the ingredients such as protein, sugar and air content play a significant role in the overall quality of ice cream (Frost, Heymann, Bredie, Djksterhuis, & Martens, 2005).

Viscosity of Ice Cream

The viscosity of cow and camel milk ice cream is mainly affected by the total solids (TS) especially MSNF and size of fat particles (Abu-Lehia et al., 1989; Goff et al., 1995). Camel milk due to its small fat droplets seems to be suitable for ice cream manufacturing (Abu-Lehia et al., 1989). The higher the concentration of fat droplets, the better the effect on the final product creaming, body, and texture (Deosarkar et al., 2016). Furthermore, water absorption, which play a key role in the arrangement of ice crystals around sugars, also found to affect the viscosity of ice cream made from camel milk (Salem et al., 2017). The crystallization around glucose and fructose rather than sucrose play a positive role in viscosity (Smith, Bakshi, & Lomauro, 1984).

The addition of soluble or insoluble fiber sources such as dates to ice cream mixture increase the viscosity and enhance body and liquefaction of ice cream produced from camel milk. This is due to the increase in total dissolved solids and the water holding capacity of soluble fiber leading to desirable effects on the three-dimensional conformation of the hydrated biopolymers (Khalil & Blassy, 2009; Salem et al., 2017). This is also reported with ice cream made form cow milk (Soukoulis, Lebesi, & Tzia, 2009). For instance, Akalın et al., (2018) showed a significant increase in viscosity of cow milk ice cream (enriched with probiotics) after the addition of different sources of fiber such as apple, orange, oat, bamboo, and wheat. Some producers were also reported to improve the quality of ice cream manufactured from camel milk including modification of whipping time (Abu-Lehia et al., 1989); and using modified starch and polysaccharides as stabilizers (Soukoulis et al., 2010).

Similarly, Salem et al. (2017) manufactured and studied the sensory characteristics of ice cream from camel milk. The researchers enhanced the ice cream viscosity by adding 5% and 10% date palm fruit (*Khalas* and *Sukkari* varieties) pieces, paste, or molasses. The addition of date palm fruit pastes and pieces (of both types) enhanced the viscosity more than molasses. The researchers also showed that the addition of soluble fiber (dates) to ice cream mixtures has enriched the viscosity, this is partially due to the restoration of water (Soukoulis et al., 2009).

In another study, Ahmed and El Zubeir (2015) manufactured ice cream from camel milk using the following ingredients (honey, sugar, skim milk powder and gum Arabic), among all tastes, combination of vanilla and coconut showed higher acceptability. While, microbial counts found to be different and depend on added flavors to the ice cream. The flavor of skim ice cream from camel milk significantly affected by texture, color, taste, and the overall acceptability (Arbuckle, 1966; El Owni & Khater, 2010).

Overrun of Ice Cream

The overrun is the increase of ice cream size during freezing due to air incorporation. The desirable overrun is 100% to achieve a desirable body, texture, and cost effectiveness of the ice cream (Arbuckle, 1986; Deosarkar et al., 2016). Overrun depends on the composition as well as the preparation conditions of ice cream (Karaca, Guven, Kaya, & Kahyaoglu, 2009). These two factors affect the whipping and air incorporation ability (Salem et al., 2017). The addition of fruits (fiber) to ice cream mixture manufactured from camel milk reduce the overrun to 20-30%and make whipping process harder (Abu-Lehia et al., 1989; Salem et al., 2017). On the other hand, increasing the total dissolved solid (MSNF) and total dissolved fat solids, as well as addition of ice to the ice cream mixture lead to improve overrun percentage (Abu-Lehia et al., 1989).

Rheological Properties of Ice Cream

Ice cream construction is measured by the ice cream foam stability as well as melting liquid (Salem et al., 2017). Ice cream stability has to reduce adhesion or docking, suitable freezing temperature, leading to high-quality foam (Salem et al., 2017). The stability of milk proteins (casein and whey protein) in the MSNF has a great impact on the ice cream texture; MSNF in the ice cream mixture should not be less than 2.5%. The instability of milk proteins leads to mixture destabilization, milk curdling, separation of milk serum, and fat churning. Milk proteins destabilize upon heat treatment of the MSNF and increase the pH of ice cream mixture (Bajad, Kalyankar, Dehmukh, Bachanti, & Bajad 2016). Jafarpour (2017) investigated the physiochemical properties of ice cream manufactured from camel milk and compared the results with those manufactured from cow milk. The results showed no significant differences between both milks in the physiochemical properties of final product. The researchers concluded that the use camel milk in ice cream manufacturing is feasible and sensibly acceptable.

Melting Properties of Ice Cream

Melting characteristics of ice cream is related melting resistance. Melting resistance is a desired characteristic (Thompson, Reniers, Baker, & Siu, 1982) and usually measured in minutes after freezing and storage for a certain period (Salem et al., 2017). Melting resistance is strongly correlated with the rheological properties (Salem et al., 2017). The more the incorporated air within the ice cream, the higher the melting resistance (Salem et al., 2017; Abu-Lehia et al., 1989). Melting resistance is associated negatively with the storage time (Sofjan & Hartel, 2011).

Large ice crystals cause poor behavior upon thawing. Additionally, when the total solids of the mixture increase, the freezing temperature become lower (Keeney & Kroger, 1974). Nonetheless, sugar content has the main effect on melting (Salem et al., 2017). The gelling ability as well as the freezing point also found to affect the melting resistance (Hartel, 2001). Therefore, the addition of fruit pieces to ice cream manufactured from camel milk can improve the melting resistance. This is due to the water holding capacity of fiber and the subsequent stabilization of the structure. Furthermore, better overrun results in significant improvement in melting resistance (Salem et al., 2017). Moreover, the melting resistance is impacted positively by fat content of the ice cream mixture as well as the non-fat solid percentage. Interestingly, the increase in non-fat solid content of the ice cream mixture up to 13% increased the melting resistance significantly from 4% to 12% in ice cream manufactured from camel milk (Salem et al., 2017).

The regulation of air arrangement as well as air incorporation during whipping at the latter stages of camel ice cream manufacturing unregulated air incorporation leading to overlapping of air pockets upon storage were found to result in poor melting resistance (Salem et al., 2017).

Frozen Yogurt

Frozen yogurt is a flavored or unflavored yogurt, which is frozen, in ice cream, freezers to obtain 50% overrun (Abu Lehia & Abu Tarboush, 1995). The quality of the final product occurs between yogurt and ice cream (Kavas & Kavas, 2016) and greatly depends on the quality of the raw material (Rea, 1983). Manufacturing frozen yogurt passes generally through nine steps where MSNF, gelatin, sucrose are blended and mixed with the fluid milk, pasteurized at 80°C for 30 minutes, inoculated with the yogurt started culture, incubated at 40°C for 4 hours, cooled at 5°C for 24 hours, flavoring, freezing, packaging, and hardening at -25°C for 24 hours (Nadia, 2007).

Kavas and Kavas (2016) produced frozen yogurt from camel milk fermented with yogurt culture (*Streptococcus thermophilus* + *Lactobacillus bulgaricus* (*Lb. bulgaricus*) and enriched with probiotic bacteria (*Lactobacillus acidophilus* and *Bifidobacterium* ssp.). The main ingredient was skim camel milk powder (5% weight/volume), *Sahlep* (*L. Orchis sancta*) as a stabilizer (2% weight/volume), and fruits (strawberry and guava mixture-20% weight/volume). Frozen ice cream was prepared by producing the ice cream then fermented with starter culture (Şireli & Orhan, 2015). The researchers found a significant ($P<0.05$) relationship between *Sahlep* and fruit fortification with the physiochemical and microbiological properties. For instance, titratable acidity, dry matter, viscosity, overrun, and melting resistance increased with *Sahlep* fortification. Additionally, the addition of the fruit pulp, *Sahlep,* affected the fat content of the final product. The fat content of the final products impacted the sustainability of the microbial viability of the final product during storage. For instance, *Lb. bulgaricus* had the highest viability followed by *Lb. acidophilus*, *Bifidobacterium* ssp. and *Str. thermophilus*, in a descending order. Nutritionally, vitamin C affected by pasteurization process. Nonetheless, the loss of vitamin C was the lowest ($P < 0.05$) in the guava probiotic frozen yogurt.

Several attempts were made to produce frozen yogurt from camel milk at the experimental scale (Ahmed, Haroun, & Eisa, 2010; Kavas & Kavas, 2016). Ahmed et al., (2010) examined the chemical and sensory characteristics of the frozen yogurt after adding three concentration of banana (10%, 12%, and 14%). Chemically, there were no significant differences among the three levels in terms of pH as well as chemical composition. The highest over run percentage (47.4±0.52%) was obtained using 10%

banana. Moreover, the use of 14% banana showed the highest ($P<0.05$) specific gravity (0.977 ± 0.27) and tended ($P>0.05$) to show the highest acceptability and palatability. The authors concluded that the manufacture of frozen yogurt from camel milk is possible if the following ingredients used; 5% fat, 13% sugar, 0.5% gelatin, 14% solid nonfat, and 14% banana.

CHOCOLATE BARS

Chocolate is a product manufactured from cocoa butter, cocoa liquor, sugar, and milk. The manufacturing of chocolate passes through five steps i, e. mixing, refining, paste coching, tempering and depositing, and molding and demolding (Shafi, Reshi, Bashir, & Bashir, 2018). Mixing of ingredients is a fundamental step, which is highly sensitive to temperature and duration. Mixing should occur continuously for 12-15 minutes at 40-50 °C. Fortunately, camel milk proteins remain stable during chocolate mixing of i.e. < 90°C. The second step of chocolate manufacturing is refining, where cocoa liquor and sugar are mixed and refined to have an overall fat content of 8-24% and fat particle size should not be more than 30μm. The final particle size plays a key role in rheological and sensory properties of chocolate (Shafi et al., 2018). Fortunately, half of the camel milk fat globule particle size of ranges between 1-5 μm and the other half ranges between 2-3 μm (Farah, 1993). It is expected, that chocolate manufactured from camel milk needs less refining.

The third step in chocolate manufacturing is conching, where chocolate is exposed to high temperature of 49-52°C for10-16 hours to reduce viscosity by removing water and some volatile compounds such as acetic acid to improve the flavor. Caution must be taken in the sense that replacing whole milk with skim milk increases conching temperature up to 79°C. Within the same context, conching liquefies chocolate and usually necessitates the addition of lecithin and extra cocoa butter (Shafi et al., 2018).

Usually, chocolate ingredient particles crystalize in 6 different sizes and shapes. Without the fourth and final step of chocolate manufacturing, the tempering, chocolate surface will appear mottled and matted. During this step, chocolate is exposed to heat (45°C) with stirring to melt all the formed crystals, then re-cooled to 36°C. During the cooling process, chocolate crystallization occurs uniformly into glossy, firm, of best snap, which melts at body temperature (37°C) (Shafi et al., 2018).

Nowadays, chocolate bars are being manufactured from camel milk at industrial scale, which is still in its initial stages.

Chocolate from camel milk is being manufactured by a number of manufacturers, the most famous ones are:

1. MILLER® chocolate: the plant is in Chambersburg/Pennsylvania/USA. The milk is usually imported from niche Smith camel farms in Netherlands (Russo, 2019).
2. Al Nassma Chocolate LLC: the plant is in Dubai/UAE launched in 2008. Milk is locally produced in UAE (European food, 2019). In addition, the chocolate products are being currently sold by the Oasis Camel Dairy® in Ramona/California/USA (Oasis Camel Dairy®, 2019).
3. Aadvik® camel milk is the first plant to manufacture chocolate from camel milk in India where chocolate manufactured with different flavors such as chilli, herbs, dates, almonds, crunch, and butterscotch. (Aadvik®, 2019).

COOKIES

The word "cookies" refers to the cracker-like products that contain flour, fat, sugar, milk powder, salt, acidulant and alkaline, water, and flavoring. The manufacturing of cookies passes through several processes such as: molding, extrusion, mixing and fermentation, sheeting, laminating, and cutting (Cauvain, Train, & Witney, 2016). The quality of cookies can be determined physically in terms of flour bulk density, wettability, viscosity, foam capacity and stability, gelation temperature, emulsification capacity, gelatinization temperature, liquid absorption capacity, swelling index, and pH). While chemically determined in terms of water and proximate composition, and sensibly (Ikechukwu et al., 2017). Manufacturing cookies from camel milk is only available from Camel cookies® of Abu Dhabi/UAE since 2013 (Camel cookies®, 2019) with different flavors such as red velvet, chocolate, pistachios, dates and saffron, saffron, and raffaello. The related scientific studies on evaluating the final product are absent and are highly recommended.

FUTURE RESEARCH DIRECTIONS

Future research is required to optimize the manufacturing conditions and overcome challenges for camel milk products in terms of heat treatment temperature, pressure, fermentation, incubation, hygienic conditions, as well as storage conditions. On the other hand, the manufacturing of different versions of camel milk products are encouraged such as skim, low fat, and those with different flavors and products for special dietary uses or medical conditions.

CONCLUSION

Camel milk and its products are good source of nutrition and income for people living in desert. Nowadays, some dairy products and non-dairy products are successfully manufactured from camel milk at the experimental level or commercial levels. Nonetheless, other products still facing processing challenges and encountering many difficulties compared with cow and sheep milk such as the sensitivity of camel milk to high temperature treatment, hygienic conditions, poor stability, and short shelf life. Dairy products manufactured from camel milk include camel milk powder, fermented products (such as yogurt, *Labneh*, kefir, Chal, Gariss, Suusac, Hurunge, Shemen, and other fermented dairy products), non-fermented products (such as ghee, cream), and desserts (such as ice cream and frozen yogurt, chocolate bars, and cookies).

ACKNOWLEDGMENT

Authors would like to thank Dr. Omar Alhaj for his convenient remarks on this chapter.

REFERENCES

Aadvik. (2019). *Welcome to Aadvik foods*. Retrieved in 22nd May, 2019 from https://www.indiamart.com/aadvikfoodsproducts/

AbdAlmageed, E. (2005). *Properties of milk powder made from the milk of cow, goat and camel* (Unpublished MSc. thesis). Umdurman Islamic University, Sudan.

Abdel-Rahman, I. (2007). *Biochemical changes in camel milk fermented by bacterial starter cultures* (Unpublished doctoral dissertation). University of Khartoum, Sudan.

Abdelgadir, W., Dennis, S., Nielsen, D., Hamad, S., & Jakobsen, M. (2008). A traditional Sudanese fermented camel's milk product, Gariss, as a habitat of *Streptococcus infantarius* subsp. *Infantarius*. *International Journal of Food Microbiology*, *127*(3), 215–219. doi:10.1016/j.ijfoodmicro.2008.07.008 PMID:18774196

Abirached, C., Medrano, C., Araujo, A., Moyna, P., Añón, M., & Panizzolo, L. (2012). Comparison of interfacial and foaming properties of soy and whey protein isolates. *Journal of Food Science and Engineering*, *2*, 376–381.

Abu Lehia, I., & Abu Tarboush, H. (1995). Milk fat products and ice cream. Academic Press.

Abu-Lehia, I., Al-Mohiezea, I., & El-Behry, M. (1989). Studies on the production of ice cream from camel milk products. *Australian Journal of Dairy Technology*, *44*, 31–34.

Accolas, J., Deffontaines, J., Aubin, F., Grosclaude, F., Kuzdzal-Savoie, S., Langlois, D., & Jeunet, R. (1975). Rural activities in the Mongolian Peoples' Republic II Dairy Products (Fr.). *Etudes Mongoles*, *6*, 7–98.

Adugnaa, M., Seifub, E., Kebededd, A., & Doluschitze, R. (2013). Quality and safety of camel milk along the value Chain in Eastern Ethiopia. *International Journal of Food Studies*, *2*(2), 150–157. doi:10.7455/ijfs/2.2.2013.a2

Afolabi, L., Onilude, H., & Afolabi, M. O. (2013). Assessment of microbiological quality of yogurt sold by street vendors in Onitsha metropolis, Anambra state, Nigeria. *British Microbiology Research Journal*, *3*(2), 198–20. doi:10.9734/BMRJ/2013/1801

Ahmed, A., & El Zubeir, I. (2015). Microbiological and sensory properties of low fat ice cream from camel milk using natural additives. *Annals. Food Science and Technology (Valahia University of Târgoviste)*, *16*(1), 236–244.

Ahmed, A. I., Mohamed, B. E., Eyousif, N. M., Faye, B., Loiseau, G., & Montet, D. (2015). Effect of production site, seasonality and age of fermented camel (Camelus dromedarius) milk gariss on fatty acids profile. *Journal of Advances in Food Science & Technology*, *2*(1), 1–8.

Ahmed, A. I., Mohamed, B. E., Yousif, N. M. E., Faye, B., & Loiseau, G. (2012). Antimicrobial activity and antibiotic resistance of LAB isolated from Sudanese traditional fermented camel (*Camelus dromedarius*) milk *gariss*. *International Journal of Biosciences*, *2*(11), 129–136.

Ahmed, S., Haroun, R., & Eisa, M. (2010). Banana frozen yogurt from camel milk. *Pakistan Journal of Nutrition, 9*(10), 955–956. doi:10.3923/pjn.2010.955.956

Akalın, A., Kesenkas, H., Dinkci, H., Unal, G., Ozer, E., & Kınık, O. (2018). Enrichment of probiotic ice cream with different dietary fibers: Structural characteristics and culture viability. *Journal of Dairy Science, 101*(1), 37–46. doi:10.3168/jds.2017-13468 PMID:29103712

Akanova, A., Kikebayev, N., Shaikenova, K., Seiitkazhy, Z., & Okuskhanov, E. (2017). Nutritive and Biological Value of Mares Milk Ice Cream. *Pakistan Journal of Nutrition, 16*(6), 457–462. doi:10.3923/pjn.2017.457.462

Akhmetsadykova, Sh., Baubekova, A., Konuspayeva, G., Akhmetsadykov, N., Faye, B., & Loiseau, G. (2015). Lactic acid bacteria biodiversity in raw and fermented camel milk. *African Journal of Food Science and Technology, 6*(3), 84–88.

Al haj, O. A., & Al Kanhal, H. A. (2010). Compositional, technological and nutritional aspects of dromedary camel milk. *International Dairy Journal, 20*, 811-821.

Al-Saleh, A. (1996). Heat coagulation of camel milk. *Journal of King Saud University, 8*, 107–117.

Al-Zoreky, N. S., & Al-Otaibi, M. M. (2015). Suitability of camel milk for making yogurt. *Food Science and Biotechnology, 24*(2), 601–606. doi:10.100710068-015-0078-z

Algruin, K., & Konuspayeva, G. (2015). Making leben with camel milk. *Scientific and Practical Journal Veterinariya, 2*(42), 398

Alhaj, O., Metwalli, A., & Ismail, E. (2011). Heat stability of camel milk proteins after sterilisation process. *Journal of Camel Practice and Research, 18*, 277–282.

Altay, F., Karbancıoglu-Güler, F., Daskaya-Dikmen, C., & Heperkan, D. (2013). A review on traditional Turkish fermented non-alcoholic beverages: Microbiota, fermentation process and quality characteristics. *International Journal of Food Microbiology, 167*(1), 44–56. doi:10.1016/j.ijfoodmicro.2013.06.016 PMID:23859403

Anema, S. G., & Li, Y. (2003). Association of denatured whey proteins with casein micelles in heated reconstituted skim milk and its effect on casein micelle size. *The Journal of Dairy Research, 70*(1), 73–83. doi:10.1017/S0022029902005903 PMID:12617395

Angulo, L., Lopez, E., & Lema, C. (1993). Microflora present in kefir grains of the Galician region (north-west of Spain). *The Journal of Dairy Research, 60*(2), 263–267. doi:10.1017/S002202990002759X PMID:8320374

Anonymous. (1986). *A/S Niro Atomizer: Technical doc.* Copenhagen: Wilentation.

Arbuckle, W. (1966). Ice cream. Avi Publ. Co. Inc.

Arbuckle, W. S. (1986). Calculating Cost and Percentage of Overrun. In *Ice Cream*. Boston, MA: Springer. doi:10.1007/978-1-4615-7222-0_10

Ashmaig, A., Hasan, A., & El Gaali, E. (2009). Identification of lactic acid bacteria isolated from traditional Sudanese fermented camel's milk (Gariss). *African Journal of Microbiological Research, 3*(8), 451–457.

Asresie, A., Eyassu Seifu, E., & Kurtu, M. (2013). Churning efficiency and microbial quality of butter made from camel milk alone and blending it with goat milk. *Net Journal of Agricultural Science, 1*(3), 75–80.

Aswal, P., Shukla, A., & Priyadarshi, S. (2012). Yoghurt: Preparation, characteristics and recent advancements. *Cibtech Journal of Bio-Protocols, 1*(2), 32–44.

Attia, H., & Dhouib, N. (2001). Dromedary milk lactic acid fermentation: Microbiological and rheological characteristics. *Microbial Biotechnology, 26*(5), 263–270. doi:10.1038j.jim.7000111 PMID:11494100

Attia, H., Kherouatou, N., Fakhfakh, N., Khorchani, T., & Trigui, N. (2000). Dromedary milk fat: Biochemical, microscopic and rheological characteristics. *Journal of Food Lipids, 7*(2), 95–112. doi:10.1111/j.1745-4522.2000.tb00164.x

Augustin, M. A. (2000). Mineral salts and their effect on milk functionality. *Australian Journal of Dairy Technology, 55*, 61–64.

Awad, H., El Zubeir, I., & Babiker, S. (2006). Microbiology of camel fermented milk (Gariss) in Sudan. *Research Journal of Microbiology, 1*(2), 160-165.

Baba, A. (2019). *Emirates Industry for camel milk & products factory*. Retrieved in 22nd May, 2019 from: https://ae1043581272.fm.alibaba.com/company_profile.html?spm=a2700.9099375.35.3.5e2b762cUmDTL4#top-nav-bar

Bajad, D., Kalyankar, S., Dehmukh, M., Bachanti, P., & Bajad, G. (2016). Impact of physico-chemical properties of mix on the final quality of ice-cream. *Asian Journal of Dairy & Food Reserch, 35*(4), 293–297.

Benabdelkamel, H., Masood, A., Alanazi, I. O., Alzahrani, D. A., Alrabiah, D. K., AlYahya, S. A., & Alfadda, A. A. (2017). Proteomic profiling comparing the effects of different 121 heat treatments on camel (*Camelus dromedarius*) milk whey proteins. *International Journal of Molecular Sciences, 18*(4), 2–15. doi:10.3390/ijms18040721 PMID:28350354

Berhe, T., Seifu, E., Ipsen, R., Kurtu, M. Y., & Hansen, E. B. (2017). Processing Challenges and Opportunities of Camel Dairy Products. *International Journal of Food Sciences, 2017*, 1–8. doi:10.1155/2017/9061757 PMID:29109953

Bernard, F., & Pascal, B. (2012). Camel sciences and economy in the world: current situation and perspectives. *Proc. 3rd ISOCARD Conference. Keynote Presentations, 2*–15.

Biratu, K., & Seifu, E. (2016). Chemical composition and microbiological quality of Dhanaan: Traditional fermented camel milk produced in eastern Ethiopia. *International Food Research Journal, 23*(5), 2223–2228.

Birchal, V., Passos, M., Wildhagen, G., & Mujumdar, A. (2005). Effect of spray-dryer operating variables on the whole milk powder quality. *Drying Technology*, *23*(3), 611–636. doi:10.1081/DRT-200054153

Brezovečki, A., Cagalj, M., Dermit, Z. F., Mikulec, N., Ljoljić, D., &Antunac, N. (2015). *Camel milk and milk products. Mljekarstvo/Dairy*, *65*(2), 81-90.

Bylund, G. (1983). Dairy Processing Handbook. Tetra Pack Processing Systems.

Camel, O. Dairy®. (2019). *Camel Milk Soap, Skincare and Chocolate*. Retrieved in 13th May, 2019 from: https://cameldairy.com/shop?olsPage=products

Camel cookies®. (2019). *Camel cookies*. Retrieved in 19th May from https://web.facebook.com/pg/camelcookiespage/about/?ref=page_internal

Camel milk South Africa®. (2019). *Organic camel milk*. Retrieved from https://camelmilksouthafrica.co.za/

Camelait®. (2019*). Al Ain – the leading producer of Camel Milk in the UAE*. Retrieved in 22nd May, from: http://camelait.asia/

Camilk®Dairy. (2019). *About camel milk & all natural camel milk products*. Retrieved in 22nd May, 2019 from: https://www.camilkdairy.com/pages/faq

Cauvain, S. P. (2016). Cookies, Biscuits and Crackers: Formulation, Processing and Characteristics. In C. Wrigley, H. Corke, K. Seetharaman, & J. Faubion (Eds.), *Encyclopedia of Food Grains* (2nd ed.; pp. 37–43). Oxford, UK: Academic Press. doi:10.1016/B978-0-12-394437-5.00119-4

Contarini, G., Povolo, M., Leardi, R., & Toppino, P. M. (1997). Influence of heat treatment on the volatile compounds of milk. *Journal of Agricultural and Food Chemistry*, *45*(8), 3171–3177. doi:10.1021/jf960849s

Corrieu, G., & Béal, C. (2016). Yogurt: The Product and its Manufacture. In Encyclopedia of Food and Health (Vol. 5, pp. 617–624). Elsevier. doi:10.1016/B978-0-12-384947-2.00766-2

Deosarkar, S., Khedkar, C., Kalyankar, S., & Sarode, A. (2016). Ice cream: uses and method of manufacture. In B. Caballero, P. Finglas, & F. Toldrá (Eds.), *The Encyclopedia of food and health* (pp. 391–397). Oxford, UK: Academic Press. doi:10.1016/B978-0-12-384947-2.00384-6

Desert farms®. (2019). *Desert farms camel milk*. Retrieved in 22nd May, 2019 from: https://desertfarms.com/pages/our-practices

Desouky, M., Shalaby, M., & Soryal, K. (2013). Compositional, rheological and organoleptic qualities of camel milk *Labneh* as affected by some milk heat treatments. *World Journal of Dairy & Food Sciences*, *8*(2), 118–130.

Desrosier, N. (2008). *Food Preservation Technology* (M. Mulyoharjo & D. Wijoyono, Trans.). Jakarta: University of Indonesia Press.

El-Agamy, E. (2000). Effect of heat treatment on camel milk proteins with respect to antimicrobial factors: A comparison with cows' and buffalo milk proteins. *Food Chemistry*, *68*(2), 227–232. doi:10.1016/S0308-8146(99)00199-5

El-Bashir, O. M. (1997). *Physiological characters and Diseases of camel in the Sudan*. Omdurman Islamic University. (in Arabic)

El Owni, O., & Khater, Z. (2010). Effect of type of flavor on sensory characteristics of ice cream from Factories and Machines. *Australian Journal of Basic and Applied Sciences, 4*(8), 3257-3260.

European food. (2019). *Al Nassma Chocolate LLC*. Retrieved in 13th May, 2019 from: https://www.european-food.com/al-nassma-chocolate-llc/interview/camel-milk-chocolate-an-arab-superfood/

Farah, Z. (1993). Composition and characteristics of camel milk. *The Journal of Dairy Research, 60*(4), 603–626. doi:10.1017/S0022029900027953 PMID:8294611

Farah, Z., & Atkins, D. (1992). Heat coagulation of camel milk. *The Journal of Dairy Research, 59*(2), 229–231. doi:10.1017/S002202990003048X

Farah, Z., & Rüegg, M. (1991). The Creaming Properties and Size Distribution of Fat Globules in Camel Milk. *Journal of Dairy Science, 74*(9), 2901–2904. doi:10.3168/jds.S0022-0302(91)78472-5

Farah, Z., Streiff, T., & Bachmann, M. (1990). Preparation and consumer acceptability tests of fermented camel milk in Kenya. *The Journal of Dairy Research, 57*(2), 281–283. doi:10.1017/S002202990002690X

Faye, B. (2016). The camel, new challenges for a sustainable development. *Tropical Animal Health and Production, 48*(4), 689–692. doi:10.100711250-016-0995-8 PMID:26922737

Faye, B., Br, B., & ElRouili, H. (2014). Camel milk value chain in Northern Saudi Arabia. *Emirates Journal of Food and Agriculture, 26*(4), 359. doi:10.9755/ejfa.v26i4.17278

Faye, B., & Konuspayeva, G. (2016). Innovations in camel milk processing: The new challenges for marketing camel dairy products and the consequences on genetic selection. In *Regional conf. for animal genetic resources conservation. Towards Sustainable Utilization*. Available on: https://oapgrc.gov.om/Documents/The new challenges for marketing camel dairy products and the consequences on genetic selection_Bernard Fye.pdf

Fitzpatrick, J., Barry, K., Cerqueira, P., Iqbal, T., O'Neill, J., & Roos, Y. (2007). Effect of composition and storage conditions on the flowability of dairy powders. *International Dairy Journal, 17*(4), 383–392. doi:10.1016/j.idairyj.2006.04.010

Fonseca, F., Passot, S., Cunin, O., & Marin, M. (2004). Collapse temperature of freeze-dried *Lactobacillus bulgaricus* suspensions and protective media. *Biotechnology Progress, 20*(1), 229–238. doi:10.1021/bp034136n PMID:14763847

Food and Agricultural Organization. (1982). *Camel and camel milk*. Rome: Author.

Frost, M., Heymann, H., Bredie, W., Djksterhuis, G., & Martens, M. (2005). Sensory Measurement of Dynamic Flavor Intensity in Ice Cream with Different Fat Levels and Flavorings. *Food Quality and Preference, 16*(4), 305–314. doi:10.1016/j.foodqual.2004.05.009

Galeboe, O., Seifu, E., & Sekwati-Monang, B. (2018). Production of camel milk yoghurt: Physicochemical and microbiological quality and consumer acceptability. *International Journal of Food Studies, 7*(2), 51–63. doi:10.7455/ijfs/7.2.2018.a5

Gemechu, A. T., & Tola, Y. B. (2017). Traditional butter and ghee production, processing and handling in Ethiopia: A review. *African Journal of Food, Agriculture, Nutrition and Development, 11*(4), 95–105.

Goff, H. (1997). Colloidal Aspects of Ice Cream—A Review. *International Dairy Journal, 7*(6-7), 363–373. doi:10.1016/S0958-6946(97)00040-X

Goff, H., Freslon, B., Sahagian, M. E., Hauber, T. D., Stone, A. P., & Stanley, D. W. (1995). Structural Development in Ice Cream—Dynamic Rheological Measurements. *Journal of Texture Studies, 26*(5), 517–536. doi:10.1111/j.1745-4603.1995.tb00801.x

Gorelik, O., Shatskikh, Y., Rebezov, M., Kanareikina, S., Kanareikin, V., Lihodeyevskaya, O., ... Okuskhanova, E. (2017). Study of Chemical and Mineral Composition of New Sour Milk Bio-product with Sapropel Powder. *Annual Research & Review in Biology, 18*(4), 1–5. doi:10.9734/ARRB/2017/36937

Guzel-Seydim, Z., Kök-Tas, T., & Greene, A. K. (2010). Kefir and koumiss: microbiology and technology. In F. Yildiz (Ed.), *Development and Manufacture of Yogurt and Functional Dairy Products* (pp. 143–163). Boca Raton, FL: CRC Press.

Guzel-Seydim, Z., Seydim, A., Grenee, A., & Bodine, A. (2000). Determination of organic acids and volatile flavour substances in kefir during fermentation. *Journal of Food Composition and Analysis, 13*(1), 35–43. doi:10.1006/jfca.1999.0842

Habtegebriel, H., Edwardb, D., Wawire, M., Silaa, D., & Seifu, E. (2018). Effect of operating parameters on the surface and physico-chemical properties of spray-dried camel milk powders. *Food and Bioproducts Processing, 1*(12), 137–149.

Habtegebriel, H., Wawire, M., & Sila, D. (2018). The effect of pretreatment (spray drying) on the yield and selected nutritional components of whole camel milk powder. *Food Science, 83*(12), 2983–2991. doi:10.1111/1750-3841.14361 PMID:30440084

Hal, J., & Hedrick, T. (1975). *Drying of milk and milk products*. Westport, CT: AVI Publ. Co. Ltd.

Ham, J. S., Shin, J. H., Noh, Y. B., Jeong, S. G., Han, G. S., Chae, H. S., ... Jo, C. (2008). Chemical and microbiological quality, capillary electrophoresis pattern, and rennet coagulation of UHT-treated and irradiated milk. *Food Science and Biotechnology, 17*, 58–65.

Hashim, I. B., Khalil, A. H., & Habib, H. (2009). Quality and acceptability of a set-type yogurt made from camel milk. *Journal of Dairy Science, 92*(3), 857–862. doi:10.3168/jds.2008-1408 PMID:19233778

Hassan, R., El Zubeir, I., & Babiker, S. (2006). Microbiology of camel fermented milk (Gariss) in Sudan. *Research Journal of Microbiology, 1*(2), 160–165. doi:10.3923/jm.2006.160.165

Hassan, R. A., El Zubei, I. E. M., & Babiker, S. A. (2007). Effect of Pasteurization of Raw Camel Milk and StorageTemperature on the Chemical Composition of Fermented Camel Milk. *International Journal of Dairy Science, 2*(2), 166–171. doi:10.3923/ijds.2007.166.171

Hazra, T., & Parmar, P. (2014). Natural Antioxidant Use in Ghee-A Mini Review. *Journal of Food Research and Technology, 2*(3), 101–105.

Hertzler, S., & Clancy, S. (2003). Kefir improves lactose digestion and tolerance in adults with lactose maldigestion. *Journal of the American Dietetic Association, 103*(5), 582–587. doi:10.1053/jada.2003.50111 PMID:12728216

Ho, T., Chan, S., Yago, A., & Shravya, R. (2019). Changes in physiochemical properties of spray-dried camel milk powder over accelerated storage. Food Chemistry. (Accepted for publication)

Hussen, M., Selamawit, H., Ashenafi, G., Fikre, Z., & Ashenafi, F. (2016). Assessment on Safety Status of Camel Raw Milk Marketed in Samara-Logia Town of Afar National Regional State, Northeast Ethiopia. *Food Science and Quality Management*, *49*, 88–88.

Hynd, J. (1980). Drying of whey. *International Journal of Dairy Technology*, *33*(2), 52–54. doi:10.1111/j.1471-0307.1980.tb01471.x

Ibrahem, S. A., & El Zubeir, I. E. M. (2016). Processing, composition and sensory characteristic of yoghurt made from camel milk and camel–sheep milk mixtures. *Small Ruminant Research*, *136*, 109–112. doi:10.1016/j.smallrumres.2016.01.014

Ibrahim, A. H., & Khalifa, S. A. (2015). The effects of various stabilizers on physiochemical properties of camel milk yoghurt. *The Journal of American Science*, *11*(1).

Ikechukwu, P., Okafor, D., Kabuo, N., Ibeabuchi, J., Odimegwu, O., Alagbaoso, E., ... Mbah, N. (2017). Production and evaluation of cookies from whole wheat and date palm fruit pulp as sugar substitute. *International Journal of Advancement in Engineering Technology Management and Applied Science*, *4*(4), 1–31.

International livestock Institute. (2013). *Camel milk, a practical guid to hygenic production and handling for improved market access*. Author.

Irigoyen, A., Arana, I., Castiella, M., Torre, P., & Ibànez, F. (2005). Microbiological, physicochemical, and sensory characteristics of kefir during storage. *Food Chemistry*, *90*(4), 613–620. doi:10.1016/j.foodchem.2004.04.021

Jafarpour, A. (2017). Feasibility of manufacture and investigation of physicochemical properties of camel milk – based ice cream. *Journal of Scientific Agriculture*, *1*, 300–302. doi:10.25081/jsa.2017.v1.838

Jagtiani, H. C., Jr., & Sakai, W. (1998). Tropical Fruit Processing (Food Science and Technology). London: Academic Press Inc.

Jouppila, K., & Roos, Y. (1994). Water sorption and time-dependent phenomena of milk powders. *Journal of Dairy Science*, *77*(7), 1798–1808. doi:10.3168/jds.S0022-0302(94)77121-6

Kalyankar, S., Deshmukh, M., Chopde, S., Khedkar, C., Lule, V., & Deosarkar, S. (2016). Milk Powder. In B. Caballero, P. Finglas, & F. Toldrá (Eds.), *The Encyclopedia of Food and Health*. Oxford, UK: Academic Press. doi:10.1016/B978-0-12-384947-2.00465-7

Karaca, O., Guven, M., Kaya, S., & Kahyaoglu, A. (2009). The Functional, Rheological and Sensory Characteristics of Ice Creams with Various Fat Replacers. *International Journal of Dairy Technology*, *62*(1), 93–99. doi:10.1111/j.1471-0307.2008.00456.x

Karaman, S., Toker, Ö., Yüksel, F., Çam, M., Kayacier, A., & Dogan, M. (2014). Physicochemical, bioactive, and sensory properties of persimmon-based ice cream: Technique for order preference by similarity to ideal solution to determine optimum concentration. *Journal of Dairy Science*, *97*(1), 97–110. doi:10.3168/jds.2013-7111 PMID:24268400

Kavas, G. (2015). Kefirs manufactured from camel (*Camelus dramedarius*) milk and cow milk: Comparison of some chemical and microbial properties. *Italian Journal of Food Science*, *27*, 357–365.

Kavas, N., & Kavas, G. (2016). Probiotic frozen yoghurt production using camel milk (*Camelus dromedarius*) with improved functions by strawberry guava (*Psidium littorale* var. *cattleianum*) fortification. *British Journal of Applied Science and Technology*, *14*(5), 1–12. doi:10.9734/BJAST/2016/23683

Keeney, P., & Kroger, M. (1974). *Fundamentals of dairy chemistry* (2nd ed.). Westport, CT: AVI Publishing Co.

Khalil, R., & Blassy, K. (2011). The Use Modified Date Pulp Fibers in Functional Low Fat Ice Cream. *Egyptian Journal of Dairy Science*, *39*, 275–283.

Kieselev, N. (1956). Bacteriological examination of chal (Ru). *Mol. Prom*, *17*, 31–34.

Knoess, K. H., Makhudum, A. J., Rafiq, M., & Hafeez, M. (1986). Milk production potential of the dromedary with special reference to the province of Punjab, *Pakistan World Anim. Rev. FAO Rome*, *57*, 11–21.

Konuspayeva, G., Faye, B., Loiseau, G., & Levieux, D. (2007). Lactoferrin and immunoglobulin contents in camel's milk (*Camelus bactrianus, Camelus dromedarius* and Hybrids) from Kazakhstan. *Journal of Dairy Science*, *90*(1), 38–46. doi:10.3168/jds.S0022-0302(07)72606-1 PMID:17183073

Konuspayeva, G., Faye, B., & Serikbaeva, A. (2003). Les produits laitiers traditionnels à base de lait de chamelle en Asie Centrale. In Atelier Intl. sur le lait de chamelle en Afrique. FAO-CIRAD-KARKARA. FAO Publ.

Korlepara, R., Kalla, A., Manthani, V., & Keerthi, S. (2017). Camel milk a white gold of dessert- a review. *International Archive of Applied Sciences and Technology*, *8*(3), 74–83.

Koroleva, N. S. (1991). Starters for fermented milks. Section 4, Kefir and kumis starters. *IDF Bulletin*, *227*, 35–40.

Kumar, M., Pandya, H. B., Dodiya, K. K., Bhatt, R., & Mangukiya, M. (2017). Advancement in industrial method of ghee making process at sarvottam dairy, Bhavnagar, Gujarat (India). *International Journal of Science. Environment ISSN*, *6*(3), 1727–1736.

Kumar, P., & Mishra, H. (2004). Yoghurt powder- a review of process technology storage and utilization. *Food and Bioproducts Processing*, *82*(2C2), 133–142. doi:10.1205/0960308041614918

Lakosa, I., & Shokin, V. (1964). Milk production. In Camels (pp. 113–120). Science. Technical Agricultural Publ.

Lore, T. A., Mbugua, S. K., & Wangoh, J. (2005). Enumeration and identification of microflora in suusac, a Kenyan traditional fermented camel milk product. *Lebensmittel-Wissenschaft + Technologie*, *38*(2), 125–130. doi:10.1016/j.lwt.2004.05.008

Mal, G., & Pathak, K. (2010). *Camel milk and milk products*. National Research Center on Camel.

Mehta, B., Jain, A., Patel, D., & Aparnathi, K. (2019). Camel Milk: Opportunity and Challenges. National Seminar on "Indian Dairy Industry - Opportunities and Challenges". *National Seminar on "Indian Dairy Industry - Opportunities and Challenges"*. Retrieved from http://www.dairyknowledge.in/sites/default/files/ch9_0.pdf

Mirghani, A. (1994). *Microbial and biochemical properties of fermented camel's milk (gariss)* (Unpublished MSc thesis).

Mistry, V. (2004). Fermented liquid milk products. In Y. H. Hui, L. Meunier-Goddik, Ö. S. Hansen, J. Josephsen, W. Nip, P. S. Stanfield, & F. Toldra (Eds.), *Handbook of Food and beverage fermentation technology* (pp. 939–957). New York: Marcel Dekker. doi:10.1201/9780203913550.ch45

Mohsin, A. (2019). Qualitative Improvement of Camel Milk Date Yoghurt by Addition of Biosynthesized Xanthan from Orange Waste. *Food Science and Technology (Campinas)*, *108*, 61–68.

Mounir, S. (2017). Foam Mat Drying. In *Drying technologies for foods-fundamentals and applications*. CRC Press.

Mourad, K., & Nour-Eddine, K. (2006). Physicochemical and microbiological studies of 'Shmen' a traditional butter made from camel milk in the Sahara (Algeria); isolation and identification of lactic acid bacteria and yeast. *Journal of Animal Science*, *12*, 45–65.

Mudgil, P., & …. (2018). Rheological, Micro-Structural and Sensorial Properties of Camel Milk Yogurt as Influenced by Gelatin. *Food Science and Technology (Campinas)*, *98*, 646–653. Retrieved from https://linkinghub.elsevier.com/retrieve/pii/S0023643818307400

Nadia, A. (2007). *Ice cream between health and disease* (1st ed.). Aleskandaria, Egypt: AlMaaref Alhaditha Library. (In Arabic)

Newton, A. E., Fairbanks, A. J., Golding, M., Andrewes, P., & Gerrard, J. A. (2012). The role of the Maillard reaction in the formation of flavour compounds in dairy products – not only a deleterious reaction but also a rich source of flavour compounds. *Food & Function*, *3*(12), 1223–1326. doi:10.1039/c2fo30089c PMID:22948260

Nijdam, J., Ibach, A., & Kind, M. (2008). Fluidisation of whey powders above the glass-transition temperature. *Powder Technology*, *187*(1), 53–61. doi:10.1016/j.powtec.2008.01.013

Nikkhah, A. (2011). Science of Camel and Yak Milks: Human Nutrition and Health Perspectives. *Food and Nutrition Sciences*, *2*(06), 667–673. doi:10.4236/fns.2011.26092

Nuñez, M. (2016). Existing Technologies in Non-cow milk processing and traditional non-cow milk products. In E. Tsakalidou & K. Papadimitriou (Eds.), *Non-Bovine Milk and Milk Products*. Elsevier.

Odongo, N., Lamuka, P., Matofari, J., & Abong, G. (2016). Risk factors associated with the post-harvest loss of milk along camel milk value chain in Isiolo County, Kenya. *African Journal of Agricultural Research*, *11*(8), 674–682. doi:10.5897/AJAR2015.9988

Omar, A., Harbourne, N., & Oruna-Concha, M. J. (2018). Effects of industrial processing methods on camel skimmed milk properties. *International Dairy Journal*, *84*, 15–22. doi:10.1016/j.idairyj.2018.03.011

Otles, S., & Cadingi, O. (2003). Kefir: A probiotic dairy-composition, nutritional and therapeutic aspects. *Pakistan Journal of Nutrition*, *2*(2), 54–59. doi:10.3923/pjn.2003.54.59

Park, Y. W., Juárez, M., Ramos, M., & Haenlein, G. F. W. (2007). Physico-chemical characteristics of goat and sheep milk. *Small Ruminant Research*, *68*(1–2), 88–113. doi:10.1016/j.smallrumres.2006.09.013

Parmar, N. B. (2013). *Characterization of ghee prepared from camel milk and evaluation of its shelf life during storage* (Master Thesis). SMC College of Dairy Science, Anand Agricultural University, Anand, Gujarat, India.

Perkins, M. L., D'Arcy, B. R., Lisle, A. T., & Deeth, H. C. (2005). Solid phase microextraction of stale flavour volatiles from the headspace of UHT milk. *Journal of the Science of Food and Agriculture*, *85*(14), 2421–2428. doi:10.1002/jsfa.2243

Quan, S., Burentegusi, Y., & Miyamoto, T. (2006). Microflora in traditional starter cultures for fermented milk, Hurunge, from inner Mongolia. *China Journal of Animal Science Journal*, *77*(2), 235–241. doi:10.1111/j.1740-0929.2006.00343.x

Rafiq, S., Huma, N., Pasha, I., Sameen, A., Mukhtar, O., & Khan, M. (2016). Chemical composition, nitrogen fractions and amino acids profile of milk from different animal species. *Asian-Australasian Journal of Animal Sciences*, *29*(7), 1022–1028. doi:10.5713/ajas.15.0452 PMID:26954163

Rea, H. (1983). *Studies on the Manufacture of Frozen Yogurt* (Unpublished MSc thesis). Ein Shams University, Egypt.

Russo, C. (2019). *Meet the Camels behind the Celebrated Camel Milk Chocolate*. Retrieved in 13th May, 2019 from: https://millerchocolate.com/blogs/news/the-story-of-the-camel-milk-chocolate-bar

Sagar, S., Mehta, B., Wadhwani, K., Darji, V., & Aparnathi, K. (2017). Evaluation of camel milk for selected processing related parameters and comparisons with cow and buffalo milk. *International Journal of Health, Animal Science and Food Safety, 3*, 27 – 37.

Saito, Z. (1985). Particle structure in spray-dried whole milk and in instant skim milk powder as related to lactose crystallization. *Food Microstructure*, *4*, 333–340.

Salem, S., Fardous, M., Meead, G., & El-Rashody, H. (2017). Effect of Camel Milk Fortified with Dates in Ice Cream Manufacture on Viscosity, Overrun, and Rheological Properties during Storage Period. *Food and Nutrition Sciences*, *8*(05), 551–564. doi:10.4236/fns.2017.85038

Saljooghi, S., Mansouri-Najand, L., Ebrahimnejad, H., Doostan, F., & Askari, N. (2017). Microbiological, biochemical and organoleptic properties of fermented probiotic drink produced from camel milk. *Veterinary Research Forum: An International Quarterly Journal*, *8*(4), 313–317. PMID:29326790

Sawaya, W. N., Khalil, J. K., Al-Shalhat, A., & Al-Mohammad, H. (1984). Chemical composition and nutritional quality of camel milk. *Journal of Food Science*, *49*(3), 744–747. doi:10.1111/j.1365-2621.1984.tb13200.x

Shafi, F., Reshi, M., Bashir, A., & Bashir, I. (2018). Chocolate processing. *International Journal of Advanced Biological Research*, *8*(3), 408–419.

Shamsia, S. M. (2009). Nutritional and therapeutic properties of camel and human milks. *International Journal of Genetics and Molecular Biology*, *1*(2), 52–58.

Shewangizaw, A. (2016). Review on the dual functions of camel milk processing and marketing for unmet demand. *Middle East Journal of Scientific Research*, *24*(10), 3058–3066.

Shori, A. (2012). Comparative study of chemical composition, isolation and identification of micro-flora in traditional fermented camel milk products: Gariss, Suusac, and Shubat. *Journal of the Saudi Society of Agricultural Sciences*, *11*(2), 79–88. doi:10.1016/j.jssas.2011.12.001

Shori, A., & Baba, A. (2014). Comparative antioxidant activity, proteolysis and in vitro-amylase and glucosidase inhibition of Allium sativum yogurts made from cow and camel milk. *Journal of Saudi Chemical Society*, *18*(5), 456–463. doi:10.1016/j.jscs.2011.09.014

Şireli, U., & Orhan, C. (2015). Frozen yogurt. *Turkish Food Journal*, *40*(3), 179–185.

Smith, D., Bakshi, A., & Lomauro, C. (1984). Changes in Function of Sweetener System and Whey Substitution. *Milchwissenschaft. Milk Science International*, *39*, 455.

Sofjan, R., & Hartel, R. (2004). Effects of overrun on structural and physical characteristics of ice cream. *International Dairy Journal*, *14*(3), 255–262. doi:10.1016/j.idairyj.2003.08.005

Solanki, D., & Hati, S. (2018). Fermented camel milk: A Review on its bio-functional properties. *Emirates Journal of Food and Agriculture*, *30*(4), 268–274. doi:10.9755/ejfa.2018.v30.i4.1661

Soleymanzadeh, N., Mirdamadi, S., & Kianirad, M. (2016). Antioxidant activity of camel and bovine milk fermented by lactic acid bacteria isolated from traditional fermented camel milk (Chal). *Dairy Science Technology*, *96*(4), 443-457. ff.ffhal01532393 doi:10.100713594-016-0278-1ff

Soukoulis, C., Lebesi, D., & Tzia, C. (2009). Enrichment of Ice Cream with Dietary Fiber: Effects on Rheological Properties, Ice Crystallization and Glass Transition Phenomena. *Food Chemistry*, *115*(2), 665–671. doi:10.1016/j.foodchem.2008.12.070

Soukoulis, C., Lyroni, E., & Tzia, C. (2010). Sensory Profiling and Hedonic Judgment of Probiotic Ice Cream as a Function of Hydrocolloids, Yogurt and Milk Fat Content. *Lebensmittel-Wissenschaft + Technologie*, *43*(9), 1351–1358. doi:10.1016/j.lwt.2010.05.006

Stahl, T., Sallmann, H. P., Duehlmeier, R., & Wernery, U. (2006). Selected vitamins and fatty acid patterns in dromedary milk and colostrums. *Journal of Camel Practice and Research*, *13*(1), 53–57.

Sulieman, A., Elamin, O., Elkhalifa, E., & Laleye, L. (2018). A comparative study of physicochemical properties of freeze-dried camel's milk and cow's milk powder. *Discourse Journal of Agriculture and Food Sciences*, *6*(2), 11–16.

Sulieman, A. M., Ilayan, A. A., & Faki, A. E. (2006). Chemical and microbiological quality of *Garris*, Sudanese fermented camel's milk product. *International Journal of Food Science & Technology*, *41*(3), 321–328. doi:10.1111/j.1365-2621.2005.01070.x

Tay, T., & Chua, Y. (2015). High temperature short time (HTST) camel milk pasteurization pilot plant. *Journal of Engineering and Applied Sciences (Asian Research Publishing Network)*, *10*(15), 6241–6245.

Temerbayeva, M., Rebezov, M., Okuskhanova, E., Zinina, O., Gorelik, O., Vagapova, O., ... Yessimbekov, Z. (2018). Development of Yogurt from Combination of Goat and Cow Milk. *Annual Research & Review in Biology*, *23*(6), 1–7. doi:10.9734/ARRB/2018/38800

Thompson, L., Reniers, D., Baker, L., & Siu, M. (1982). Succinylated whey protein concentrates in ice cream and instant puddings. *Journal of Dairy Science*, *66*(8), 1630–1637. doi:10.3168/jds.S0022-0302(83)81985-7

Toba, T., Arihara, K., & Adachi, S. (1987). Comparative study of polyssacharide from kefir grains, an encapsuled homofermentative Lactobacillus species and Lactobacillus kefir. *Milchwissenschaf*, *42*, 565–568.

Vasbinder, A. J., Rollema, H. S., & Kruif, C. G. (2003). Impaired rennetability of heated milk; study of enzymatic hydrolysis and gelation kinetics. *Journal of Dairy Science*, *86*(5), 1548–1555. doi:10.3168/jds.S0022-0302(03)73740-0 PMID:12778565

Vazquez-Landaverde, P. A., Torres, J. A., & Qian, M. C. (2006). Effect of high-pressuremoderate-temperature processing on the volatile profile of milk. *Journal of Agricultural and Food Chemistry*, *54*(24), 9184–9192. doi:10.1021/jf061497k PMID:17117808

Vazquez-Landaverde, P. A., Velazquez, G., Torres, J. A., & Qian, M. C. (2005). Quantitative determination of thermally derived off-flavor compounds in milk using solid-phase microextraction and gas chromatography. *Journal of Dairy Science*, *88*(11), 3764–3772. doi:10.3168/jds.S0022-0302(05)73062-9 PMID:16230682

Weerathilake, W. A. D. V., Rasika, D. M. D., Ruwanmali, J. K. U., & Munasinghe, M. A. D. D. (2014). The evolution, processing, varieties and health benefits of yogurt. *International Journal of Scientific and Research Publications, 4*(4), 1–10. Retrieved from http://www.ijsrp.org/research-paper-0414/ijsrp-p2855.pdf

Wernery, U. (2007). Camel milk–new observations. In T.K. Gahlot (Eds.). *Proceedings of the International Camel Conference* (pp: 200-204). CVAS.

Wernery, U. (2008). Camel milk-new observations. In *Conference proceedings: International Camel conference. Recent trends in camel research and future strategies for saving camels* (pp. 200-204). Bikaner.

Wu, Y., Huang, P., Li, Y., Zhang, X. Y., Xu, Z. Z., Wang, B. F., & Shi, J. (2011). Molecular biological identification of lactic acid bacteria in fermented camel milk as a Kazakh traditional food in Xinjiang. *Food Science*, *32*(1), 173–176.

Yagil, R., & Etzion, Z. (1979). Antidiuretic hormone and aldosterone in the dehydrated and rehydrated camel. *Comparative Biochemistry and Physiology*, *63A*(2), 275–278. doi:10.1016/0300-9629(79)90159-2

Yam, B., Khomeiri, M., Mahounak, A., & Jafari, S. (2014). Hygienic quality of camel milk and fermented camel milk (Chal) in Golestan Province, Iran. *Journal of Microbiology Research (Rosemead, Calif.)*, *4*(2), 98–103.

Yazdanpanah, N., & Langrish, T. (2011). Fast crystallization of lactose and milk powder in fluidized bed dryer-crystallizer. *Dairy Science & Technology*, *91*(3), 323–340. doi:10.100713594-011-0015-8

Yoganandi, J., Mehta, B., Wadhwani, K. N., Darji, V. B., & Aparnathi, K. D. (2014). Comparison of physico-chemical properties of camel milk with cow milk and buffalo milk. *Journal of Camel Practice and Research*, *21*(2), 253–258. doi:10.5958/2277-8934.2014.00045.9

Yuksekdag, Z. N., Beyatli, Y., & Aslim, B. (2004). Determination of some characteristics coccoid forms of lactic acid bacteria isolated from Turkish kefirs with natural probiotic. *Lebensmittel-Wissenschaft + Technologie*, *37*(6), 663–667. doi:10.1016/j.lwt.2004.02.004

Zahedi, M., Salami, M., & Moslehishad, M. (2016). Fermented camel milk (Chal): Chemical, microbial and functional properties. *Journal of Pharmaceutical and Health Sciences*, *4*(3), 193–204.

Zayas, J. F. (1997). Foaming properties of proteins. In J.F. Zayas (Ed.), Functionality of proteins in food (pp. 260-309). Springer - Verlag. doi:10.1007/978-3-642-59116-7_6

Zibaee, S., Hosseini, S. M., Yousefi, M., Taghipour, A., Kiani, M. A., & Noras, M. R. (2015). Nutritional and Therapeutic Characteristics of Camel Milk in Children: A Systematic Review. *Electronic Physician*, *7*(7), 1523–1528. doi:10.19082/1523 PMID:26767108

Zouari, A., Perrone, T., Dolivet, A., Schuck, P., Gaucheron, F., Attia, H., & Ayadi, M. (2018). Physicochemical properties of spray dried camel milk powder: comparative study with cow milk powder. In *EuroDrying'2017 – In 6th European Drying Conference* (p. 19-21). Liège: Belgium: Academic Press.

Zubeir, I. (2015). Fluid milk processing and marketing for sustainable development of the camels' herders communities. *SUST Journal of Agricultural and Veterinary Sciences*, *16*(1), 1–13.

Chapter 6
Manufacture and Challenges of Camel Milk Cheese

Gaukhar Konuspayeva
Al-Farabi Kazakh National University, Kazakhstan

ABSTRACT

The difficulties in camel milk coagulation due to low concentration in κ-casein was the main obstacle for its processing into cheese. Thus, for 80 years, camel scientists concentrated their efforts on improving coagulation by different methods including use of plant or camel calf abomasum extracts. However, in all cases, poor cheese yield and organoleptic properties were obtained. The recent introduction of the CHY-Max – M1000®, on market solved the problem of clotting. Obtained by genetic engineering, this camel rennet allows high cheese yield. However, other challenges must be met: (1) investigation by fundamental studies of the "behavior" of camel milk during the different steps of cheese processing, (2) to set up final products corresponding to food preferences of local consumers, (3) to ensure transfer of camel cheese technology to camel dairy industry. Based on experiences in different camel countries, the chapter is taking stock of the challenges regarding technological development, cultural satisfaction, and commercialization of camel cheese.

INTRODUCTION

Cow, ewe, goat or buffalo milk was processed into cheese for centuries, or even millennium. At the reverse, despite the popularity of camel milk among pastoralists all over the world, traditional camel cheese has never existed. Camel milk is consumed in raw or fermented form in most of the camel milk producing countries. Especially, fermented milk as *shubat* (Kazakhstan), *khoormog* (Mongolia), *gariss* (Sudan) or *suussac* (Kenya) is the most common form for keeping camel milk beyond a few hours in the absence of a cold chain (see Chapter 3 and 5). Indeed, all along the history, camel milk was not processed into high variable dairy products in comparison to the milk from other dairy species (Faye & Konuspayeva, 2012).

The physio-chemical properties of camel milk make it difficult to coagulate, especially if bovine rennet is used as it has been done with the first trials (Ramet, 1989). Therefore, this difficulty to get a clot led researchers to focus their investigations first in order to find a technological solution, then in a

DOI: 10.4018/978-1-7998-1604-1.ch006

Table 1. Proportion of casein fractions in milk from different species

Species	κ-casein	α_{S1}-casein	α_{S2}-casein	β-casein	References
Bactrian	3.1 ± 1.9	36.1 ± 2.3	7.1 ± 1.5	53.7 ± 2.1	Ryskaliyeva, Henry., Miranda, Faye, Konuspayeva & Martin et al., 2018
Dromedary	3.6 ± 2.1	37.4 ± 3.9	5.8 ± 1.0	53.2 ± 3.5	Ryskaliyeva et al., 2018
Cow	15	40	5	40	McMahon & Brown, 1984
Goat	13	38	11	38	Boulanger, Grosclaude & Mahé, 1984
Ewe	9.1 – 10.8	33.9 – 39.9	12 – 16.4	37 – 42.3	Moatsou, Samolada, Katsabeki & Anifantakis, 2004
Buffalo	10.6	22.8	13.0	53.6	Feligini, Bonizzi, Buffoni, Consenza & Ramunno., 2009

second step, to understand the behavior of the matrix "camel milk" and its evolution under the effect of different starters. However, recent advances were obtained in camel cheese processing in different parts of the world. These recent and significant advances are presented in the present chapter.

Why Camel Milk Does Not Coagulate Traditionally?

Milk clotting is caused by the enzymatic hydrolysis of the protein bonds within the casein micelles causing aggregation of these micelles, then lead to the formation of curd. However, although the types of casein fractions in camel milk is comparable to that of cow's milk (see Chapter 2), the proportions of the different caseins are not similar (Table 1).

The low concentration of κ-casein in camel milk should be the main explanation (3-4% only against 13-15% in cow's milk according to Kappeler, Farah and Puhan, (2003) of its clotting difficulties (see Chapter 2). In addition, bovine chymosin (the main enzyme of the rennet) used in the dairy industry does not allow the optimal clotting of casein micelles of camel milk, leading to a weak curd for a similar time than for bovine milk (also see Chapter 10). Indeed, bovine rennet is cutting camel caseins at different locations than for cow milk leading to a slow reaction of the casein micelles bounds to constitute a clot.

THE FIRST CHALLENGE: GETTING FIRM COAGULUM

The difficulties to get a firm coagulum explain why most of the researches regarding camel cheese making was focused on the clotting step. The first tests achieved in the laboratory used bovine rennet with similar concentrations than that used for cow milk (Farah & Bachmann, 1987). The obtained coagulum was a precipitate in the form of flocks without clot. Moreover, the coagulation time for camel milk was 2-3 times longer than for cow milk and such difference persisted whatever the decreasing pH, increasing temperature or added calcium. The first large-scale work on the cheese-making capacity of camel milk was performed by J.P. Ramet, Professor at ENSAIA-Nancy (Ramet, 1989). To improve the coagulation of camel milk, this author used 3 components: (i) rennet extracted from cow-calf stomach, (ii) a coagulant preparation resulting from a mold classically used in the dairy industry *Rhizomucor miehei*, and (iii) chloride and calcium phosphate. But the amount of the rennet had to be 4 times more important than for the same amount of cow's milk, and the coagulum obtained was fragile and brittle

(Ramet, 1989). In consequence, the direct placing in molds was almost impossible due to a large loss of curd. Finally, a low cheese yield (number of liters of milk to get one kg of cheese) was obtained: 5-7% only depending on the type of cheese while cheese yield with cow milk is 10-12%. Moreover, the loss of fat in whey was 3 times more important than that in cow's milk, which led to less unctuous products in the mouth (Ramet, 1989).

Other tests carried out elsewhere at the same time faced the same problems (Mehaia, 1993); low yield, fat loss in whey, lower consumer acceptability. However, Ramet's work in 1989 led to the commercialization of a bovine-based preparation under the commercial name Camifloc®, made by the French company Bioserae©. This preparation was used by various researchers in the laboratory (Ramet, 2001; El-Zubeir & Jabreel, 2008; Ahmed & El-Zubeir, 2011) to test different types of cheese. It was distributed also in different development projects among camel pastoralists in Kenya, Mali, Mongolia and Niger (Vias et al., 2003; Faye & Vias, 2004). However, except for the cheese "caravan®" commercialized by the dairy plant Tiviski in Mauritania (Abeiderrahmane, 1997), Camifloc® was no longer used in the dairy industry.

In Algeria, several authors tested abomasum extracts from young or adult camel on the clotting activity of camel milk (Siboukeur, Mati & Hessas, 2005), the best clotting activity being obtained with extracts from adult camel (Boudjenah-Haroun et al. 2011). However, this method requires to collect a large amount of abomasum at slaughterhouse and is difficult to spread it at the industrial level. Moreover, the cheese yield and the acceptability of the final product were not assessed.

Due also to the difficulty to provide remote areas in such Camifloc® preparation, several scientists tested other coagulants easily available on the local market or in the proximate environment. It includes the use of plant extracts, for example, in Ethiopia, Hailu, Hansen, Seifu, Eshetu and Ipsena (2014) used extracts of ginger (*Zingiber officinale*), but the yield was still low compared to cow milk (8.7±1.2%) and the acceptability by consumers was not optimal. Clotting activity of extracts from *Moringa oleifera* was also tested in Ethiopia (Terefe, Kebede & Kebede, 2017) with an apparent good curd firmness at pH 5, 65°C temperature and partially purified extract concentration of 10% for both seeds and leaves. However, no data on cheese yield was reported. Acid coagulation was also tested with acetic acid (Mohamed, Babiker & Mohamed, 2013), citric acid (Mal, Biakhat, Suchitra, Sena & Pathak, 2010) or directly lemon juice (Mihretie, Tadesse, Amakelew & Fikru, 2018) but with obvious consequences on the organoleptic properties of the final product. The addition of calcium chloride and hydrogen phosphate dehydrate in acid-induced gel was investigated. The results showed that the comparative storage modulus (measuring the strength rigidity of the gel) and loss modulus (measuring the resistance to deformation) of camel milk gels were significantly lower than those of cow milk gels despite the slight improvement with the addition of calcium chloride (Kamal, Foukani & Karoui, 2017a). Enzymatic extract from kaolin layer in chicken gizzard was also tested (Hamidi, Choukri & Hachi, 2017) with a good apparent cheese yield (12.2±1.2%) with a certain between-breed variability, but the acceptability of the cheese was not assessed. In summary, getting a coagulum is not enough to get cheese.

The solution to getting a firm curd was found as a result of the fundamental study of Kappeler et al., (2006) in Switzerland on the sequencing of camel chymosin. By introducing the coding gene for camel chymosin into a mold (*Aspergillus Niger*), it was possible to obtain a specific recombinant enzyme for camel milk, having much better coagulant properties not only for camel milk but also for bovine milk. Indeed, camel chymosin appeared to have a 70% higher clotting activity toward cow milk (Kappeler et al., 2006) due to some molecular specificities (Sorensen, Palmer, Qvist & Schiott, 2011). This recombinant enzyme was produced later at the industrial scale and commercialized from 2008 under the trade name Chymax-M1000® by Chr. Hansen ©. Therefore, the cheese yield could be compared to that obtained with cow's or small ruminants' milk and the quality of the coagulum (firmness) better compatible with a quality cheese processing. The performance of this camel rennet was assessed also to make cow cheese showing a comparative efficiency with bovine rennet (Alinovi et al., 2018; Gumus & Hayaloglu, 2019). However, even if the challenge for getting firm clotting of camel milk was finally achieved, is it possible to make "good" camel cheeses that meet the tastes of consumers? It was the second challenge for researchers.

A SECOND CHALLENGE: CAMEL CHEESE PROCESSING AT LARGE-SCALE INDUSTRY

In most cases, the manufacture of camel cheese was achieved by researchers in their laboratory (Ahmed & El-Zubeir, 2011; Mohamed et al. 2013) rather than by professional cheese technicians at small or industrial scale with few exceptions (Jones-Abeiderrhamane, 2013). The challenge nowadays for the camel dairy industry and the researchers is to define the adapted technologies for a large-scale cheese processing in order to respond to consumers' demand. Indeed, the camel "protein-lipid matrix" behavior differs widely from other milk used in the cheese industry. Different technological parameters have been tested to determine cheese properties using gruyere (Konuspayeva, Faye, Baubekova & Loiseau, 2012), mozzarella (Konuspayeva, Camier, Gaucheron & Faye, 2014a), feta and halloumi technologies (Konuspayeva et al., 2017), but the final product has proved to be different from what was expected in terms of texture, taste and flavor. Therefore, it is essential to understand the behavior of the "camel milk" matrix during cheese processing, but also to adapt the cheese technology to get product corresponding to the consumers' tastes and to organize the diffusion of the camel milk manufacturing technologies at a large scale to get camel cheese out of the laboratories.

Understanding the "Behavior" of Camel Milk

Getting coagulum is the first step in cheese processing. The processes of acidification, renneting draining, brining, syneresis and possible thermal treatments also require thorough investigation to understand the behavior of camel milk during the various stages leading liquid milk to cheese. Due to the recent achievement of camel cheese, rheological studies were performed on few occasions (Shahein, Hassanein & Zayan, 2014; Hailu et al., 2016; Soltani, Boran & Hayaloglu, 2016; Ayyash, Abu-Jdayil, Hamed & Shaker, 2018; Hailu et al., 2018).). Some texture measurements of soft camel cheese for assessing hardness (resistance to compression expressed as Newton) or adhesiveness (expressed as Newton second) were recently described (Mohammed et al., 2019). Mostly, the studies indicated that firmness of soft cheese was increased at both 4°C and 18°C storage temperatures for 22 days but then decreased. The adhesiveness of cheese samples stored at refrigerated temperature also significantly increased as storage time progressed (Mohammed *et al.*, 2019). Comparing various blends of milk coagulants (*Rhizomucor miehei* protease and camel chymosin) on microstructure and rheological properties of Iranian white cheese ripened over 90 days, Soltani et al. (2016), reported a more compact protein network and firmer structure in the cheeses made with camel chymosin. Increasing levels of camel chymosin in the coagulant blends provided less protein breakdown and a more solid-like viscoelastic structure. The pre-heating of camel milk at 50°C affected negatively the gelation properties, and at 70°C prevented the formation of rennet-induced milk gels while no effect was observed on the gelation properties of cow milk gels (Kamal, Foukani, & Karoui, 2017b). Such results emphasize the difficulties to get camel cheese with pasteurized milk. The effect of different processing methods on camel milk composition will be discussed in Chapter 10.

To compare the behavior of camel with cow milk during cheese processing, Konuspayeva et al. 2017 used adjusted cow milk to obtain similar fat and total nitrogen concentrations. They got similar cheese raw yields (7.4±0.15 vs 7.3±0.55 kg/100 kg for camel and cow milk, respectively). The total nitrogen recovery appeared higher in camel cheese and fat recovery was higher in cow cheese while calcium recovery was the same in both kinds cheese. Moreover, in camel whey, fat and total nitrogen content were higher (9.0±1.73 g/ kg and 9.21±0.23 g/ kg, respectively) than in cow whey (7.7±1.61 g/ kg and 7.30±0.02 g/ kg, respectively) despite similar dry matter (68.9± 3.2 and 68.1± 1.15% in camel and cow whey, respectively).

Another point to be investigated is the rate of curd syneresis (Camier, Beaucher, Gaucheron, Konuspayeva & Faye, 2014). In cow milk, after curd formation, ripening is starting and crust is appearing, and no wetter lost is observed. In the camel curd, crust formation is very weak, and serum is continuously going out of the curd which becomes too dry for correct ripening (personal observation). Probably, this property can be seen in a positive way (for example to make Feta type cheese which requires more humidity) and could be used to find better cheese type made from camel milk.

One of the technological difficulties associated with camel milk is its slow acidification (10 hours to decrease from pH 6.6 to 5) compared to cow's milk (Farah & Bachmann, 1997), even if it can be improved at 36°C compared to 20°C (Konuspayeva *et al*, 2014a). It is, therefore, necessary to use starters with high-acidifying power (for example thermophilic starters containing *Lactobacillus helveticus*, and *Lactobacillus lactis* or *Streptococcus thermophilus*) allowing rapid acidification to strengthen the coagulum (Konuspayeva *et al.*, 2014). Globally, few types of lactic starters have been tested in the literature and they are all starters used for cow's milk (Konuspayeva *et al.*, 2014a). Some studies were carried out on the identification of the specific lactic flora of camel milk (Akhmetsadykova *et al.*, 2015), but their potential use in the manufacture of cheeses having typicality proper to camel milk was never explored. Yet, studies on camel milk microflora would be of high interest for different reasons: (i) to identify the strains specific to camel milk able to provide specific aroma for camel cheese, (ii) to contribute to the knowledge of the lactic bacteria biodiversity as a large number of microorganisms in camel milk was not identified (Jans, Bugnard, Njage, Lacroix & Meile, 2012; Akhmesadykova *et al.*, 2015), (iii) to develop a large variety of camel cheese. The microbial aspect of lactic acid bacteria isolated from camel milk was discussed in details in Chapter 4.

The impact of the lactation stage was evaluated, which allowed to give 25 postpartum days as the minimum limit from which the camel milk can coagulate optimally. In addition, the use of camel chymosin does not require the addition of phosphate or calcium chloride, as no effect was observed (Konuspayeva et al., 2014a) contrary to acid-induced gelation (Kamal et al., 2017a) and contrary to cow milk (Wolfschoon, 1997).

To our knowledge, no analysis of volatile organic compounds responsible for flavor was undertaken for camel cheese while it is achieved regularly in cow cheese (Gioacchini, De Santi, Guescini, Brandi & Stocchi, 2010). However, recently, aroma compounds formed in soft ripened camel milk cheese were investigated, showing that those aroma were affected by ripening time, coagulant and NaCl levels (Hailu et al., 2018). Therefore, many fields of investigation need to be implemented by basic research for better control of camel cheese processing.

Products that Meet the Needs of Consumers

As well in Saudi Arabia (Konuspayeva et al., 2012, 2014a, 2014b and 2015) as in Mauritania (Jones-Abeiderrhamane, 2013), the temptation was great to make cheeses resembling to the known cow cheeses like Camembert, Gruyere, Tomme, Feta, Mozzarella or Saint-Paulin. However, most of the time, the results were disappointing because of the specific properties of camel milk as mentioned above. Overall, the acceptance of these products by local consumers who are not accustomed to consuming "typed" cheeses like for example consumers from southern Europe, could be an important constraint for the development of a local market. So, the orientation was made towards cheeses with a rather neutral taste (feta or halloumi type) requiring no ripening and closer to consumption habits of local people (Konuspayeva et al., 2017), especially in the Middle East, where successful cheeses are closed to spreadable cheese ("vache-qui-rit" © type) or white soft cheese. Some proposals for setting up spreadable cheese (El-Sayed, El-Shafei & Khalifa, 2018) or white soft cheese (El-Zubeir, & Jabreel, 2008) were done in the literature (figure 1 and 2), but the acceptability was variable and required often to mix with milk (Qadeer, Huma, Sameen & Iqbal, 2015) or cheese (El-Sayed et al., 2018) from other species to improve the organoleptic properties.

However, as said above, most laboratory tests have not resulted in scale production, and few studies were achieved on the sensory analysis of camel cheeses. Moreover, few publications are based on trained panels of tasters, accustomed or not to the consumption of cheese (Konuspayeva et al., 2017). The challenge now for the camel cheese makers is to find the best cheese allowing a popular acceptation of the products, not only for degustation of the cheese itself, but also to integrate it in different local recipes or special culinary preparations. Such investigations are necessary to ensure a convenient cheese production development at a larger scale.

Industrial Development and Future Trend

For the moment, camel milk production does not go out of its marginality. Few initiatives have emerged outside the laboratory tests. Tiviski dairy plant in Mauritania, a pioneer in this field, produces its cheese on-demand only due to the narrowness of its internal market and its difficulties in export (Jones-Abeiderrhamane, 2013). The cheese made in the Camelicious farm in Dubai is using traditional acid-induced coagulation technology (using lemon juice) with unconvincing organoleptic results. In Morocco, Egypt or Tunisia, the marketing of fresh white cheeses is remaining confidential and the products offered are of varying quality. In Saudi Arabia, although industrial dairy testing has been conducted and training of technologists from dairy plants was performed (Faye & Konuspayeva, 2014), development towards the private sector remained limited (Konuspayeva et al., 2017).

In fact, the diffusion of camel cheese faces two main constraints:

- Beyond the technological difficulties widely mentioned above, the hygienic quality of the milk used for cheese processing remains an important challenge, especially as the use of pasteurized camel milk leads to clotting difficulties, that makes raw milk preferred (personal observation). Indeed, several surveys showed that the hygienic status of raw camel milk is often insufficient. For example, in Kenya, Kaindi et al., (2011) reported that 75% of bulked camel milk at the final market exceeded the acceptable limit of 10^6CFU/ml for the total bacterial count and 5 x 10^4 cfu/ml for the enterobacteria. In Ethiopia, Adugna, Seifu, Kededed & Doluschitze, 2013 observed total bacterial

Figure 1. Technological chain of preparation of soft cheese from camel milk ("Feta" technology from after Konuspayeva et al., 2017)

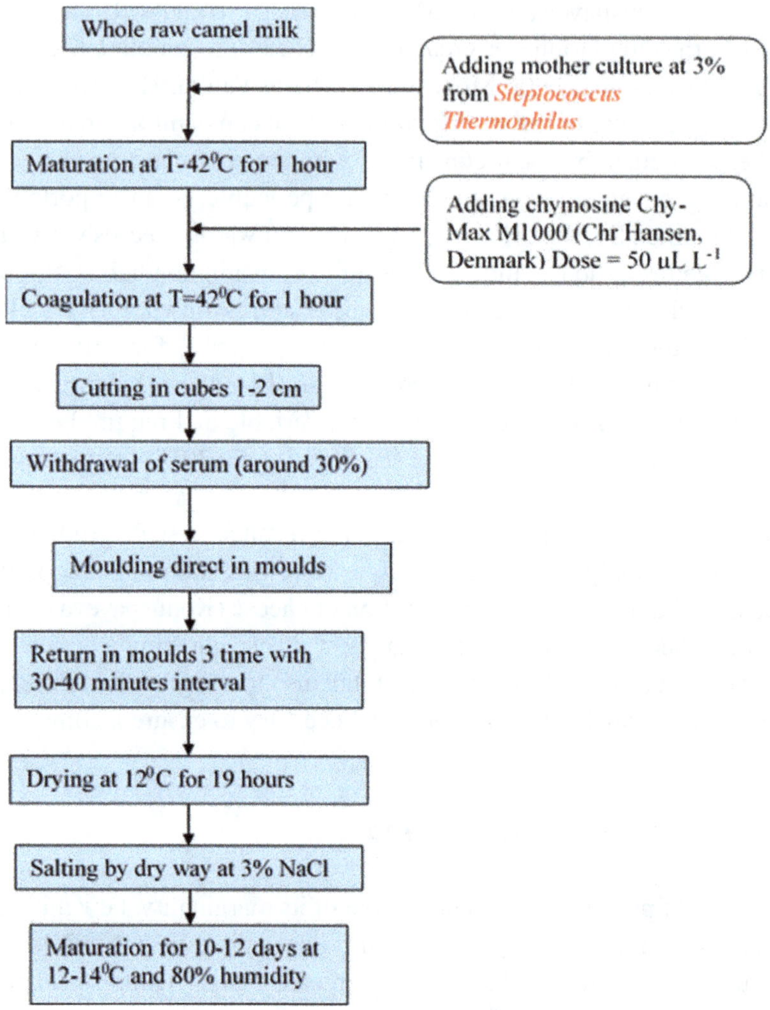

count and coliform of log 5.2± 1.9 and 2.9± 2.3 CFU/ml respectively which shows insufficient hygiene. The poor hygienic status of camel milk is linked to bad milking practices (Tourette, Messad & Faye, 2002) but also to the conditions of storage and transport (Yam, Khomeiri, Mahounak & Jafari, 2014). The manufacture of camel cheese according to halloumi technology (Konuspayeva et al, 2017) is an interesting alternative for processing low contaminated milk because in the final phase of the cheese making, the product undergoes heat treatment. Indeed, the coagulum is pasteurized in whey at 80°C during processing.

- However, the main difficulty is probably linked to the cost of the final product. The price of camel milk is high, often 2 to 3 times more than cow's milk. In Algeria, it could reach almost 10 times of cow milk's price (Faye, Jaouad, Bhrawi, Senoussi & Bengoumi, 2014). Even if cheese yield is nowadays comparable to that of other kinds of milk, the cost of the raw material used to make cheese contributes to increasing significantly the price of the cheese. Except in the Gulf

Figure 2. Technological chain of preparation of hard cheese from camel milk ("gruyere" technology from after Konuspayeva et al., 2012)

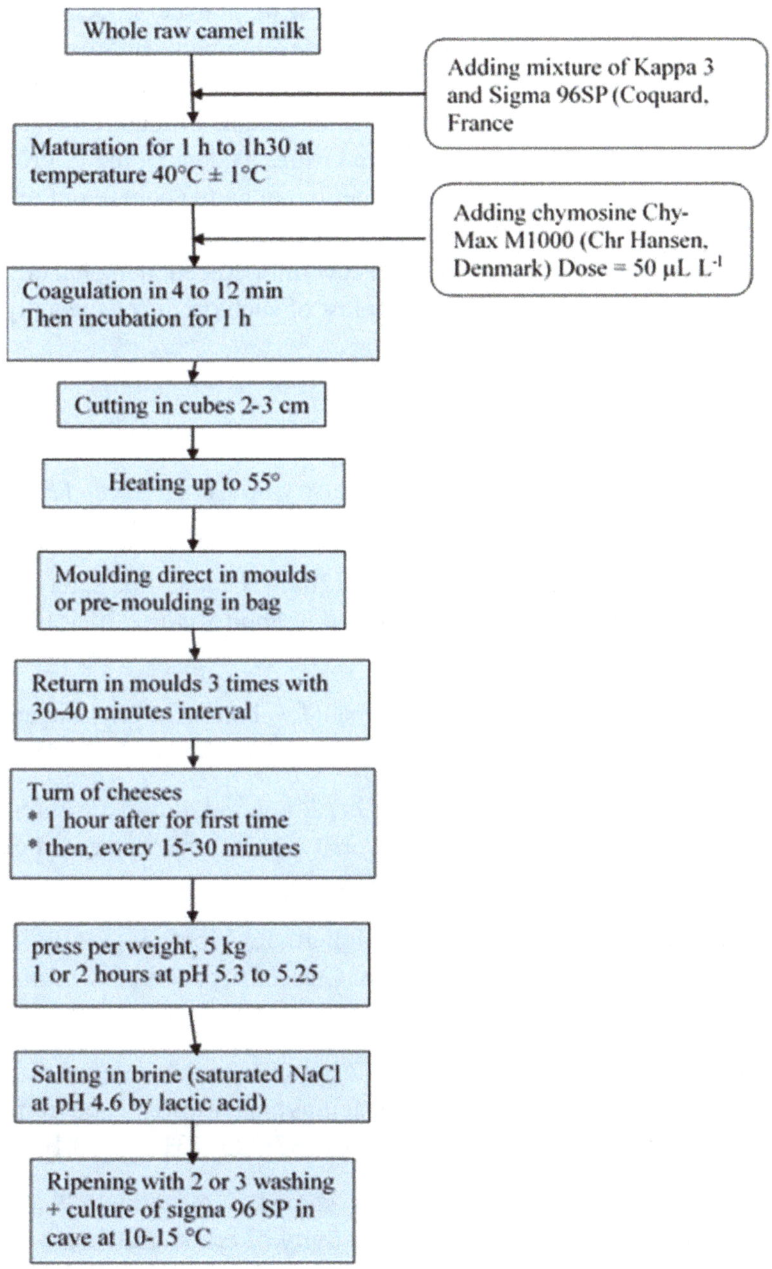

countries, producers of camel milk are living often in poor countries or in marginalized areas. Therefore, camel Cheese remains almost a luxury product, affordable only with low weight packaging. Moreover, its export to the western countries is confronted with sanitary barriers as shown in the example of the dairy plant Tiviski in Mauritania (Grandval, 2012).

CONCLUSION

If the cheese made from cow or sheep's milk can avail itself of an experience of several millennia, the camel cheese is only at the beginning of its history and its development. But to do this, if recent technological advances have been made, it is important today to fill gaps in the knowledge of the different steps at cheese processing in order to meet better the cultural and financial requirements of consumers. The ' exoticism ' of the camel cheese will be not enough to ensure its development. Producers, developers, dairy plants managers, and scientists must work together to put camel cheese out of its present marginality. One way for solving the problem of the high cost of camel cheese could be the valorization of the whey, which contains more valuable components than cow milk. Recent personal observations achieved in Mauritania show the nutritive and organoleptic interest of such product especially in arid lands.

REFERENCES

Abeiderrahmane, N. (1997). Camel milk and modern industry. *Journal of Camel Practice and Research*, *4*(2), 223–228.

Adugna, M., Seifu, E., Kebeded, A., & Doluschitze, R. (2013). Quality and safety of camel milk along the value chain in Eastern Ethiopia. *International Journal of Food Studies*, *2*(2), 150–157. doi:10.7455/ijfs/2.2.2013.a2

Ahmed, N. A. A., & El-Zubeir, E. M. (2011). Effect of salt level on some physical and chemical properties and acceptability of camel milk cheese. *Journal of Camelid Science*, *4*, 40–48.

Akhmetsadykova, Sh., Baubekova, A., Konuspayeva, G., Akhmetsadykov, N., Akhmetsadykov, N., Faye, B., & Loiseau, G. (2015). Lactic acid bacteria biodiversity in raw and fermented camel milk. *African Journal of Food Science and Technology*, *6*(3), 84–88.

Alinovi, M., Cordioli, M., Francolino, S., Locci, F., Ghiglietti, R., Monti, L., ... Giraffa, G. (2018). Effect of fermentation-produced camel chymosin on quality of Crescenza cheese. *International Dairy Journal*, *84*, 72–78. doi:10.1016/j.idairyj.2018.04.001

Ayyash, M., Abu-Jdayil, B., Hamed, F., & Shaker, R. (2018). Rheological, textural, microstructural and sensory impact of exopolysaccharide-producing Lactobacillus plantarum isolated from camel milk on low-fat akawi cheese. *Lebensmittel-Wissenschaft + Technologie*, *87*, 423–431. doi:10.1016/j.lwt.2017.09.023

Boudjenah-Haroun, S., Laleye, L., Moulti-Mati, F., Si Ahmed, S., Mahboub, N., Siboukeur, O. E., & Mati, A. (2011). Comparative study of milk clotting activity of crude gastric enzymes extracted from camels' abomasum at different ages and commercial enzymes (rennet and pepsin) on bovine and camel milk. *Emirates Journal of Food and Agriculture*, *23*, 301–310.

Boulanger, A., Grosclaude, F., & Mahé, M. F. (1984). Polymorphisme des caséines αs1 et αs2 de la chèvre (Capra hircus). *Génétique, Sélection. Evolution; International Journal of Organic Evolution*, *16*(2), 157–176.

Camier, B., Beaucher, E., Gaucheron, F., Konuspayeva, G., & Faye, B. (2014). Fabrication et caractérisation physico-chimique d'un fromage « blanc » fabriqué à partir de lait de chamelle-une comparaison avec le lait de vache. Actes des 1ères rencontres internationales "le lait, vecteur de développement", 105.

El-Sayed, M. A., El-Shafei, S. M. S., & Khalifa, S. A. (2018). Manufacture of processed cheese spread from camel cheese based: Evaluation of cheese characteristics. *American Journal of Food Science and Nutrition Research*, *5*(4), 76–86.

El-Zubeir, I. E. M., & Jabreel, S. O. (2008). Fresh cheese from camel milk coagulated with Camifloc. *International Journal of Dairy Technology*, *61*(1), 90–95. doi:10.1111/j.1471-0307.2008.00360.x

Farah, Z., & Bachmann, M. R. (1987). Rennet coagulation properties of camel milk. *Milchwissenschaft. Milk Science International*, *42*, 689–692.

Faye, B., Jaouad, J., Bhrawi, K., Senoussi, A., & Bengoumi, M. (2014). Elevage camelin en Afrique du Nord: État des lieux et perspectives. *Revue d'Élevage et de Médecine Vétérinaire des Pays Tropicaux*, *67*(4), 213–221. doi:10.19182/remvt.20563

Faye, B., & Konuspayeva, G. (2012). The sustainability challenge of the dairy sector- The growing importance of the non-cattle milk production worldwide. *International Dairy Journal*, *24*(2), 50–56. doi:10.1016/j.idairyj.2011.12.011

Faye, B., & Konuspayeva, G. (2015). *Camel cheese making workshop: short report. Rapport FAO, projet UTF/SAU/044/SAU*. Riyadh: FAO Publ.

Faye, B., & Vias, G. (2004). Scientific support of the camel sub-sector development project in Niger. *Proceedings of International Conference. On « Saving the camel and peoples' livelihood »*, 64-70.

Feligini, M., Bonizzi, I., Buffoni, J. N., Consenza, G., & Ramunno, L. (2009). Identification and quantification of α-s1, α-s2, β, and κ-caseins in water buffalo milk by reverse phase-high performance liquid chromatography and mass spectrometry. *Journal of Agricultural and Food Chemistry*, *57*(7), 2988–2992. doi:10.1021/jf803653v PMID:19256489

Genene, A., Hansen, E., Eshetu, M., Hailu, Y., & Ipsen, R. (2019). Effect of heat treatment on denaturation of whey protein and resultant rennetability of camel milk. *LWT*, *101*, 404–409. doi:10.1016/j.lwt.2018.11.047

Gioacchini, A. M., De Santi, M., Guescini, M., Brandi, G., & Stocchi, V. (2010). Characterization of the volatile organic compounds of Italian 'Fossa' cheese by solid-phase microextraction gas chromatography/mass spectrometry. *Rapid Communications in Mass Spectrometry*, *24*(23), 3405–3412. doi:10.1002/rcm.4782 PMID:21072795

Grandval, F. (2012). Tiviski: une entreprise de valorisation du lait local en Mauritanie. *Inter-réseaux, développement rural*, 5. Retrieved from http://www.inter-reseaux.org/IMG/pdf/Note_Tiviski_final.pdf

Gumus, P., & Hayaloglu, A. A. (2019). Effects of blends of camel and calf chymosin on proteolysis, residual coagulant activity, microstructure, and sensory characteristics of Beyaz peynir. *Journal of Dairy Science*, *102*(7), 5945–5956. doi:10.3168/jds.2018-15671 PMID:31079909

Hailu, Y., Hansen, E., Seifu, Y., Eshetu, M., Agerlin, M., Petersen, M. A., ... Ipsen, R. (2018). Rheological and sensory properties and aroma compounds formed during ripening of soft brined cheese made from camel milk. *International Dairy Journal, 81*, 122–130. doi:10.1016/j.idairyj.2018.01.007

Hailu, Y., Hansen, E. B., Seifu, E., Eshetu, M., & Ipsena, R. (2016). Factors influencing the gelation and rennetability of camel milk using camel chymosin. *International Dairy Journal, 60*, 62–69. doi:10.1016/j.idairyj.2016.01.013

Hailu, Y., Seifu, E., & Yilma, Z. (2014). Physicochemical properties and consumer acceptability of soft unripened cheese made from camel milk using crude extract of ginger (*Zingiber officinale*) as coagulant. *African Journal of Food Science, 8*(2), 87–91. doi:10.5897/AJFS2013.1102

Hamidi, M., Choukri, A., & Hachi, M. (2017). Influence de la race cameline sur la production fromagère avec un extrait de kaolin du gésier de poulet en Algérie; étude préliminaire. *Livestock Research for Development, 29*(5). Retrieved from http://www.lrrd.org/lrrd29/5/med29085.html

Jans, C., Bugnard, J., Njage, P., Lacroix, C., & Meile, L. (2012). Lactic acid bacteria diversity of African raw and fermented camel milk products reveals a highly competitive, potentially health-threatening predominant. *Lebensmittel-Wissenschaft + Technologie, 47*(2), 371–379. doi:10.1016/j.lwt.2012.01.034

Jones-Abeiderrhamane, N. (2013). *Camel cheese: seemed like a good idea*. Nouakchott, Mauritania: Nancy Jones-Abeiderrahmane.

Kaindi, D.W.M., Schelling, E., Wangoh, J., Imungi, J.K., Farah, Z. & Meile, L. (2011). Microbiological quality of raw camel milk across the Kenya market chain. *Food, 5*(1), 79-83.

Kamal, M., Foukani, M., & Karoui, R. (2017a). Rheological and physical properties of camel and cow milk gels enriched with phosphate and calcium during acid-induced gelation. *Journal of Food Science and Technology, 54*(2), 439–446. doi:10.100713197-016-2480-9 PMID:28242943

Kamal, M., Foukani, M., & Karoui, R. (2017b). Effects of heating and calcium and phosphate mineral supplementation on the physical properties of rennet-induced coagulation of camel and cow milk gels. *The Journal of Dairy Research, 84*(2), 220–228. doi:10.1017/S0022029917000152 PMID:28524011

Kappeler, S., Farah, Z., & Puhan, Z. (2003). 5′-Flanking regions of camel milk genes are highly similar to homologue regions of other species and can be divided into two distinct groups. *Journal of Dairy Science, 86*(2), 498–508. doi:10.3168/jds.S0022-0302(03)73628-5 PMID:12647956

Kappeler, S. R., Van den Brink, H. J., Rahbek-Nielsen, H., Farah, Z., Puhan, Z., Hansen, E. B., & Johansen, E. (2006). Characterizations of recombinant camel chymosin reveals superior properties for the coagulation of bovine and camel milk. *Biochemical and Biophysical Research Communications, 342*(2), 647–654. doi:10.1016/j.bbrc.2006.02.014 PMID:16488399

Konuspayeva, G., Al-Hammad, K., Algruin, K., Alshammari, F., Al-Rasheedi, F. S., & Faye, B. (2015). Manufacturing camel cheese: the experience of Saudi Arabia. *Scientific and Practical Journal Veterinariya, 2*(42), 203-205.

Konuspayeva, G., Camier, B., Aleilawi, N., Al-Shumeimyri, M., Al-Hammad, K., Algruin, K., ... Faye, B. (2017). Manufacture of dry- and brine-salted soft camel cheeses for the camel dairy industry. *International Journal of Dairy Technology*, *70*(1), 92–101. doi:10.1111/1471-0307.12319

Konuspayeva, G., Camier, B., Gaucheron, F., & Faye, B. (2014a). Some parameters to process camel milk into cheese. *Emirates Journal of Food and Agriculture*, *26*(4), 354–358. doi:10.9755/ejfa.v26i4.17277

Konuspayeva, G., Faye, B., Baubekova, A., & Loiseau, G. (2012). Camel gruyere cheese making. *Proceedings of the 3rd ISOCARD conference*, 218-219.

Konuspayeva, G., Shomamrey, M., Aleliwi, N., Camier, B. & Faye, B. (2014b). New trials to make camel mozzarella. *Bulletin of Al-Farabi University, Série biologie*, *1/2*(60), 138-140.

Mal, G., Bjakhat, C., Suchitra Sena, D., & Pathak, K. M. L. (2010). Effect of coagulants on preparation of camel milk paneer. *Journal of Camel Practice and Research*, *17*(2), 181–184.

Mc Mahon, D. J., & Brown, R. J. (1984). Composition, structure and integrity of casein micelles: A review. *Journal of Dairy Science*, *67*(3), 499–512. doi:10.3168/jds.S0022-0302(84)81332-6

Mehaia, M. A. (1993). Fresh soft white cheese (Domiati-type) from camel milk: Composition yield and sensory evaluation. *Journal of Dairy Science*, *76*(10), 2845–2855. doi:10.3168/jds.S0022-0302(93)77623-7

Mihretie, Y., Tadesse, N., Amakelew, S., & Fikru, S. (2018). Cheese production from camel milk using lemon juice as a coagulant. *Journal of Environmental and Agricultural Sciences*, *17*, 11–19.

Moatsou, G., Samolada, M., Katsabeki, A., & Anifantakis, E. (2004). Casein fraction of ovine milk from indigenous Greek breeds. *Dairy Science & Technology*, *84*(3), 285–296. doi:10.1051/lait:2004006

Mohamed, A. E., Babiker, I. A., & Mohamed, T. E. (2013). Preparation of fresh soft cheese from dromedary camel milk using acid and heat method. *Research Opinions in Animal & Veterinary Sciences*, *3*, 289–292.

Mohammed, S., Eshetu, M., Tadesse, Y., & Hailu, Y. (2019). Rheological properties and shelf life of soft cheese made from camel milk using camel chymosin. *Journal of Dairy & Veterinary Sciences*, *10*(4), 555794. doi:10.19080/JDVS.2019.10.555794

Qadeer, Z., Huma, N., Sameen, A., & Iqbal, T. (2015). Camel milk cheese: Optimization of processing conditions. *Journal of Camelid Science*, *8*, 18–25.

Ramet, J. P. (1989). L'aptitude fromagère du lait de dromadaire. *Revue d'Élevage et de Médecine Vétérinaire des Pays Tropicaux*, *42*(1), 105–111.

Ramet, J. P. (2001). The technology of making cheese from camel milk (Camelus dromedarius). In *Animal production and health paper n°113*. Rome, Italy: FAO.

Ryskaliyeva, A., Henry, C., Miranda, G., Faye, B., Konuspayeva, G., & Martin, P. (2018). Combining different proteomic approaches to resolve complexity of the milk protein fraction of dromedary, Bactrian camels and hybrids, from different regions of Kazakhstan. *PLoS One*, *13*(5), e0197026. doi:10.1371/journal.pone.0197026 PMID:29746547

Shahein, M. R., Hassanein, A. M., & Zayan, A. F. (2014). Evaluation of soft cheese manufactured from camel and buffalo milk. *World Journal of Dairy Food Science*, *9*(2), 213–219.

Siboukeur, O., Mati, A., & Hessas, B. (2005). Amélioration de l'aptitude à la coagulation du lait cameline (Camelus dromedarius): Utilisation d'extraits enzymatiques coagulants gastriques de dromadaires. *Cahiers Agricultures*, *14*(5), 473–478.

Soltani, M., Boran, O. S., & Hayaloglu, A. A. (2016). Effect of various blends of camel chymosin and microbial rennet (*Rhizomucor miehei*) on microstructure and rheological properties of Iranian UF White cheese. *Lebensmittel-Wissenschaft + Technologie*, *68*, 724–728. doi:10.1016/j.lwt.2016.01.028

Sorensen, J., Palmer, D. S., Qvist, K. B., & Schiott, B. (2011). Initial stage of cheese production: A molecular modeling study of bovine and camel chymosin complexed with peptides from the chymosin-sensitive region of κ-casein. *Journal of Agricultural and Food Chemistry*, *59*(10), 5636–5647. doi:10.1021/jf104898w PMID:21476511

Terefe, M. A., Kebede, A., & Kebede, M. (2017). Clotting Activities of Partially Purified Extracts of *Moringa oleifera L.* on Dromedary Camel Milk. *East African Journal of Sciences*, *11*(2), 117–128.

Tourette, I., Messad, S., & Faye, B. (2002). Impact des pratiques de traite des éleveurs sur la qualité sanitaire du lait de chamelle en Mauritanie. *Revue d'Élevage et de Médecine Vétérinaire des Pays Tropicaux*, *55*(3), 229–233. doi:10.19182/remvt.9827

Vias, G., Bonfoh, B., Garba, M., Ilou, I., Kamil, H., & Faye, B. (2003). Valorisation du lait de chamelle au Sahel: opération " fromages camélins " dans le Tadsit (Niger) et à Tombouctou (Mali). Séminaire sous-régional " lait sain pour le Sahel ", 24 fev.-3 mars 2003, Bamako. *Etudes et recherches sahéliennes, 8-9*, 39-46.

Wolfschoon, A. (1997). Influence of calcium chloride addition to milk on the cheese yield. *International Dairy Journal*, *7*(4), 249–254. doi:10.1016/S0958-6946(97)00005-8

Yam, B. A. Z., Khomeiri, M., Mahounak, A. S., & Jafari, S. M. (2014). Hygienic Quality of Camel Milk and Fermented Camel Milk (Chal) in Golestan Province, Iran. *Journal of Microbiology Research (Rosemead, Calif.)*, *4*(2), 98–103.

Chapter 7
Exploring Potential Therapeutic Properties of Camel Milk

Omar Amin Alhaj
University of Petra, Jordan

ABSTRACT

This chapter highlights the potential health benefits of camel milk including antioxidant, anti-cancer activity, antihypertensive properties, antidiabetic activity, antimicrobial activity, hypoallergenicity activity, and anti-Crohn's disease. In addition to the most recent identified functional properties of camel milk. The bioactivity of conjugated linoleic acid (CLA), D and L amino acid, as well as oligosaccharide in camel milk will be also discussed. The proposed mechanisms behind these properties and potential health benefits are explained. This chapter also describes composition and nutritive value of camel milk and their association to functional properties. The current available information in the literature on camel milk is covered too.

INTRODUCTION

Over thousands of years, food has provided energy and nutrients to sustain life. During the last few decades, human dietary behaviour has changed and become more informative and complex. This change has been accompanied with a change in life style, food hygiene, with more emphasis to reduce the use of artificial additives including antimicrobial agents and the use of antibiotics and other antimicrobial substances, hence a new concept of food has been introduced to provide nutritious food with certain functionality to improve human health and welfare.

Traditional foods are those that are usually eaten to fulfil basic nutrients to body as well as cultural and social wellbeing; while functional foods are those, which provide health benefits beyond basic nutritional needs by virtue of some ingredients. The term (functional food) emerged in the middle of last century (Doyon, 2008). Camel milk has been used by the locals in Somalia for its perceived health benefits such as tuberculosis, fever, malaria and many others illnesses without real evidence for its real health benefits (Asresie & Yusuf, 2014). The Food and Agricultural Organization statistics (FAOSTAT) in 2019 reported that the annual production value of camel milk worldwide in US$ doubled between

DOI: 10.4018/978-1-7998-1604-1.ch007

2006 to 2016, and expected to increase in the future as shown in Figure 1. This chapter aims to study the potential health benefits of camel milk including antioxidant, anti-cancer activity, antihypertensive properties, anti-diabetic activity, antimicrobial activity, hypoallergenicity activity, and anti-Crohn's disease.

BACKGROUND

Camel Milk Composition

Long time ago, camel milk has been used as essential food in arid regions worldwide. Camel milk is described as an opaque-white, frothy, indeed have a sweet, sharp, and salty in taste (Al haj & Al Kanhal, 2010). This sense of taste description is general and varies slightly according to the type of feed and water accessibility (Farah, 1996). For example, when camel has free access to water, the water content of camel milk corresponds to 87% (Sisay & Awoke, 2015). Conversely, when water is scarce, the water content of camel milk increases to 91% due to the secretion of antidiuretic hormone, decrease of fat content, and type of eaten forage (FAO, 2013).

The major components of camel milk proteins are casein (β-casein followed by αs1-casein, and αs2-casein), and whey protein (α-lactalbumin (α-LA), lacto(trans)ferrin(LF), and lactophorin (Groenen, Dijkhof, & Van der Poel, 1995), peptidoglycan acidic protein (Kappeler, Heuberger, Farah, & Puhan, 2004; Sharma et al., 2011), whey acidic protein (WAP), glycosylation-dependent cell adhesion molecule 1 (GlyCAM-1, lactophorin, PP3), in addition to peptidoglycan recognition protein short variant (PGRP-S), lactoperoxidase (LP), and obviously immunoglobulins (Kappeler, Farah, & Puhan, 1998). Additionally, camel milk contains the immune proteins peptidoglycan recognition protein (PGRP), lactoferrin, lysozyme, and lactoperoxidase, and insulin-like compounds (Gul, Farooq, Anees, Khan, & Rehan, 2015). Moreover, annotated genome sequences have been published for camels, and can be utilized for proteomic analysis (Wu et al. 2014). Compared to other mammalian milks, camel milk shows

Figure 1. The gross production of whole fresh camel milk (estimated as current million USD) change between 1991 to 2016 (FAOSTAT, 2019). Reproduced with permission of Food and Agriculture Organization of the United Nations.

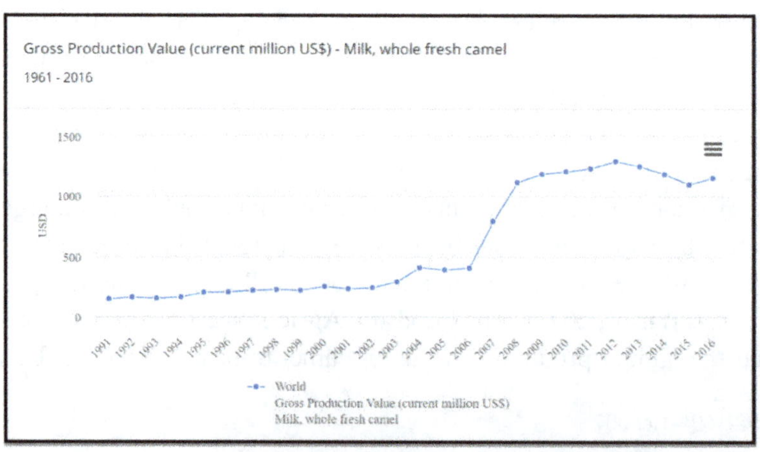

some similarities and differences in their composition, specifically in the content of β-Lactoglobulin, β-casein, κ-casein and αs-casein contents (see Chapter 2).

The variation in the macro composition of camel milk compared to other mammalian milks is shown in Table 1. Whereas, fat content of buffalo and sheep milks is higher than that of camel milk; similarly lactose content of human milk is higher than that of camel milk. On the other hand, variations were also found in camel milk composition in the literature due to the method of analysis, geographical location of the drawn sample, lactation stage, age, feed, and breed (Al haj & Al Kanhal, 2010). The composition of camel milk (mean values) from 45 references of different parts of the world as follows: 88% water, 4.4% lactose, 3.5% fat, 3.1% protein, and 0.79% ash (Al haj & Al Kanhal, 2010). The composition and nutritional value of camel milk have been discussed in Chapter 2.

FUNCTIONALITY OF CAMEL MILK

Historically, camel milk has been used for the treatment of many ailments including: tuberculosis, dropsy, asthma jaundice, leishmaniasis (Shalash, 1984; Abdelgadir, Ahmed, & Dirar, 1998) and respiratory insufficiency (Yagil, 1987). The functional properties of camel milk have been reviewed recently by Izadi, Khedmat, & Mojtahedi (2019) and previously by Al haj & Al Kanhal (2010).

Camel milk considered as a functional food by virtue of many bioactive ingredients. These bioactive compounds either naturally exist in camel milk including immunoglobulins, and other antimicrobial compounds mentioned later (El-Agamy, Ruppanner, Ismail, Champagne, & Assaf, 1992; Agrawal, Budania, Sharma, Gupta, & Kochar, 2007) or those which can be released upon digestion with proteolytic bacterial enzymes, and enzymatic hydrolysis whether at the *in vivo* or *in vitro* level (Alhaj, Kanekanian, Peters, & Tatham 2010; Salami et al., 2010; Salami, Moosavi-Movahedi, Moosavi-Movahedi, Ehsani, & Yousefi, 2011; Moslehishad *et al.*, 2013; Kumar, Chatli, Singh, Mehta, & Kumar, 2016a; Alhaj, Metwalli, Ismail, Ali, Al-khalifa, & Kanekanian, 2018).

Park (2009) defined bioactive compounds as either naturally occurring compounds or those which are formulated during food processing. For example, bioactive peptides of camel milk can be either generated through fermentation with proteolytic bacterial enzymes (Alhaj et al, 2018), enzymatic hydrolysis with either purified specific proteases or with a mixture of pepsin and pancreatin (Mati et al., 2017) or enriched by addition of starter culture (Kuwabara et al., 1995; Alhaj et al., 2018). For instance, the addition of *Lactobacillus helveticus* or *Lactobacillus acidophilus* solely or in combination with camel milk was

Table 1. The macro composition of different types of mammalian milks

	Water	Protein	Fat	Ash	Lactose
Camel	86-88	2.15-4.9	1.2-6.4	0.6-0.9	2.4-5.8
Cow	85-87	3.2-3.8	3.7-4.4	0.7-0.8	4.8-4.9
Buffalo	82-84	3.3-3.6	7.0-11.5	0.8-0.9	4.5-5.0
Sheep	79-82	5.6-6.7	6.9-8.6	0.9-1.0	4.3-4.8
Goat	87-88	2.9-3.7	4.0-4.5	0.8-0.9	3.6-4.2
Human	88-89	1.1-1.3	3.3-4.7	0.2-0.3	6.8-7.0

Data adapted from Al haj & Al Kanhal, (2010); Rafiq *et al.*, (2016)

reported to release ACE-inhibitory peptides (Alhaj, 2017), antioxidant peptides (Al-Saleh, et al., 2014), and antimicrobial peptides (Alhaj et al., 2018). Bioactive compounds are thought to have physiological and/or biochemical functions when consumed by humans. What is interesting about the bioactive compounds of camel milk is that some of them are stable upon heat treatment; even after sterilization and provide functionality such as: angiotensin converting enzyme (ACE)-inhibitory activity, antimicrobial, anticancer and antioxidant effect (Al-Saleh, Metwalli, Ismail, & Alhaj 2014; Alhaj, 2017; Amr, Takruri, Shomaf, Alhaj, Faris & Abdel-Rahman, 2018). On the other hand, some of the bioactive compounds such as lactoferrin could be inactivated by lower temperatures such as pasteurization (Claeys et al., 2014).

POTENTIAL FUNCTIONAL INGREDIENTS OF CAMEL MILK

D and L Amino Acids

The functionality of camel milk protein is attributed to its amino acid content, which might contain up to 23 amino acid residues (Otte, Shalaby, Zakora, & Neilsen, 2007). Apart from these proteins, bioactive peptides are protein fragments having positive impact on body functions or conditions (Kitts & Weiler, 2003). Amino acids are the basic structural and functional units of proteins. Essential amino acids are those which either can't be synthesized sufficiently within the human body or synthesized in limited amounts to meet the body needs. Kappeler et al. (1998) has studied the amino acid sequence of camel milk casein, the number of amino acid residues in caseins sequences was reported as follows: αs1-casien, 207; αs2-casein178; β-casein, 217; κ-casein, 162.

Bovine milk and camel milk both contain the essential amino acids threonine, valine, methionine, leucine, isoleucine, phenylalanine, histidine, and lysine. On the other hand, camel milk is rich in some important amino acids such as leucine, lysine, threonine, methionine, isoleucine, histidine, phenylalanine, valine, and aspartic acid (see Chapter 2). Among different animal species (buffalo, cow, sheep, goat, sheep, and camel), the content of Leucine in milk caseins was highest in cow, camel and buffalo, respectively. While, the goat milk caseins showed the highest concentrations of histidine, phenylalanine, and isoleucine (Rafiq et al., 2016). On the other hand, glycine and cystine was found to be higher in bovine milk casein compared to camel milk casein (Farah & Rüegg, 1989).

Most amino acids in milk occur is in the L-form. On the other hand, the corresponding stereoisomers are D-form of amino acids (Brueckner & Hausch, 1990). Recently, D-forms of amino acids have been used extensively in pharmaceutics. For instance, D-Asp was found to stimulate the synthesis of testosterone, increases human sperm count, enhance sperm mobility, involved in human pre-ovulatory follicular fluid (D'Aniello et al., 2007, Topo, Soricelli, D'Aniello, Ronsini, & D'Aniello, 2009), and has probable relationship with the prevention of autoimmune diseases (Aswad, Paranandi, & Schurter, 2000).

It has been thought for long time that the presence of D-form of amino acids in dairy products was attributed to the presence of some active bacteria (Brueckner & Hausch, 1990). On the other hand, free D-amino acids are found in camel milk but in low amounts, which has been attributed to bacterial digestion and autolysis. For example, the presence of anaerobic bacterial strains in raw camel milk includes *Bacterioides, Ruminococcus* and *Butyrivibrio* (Brückner & Fujii, 2010).

Indeed, the addition of certain bacterial strains to camel milk was found to enhance the D-amino acid content. For instance, the addition of lactic acid bacteria such as *Lactobacillus acidophilus* and *Streptococcus thermophilus;* or *Lactobacillus helveticus* and *Streptococcus thermophilus; and Lactobacillus bulgaricus* and *Streptococcus thermophilus* have remarkably increased the content of D- Ala, D-Val, D-Orn, D-Lys and D-Arg in camel milk due to fermentation (Alhaj, Al-Khalifa, Metwalli, Ismail, & Ali 2017).

OLIGOSACCHARIDES

Similar to other mammalian milks, lactose predominates camel milk sugars as it comprises 4.4% of total milk composition (Al haj & Al Kanhal, 2010). Other sugars were identified in camel milk such as neutral and acidic oligosaccharides, glucose, fructose, and glucosamine (Fox & McSweeney, 1998).

Oligosaccharides are polymerized carbohydrates into 3-14 sugars containing lactose residues and some N-acetyl groups (Walstra, Wouters, & Geurts, 2008). Alhaj et al. (2013) detected the prebiotic 3'-GL oligosaccharide which is usually added to the infant formula (Urashima, Kitaoka, Asakuma, & Messer, 2009). Oligosaccharides are thought to modulate intestinal flora, ameliorate gastrointestinal activities, enhance mineral absorption, reduce intestinal adhesion of pathogenic bacteria, and enhance the growth of the beneficial bacterial strain *Bifidobacterium bifidum*, and enhance the immune system (Boehm & Stahl, 2007; Kunz & Rudloff, 2006).

Nonetheless, human milk is superior over other mammalian milks including camel milk in terms of the number as well as the concentration of oligosaccharides (Urashima, Murata, & Nakamura, 1997; Fukuda et al., 2010; Alhaj et al., 2013). For instance, Boehm & Stahl (2003) find 87 oligosaccharides in human milk compared to 13 in Bactrian camel milk /colostrum (Fukuda et al., 2010) and 7 in Dromedary camel milk (Alhaj et al., 2013). Additionally, camel and bovine milk oligosaccharides were found to decrease during lactation compared to human milk (Finke, 2000; Martin, Martin-Sosa, Garcia-Pardo, & Hueso, 2001; Fukuda, et al., 2010). The composition and health benefits of colostrum will be discussed in details in Chapter 11.

Interestingly, significant homology and heterogeneity in the oligosaccharides structures of human and camel milk were reported (Mehra & Kelly, 2006; Fukuda et al., 2010; Alhaj et al., 2013). For instance, two oligosaccharides were identified only in camel milk including sialyl -3'-galactosyllactose and sialyllacto-N-novopentaose-a. On the other hand, the oligosaccharides 3'-GL, lacto-N-neotetraose (LNnH), 3'-SL, 6'-SL and MSLNnH oligosaccharides were detected in dromedary camel and human milk as reported by Alhaj et al., (2013). Moreover, the oligosaccharides sialyllacto-N-novopentaose-a, LNnH and MFLNnH, that contain Gal(β1–4) GlcNAc(N-acetyllactosamine, are categorized as Type II oligosaccharides. Those were only found in camel milk (Alhaj et al., 2013) and will probably represent a significant dissimilarity between human milk and camel milk as stated by Fukuda et al., (2010).

FATTY ACIDS (FA)

In a well-balanced diet, saturated fat intake is allowed to contribute to 10% of total fat intake (Rolfes, Pinna, & Whitney, 2015). Camel milk contains various milk fat globule membrane proteins, FA synthase, xanthine dehydrogenase/oxidase, butyrophilin, in addition to lactadherin, milk fat globule- epidermal growth factor 8, and adipophilin (Saadaoui et al. 2013). In recent *in vitro* study (Al-Nasseri et al. 2019), camel milk lipids were found to have the ability to regulate gBSA-induced macrophage inflammation which could be an advantage in diabetes and other inflammatory conditions. In the same publication, researchers attributed the mechanism behind this action to modulating the expression of key inflammatory regulators including NF-KB and NLRP3 inflammasome subunit. Furthermore, camel milk was found to contain many important FAs such as linoleic acid, linolenic acid and oleic acid as shown in Table 2. Compared with bovine milk fat, the content in camel milk was higher (43% vs. 32%); while human milk fat contains higher amount of unsaturated FAs (up to 50%) especially those corresponding to essential FAs linoleic and linolenic fatty acids (Koletzko, 2016; Al haj & Al Kanhal, 2010; Haddadin, Gammoh, & Robinson, 2008; Sawaya, Khalil, Al-Shalhat, & Al-Mohammad, 1984). In recent study (Maqsood et al., 2019), camel milk lipids were found to have higher amount of monounsaturated fatty acids compared to lipids content in cow milk (29.2% vs. 23.79%, respectively). On the other hand, human milk fat contains a higher amount of unsaturated fatty acids compared with that of camel milk fat (Konuspayeva, Lemarie, Faye, Loiseau, & Montet, 2008). Other fatty acids that occur in camel milk include vaccenic acid, butyric acid. In addition to Sphingolipids, 13-methyltetradecanoic acid, stearic acid, ether lipids, and omega-3, 6 FAs (Table 2) as well as vitamins A, D occur in camel milk too (Bauman, Mather, Wall, & Lock, 2006). On the other hand, bovine milk exhibited considerable amounts of short chain FAs including butyric, caproic, carprylic and capric acids; while these FAs which were classified as atherosclerosis promoter not detected in camel milk (Maqsood et al., 2019).

Recently, Mohamed and Mustafa (2016) analyzed the fatty acid profile of camel milk from farming and pastoral system of Sudan. The authors found that camel milk contains essential fatty acids (Table 2). Based on the adequate intakes of linoleic, linolenic, and saturated FAs specified in this table, camel milk is a rich source of these fats since each serving of camel milk provides 10-19% of the adequate intake of these FAs. Noteworthy that saturated FA content of camel milk is less than those of bovine, goat, and sheep but higher than that of human milk as shown in Table 2. Konuspayeva et al., (2008) reported that the percentage of saturated acids in camel milk fat is lower (67.7%) compared to bovine milk fat (69.9%). Four Fatty acids were found to represent more than 75% of total FAs in camel milk including palmitic 35.97%, oleic 16.34%, myristic 15.84% and stearic acid 11.55% (Maqsood et al., 2019).

Table 2. Fatty acid contents (g/100 g) of camel milk compared to other mammalian milks and average value for adult males and females (g/day)

Fatty acid (FA)	Camel	Goat	Sheep	Cow	Human
Oleic acid (C18:1ω9c)	1.035	18.65	20.18	22.36	30.56
Linoleic acid (C18:2ω6c)	1.405	2.25	2.32	2.57	3.88
Linolenic acid (C18:3ω3)	0.135	0.77	0.92	0.5	0.16
Total FAs	8.499	4.27	6.09	3.76	3.20
Saturated FAs	55.80	68.79	64.23	68.72	39
ω-3 FAs	2.40	0.44	1.31	0.56	0.48
ω-6 FAs	1.415	1.78	2.97	2.83	12.8
ω-3/ω-6	5.84	5	2.31	6.01	2.54

Data adopted from Borschell et al., 1986; Markiewicz-Kęszycka, Czyżak-runowska, Lipińska, & Wójtowski (2013); Rolfes et al., (2015); Koletzko (2016); Mohamed & Mustafa (2016).

Conjugated linoleic acid (CLA) was also found in camel milk in higher amounts than those in bovine milk (4.56 vs. 1.07 mg/g) (Cardak, Yetismeyen, & Bruckner, 2003; Al-khdier, Al-Saleh, Abu-Tarboush, Ismail, & Metwalli, 2014). This concentration was found to be enhanced upon the inoculation of camel milk with the bacterial cultures of *Bifidobacterium angulatum*, *Bifidobacterium longum* subsp. *infantis* and *Lactobacillus delbrueckii* subsp. *bulgaricus* (Al-khdier et al., 2014). Many functional properties were attributed to CLA such as anticancer, enhancement of immunity, anti-inflammatory, anti-diabetic, and anti-atheroschlerotic effects (Gnädig, Xue, Berdeaux, Chardigny, & Sebedio, 2003).

POTENTIAL HEALTH EFFECT OF CAMEL MILK

Antioxidant

Free radicals can be created within the human body either naturally during cell respiration of mitochondria (Virtanen, Pihlanto, Akkanen, & Korhonen, 2007) or synthetically due to the exposure to light, heat, or smoking. Free radicals can attack the weak molecules of the body such as polyunsaturated fats, proteins, and nucleic acids causing their damage (Sah, Vasiljevic, McKechnie, & Donkor, 2014). The body has its own mechanisms to get rid of free radicals (Virtanen et al., 2007). When the body capacity of forming free radicals exceeds that of getting rid of these radicals, oxidative stress ailments occur. It has been thought for long time that diabetes type I, cardiovascular disease, cataracts, and some types of cancers are related to prolonged oxidative stress. As well, aging process is thought to be related to the body oxidative status (Sah et al., 2014; Shori, 2013). The International Food Information Council Foundation (2019) reported that only about 34% of the worldwide consumers ingest enough foods containing potential antioxidant effect.

Indeed, camel milk has been reported to have antioxidant activity *in vitro* (Salami et al., 2011; Shori, 2013; Al-Saleh et al., 2014; Jrad et al., 2014) as well as *in vivo* (AL-Ayadhi & Elamin, 2013). At the *in vitro* level, Al-Saleh et al. (2014) showed that camel milk contains total polyphenols in amounts higher than that of hydrolysate cow casein and un-hydrolysed camel casein. Similarly, Jrad et al. (2014) showed that the free radical scavenging capacities (measured as trolox equivalent and by DPPH assay) of camel milk casein and camel milk casein hydrolysate were higher than those of camel milk protein or camel milk protein (casien) hydrolysate alone. Moreover, camel milk proteins hydrolysates from simulated gastric and intestinal digestion shown to have greater antioxidant activity compared to bovine milk proteins (Maqsood et al., 2019).

The antioxidant activity of camel milk casein reported to increase significantly with degree of hydrolysis and hydrolysis time when assessed by ABTS, DPPH and FRAP assays (Kumar et al., 2016a). Furthermore, the antioxidant properties of camel milk are thought to be attributed to chymotrypsin-hydrolysed β-casein (Salami et al., 2011) and amino acid residues including phenylalanine, tyrosine, cysteine, tryptophan and methionine (Moure, Domínguez, & Parajó, 2006).

Additionally, antioxidant peptides have been found to exhibit antioxidant properties of camel milk. Antioxidant peptides are food-derived peptides containing 5-16 amino acid residues which can be easily absorbed in the small intestine. Antioxidant peptides can be derived from milk and dairy products. They are considered safe and cheap (Sarmadia & Ismail, 2010).

Obviously, the fermentation of camel milk into yogurt resulted in the production of more peptides due to proteolytic activity and exerted further antioxidant capacity (Moslehishad et al., 2013). Recently, Tak, Bais, Singh, Singh, & Nayak (2018) examined the antioxidant content and capacity of camel yogurt (fermented by *Lactobacillus fermentum* for 8 hours) and found that this yogurt has exhibited antioxidant properties probably by virtue of reduced pH value. Similarly, Zahedi, Salami, & Moslehishad (2016) found that the fermented camel milk product (*Chal*) exerted antioxidant effect at the *in vitro* level too.

Furthermore, Ayyash and colleagues (2018) showed that camel milk fermented with indigenous probiotic lactic strains *Lactobacillus reuteri*, *Lactobacillus plantarum* or *Lactococcus lactis* (Ayyash, Al-Dhaheri, Al Mahadin, Kizhakkayil, & Abushelaibi, 2018) showed antioxidant activity higher than that of bovine milk.

In another study, Al-Shamsi, Mudgil, Hassan, and Maqsood (2018) showed that even camel milk protein hydrolysates showed antioxidant properties at the *in vitro* level and within the food system, however, caution must be taken as the shelf life of this yogurt decreases with time which might cause further analysis of antioxidant bioactive peptides by yogurt culture. On the other hand, the type of enzymes hydrolysates exhibit different antioxidant activities *in vitro*. For example, papain showed greater (2,2'-azino-bis-3-ethylbenzthiazoline-6-sulphonic acid) ABTS radical scavenging activity than alcalase, and bromelain enzyme (Al-Shamsi et al., 2018). Moreover, α-chymotrypsin enzyme showed greater antioxidant activity as compared to alcalase and papain enzymes (Kumar et al., 2016a).

Unfortunately, it should be taken into consideration that pasteurization of camel milk at 63°C/10 minutes has been found to reduce the antioxidant activity significantly when determined by *in vitro* analysis (Ajlouni, Michelle, Senaka, & Timothy, 2017). On the other hand, caution must be taken regarding the consumption of fresh unpasteurized camel milk as it possesses high microbiological risk to the consumer (Bulca, 2017).

ANTICANCER

According to the World Health Organization (WHO, 2019) cancer is one of the top ten leading causes of death worldwide, causing 6.9 million deaths in 2018. Lung, mammary, and colorectal cancers are the top three cancer types in terms of incidence. These three cancers are responsible for one third of the cancer incidence and mortality burden worldwide. Cancers can be attributed to the interaction between genetic factors as well as environmental factors. Among the environmental factors is the dietary behaviors. Many studies evaluated the relationship between dietary factors and certain types of cancers.

Camel milk has been favored over bovine milk by Mediterranean cancer patients (Quita & Kurdi, 2010). Additionally, camel milk has been found additionally to inhibit the tumors of liver, blood, and lung *in vitro* (Abdel Galil, Abdel Gader, & Alhaider, 2016).

Regarding colorectal cancer, some studies showed no effect of dairy product consumption and specifically camel milk, while others showed that the consumption of dairy products decreased the risk for the incidence of colorectal cancer (Quita & Kurdi, 2010; Korashy et al., 2012; Amr et al., 2018). The chemopreventive effects of camel milk have been suggested by studying its effects on cancer biomarkers. These effects were attributed to the functional compounds such as conjugated linoleic acid, sphingolipids, calcium, lactoferrin, casein or the addition of probiotic and prebiotic (Gill & Rowland, 2003). In Fischer rats, fermented camel milk inhibited colon carcinogenesis (Amr et al., 2018). Furthermore, camel milk cancer cell proliferation and angiogenesis inhibition (Kula, 2016). An interesting mechanism that has been demonstrated by Levy et al. (2013) is that camel milk antibodies bind selectively to the tumors and kill them.

At the *in vitro* level, the water extracts of fermented camel milk had exerted potent anti-cancer effects against MCF-7, Caco-2 and HELA cancer cell lines more than those of fermented bovine milk by reducing cell proliferation significantly (Ayyash et al., 2018a). Similarly, Keykanlu et al., (2016) found that camel milk lactoferrin specifically inhibited MCF-7 breast cancer cell line. Interestingly, these researchers also showed that the lactoferrin-extracted camel milk and encapsulated nanoparticles also exerted the same effect in a dose dependent manner; a finding which initiated the pharmaceutical use of camel milk. Lactoferrin is thought to be able to reduce carcinogenesis by altering activating proteins, induction of cell apoptosis, and activation of natural killer cells (Keykanlu et al., 2016).

Lead contamination is common among cancer patients (Akhmetsadykova et al., 2009). By virtue of lactic acid bacteria within the fermented camel milk product (Shubat), Singh, Mal, Kumar, Patil, & Pathak (2017) hypothesized that camel milk can help cancer patients in absorbing lead to be excreted in the feces. Within the same context, camel milk was found to improve the histopathological appearance of renal tissue of rats after induced cadmium toxicity (Oudah, 2016).

Indeed, a recent meta-analysis by Mihic, Rainkie, Wilby, & Pawluk (2016) evaluated the strength of scientific evidence related to the anticancer activity of camel milk on cancer showed that camel milk has antiangiogenic, anticytotoxic, and antigenotoxic effects of cisplatin therapy against cancer. Nonetheless, the available scientific evidence is still preliminary and thus, researches are recommended to explore the oncological aspects of camel milk. Additionally, the same authors highlighted the importance of testing the effect of camel milk on toxicity in humans. The effect of camel milk on cancer as a chronic disease will be discussed in details in Chapter 8.

ANTIHYPERTENSIVE PROPERTIES

Renin-angiotensin enzyme system is a physiological system regulated by pituitary hormones. This system regulates blood pressure (Rolfes et al., 2015). One of the essential enzymes of this system is the angiotensin-I-converting enzyme (ACE) which is an exopeptidase that cleaves dipeptides from the C-terminal ends of various peptide substrates and regulates the activity of several endogenous bioactive peptides (Pan, Luo, & Tanokura, 2005). *In vivo*, ACE acts on angiotensin-I in renin angiotensin system to hydrolyze the dipeptide (His-Leu) from its C-terminal leading to the conversion into the potent vasoconstrictor angiotensin II (Tagliazucchi, Shamsia, & Conte, 2016). The slight reduction of blood pressure caused by angiotensin-II by 5 mm Hg is known to reduce the risk of cardiovascular disease by 15% (Meisel, Walsh, Murray, & FitzGerald, 2006).

It is well demonstrated the hypertension diseases is based on controlling of Na^+/K^+-ATPase balance. Insulin and catecholamine hormones, which are highly present in camel milk (Agarwal et al., 2003; Zagorski et al., 1998) are the principal mediators of acute hormonal control of Na^+/K^+-ATPase. Insulin is a major regulator of potassium homeostasis and has multiple effects on sodium pump activity. Within minutes of elevated insulin secretion, pumps containing alpha-1, and 2 isoforms have increased affinity for sodium and increased turnover, which hemostat blood pressure (Soetikno et al., 2011). Moreover; the activities of total ATPase's (Na^+/K^+)-ATPase, Ca^{2+}/ATPase, and Mg^{2+}/ATPase were significantly decreased in erythrocytes, liver, and kidney of diabetic rats fed routinely on camel milk (Al-Numair, Chandramohan, Kamalakkannan, Alsaif, & Sundaraselvan, 2010).

The ACE-inhibitory bioactive peptides occur naturally in the primary structures of food proteins such as camel milk proteins (Li et al., 2004; Jang & Lee, 2005; Meisel et al., 2006) or released depending on the degree of camel milk protein hydrolysis, and amino acid sequence of proteins (Salami et al., 2011), and type of proteolytic enzyme such as trypsinolysis alone or trypsinolysis followed by pepsinolysis (Salami et al., 2010). The functional properties of camel whey proteins including ACE-inhibitory activity, antioxidant and antimicrobial effects has been found to improve by adding proteolytic enzymes such as trypsin, pepsin, and chymotrypsin (Salami et al., 2010; 2011).

Moreover, ACE-inhibitory bioactive peptides can be released using either individual or combined cultures. Donker, Henriksson, Singh, Vasiljevic, & Shah (2007) showed that the most potent ACE-inhibitory peptides can be originated from β-casein representing 65% of whole camel milk caseins as reported by Kappeler, Farah, & Puhan (2003). Twelve ACE-inhibitory peptides were identified (Alhaj, 2017) from camel milk (dromedary) fermented with *L. acidophilus* and *L. helveticus* strains solely. Seven of them released from camel milk protein using *L. helveticus* strain as follows: three peptides were released from sequences 1 (LSLSQF, SLSQF or SQF) KVLPVPQ, the second three were released from protein sequences 2 (TDLEN, DLEN or LEN) LHLPLPL, and finally one ACE-inhibitory peptide was released from sequence 3 KVLPVPQQMVPYPQ. The data of expasy proteomics server (Bioinformatics Resource Portal) showed that the sequence 1 and 3 are corresponding to amino acid positions of 178–198, while sequence 2 to positions 144-155 in β-casein of dromedary camel milk proteins. Additionally, camel milk fermented with *L. acidophilus* strain solely released only three ACE-inhibitory peptides from water soluble permeates (WSP) of camel milk (Alhaj, 2017) due to slow growth *L. acidophilus* strain compared to *L. helveticus*. The identified ACE-inhibitory peptides of camel milk fermented with *L. acidophilus* strain were as follow: one peptide belongs to the sequence 4 VLPFQEPVPDPVRG; one peptide belongs to the sequence 5 FQEPFPDPVR and finally one peptide belongs to the sequence 6 VMVPFLQPK. Whereas, sequences 4 and 5 corresponding to positions 206–219; and finally sequence 6 corresponding to position 98–107. All identified ACE-inhibitory peptides (Alhaj, 2017) were corresponding to β-casein of camel (*Camelus dromedarius*) milk. In another study (Nongonierm, Paolella, Mudgil, Maqsood, & FitzGerald, 2018), nine ACE-inhibitory peptides were identified from camel milk proteins (corresponding to β-casein and αs1-casein) hydrolyzed using trypsin enzyme as follow; FLQY, FQLGASPY, ILDKEGIDY, ILELA, LLQLEAIR, LPVP, LQALHQGQIV, MPVQA and SPVVPF. On the other hand, ACE-inhibitory proteins corresponding to IPP and VPP have been released by Pan and Guo, (2010); and Yamamoto, Akino, & Takano (1994) within water soluble fractions of fermented bovine milk products using *L. lactis* (Rodríguez-Figueroa et al., 2010) and *L. jensinii* (Philanto, Virtanen, & Korhonen, 2010) such as sour milk (Nakamura et al., 1995a, Nakamura, Yamamoto, Sakai, & Takano, 1995), soft hard cheeses (Bütikofer, Meyer, Sieber, & Wechsler, 2007; Meyer, Butikofer, Walther, Wechsler, & Sieber, 2009), and yogurt (Kajimoto et al., 2002). Moreover, camel milk proteins hydrolysates from simulated gastric and intestinal digestion shown to have greater ACE inhibitory properties compared to bovine milk proteins (Maqsood et al., 2019).

In another study, Moslehishad et al. (2013) released ACE-I polypeptide from camel milk proteins using *L. rhamnosus*. Moreover, the polypeptide (Ala-Ile-Pro-Pro-Lys-Lys-Asn-Gln-Asp) was identified from Mongolia camel milk in the presence of *L. helveticus* (Quan, Tsuda, & Miyamoto, 2008). In recent study, Solanki, Hati, & Sakure, (2017) identified 26 peptides corresponding to ACE-inhibitory activity from different food sources.

All identified ACE-inhibitory peptides from dromedary camel milk proteins were corresponding to β-casein and some contain at least one proline (P) residue at their C-terminal position (Alhaj, 2017). The amino acids which have hydrophobic properties such as tryptophan (W), phenylalanine (F), tyrosine (Y) and especially proline (P) probably contributed to the ACE-inhibitory peptide properties (Li, Le, Shi, & Shrestha, 2004; López-Fandiño, Otte, & Van Camp, 2006; Moslehishad et al., 2013). Additionally, the casein macropeptide (CMP); a hydrolysis product of κ-casien has been found to regulate blood flow (Dziuba & Dziuba, 2014). Moreover, Dziuba & Dziuba (2014) found ACE-inhibitory tripeptides composed of Val-Pro-Pro and Ile-Pro-Pro. Recently, Alhaj et al., (2018) have reported that ACE-inhibitory activity of camel milk proteins using *Lactobacillus acidophilus* and *Streptococcus thermophilus* or *Lactobacillus helveticus* and *Streptococcus thermophilus* are time and strain dependent. Moreover, the balance between the formation of ACE-inhibitory peptides and subsequent degradation is the potential factor for camel milk blood pressure lowering effect (Fallah et al., 2019).

At the *in vivo* level, Yahya, Alhaj, & Al-Khalifah (2017) studied the effect of feeding skim fermented and unfermented camel milk on spontaneous hypertension rat model. The hypotensive effect of fermented skim camel milk was found to be dose-dependent using *L. helveticus* and *S. thermophillus* in short and long-term study. On the other hand, fermented camel milk exhibited insignificant antihypertensive effects on obese adolescents (Fallah et al., 2019) and patients with type 2 diabetes (Ejtahed et al., 2015).

ANTIDIABETIC

Type I diabetes mellitus (T1DM) is a disorder that is characterized by an autoimmune reaction which destroys the pancreas and reduces or even hinders insulin secretion (Rolfes et al., 2015). Revising correlational types of epidemiological research, the prevalence of diabetes communities that consume higher amounts of camel milk was found to be lower than in those which consume lower amounts (Agrawal, Jain, Shah, Chopra, & Agarwal, 2011) such as Raica community of India (Agrawal, Budania, Sharma, Gupta, & Kochar, 2007). The effect of camel milk on diabetes mellitus as a chronic disease will be discussed in details in Chapter 8 and 9.

Long time ago, Yagil (1987) reported that camel milk probably stabilized T1DM. Recently, Khan, Alzohairy, & Mohieldein (2013) reported that this stabilization had occurred within 30 days in experimental rats. In another research, camel milk consumption was found to reduce insulin requirements (Agrawal et al., 2011; Agrawal et al., 2003; Khan et al., 2013) to zero (Khan & Alzohairy, 2011) in T1DM patients. Additionally, camel milk was found to improve renal and hepatic functions in diabetic patients (El-Sayed, AL-Shoeibi, Abd El-Ghany, & Atef, 2011).

Insulin like proteins present in camel milk in high concentration (150 U/ml) (Gizachew, Teha, & Birhanu, 2014). Unlike to other mammalian insulins, camel milk insulin doesn't coagulate in the acidic medium of the stomach (Agrawal et al., 2003; Abdel Galil et al., 2016) and is protected from proteolysis in the upper GIT (Mullaicharam, 2014) probably because camel milk insulin has been thought to be microencapsulated by camel milk nano lipid droplets (Malik, Al-Senaidy, Jankun, & Jankun, 2012).

Asha, Pareek, & Shah (2016) attributed the heat stability, the coagulation resistance, and the efficacy in reaching the circulator system unchanged due to the fact that camel milk insulin has a higher affinity toward alanine incorporation toward its primary structure during the biological evolutionary process of camel milk compared to that of human milk. Additionally, camel milk has been found to contain tissue repairing proteins; a mechanism that has been suggested to the antidiabetic activity of camel milk (Abbas, Ashraf, Nazir, & Sarfraz, 2013; Gul, Farooq, Anees, Khan, & Rehan, 2015). On the other hand, the C-lobe of lactoferrin has been found to have affinity to different sugars such as glucose, sucrose, galactose, and mannose (Sharma, Sinha, Kaushik, Kaur, & Singh, 2013). This is probably responsible for the antidiabetic properties of camel milk. Compared to bovine milk, the inhibition percentages of α-amylase in fermented camel milk using *Lactococcus lactis* during prolonged storage were greater (Ayyash et al., 2018b).

In animals (diabetic Albino rats), supplementation with camel milk reduced blood glucose concentration as shown by Baragob (2015) and diabetic dogs as reported by Sboui et al.,(2010), effect were dose-dependent. Similar results were found in Alloxan-induced diabetic rats after feeding camel milk for 4 weeks by Kebir, Aichouni, & Zahzeh (2017). Furthermore, these researchers found improvements in blood lipid profile. It has been thought that the anti-diabetic functionality of camel milk is related to the presence of insulin-like compounds such as half-cystien, immunoglobulins (Breitling, 2002), and lactoferrin (Kula, 2016).

Conversely, Kumar, Venu, & Manchala (2016) found no effect of feeding camel milk (raw, pasteurized, or boiled) on blood glucose concentration, fasting insulin concentration, neither blood lipid profile compared to bovine's milk for 30 days in streptozotocin-induced diabetes; a representative model of diabetes type I in rats. Nonetheless, the effect started after 60 days of feeding. For the first time, these authors have found that feeding rats 65% sucrose diet (which is representative to glucose intolerance test; a risky stage which might induce type II diabetes) with raw camel milk only reduced significantly blood glucose concentration indicating that some heat-labile antihyperglycemic agents(s) present in camel milk. In both models, camel milk improved blood lipid profile of rats.

Recently, Ebaid (2015) found that camel milk peptides was an effective antioxidant and immune stimulant as it induced oxidative stability and speeded up wound healing in diabetic model animals. These results were thought to make camel milk a potential adjuvant in improving wound healing in those with diabetic conditions.

Interestingly, El-Abd, Abdel-Hamid, Ahmed-Farid, El-demerdash, & Mohamed (2018) found an ameliorative effect of fermented camel milk using *Lactobacillus delbrueckii* subsp. *bulgaricus* and *Streptococcus salivarious* subsp. *thermophilus* on non-alcoholic fatty liver disease of Sprague-Dawly rats. Noteworthy, the ameliorative effect was accompanied with a significant improvement in serum glucose concentration, tumor necrosis factor alpha (TNFα), nitrous oxide, total cholesterol, low density lipoprotein cholesterol (LDL-C), triglycerides (TG), malonaldehyde (MAD), the liver enzymes aspartate aminotransferase (AST), alanine aminotransferase (ALT), and oxidized glutathione (GSSG).

A recent meta-analysis for human and animal trials on the effect of camel milk on diabetes mellitus by Mihic et al. (2016) showed that camel milk tended to improve glycemic control, liver function, dyslipidemia, and diabetic nephropathy in synthetically induced diabetes. On the other hand, the related human studies showed improvements in blood glucose and insulin concentrations but not blood lipid profile. These studies were limited by the experimental designs as well as the lack of control groups. Accordingly, camel milk was not recommended as a therapeutic agent against diabetes. However, there is no contraindication of the use of camel milk for diabetics as a part of a healthy life style. The authors emphasized the importance of performing randomized clinical human trials on diabetic patients.

ANTIMICROBIAL

Several researches reported that camel milk contains many antimicrobial compounds such as immunoglobulins, lactoperoxidase, lactoferrin, hydrogen peroxide, lysozyme (Al-Juboori, Mohammed, Rashid, Kurian, & El Refaey, 2013) in amounts greater than those of other mammalian milks including bovine, buffalo, goat, and ewe as shown in Table 3 (Kappeler, Farah, & Puhan, 1999; Abrhaley & Leta, 2018). Lysozymes are usually specialized in enhancing immunity against invading pathogens while immunoglobulins are related to body infections (Jilo, 2016).

Additionally, camel milk contains xanthine oxidoreductase (XOR) protein (Harrison, 2006) and peptidoglycan recognition protein (PGRP) as shown by Kappeler et al., (1999), immunoglobulins (Abd El-Salam & El-Shibiny, 2013). These peptides could be released upon the exposure to digestive enzymes (Gobbetti, Minervini, & Rizzello, 2004). Furthermore, the casein macropeptide (CMP); a hydrolysis products of κ-casien has been found to exert antimicrobial activity against *E. coli*, inhibit bacterial and viral adhesion, enhance the growth of *Bifidobacteria* and to modulate immunity (Dziuba & Dziuba, 2014). Moreover, the N-lobe of lactoferrin with its unique amino acid sequencing is thought to be responsible for camel milk antimicrobial activity (Sharma et al., 2013).

Camel milk contains minor amounts of PGRP which work as protective antibiotic protein (El-Agamy, 2000; Merin et al., 2001; Kappeler, Heuberger, Farah, & Puhan 2004; El-Hatmi, Girardet, Gaillard, Yahyaoui, & Attia, 2007). This protein is secreted from white blood cells having a depolarizing properties against cell membranes of Gram positive and Gram negative bacteria. Additionally, PGRP is known to induce metal, thiol, and oxidative stress within the bacterial cells (Kashyap et al., 2014)

Interestingly, camel milk lactoperoxidase was found to stimulate the non-immune host defense. Additionally, camel milk lactoperoxidase has a close (71%) similarity to human thyroid peroxidase in terms of iodination, coupling, and formation of human thyroid hormone (Mullaicharam, 2014).

Camel milk was found to have antimicrobial activity against pathogenic bacteria such as *E. coli* and *L. monocytogens* (Benkerroum, Mekkaoui, Bennani, & Kamal, 2004). What is noteworthy to mention

Table 3. Shows the average concentrations of antimicrobial compounds such as lactoferrin, lysozyme and immunoglobulins G in different species of milk (mg/l)

Specification	Lactoferrin	Lysozyme	Immunoglobulins G
Human	700-2000	100-890	40-54
Cow	80-500	0.73-0.60	100-800
Buffalo	50-320	0.13-0.15	460-1300
Camel	200-728	0.73-5.00	2000
Goat	98-150	0.25	100-400
Ewe	140	1-4	500
Mare	820	400-890	390

Data adapted from Król, Brodziak, Litwińczuk, & Barłowska (2012)

that this property is more obvious in raw camel milk than heat-treated milk (80°C for 4 seconds or 67°C for 1 minute) probably due to the fact that lysozyme is sensitive to heat treatment (Benkerroum et al., 2004). In another study, synergistic effect was reported between camel milk and ciprofloxacin against the growth of *E. coli* and *S. aureus* (Yassin, Soliman, Mostafa, & Ali, 2015). The effect of different heat treatment methods on camel milk composition and health properties are discussed in Chapter 10.

These compounds have been thought to have antibacterial properties against pathogenic bacterial strains such as *Staphylococcus aureus*, *Listeria monocytogenes*, *Salmonella typhimurium* and *Escherichia coli* (El-Agamy et al., 1992; Benkerroum et al., 2004), *Lactococcus lactis* subsp. *cremoris*, *Escherichia coli*, *Staphylococcus aureus*, *Salmonella typhimurium* (Al-Majali, Ismail, & Al-Hami, 2007), *Pseudomonas eruginosa* (Mehrin et al., 2011) and rotavirus (Al-Majali et al., 2007; Singh et al., 2017). In contrast, Mihic et al. (2016) showed a limited scientific evidence on the antibacterial effect of camel milk against *Salmonella* infections.

Among other mammalian milk (except for human and mare milk), camel milk contains the highest amount of lactoferrin. Lactoferrin occurs in camel milk (mg/l) (200-728) in amounts about 1.5 times greater than that of bovine milk (80-500) and about 4 times greater than that of goat milk (98-150). Camel milk showed anthelmintic activity against *Haemonchus contortus in vitro*, this was significantly dose-dependent and due to the presence of lactoferrin and vitamin C in whole camel milk (Alimi et al., 2016). Furthermore, when camel milk was compared with other mammalian milks (bovine, ewe and goat), it showed to have an inhibitory effect on egg hatching.

Król et al., (2012) reported that lysozyme occurs in camel milk in amounts (mg/l) (0.73-5.00) higher than those in bovine milk (0.73-0.60), goat milk (0.25), and ewe milk (1-4). Furthermore, camel milk contains 2000 mg/L immunoglobulin which is higher than that of buffalo (460-1300) and much more than human milk does (40-54).

The immunoglobulins in camel milk offer a natural protection of the gut membrane of the newly born infant. For instance, the innumnoglobulin PGRP inactivate the pathogenic bacteria by binding to the peptidoglycan structures of the bacterial cell wall (Abd El-Salam & El-Shibiny, 2013). On the other hand, lactoferrin of camel milk binds iron and hinders its availability to the bacteria such as *S. typhimurium* (Abd El-Salam & El-Shibiny, 2013). Furthermore, among different mammal's species (Sheep, goat, alpaca, and human), camel lactoferrin exhibited the highest activity against *E. coli* O157:H7 followed by goat and sheep, while human and alpaca lactoferrins showed the least activity (Conesa et al., 2008). Interestingly, camel milk lysozymes have been shown to prolong the milk gelatinization into yogurt because of the delay in the bacterial culture growing (Jumah, Shaker, & Abu-Jadayil, 2001). On the other hand, the antimicrobial substances of camel milk have been shown to lose their activity upon heating at 100 °C for 30 min (El-Agamy, 2000; Singh *et al.*, 2017).

The antimicrobial peptide activity of camel milk depends greatly on the strain, incubation time and peptide amino acid sequence. Additional factors including structural activity were also found to enhance the antimicrobial effect (Gobbetti et al., 2004). Likewise, the replacement of Asp (D) with Arg (R) and adding Lys (K) residues to the *C*-terminus of antimicrobial peptide was found to enhance the antimicrobial activity against Gram-negative bacteria (Pellegrini, Dettling, Thomas, & Hunziker, 2001).

Interestingly, the inoculation of camel milk with bacterial cultures enhanced the antibacterial properties of camel milk peptides. Alhaj et al., (2018) inoculated camel milk with the combined culture of *Lactobacillus acidophilus* and *Streptococcus thermophilus* or *Lactobacillus helveticus* and *Streptococcus thermophilus* and found an enhancement of the antimicrobial activity against *Bacillus cereus*, *S. typhimurium* and *S. aureus;* while no antimicrobial effects was found using unfermented camel milk against any of the tested pathogens. The antimicrobial activity of camel milk was found to be strains dependent. Alhaj et al., (2018) reported that the antimicrobial activity of camel milk containing *L. helveticus* and *S. thermophilus* was higher than that exhibited in camel milk containing *L. acidophilus* and *S. thermophiles*. This has been attributed to the proteolytic system of *L. helveticus*, which generate more antimicrobial peptides during fermentation (Alhaj et al., 2018). Recently, Muhialdina and Algboory (2018) identified 32 peptides from fermented camel milk (*Lactobacillus plantarum*) having antimicrobial activity against *Staphylococcus faecalis*, *Shigella dysenteriae*, *Staphylococcus aureus* and *E. coli*. The identified antimicrobial peptides belong to various proteins of camel milk as follow: six peptides belong to Lactophorin; seven peptides belong to α-S2-casein; nine peptides belong to β-casein; and the higher number of antimicrobial peptides of 10 belonged to α-S1- casein. On the other hand, the type of enzyme reported to exhibit different antimicrobial effect against tested pathogens. For example, Alcalase and α-Chymotrypsin found to produce greater antimicrobial activity than Papain (Kumar, Chatli, Singh, Mehta, & Kumar, 2016b). Furthermore, whole hydrolysates showed significantly greater antimicrobial effect than its fractions against tested pathogens.

HYPOALLERGENIC EFFECT

Food sensitivity usually occurs due to the reaction between food antigens and somatic antibodies. Human milk is usually the ideal food to the neonate for the first six months of life (Rolfes et al., 2015). However, 10% of infants show sensitization against mammalian milk proteins as well as soy protein (Businco, Bruno, Giampietro, & Cantoni, 1992; Maldonado, Gil, Narbona, & Molina, 1998; El-Agamay, Nawar, Shamsia, Awad, & Haenlein, 2009). Additionally, some infants need infant formula to complete their energy and nutrient needs (El-Agamy, 2007). Usually, the sensitizing components of bovine milks are β-lactoglobulin (El-Agmay, 2007) and αs-casein (Taylor, 1986). Similar to human milk, camel milk is thought to be hypoallergic due to the high content of β-casein, in addition to low content of αs- casein (El-Agamay et al., 2009). Moreover, similarity of immunoglobulins content (Shabo, Barzel, Margoulis, & Yagil, 2005) and lacking of β-lactoglobulin (Kappeler, Farah, & Puhan, 1998). Additionally, the digestibility of camel milk is partially attributed to the small diameter of fat droplets allowing greater surface area for stomach digestive enzymes (Kula, 2016). Furthermore, it has been thought that the high percentage of β-casein (in a concentration near to that of human milk) improves camel milk digestibility (El-Agamy et al., 2009).

Another sensitizing compound of milk is lactose (Ehlayel, Hazeima, Al-Mesaifri, & Bener, 2011). Indeed, camel milk is low in lactose and specifically the L-type (Baubekova, Kalimbetovaa, Akhmetsadykova, Konuspayeva, & Faye, 2015), humans with lactose intolerance can digest camel milk with minimal expression of lactose intolerance symptoms (Shabo et al., 2005) with an excellent acceptance rate of 23 out of 25 lactose intolerant patients (Kaskous, 2016). This occurs probably because camel milk produces casomorphin which stimulates intestinal activity leaving lactose more exposed to lactase enzyme action (Cardoso, Santos, Cardoso, & Carvalho, 2010).

It has been found that among goat, bovine, sheep, buffalo and human milks, camel milk has the highest concentration of immunoglobulins G (El-Agamy, 2009). Due to their reduced size relative to those of human milk, they can be digested easily and move across the blood brain barrier (Abdel Galil et al., 2016). Camel milk was recently reported (Navarrete-Rodríguez et al., 2018) to be safe and suitable for pediatric patients above one year old with bovine milk allergy.

OTHER FUNCTIONAL ASPECTS OF CAMEL MILK

Nowadays, lactoferrin is one of the essential biopharmaceutical choices against hepatitis C virus infection (Redwan & Tabll, 2007). Researchers showed that the incubation of hepatitis C virus with camel milk lactoferrin has no evidence to kill the virus. Nevertheless, direct interaction between hepatitis C virus and lactoferrin lead to inhibit the virus's entry in to the cells after 7 day incubation. Noteworthy, the C-lone of lactoferrin and immunoglobulin G are the responsible part for the anti-hepatitis C activity of lactoferrin (Sharma et al., 2013; Kaskous, 2016).

Interestingly, camel milk has been found to inhibit other viruses such as Cytomegalovirus (CMV), human immunodeficiency virus (HIV, the virus responsible for AIDS) and herpes simplex virus-1, as well as fungi such as *Candida albicans* (Abrhaley & Leta, 2018). Additionally, a fermented camel milk product (*shubat*) which is used traditionally in Kazakhstan, has been shown to exhibit antiviral properties due to the presence of the metabolic products of lactic acid bacteria and yeast (Chuvakova et al., 2000).

In 2010, Mona showed that camel milk has stopped diarrhea in rats with *Rota virus* and hypothesized that this was due to the sodium and potassium contents of camel milk (Mona, 2010).

Studies related to the presence and/or beneficial effects of probiotic bacteria from camel milk started by Yateem, Balba, Al-Surrayai, Al-Mutairi, & Al-Daher, since 2008 then, the related literature has accumulated (Maurad & Meriem, 2008; Mutlag et al. 2013; Abbas & Mahasneh, 2014). Recently, Saljooghi, Mansouri-Najand, Ebrahimnejad, Doostan, and Askari (2017) showed the survival of lactic acid bacteria (10^6 CFU/ml) with acceptable organoleptic properties till the 9th day of fermented camel milk storage. The microbial aspect of lactic acid bacteria isolated from camel milk has been discussed in Chapter 4.

Additionally, the immunoglobulins of the G type (IgG) of camel milk were known to recognize hepatitis C virus peptides where human IgG cannot at all (El-Fakharany et al., 2012). Furthermore, camel milk enhanced immune response of hepatitis B patients and inhibited hepatitis B DNA replication (Saltanat et al., 2009).

The improvement of tuberculosis patients in terms of serum Fe and Zn concentrations, weight gain (Singh et al., 2017), cough, sputum, and chest pain after supplementation with 1L camel milk/day for a month has been recorded by Wernery and Yagil (2012).

Recently, camel milk has been shown to have antiulcer effects due to the presence of Mg which has been shown to enhance the antioxidant activity (Markiewicz-Górka, Zawadzki, Januszewska, Hom.bek-Urban, & Pawlas, 2011). Additionally, it has been shown by Al-Wabel, Hassan, Abbas, & Muosa, (2012) that camel milk consumption induced the production of nitric oxide and mucous, inhibited neutrophil adherence to the endothelial cells, and increased blood flow to the gastric cells (Markiewicz-Górka et al., 2011). However, the up-to-date scientific evidence regarding this issue is still intriguing and warrant and human studies are highly recommended in this issue (Mihic et al., 2016).

Crohn's disease is thought to be an autoimmune disease in which the digestive system passes through systematic inflammation (Rolfes et al., 2015). On the other hand, the infection of the digestive system with the bacteria *Mycobacterium avium subspecies: paratuberculosis* (MAP) cause secondary Crohn's disease. Knowing the fact that camel milk has many antibacterial properties and might restore the immune function, Shabo, Barzel, & Yagil, (2008) found that pasteurized camel milk treated the symptoms of the alimentary tract including Crohn's disease.

By virtue of many functional constituents, camel milk is now recognized as an antiaging food (Kula, 2016). Due to the fact that this milk is rich source of vitamin C and short peptides. Vitamin C is a strong antioxidant. Additionally, it aids in the formation of the protein collagen which firms the skin probably by the efficacy of the C-lobe of lactoferrin protein to aid in collagen contractibility (Takayama, Mizumachi, & Takezawa, 2002). The short peptides produced after camel milk digestion are thought to have antioxidant effect (Salami et al., 2011). Within the same context, Choi, Park, Kim, Lee, & Kim (2013) found that camel milk contains α-hydroxyl acids that plumps the epidermis and smooth fine lines. Additionally, these acids aid in creating new younger cells by breaking down the sugars that adhere aged cells together.

CONCLUSION AND FUTURE RESEARCH DIRECTIONS

Camel milk is recognized nowadays as a functional food by virtue of many bioactive ingredients. Despite the fact that many bioactive compounds were identified in camel milk and their mechanisms of bioactivity were identified, future research is recommended to search for other functional ingredients of this food as well as to elucidate other functionalities and their related mechanisms. The scientific evidence on the effect of camel milk on health on both humans and animals need to be enriched and strengthened through the use of controlled human clinical trials. Additionally, the effect of extracting the bioactive compounds of camel milk on their functionality upon use in pharmaceutical preparations need to investigated thoroughly.

ACKNOWLEDGMENT

I would like to thank Dr. Hiba Al-Sayyed for her convenient remarks on this chapter. I would like to thank the Food and Agricultural Organization (FAO) for their permission of adopting the figure.

REFERENCES

Abbas, M., & Mahasneh, A. (2014). Isolation of Lactobacillus strains with probiotic potential from camel's milk. *African Journal of Microbiological Research*, *8*(15), 1645–1655. doi:10.5897/AJMR2013.6598

Abbas, S., Ashraf, H., Nazir, A., & Sarfraz, L. (2013). Physico-chemical analysis and composition of camel Milk. *Intestinal Research*, *2*, 85–98.

Abd El-Salam, M. H., & El-Shibiny, S. (2013). Bioactive Peptides of Buffalo, Camel, Goat, Sheep, Mare, and Yak Milks and Milk Products. *Food Reviews International*, *29*(1), 1–23. doi:10.1080/87559129.2012.692137

Abdel Galil, M. (2016). The unique medicinal properties of camel products: A review of the scientific evidence. *Journal of Taibah University Medical Sciences*, *11*(2), 98–103. doi:10.1016/j.jtumed.2015.12.007

Abdelgadir, W., Ahmed, T., & Dirar, H. (1998). The traditional fermented milk products of the Sudan. *International Journal of Food Microbiology*, *44*(1-2), 1–13. doi:10.1016/S0168-1605(98)00090-7 PMID:9849779

Abrhaley, A., & Leta, S. (2018). Medicinal value of camel milk and meat. *Journal of Applied Animal Research*, *46*(72), 552–558. doi:10.1080/09712119.2017.1357562

Agrawal, P., Swami, S., Beniwal, R., Kochar, D., Sahani, M., Tuteja, F., & Ghouri, S. (2003). Effect of camel milk on glycemic control, risk factors and diabetes quality of life in type-1 diabetes: A randomised prospective controlled study. *Journal of Camel Practice and Research*, *10*(1), 45–50.

Agrawal, R., Budania, S., Sharma, P., Gupta, R., Kochar, D. K., Panwar, R. B., & Sahani, M. S. (2007). Zero prevalence of diabetes in camel milk consuming Raica community of northwest Rajasthan, India. *Diabetes Research and Clinical Practice*, *76*(2), 290–296. doi:10.1016/j.diabres.2006.09.036 PMID:17098321

Agrawal, R., Jain, S., Shah, S., Chopra, A., & Agarwal, V. (2011). Effect of camel milk on glycemic control and insulin requirement in patients with type 1 diabetes: 2-years randomized controlled trial. *European Journal of Clinical Nutrition*, *65*(9), 1048–1052. doi:10.1038/ejcn.2011.98 PMID:21629270

Ajlouni, S., Michelle, R., Senaka, R., & Timothy, D. (2017).. . *Archives of the International Society of Antioxidants in Nutrition and Health*, *5*(2), 1–4.

Akhmetsadykova, S., Konuspayeva, S., Loiseau, G., Baubekova, A., Kanayat, S., Akhmetsadykov, N., & Faye, B. (2012) Protection against lead contamination by strains of Lactic Acid Bacteria (LAB) from fermented camel milk. *Proceedings of the 3rd conference of the international society of camelid research and development*, 420–22. Retrieved from https://www.academia.edu/4489898/Farmers_Attitude_Towards_Interventions_Regarding_Camel_Calf_Health_Care

AL-Ayadhi, L., & Elamin, N. E. (2013). Camel milk as a potential therapy as an antioxidant in autism spectrum disorder (ASD). *Evidence-Based Complementary and Alternative Medicine*, 1–8. PMID:24069051

Al-Juboori, A., Mohammed, M., Rashid, J., Kurian, J., & El Refaey S. (2013). Nutritional and medicinal value of camel (Camelus Dromedarius) milk. *Food & Environment II, 170*, 221-232.

Al-Khdier, A. M., Al-Saleh, A. A., Abu-Tarboush, H. M., Ismail, E. A., & Metwalli, A. (2014). The ability of some starter cultures to increase the conjugated linoleic acid level in cow and camel milks. *Journal of Pure & Applied Microbiology*, *8*, 363–370.

Al-Majali, A., Ismail, Z., & Al-Hami, Y. (2007). Lactoferrin concentration in milk from camels (*Camelus dromedarius*) with and without subclinical mastitis. *International Journal of Applied Research in Veterinary Medicine*, *5*, 120.

Al-Nasseri, R. H., Al-Ruqashi, H., Al-Sabahi, J., Al-Harrasi, A., Kanekanian, A., Banerjee, Y., ... Hassan, N. (2019). Lipids derived from camel milk regulate NLRP3 inflammasome subunit-dependent inflammatory responses in human macrophages. *Functional Foods in Health and Disease*, *9*(4), 224–240. doi:10.31989/ffhd.v9i4.567

Al-Numair, S., Chandramohan, G., Kamalakkannan, N., Alsaif, M. A., & Sundaraselvan, G. (2010). Effect of camel milk on the activities of ATPases in normal and streptozotocin-diabetic rats. *Polish Journal of Food and Nutrition Sciences*, *60*(4), 375–380.

Al-Saleh, A., Metwalli, A., Ismail, E., & Alhaj, O. (2014). Antioxidative activity of camel milk casein hydrolysates. *Journal of Camel Practice and Research*, *21*(2), 229–237. doi:10.5958/2277-8934.2014.00041.1

Al-Shamsi, K., Mudgil, P., Hassan, H., & Maqsood, S. (2018). Camel milk protein hydrolysates with improved technofunctional properties and enhanced antioxidant potential in in vitro and in food model systems. *Journal of Dairy Science*, *101*(1), 47–60. doi:10.3168/jds.2017-13194 PMID:29128226

Al-Wabel, N., Hassan, A., Abbas, H., & Muosa, H. (2012). Antiulcerogenic effect of camel milk against ethanol induced gastric ulcers in rats. *WebmedCentral Veterinary Medicine*, *3*(3), WMC002804.

Alhaj, O., & Al Kanhal, H. A. (2010). Compositional, technological and nutritional aspects of dromedary camel milk. *International Dairy Journal*, *20*(12), 811–821. doi:10.1016/j.idairyj.2010.04.003

Alhaj, O., Al-Khalifa, A., Metwalli, A., Ismail, E., & Ali, H. (2017). *Method of making a fermented dairy product from camel milk*. United States Patent, Number US9,623,057B1.

Alhaj, O., Kanekanian, A., Peters, A., & Tatham, A. (2010). Hypocholesterolemic effect of *Bifidobacterium animalis* subsp. *Lactis* (Bb12) and trypsin casein hydrolysate. *Food Chemistry*, *123*(2), 430–435. doi:10.1016/j.foodchem.2010.04.061

Alhaj, O., Metwalli, A., Ismail, E., Ali, H., Al-khalifa, A., & Kanekanian, A. (2018). Angiotensin converting enzyme-inhibitory activity and antimicrobial effect of fermented camel milk (*Camelus dromedarius*). *International Journal of Dairy Technology*, *17*(1), 27–35. doi:10.1111/1471-0307.12383

Alhaj, O., Taufik, E., Handa, Y., Fukuda, K., Saito, T., & Urashima, T. (2013). Chemical characterization of oligosaccharides in commercially pasteurized dromedary camel (*camelusdromedarius*) milk. *International Dairy Journal*, *28*(2), 70–75. doi:10.1016/j.idairyj.2012.08.008

Alhaj, O. A. (2017). Identification of potential ACE-inhibitory peptides from dromedary fermented camel milk. *CYTA: Journal of Food*, *15*(2), 191–195. doi:10.1080/19476337.2016.1236353

Alhaj, O. A., Kanekanian, A., & Peters, A. (2007). Investigation on whey proteins profile of commercially aviabale milk-based probiotics health drinks using fast protein liquid chromatography (FPLC). *British Food Journal*, *109*(6), 469–480. doi:10.1108/00070700710753526

Alimi, D., Hajaji, S., Rekik, M., Abidi, A., Gharbi, M., & Akkari, H. (2016). First report of the in vitro nematicidal effects of camel milk. *Veterinary Parasitology*, *228*, 153–159. doi:10.1016/j.vetpar.2016.09.003 PMID:27692318

Amr, A., Takruri, H., Shomaf, M., Alhaj, O., & Faris, M. (2018). Fermented Camel (*Camelus dromedarius*) and Bovine Milk Attenuate Azoxymethane-induced Colonic Aberrant Crypt Foci in Fischer 344 Rats. *Pakistan Journal of Nutrition*, *17*(4), 179–189. doi:10.3923/pjn.2018.179.189

Asha, A., Pareek, K., & Shah, S. (2016). In silico physico-chemical comparative study of human and camel insulin. *IOSR Journal of Pharmacy*, *6*(11), 50–53.

Asresie, A., & Yusuf, M. (2014). Traditional Consumption, Therapeutic Value and Its Derived Dairy Products of Dromedary Camel (Camelus Dromedaries) Milk in Somali Regional State, Eastern Ethiopia: A Review. *Global Journal of Animal Scientific Research*, *3*, 240–246.

Aswad, D. W., Paranandi, M. V., & Schurter, B. T. (2000). Isoaspartate in peptides and proteins: Formation, significance, and analysis. *Journal of Pharmaceutical and Biomedical Analysis*, *21*(6), 1129–1136. doi:10.1016/S0731-7085(99)00230-7 PMID:10708396

Ayyash, M., Al-Dhaheri, A. S., Al Mahadin, S., Kizhakkayil, J., & Abushelaibi, A. (2018b). In vitro investigation of anticancer, antihypertensive, antidiabetic, and antioxidant activities of camel milk fermented with camel milk probiotic: A comparative study with fermented bovine milk. *Journal of Dairy Science*, *101*(2), 900–911. doi:10.3168/jds.2017-13400 PMID:29224862

Ayyash, M., Al-Nuaimi, S., Al-Mahadin, S., & Liu, S. (2018a). *In vitro* investigation of anticancer and ACE-inhibiting activity, α-amylase and α-glucosidase inhibition, and antioxidant activity of camel milk fermented with camel milk probiotic: A comparative study with fermented bovine milk. *Food Chemistry*, *239*, 588–597. doi:10.1016/j.foodchem.2017.06.149 PMID:28873609

Baragob, A. E. A. (2015). Composition and hypoglycemic effect of camel milk in streptozotocin–induced diabetic rats. *Biochemistry and Biotechnology Research*, *3*, 38–42.

Baubekova, A., Kalimbetovaa, S., Akhmetsadykova, O., Konuspayeva, & Faye, B. (2015). Comparison of D. Lactate and L. lactate content in cow and camel milk. *Scientific and Practical Journal Veterinarya, 2*, 397-398.

Bauman, D., Mather, I., Wall, R., & Lock, A. (2006). Major advances associated with the biosynthesis of milk. *Journal of Dairy Science*, *89*(4), 1235–1243. doi:10.3168/jds.S0022-0302(06)72192-0 PMID:16537956

Benkerroum, N., Mekkaoui, M., Bennani, N., & Kamal, H. (2004). Antimicrobial activity of camel's milk against pathogenic strains of Escherichia coli and Listeria monocytogene. *International Journal of Dairy Technology*, *57*(1), 39–43. doi:10.1111/j.1471-0307.2004.00127.x

Boehm, G., & Stahl, B. (2003). Oligosaccharides. In Functional Dairy Products (pp. 203-243). Cambridge, UK: Woodhead Publishers.

Boehm, G., & Stahl, B. (2007). Oligosaccharides from Milk. *The Journal of Nutrition*, *137*(3), 847S–849S. doi:10.1093/jn/137.3.847S PMID:17311985

Borschell, M., Elkin, R., Kirksey, A., Story, J., Galal, O., Harrison, G., & Jerome, N. (1986). Fatty acid composition of mature human milk of Egyptian and American women. *The American Journal of Clinical Nutrition*, *44*(3), 330–335. doi:10.1093/ajcn/44.3.330 PMID:3751954

Breitling, L. (2002). Insulin and anti-diabetic activity of camel milk. *Journal of Camel Practice and Research*, *9*, 43–45.

Brückner, H., & Fujii, N. (2010). *D-Amino Acids in Chemistry, Life Sciences and Biotechnology*. Weinheim, Germany: Verlag Helvetica ChimicaActa, Zürich, Switzerland and Wiley-VCH.

Brueckner, H., & Hausch, M. (1990). D-amino acids in dairy products: Detection, origin and nutritional aspects. I. Milk, fermented milk, fresh cheese and acid crude cheese. *Milchwissenschaft. Milk Science International*, *45*, 357–360.

Bulca, S. (2017). Functional properties of camel milk and their influences on technological applications. *Scientific Bulletin. Series F. Biotechnologies*, *21*, 275–283.

Businco, L., Bruno, G., Giampietro, P., & Cantoni, A. (1992). Allergenicity and nutritional adequacy of soy protein formulas. *The Journal of Pediatrics*, *121*(5), S21–S28. doi:10.1016/S0022-3476(05)81402-7 PMID:1447630

Butikofer, U., Meyer, J., Sieber, R., & Wechsler, D. (2007). Quantification of the angiotensinconverting enzyme-inhibiting tripeptides Val Pro-Pro and Ile-Pro-Pro in hard, semi-hard and soft cheeses. *International Dairy Journal*, *17*(8), 968–975. doi:10.1016/j.idairyj.2006.11.003

Cardak, A., Yetismeyen, A., & Bruckner, H. (2003). Quantitative comparison of free fatty acids in camel, goat and cow milk. *Milchwissenschaft. Milk Science International*, *58*, 127–130.

Cardoso, R., Santos, R., Cardoso, C., & Carvalho, M. (2010). 12 Consumption of camel's milk by patients intolerant to lactose. A preliminary study. 13. *Revista Alergia Mexico*, *57*, 26–32. PMID:20857626

Choi, S., Park, K., Kim, D., Lee, D., & Kim, Y. (2013). Preparation of Camel Milk Liposome and Its Anti-Aging Effects. *Journal of the Society of Cosmetic Scientists of Korea*, *40*(2), 155–161. doi:10.15230/SCSK.2014.40.2.155

Chuvakova, Z., Beisembayeva, R., Puzyrevskaya, Saubenouva, O., Shamenova, M., Glebova, M., … Baimenov, E. K. (2000). Chemical Composition, Microbial Control and Antiviral Properties of Freshly Made and Conserved Shubat "Bota." *Proc. 2nd International Camelid Conference Agro economics of Camelid Farming*, 8-12.

Claeys, W. L., Verraes, C., Cardoen, S., De Block, J., Huyghebaert, A., Raes, K., ... Herman, L. (2014). Consumption of raw or heated milk from different species: An evaluation of the nutritional and potential health benefits-review. *Food Control*, *42*, 188–201. doi:10.1016/j.foodcont.2014.01.045

Conesa, C., Sánchez, L., Rota, C., Pérez, M. D., Calvo, M., Farnaud, S., & Evans, R. W. (2008). Isolation of lactoferrin from milk of different species: Calorimetric and antimicrobial studies. *Comparative Biochemistry and Physiology-Part B. Biochemical and Molecular Biology*, *150*(1), 131–139. doi:10.1016/j.cbpb.2008.02.005 PMID:18387837

D'Aniello, G., Grieco, N., Filippo, M., Capiello, F., Topo, E., D'Aniello, E., & Ronsini, S. (2007). Reproductive implication of D-aspartic acid in human pre-ovulatory follicular fluid. *Human Reproduction (Oxford, England)*, *22*(12), 3178–3183. doi:10.1093/humrep/dem328 PMID:17951582

Donkor, O. N., Henriksson, A., Singh, T. K., Vasiljevic, T., & Shah, N. P. (2007). ACE-inhibitory activity of probiotic yoghurt. *International Dairy Journal*, *17*(11), 1321–1331. doi:10.1016/j.idairyj.2007.02.009

Doyon, M., & Labrecque, J. A. (2008). Functional foods: A conceptual definition. *British Food Journal*, *110*(11), 1133–1149. doi:10.1108/00070700810918036

Dziuba, B., & Dziuba, M. (2014). Milk proteins-derived bioactive peptides in dairy products: Molecular, biological and methodological aspects. *Acta Scientiarum Polonorum. Technologia Alimentaria*, *13*(1), 5–25. doi:10.17306/J.AFS.2014.1.1 PMID:24583380

Ebaid, H., Abdel-salam, B., Hassan, I., Al-Tamimi, J., Metwalli, A., & Alhazza, I. (2015). Camel milk peptide improves wound healing in diabetic rats by orchestrating the redox status and immune response. *Lipids in Health and Disease*, *14*(1), 132–142. doi:10.118612944-015-0136-9 PMID:26498022

Ehlayel, M., Hazeima, K., Al-Mesaifri, F., & Bener, A. (2011). Camel milk: An alternative for cow's milk allergy in children. *Allergy and Asthma Proceedings*, *32*(3), 255–258. doi:10.2500/aap.2011.32.3429 PMID:21703103

Ejtahed, H. S., Naslaji, A. N., Mirmiran, P., Yeganeh, M. Z., Hedayati, M., Azizi, F., & Movahedi, A. M. (2015). Effect of camel milk on blood sugar and lipid profile of patients with type 2 diabetes: A pilot clinical trial. *International Journal of Endocrinology and Metabolism*, 13. PMID:25745496

El-Abd, M., Abdel-Hamid, M., Ahmed-Farid, O., El-demerdash, M., & Mohamed, Z. (2018). Protective effect of synbiotic fermented camel milk on non-alcoholic fatty liver disease in rats. *Current Science International*, *7*(4), 466–480.

El-Agamy, E. (2000). Effect of heat treatment on camel milk proteins with respectto antimicrobial factors: A comparison with cows' and buffalo milk proteins. *Food Chemistry*, *68*(2), 227–232. doi:10.1016/S0308-8146(99)00199-5

El-Agamy, E. (2007). The challenge of cow milk protein allergy. *Small Ruminant Research*, *68*(1-2), 64–72. doi:10.1016/j.smallrumres.2006.09.016

El-Agamy, E., Nawar, M., Shamsia, S., Awad, S., & Haenlein, G. (2009). Are camel milk proteins convenient to the nutrition of cow milk allergic children. *Small Ruminant Research*, *82*(1), 1–6. doi:10.1016/j.smallrumres.2008.12.016

El-Agamy, E. I., Ruppanner, R., Ismail, A., Champagne, C. P., & Assaf, R. (1992). Antibacterial and antiviral activity of camel milk protective proteins. *The Journal of Dairy Research*, *59*(2), 169–175. doi:10.1017/S0022029900030417 PMID:1319434

El-Fakharany, E. N., Abedelbaky, B., Haroun, L., Sanchez, N., Redwan, E., & Redwan, E. M. (2012). Anti-infectivity of camel polyclonal antibodies against hepatitis C virus in Huh 7.5 hepatoma. *Virology Journal*, *16*(9), 201–211. doi:10.1186/1743-422X-9-201 PMID:22978304

El-Hatmi, H., Girardet, J. M., Gaillard, J. L., Yahyaoui, M. H., & Attia, H. (2007). Characterization of whey proteins of camel (Camelus dromedarius) milk and colostrum. *Small Ruminant Research*, *70*(2-3), 267–271. doi:10.1016/j.smallrumres.2006.04.001

El-Sayed, M. (2011). Effects of camels milk as a vehicle for insulin on glycaemic control and lipid profile in Type 1 diabetics. *American Journal of Biochemistry and Biotechnology*, *7*(4), 179–189. doi:10.3844/ajbbsp.2011.179.189

Fallah, Z., Feizi, A., Hashemipour, M., Namazi, N., Azarbayejani, L., & Kelishadi, R. (2019). Effect of Fermented Camel Milk on Obesity Measures and Blood Pressure of Adolescents with Metabolic Syndrome. *Journal of Pediatrics Review*, *7*, 181–189. doi:10.32598/jpr.7.3.181

FAO. (2013). *Statistical Year Book*. Rome, Italy: Food and Agriculture Organization of the United Nations.

FAOSTAT. (2019). *Food and Agricultural Organization of the United Nations/Statistics*. Retrieved from: http://www.fao.org/faostat/en/#data/QV/visualize

Farah, Z. (1996). *Camel milk properties and products*. St. Gallen, Switzerland: SKAT, Swiss Centre for Developments Cooperation in Technology and Management.

Farah, Z., & Rüegg, M. W. (1989). The size distribution of casein micelles in camel milk. *Food Microstructure*, *8*, 211–216.

Finke, B. (2000). *Isolierung und charakterisierung von oligosaccharide naushumanen und tierischenmilchen* (Ph.D. thesis). University of Giessen, Shaker Verlag, Aachen, Germany.

Fox, P., & McSweeney, P. (1998). Lactose chapter. In *Dairy Chemistry and Biochemistry* (1st ed.; pp. 21–66). Thomson Science.

Fukuda, K., Yamamoto, A., Ganzorig, K., Khuukhenbaatar, J., Senda, A., Saito, T., & Urashima, T. (2010). Chemical characterization of the oligosaccharides in Bactrian camel (Camelusbactrianus) milk and colostrums. *Journal of Dairy Science*, *93*(12), 5572–5587. doi:10.3168/jds.2010-3151 PMID:21094729

Gill, C., & Rowland, I. (2003). Cancer. In Functional Dairy Products (pp. 19-53). Cambridge, UK: Woodhead Publishers.

Gizachew, A., Teha, J., & Birhanu, T. (2014). Review on Medicinal and Nutritional Values of Camel Milk. *Nature and Science*, *12*(120), 35–40.

Gnädig, S., Xue, Y., Berdeaux, O., Chardigny, J. M., & Sebedio, J. L. (2003). Conjugated linoleic acid (CLA) as a functional ingredient. In Functional Dairy Products (pp. 263-298). CRC Press.

Gobbetti, M., Minervini, F., & Rizzello, C. G. (2004). Angiotensin I-converting enzyme-inhibitory and antimicrobial bioactive peptides. *International Journal of Dairy Society*, *57*(2-3), 173–188. doi:10.1111/j.1471-0307.2004.00139.x

Groenen, M. A. M., Dijkhof, R. J. M., & Van der Poel, J. J. (1995). Characterization of a GlyCAM1-like gene (glycosylation dependent cell adhesion molecule 1) which is 19 highly and specifically expressed in the lactating bovine mammary gland. *Gene*, *158*(2), 189–195. doi:10.1016/0378-1119(95)00138-V PMID:7607540

Gul, W., Farooq, N., Anees, D., Khan, U., & Rehan, F. (2015). Camel Milk: A Boon to Mankind. *International Journal of Research Studies in Biosciences*, *3*, 23–29.

Haddadin, M. S. Y., Gammoh, S. I., & Robinson, R. K. (2008). Seasonal variations in the chemical composition of camel milk in Jordan. *The Journal of Dairy Research*, *75*(1), 8–12. doi:10.1017/S0022029907002750 PMID:17971263

Hamed, H., El-Feki, A., & Gargouri, A. (2016). Influence of Wet and Dry Season on Milk Composition of Dromedary Camels (*Camelus dromedarius*) from Tunisia. *Iranian Journal of Applied Animal Science*, *7*(1), 163–167.

Harrison, R. (2006). Milk xanthine oxidase: Properties and physiological roles. *International Dairy Journal*, *16*(6), 546–554. doi:10.1016/j.idairyj.2005.08.016

IFIC. (2019). *Functional foods, International Food Information Council Foundation*; Retrieved January 12, 2019, from http://www.foodinsight.org

Izadi, A., Khedmat, L., & Mojtahedi, S. Y. (2019). Nutritional and therapeutic perspectives of camel milk and its protein hydrolysates: A review on versatile biofunctional properties. *Journal of Functional Foods*, *60*, 103441. doi:10.1016/j.jff.2019.103441

Jang, A., & Lee, M. (2005). Purification and identification of angiotensin converting enzyme inhibitory peptides from beef hydrolysates. *Meat Science*, *69*(4), 653–661. doi:10.1016/j.meatsci.2004.10.014 PMID:22063143

Jilo, K. (2016). Medicinal Values of Camel Milk. *International Journal of Veterinary Science and Research*, *2*(1), 18-25.

Jrad, Z., Girardet, J.-M., Adt, I., Oulahal, I., Degraeve, N., Khorchani, P., & El Hatmi, H. (2014). Antioxidant activity of camel milk casein. *Mljekarstvo*, *64*, 287–294. doi:10.15567/mljekarstvo.2014.0408

Jumah, R., Shaker, R., & Abu-Jadayil, B. (2001). Effect of milk source on therheological properties of yoghurt during the gelation process. *International Journal of Dairy Technology*, *54*(3), 89–93. doi:10.1046/j.1364-727x.2001.00012.x

Kajimoto, O., Kurosaki, T., Mizutani, J., Ikeda, N., Kaneko, K., Aihara, K., ... Nakamura, Y. (2002). Antihypertensive effects of liquid yogurts containing "lactotripeptides (VPP, IPP)" in mild hypertensive subjects. *Journal of Nutrition and Food*, *5*, 55–66.

Kappeler, S., Farah, Z., & Puhan, Z. (1998). Sequence analysis of *Camelus dromedaries* milk caseins. *The Journal of Dairy Research*, *65*(2), 209–222. doi:10.1017/S0022029997002847 PMID:9627840

Kappeler, S., Farah, Z., & Puhan, Z. (1999). Alternative splitting of lactophorin mRNA from lactating mammary gland of the camel (*Camelus dromedarius*). *Journal of Dairy Science*, *82*(10), 2084–2093. doi:10.3168/jds.S0022-0302(99)75450-0 PMID:10531593

Kappeler, S., Farah, Z., & Puhan, Z. (2003). 5′-Flanking regions of camel milk genesare highly similar to homologue regions of other species and can be divided into two distinct groups. *Journal of Dairy Science*, *86*(2), 498–508. doi:10.3168/jds.S0022-0302(03)73628-5 PMID:12647956

Kappeler, S. R., Heuberger, C., Farah, Z., & Puhan, Z. (2004). Expression of the peptidoglycan recognition protein, PGRP, in the lactating mammary gland. *Journal of Dairy Science*, *87*(8), 2660–2668. doi:10.3168/jds.S0022-0302(04)73392-5 PMID:15328291

Kashyap, D.R, Rompca, A., & Gaballa, A. (2014). Peptidoglycan recognition proteins kill bacteria by inducing oxidative, thiol, and metal stress. *PLoS Pathog*, *10*(7), 1-17.

Kaskous, S. (2016). Importance of camel milk for human health. *Emirates Journal of Food and Agriculture*, *28*(3), 158–163. doi:10.9755/ejfa.2015-05-296

Kebir, N., Aichouni, A., & Zahzeh, T. (2017). Raw camel milk properties on alloxan-induced diabetic Wistar rats. *Romanian Journal of Diabetes, Nutrition, and Metabplic Disorders*, *24*(1), 41-47. doi:10.1515/rjdnmd-2017-0005

Keykanlu, H., Zibaei, S., Ardjmand, M., & Safekordi, A. (2016). Fluorocarbon nanostructures (PFOB-NEP) as camel milk lactoferrin and its anti-cancer effects on human breast cancer cell line MCF7. *Izvestiia po Himiia*, *48*(2), 323–331.

Khan, A., & Alzohairy, M. (2011). Hepatoprotective effects of camel milk against CCl4-induced hepatotoxicity in Rats. *Asian Journal of Biochemistry*, *6*(2), 171–180. doi:10.3923/ajb.2011.171.180

Khan, A. A., Alzohairy, M. A., & Mohieldein, A. H. (2013). Antidiabetic Effects of Camel Milk in Streptozotocin-induced Diabetic Rats. *American Journal of Biochemistry and Molecular Biology*, *3*(1), 151–158. doi:10.3923/ajbmb.2013.151.158

Kitts, D., & Weiler, K. (2003). Bioactive proteins and peptides from food sources. Applications of bioprocesses used in isolation and recovery. *Current Pharmaceutical Design*, *9*(16), 1309–1323. doi:10.2174/1381612033454883 PMID:12769739

Koletzko, B. (2016). Human Milk Lipids. *Annals of Nutrition & Metabolism*, *69*(suppl 2), 28–40. doi:10.1159/000452819 PMID:28103608

Konuspayeva, G., Lemarie, E., Faye, B., Loiseau, G., & Montet, D. (2008). Fatty acid and cholesterol composition of camel's (Camelus bactrianus, Camelus dromedaries and hybrids) milk in Kazakhstan. *Dairy Science & Technology*, *88*(3), 327–340. doi:10.1051/dst:2008005

Korashy, H., Maayah, Z., Abd-Allah, A., El-Kadi, A., & Alhaider, A. (2012). Camel Milk Triggers Apoptotic Signaling Pathways in Human Hepatoma HepG2 and Breast CancerMCF7 Cell Lines through Transcriptional Mechanism. *Journal of Biomedicine & Biotechnology*, 1–9. doi:10.1155/2012/593195

Król, J., Brodziak, A., Litwińczuk, Z., & Barłowska, J. (2012). Selected Factors Determining the Content of Lactoferrin, Lysozyme and Immunoglobulins G in Bovine Milk. In *A Search for Antibacterial Agents*. IntechOpen. Available from: https://www.intechopen.com/books/a-search-for-antibacterial-agents/selected-factors-determining-the-content-of-lactoferrin-lysozyme-and-immunoglobulins-g-in-bovine-milk

Kula, J. (2016). Medicinal Values of Camel Milk. *International Journal of Veterinary Scientific Research*, *2*(1), 18-25. Doi:10.17352/ijvsr.000009

Kumar, D., Chatli, M. K., Singh, R., Mehta, N., & Kumar, P. (2016a). Enzymatic hydrolysis of camel milk casein and its antioxidant properties. *Dairy Science & Technology*, *96*(3), 391–404. doi:10.100713594-015-0275-9

Kumar, D., Chatli, M. K., Singh, R., Mehta, N., & Kumar, P. (2016b). Antioxidant and antimicrobial activity of camel milk casein hydrolysates and its fractions. *Small Ruminant Research*, *139*, 20–25. doi:10.1016/j.smallrumres.2016.05.002

Kumar, K., Venu, L., & Manchala, R. (2016). Anti-hyperglycemic activity of camel milk in rat models of diabetes / insulin resistance. *International Journal of Research Studies in Medical and Health Sciences, 1*(1), 7–14.

Kunz, C., & Rudloff, S. (2006). Health promoting aspects of milk oligosaccharides. *International Dairy Journal, 16*(11), 1341–1346. doi:10.1016/j.idairyj.2006.06.020

Kuwabara, Y., Nagai, S., Yoshimitsu, N., Nakagawa, I., Watanabe, Y., & Tamai, Y. (1995). Antihypertensive effect of the milk fermented by culturing with various lactic acid bacteria and yeast. *Journal of Fermentation and Bioengineering, 80*(3), 294–295. doi:10.1016/0922-338X(95)90834-M

Levy, A., Steiner, L., & Yagil, R. (2013). Camel milk: Disease control and dietary laws. *Journal of Health Science, 1*, 48–53.

Li, G., Le, G., Shi, Y., & Shrestha, S. (2004). Angiotensin I-converting enzyme inhibitory peptides derived from food proteins and their physiological and pharmacological effects. *Nutrition Research (New York, N.Y.), 24*(7), 469–486. doi:10.1016/S0271-5317(04)00058-2

López-Fandiño, R., Otte, J., & Van Camp, J. (2006). Review: Physiological, chemicaland technological aspects of milk-protein-derived peptides with antihypertensiveand ACE-inhibitory activity. *International Dairy Journal, 16*(11), 1277–1293. doi:10.1016/j.idairyj.2006.06.004

Mader, J., Salsman, D., Conrad, D., & Hoskin, D. (2005). Bovine lactoferricin selectively induces apoptosis in human leukemia and carcinoma cell lines. *Molecular Cancer Therapeutics, 4*(4), 612–624. doi:10.1158/1535-7163.MCT-04-0077 PMID:15827335

Maldonado, J., Gil, A., Narbona, E., & Molina, J. A. (1998). Special formulas in infant nutrition: A review. *Early Human Development, 53*, S23–S32. doi:10.1016/S0378-3782(98)00062-0 PMID:10102652

Malik, A., Al-Senaidy, A., Jankun, E., & Jankun, J. (2012). A study of the anti-diabetic agents of camel milk. *International Journal of Molecular Medicine, 30*(3), 585–592. doi:10.3892/ijmm.2012.1051 PMID:22751901

Maqsood, S., Al-Dowaila, A., Mudgil, P., Kamal, H., Jobe, B., & Hassan, H. M. (2019). In-depth characterization of protein and lipid fractions from camel and cow milk, their functionality, antioxidant and antihypertensive properties upon simulated gastro-intestinal digestion. *Food Chemistry, 279*, 328–338. doi:10.1016/j.foodchem.2018.12.011 PMID:30611498

Markiewicz-Górka, I., Zawadzki, M., Januszewska, L., Hombek-Urban, K., & Pawlas, K. (2011). Influence of selenium and/or magnesium on alleviation alcohol induced oxidative stress in rats, normalization function of liver and changes in serum lipid parameters. *Human and Experimental Toxicology, 30*(11), 1811–1827. doi:10.1177/0960327111401049 PMID:21474619

Markiewicz-kęszycka, M., Czyżak-runowska, G., Lipińska, P., & Wójtowski, J. (2013). Fatty acid profile of milk - a review. *Bulletin of the Veterinary Institute in Pulawy, 57*(2), 135–139. doi:10.2478/bvip-2013-0026

Martin, M., Martin-Sosa, S., Garcia-Pardo, L., & Hueso, P. (2001). Distribution of bovine sialoglycoconjugates during lactation. *Journal of Dairy Science*, *84*(5), 995–1000. doi:10.3168/jds.S0022-0302(01)74558-4 PMID:11384055

Mati, A., Girardet, J.-M., Xenakis, D., & Linden, G. (1991). Isolation and characterization of proteose-peptone hydrophobic fractions of cow's, ewe's and goat's milk. *Le Lait*, *71*, 259–273. doi:10.1051/lait:1991320

Mati, A., Senoussi-Ghezali, C., Ahmed Zennia, S. S., Almi-Sebbane, D., El-Hatmi, H., & Girardet, J. (2017). Dromedary camel milk proteins, a source of peptides having biological activities – A review. *International Dairy Journal*, *73*, 25–37. doi:10.1016/j.idairyj.2016.12.001

Maurad, K., & Meriem, K. (2008). Probiotic characteristics of *Lactobacillus plantarum* strains from traditional butter made from camel milk in arid regions (Sahara) of Algeria. *Grasas y Aceites*, *59*(3), 218–224. doi:10.3989/gya.2008.v59.i3.511

Mehra, R., & Kelly, P. (2006). Milk oligosaccharides: Structural and technological aspects [Review]. *International Dairy Journal*, *16*(11), 1334–1340. doi:10.1016/j.idairyj.2006.06.008

Mehrin, B., Saeid, Z., Maryam, I., Samane, L. A., Somaye, B., Mahbobe, M., & Ali, H. (2011). The extract of lactoperoxidase enzyme from camel milk using chromatography methods and its antibacterial effects on *Pseudomonas aeruginosa. Clinical Biochemistry*, *44*(13), S92–S92. doi:10.1016/j.clinbiochem.2011.08.208

Meisel, H., Walsh, D., Murray, B., & FitzGerald, R. (2006). ACE inhibitory peptides. In Y. Mine & F. Shahidi (Eds.), *Nutraceutical Proteins and Peptides in Health and Disease* (Vol. 4, pp. 269–315). Taylor & Francis Group Publisher.

Merin, U., Bernstein, S., Bloch-Damti, A., Yagil, R., van Creveld, C., Lindner, P., & Gollop, N. (2001). A comparative study of milk serum proteins in camel (*Camelus dromedarius*) and bovine colostrum. *Livestock Production Science*, *67*(3), 297–30. doi:10.1016/S0301-6226(00)00198-6

Meyer, J., Butikofer, U., Walther, B., Wechsler, D., & Sieber, R. (2009). Hot topic: Changes in angiotensin-converting enzyme inhibition and concentration of the teripeptides Val-Pro-Pro and Ile-Pro-Pro during ripening of different Swiss cheese varieties. *Journal of Dairy Science*, *92*(3), 826–836. doi:10.3168/jds.2008-1531 PMID:19233775

Mihic, T., Rainkie, D., Wilby, K., & Pawluk, S. (2016). The Therapeutic Effects of Camel Milk: A Systematic Review of Animal and Human Trials. *Journal of Evidence-Based Complementary & Alternative Medicine*, *21*(4), NP110–NP126. doi:10.1177/2156587216658846 PMID:27432772

Mohamed, E., & Mustafa, A. (2016). Fatty acids content in milk of dromedary camel (*Camelus dromedarius*) from farming and pastoral systems in Sudan. *International Journal of Science and Research*, *5*(6), 570–573.

Mona, E. (2010). Biochemical effects of fermented camel milk on diarrhea in rats. *New York Science Journal*, *3*(5), 106–111.

Moslehishad, M., Ehsani, M. R., Salami, M., Mirdamadi, S., Ezzatpanah, H., Niasari, A., & Moosavi-Movahedi, A. (2013). The comparative assessment of ACE-inhibitory and antioxidant activities of peptide fractions obtained from fermented camel and bovine milk by *Lactobacillus rhamnosus* PTCC 1637. *International Dairy Journal*, *29*(2), 82–87. doi:10.1016/j.idairyj.2012.10.015

Moure, A., Domínguez, H., & Parajó, J. (2006). Antioxidant properties of ultrafiltration-recovered soy protein fractions from industrial effluents and their hydrolysates. *Process Biochemistry*, *41*(2), 447–456. doi:10.1016/j.procbio.2005.07.014

Muhialdina, B. J., & Algboory, H. L. (2018). Identification of low molecular weight antimicrobial peptides from Iraqi camel milk fermented with *Lactobacillus plantarum. PharmaNutrition*, *6*(2), 69–73. doi:10.1016/j.phanu.2018.02.002

Mullaicharam, A. (2014). A review on medicinal properties of Camel milk. *World Journal of Pharmaceutical Science*, *2*(3), 237–242.

Mutlag, A., Al-Zoreky, N., & El-Dermerdash, H. (2013). Camel's milk as a natural source for probiotics. *Research Journal of Microbiology*, *8*, 70–80. doi:10.3923/jm.2013.70.80

Nakamura, Y., Yamamoto, N., Sakai, K., Okubo, A., Yamazaki, S., & Takano, T. (1995a). Purification and characterization of angiotensin I-converting enzyme inhibitors from sour milk. *Journal of Dairy Science*, *78*(4), 777–783. doi:10.3168/jds.S0022-0302(95)76689-9 PMID:7790570

Nakamura, Y., Yamamoto, N., Sakai, K., & Takano, T. (1995b). Antihypertensive effect of sour milk and peptides isolated from it that are inhibitors to angiotensin I-converting enzyme. *Journal of Dairy Science*, *78*(6), 1253–1257. doi:10.3168/jds.S0022-0302(95)76745-5 PMID:7673515

Navarrete-Rodríguez, E. M., Ríos-Villalobosaet, L. A., Alcocer-Arreguína, C. R., Del-Rio-Navarro, B. E., & … . (2018). Cross-over clinical trial for evaluating the safety of camel's milk intake in patients who are allergic to cow's milk protein. *Allergologia et Immunopathologia*, *46*(2), 149–154. doi:10.1016/j.aller.2017.06.005 PMID:29223706

Nongonierm, A. B., Paolella, S., Mudgil, P., Maqsood, S., & FitzGerald, R. J. (2018). Identification of novel dipeptidyl peptidase IV (DPP-IV) inhibitory peptides in camel milk protein hydrolysates. *Food Chemistry*, *244*, 340–348. doi:10.1016/j.foodchem.2017.10.033 PMID:29120791

Otte, J., Shalaby, S., Zakora, M., & Neilsen, M. (2007). Fractionation and identification of ACE-inhibitory peptides from α-lactalbumin and β-casein produced by thermolysin-catalysed hydrolysis. *International Dairy Journal*, *17*(12), 1460–1472. doi:10.1016/j.idairyj.2007.04.008

Oudah, L. (2016). The effect of camel milk in the tissue changes to the kidneys of laboratory male rats treated by cadmium. *International Journal of Animal Health and Livestock Production Research*, *1*(2), 8–14.

Pan, D., & Guo, Y. (2010). Optimization of sour milk fermentation for the production of ACE inhibitory peptides and purification of a novel peptide from whey protein hydrolysate. *International Dairy Journal*, *20*(7), 472–479. doi:10.1016/j.idairyj.2010.01.007

Pan, D., Luo, Y., & Tanokura, M. (2005). Antihypertensive peptides from skimmed milk hydrolysate digested by cell-free extract of Lactobacillus helveticus JCM1004. *Food Chemistry*, *91*(1), 123–129. doi:10.1016/j.foodchem.2004.05.055

Park, Y. (2009). Overview of bioactive components in milk and dairy products. In Y. W. Park (Ed.), *Bioactive Componentsin Milk and Dairy Products* (pp. 3–13). Blackwell Publishing. doi:10.1002/9780813821504.ch1

Pellegrini, A., Dettling, C., Thomas, U., & Hunziker, P. (2001). Isolation and characterization of four bactericidal domains in the bovine β-lactoglobulin. *Biochemicaet Biophysica Acta*, *1526*(2), 131–140. doi:10.1016/S0304-4165(01)00116-7 PMID:11325534

Philanto, A., Virtanen, T., & Korhonen, H. (2010). Angiotensin I converting enzyme (ACE) inhibitory activity and antihypertensive effect of fermented milk. *International Dairy Journal*, *20*(1), 3–10. doi:10.1016/j.idairyj.2009.07.003

Quan, S., Tsuda, H., & Miyamoto, T. (2008). Angiotensin I-converting enzyme inhibitory peptides in skim milk fermented with *Lactobacillus helveticus* 130B4 from camel milk in Inner Mongolia, China. *Journal of the Science of Food and Agriculture*, *88*(15), 2688–2692. doi:10.1002/jsfa.3394

Quita, S., & Kurdi, A. (2010). Antigenotoxic and anticytotoxic effect of camel milk in mice treated with cisplatin. *Saudi Journal of Biological Sciences*, *17*(2), 159–166. doi:10.1016/j.sjbs.2010.02.010 PMID:23961073

Rafiq, S., Huma, N., Pasha, I., Sameen, A., Mukhtar, O., & Khan, M. (2016). Chemical composition, nitrogen fractions and amino acids profile of milk from different animal species. *Asian-Australasian Journal of Animal Sciences*, *29*(7), 1022–1028. doi:10.5713/ajas.15.0452 PMID:26954163

Redwan, E., & Tabll, A. (2007). Camel lactoferrin markedly inhibits hepatitis C virus genotype 4 infection of human peripheral blood leukocytes. *Journal of Immunoassay & Immunochemistry*, *28*(3), 267–277. doi:10.1080/15321810701454839 PMID:17613672

Rodríguez-Figueroa, J. C., Reyes-Díaz, R., González-Cordoba, A. F., & Troncoso-Rojas, R. (2010). Angiotensin-converting enzyme inhibitory activity of milk fermented by wild and industrial *Lactococcus lactis* strains. *Journal of Dairy Science*, *93*(11), 5032–5038. doi:10.3168/jds.2010-3103 PMID:20965317

Rolfes, S., Pinna, K., & Whitney, E. (2015). Understanding Normal and Clinical Nutrition (10th ed.). Cengage learning.

Saadaoui, B., Henry, C., Khorchani, T., Mars, M., Martin, P., & Cebo, C. (2013). Proteomics of the milk fat globule membrane from *Camelus dromedarius*. *Proteomics*, *13*(7), 1180–1184. doi:10.1002/pmic.201200113 PMID:23349047

Sah, B., Vasiljevic, T., McKechnie, S., & Donkor, O. (2014). Effect of probiotics on antioxidant and antimutagenic activities of crude peptide extract from yogurt. *Food Chemistry*, *156*, 264–270. doi:10.1016/j.foodchem.2014.01.105 PMID:24629967

Sahani, M., Agrawal, R., Tuteja, F., Ghouri, S., Aminudeen, R., & Sena, D. (2005). Hypoglycemic activity of camel milk in straptozotocin induced hyperglycemia in rats. *The Indian Journal of Animal Sciences*, *75*, 1436–1437.

Salami, M., Moosavi-Movahedi, A., Ehsani, M., Yousefi, R., Haertlé, T., Chobert, J., ... Niasari-Naslaji, A. (2010). Improvement of the antimicrobial and antioxidant activities of camel and bovine whey proteins by limited proteolysis. *Journal of Agricultural and Food Chemistry*, *58*(6), 3297–3302. doi:10.1021/jf9033283 PMID:20175528

Salami, M., Moosavi-Movahedi, A., Moosavi-Movahedi, F., Ehsani, M. R., Yousefi, R., Farhadi, M., ... Haertlé, T. (2011). Biological activity of camel milk casein following enzymatic digestion. *The Journal of Dairy Research*, *78*(4), 471–478. doi:10.1017/S0022029911000628 PMID:21910944

Saljooghi, S., Mansouri-Najand, L., & Ebrahimnejad, F., Doostan & Askari, N. (2017). Microbiological, biochemical and organoleptic properties of fermented probiotic drink produced from camel milk. *Veterinary Research Forum: An International Quarterly Journal*, *8*(4), 313–317. PMID:29326790

Saltanat, H., Li, H., Xu, Y., Wang, J., Liu, F., & Geng, X. H. (2009). The influences of camel milk on the immune response of chronic hepatitis B. *Chinese Journal of Cellular and Molecular Immunology*, *25*(5), 431-433.

Sarmadi, B., & Ismail, A. (2010). Antioxidative peptides from food proteins: A review. *Peptides*, *31*(10), 1949–1956. doi:10.1016/j.peptides.2010.06.020 PMID:20600423

Sawaya, W. N., Khalil, J. K., Al-Shalhat, A., & Al-Mohammad, H. (1984). Chemical composition and nutritional quality of camel milk. *Journal of Food Science*, *49*(3), 744–747. doi:10.1111/j.1365-2621.1984.tb13200.x

Sboui, A., Khorchani, T., Djegham, M., Agrebi, A., Elhatmi, H., & Belhadj, O. (2010). Anti-diabetic effect of camel milk in alloxan-induced diabetic dogs: A dose–response experiment. *Journal of Animal Physiology and Animal Nutrition*, *94*(4), 540–546. doi:10.1111/j.1439-0396.2009.00941.x PMID:19906135

Shabo, Y., Barzel, & Yagil, R. (2008). Etiology of Crohn's Disease and Camel Milk Treatment. *Journal of Camel Practice and Research*, *15*, 55–59.

Shabo, Y., Barzel, R., Margoulis, M., & Yagil, R. (2005). Camel milk for food allergies in children. *Immunology and Allergies*, *7*, 796–798. PMID:16382703

Shalash, M. R. (1984). The production and utilization of camel milk. In W. R. Cockrill (Ed.), *The Camelid: An all-purpose animal* (pp. 196–208). Uppsala, Sweden: Scandinavian Institute of African Studies.

Sharma, P., Dube, D., Singh, A., Mishra, B., Singh, N., Sinha, M., ... Singh, T. P. (2011). Structural basis of recognition of pathogen-associated molecular patterns and inhibition of proinflammatory cytokines by camel peptidoglycan recognition protein. *The Journal of Biological Chemistry*, *286*(18), 16208–16217. doi:10.1074/jbc.M111.228163 PMID:21454594

Sharma, S., Sinha, M., Kaushik, S., Kaur, P., & Singh, T. (2013). C-lobe of lactoferrin: The whole story of the half-molecule. *Biochemistry Research International*, *ID271641*, 1–8. doi:10.1155/2013/271641 PMID:23762557

Shori, A. (2013). Antioxidant activity and viability of lactic acid bacteria in soybean-yogurt made from cow and camel milk. *Journal of Taibah University for Science*, *7*(4), 202–208. doi:10.1016/j.jtusci.2013.06.003

Singh, R., Mal, G., Kumar, D., Patil, D., & Pathak, K. (2017). Camel Milk: An Important Natural Adjuvant. *Agricultural Research*, *6*(4), 327–340. doi:10.100740003-017-0284-4

Sisay, F., & Awoke, K. (2015). Review on production, quality and use of camel milk in Ethiopia. *Journal of Fisheries & Livestock Production*, *3*(3), 1–4.

Soetikno, V., Watanabe, K., Sari, F. R., Harima, M., Thandavarayan, R. A., Veeraveedu, P. T., ... Suzuki, K. (2011). Curcumin attenuates diabetic nephropathy by inhibiting PKC-a and PKC-b1 activity in streptozotocin-induced type I diabetic rats. *Molecular Nutrition & Food Research*, *55*(11), 1655–1665. doi:10.1002/mnfr.201100080 PMID:22045654

Solanki, D., Hati, S., & Sakure, A. (2017). In silico and in vitro analysis of novel angiotensin I-converting enzyme (ACE) inhibitory bioactive peptides derived from fermented camel milk (Camelus dromedarius). *International Journal of Peptide Research and Therapeutics*, *23*(4), 441–459. doi:10.100710989-017-9577-5

Stenberg, M., Marko-Varga, G., & Oste, R. (2002). Enantio separation of D- and L-amino acids by a coupled system consisting of an ion-exchange column and a chiral column and determination of D-aspartic acid and d-glutamic acid in soy products. *Food Chemistry*, *79*(4), 507–512. doi:10.1016/S0308-8146(02)00215-7

Tagliazucchi, D., Shamsia, S., & Conte, A. (2016). Release of angiotensin converting enzyme-inhibitory peptides during in vitro gastro-intestinal digestion of camel milk. *International Dairy Journal*, *56*, 119–128. doi:10.1016/j.idairyj.2016.01.009

Tak, L., Bais, B., Singh, R., Singh, S., & Nayak, T. (2018). Assessment of Probiotic and Neutraceutical Properties of Camel Milk Yoghurt. *International Journal of Current Microbiology and Applied Sciences*, *7*(10), 3351–3357. doi:10.20546/ijcmas.2018.710.388

Takayama, Y., Mizumachi, K., & Takezawa, T. (2002). The bovine lactoferrin region responsible for promoting the collagen gel contractile activity of human fibroblasts. *Biochemical and Biophysical Research Communications*, *299*(5), 813–817. doi:10.1016/S0006-291X(02)02748-1 PMID:12470651

Taylor, S. (1986). Immunological and allergic properties of cows' milk proteins in humans. *Journal of Food Protection*, *49*(3), 239–250. doi:10.4315/0362-028X-49.3.239 PMID:30959730

Topo, E., Soricelli, A., D'Aniello, A., Ronsini, S., & D'Aniello, G. (2009). The role and molecular mechanism of D-aspartic acid in the release and synthesis of LH and testosterone in humans and rats. *Reproductive Biology and Endocrinology*, *7*(1), 120–131. doi:10.1186/1477-7827-7-120 PMID:19860889

Urashima, T., Kitaoka, M., Asakuma, S., & Messer, M. (2009). Milk oligosaccharides. In P. L. H. McSweeney & P. F. Fox (Eds.), *Advanced Dairy Chemistry. Lactose, Water, Salts and Minor Constituents* (Vol. 3, pp. 295–349). New York, NY: Springer Science Business Media.

Urashima, T., Murata, S., & Nakamura, T. (1997). Structural determination of monosialyltrisaccharides obtained from caprine colostrum. *Comparative Biochemistry and Physiology*, *116B*(4), 431–435. doi:10.1016/S0305-0491(96)00269-6 PMID:9149396

Virtanen, T., Pihlanto, A., Akkanen, S., & Korhonen, H. (2007). Development of antioxidant activity in milk whey during fermentation with lactic acid bacteria. *Journal of Applied Microbiology*, *102*(1), 106–115. doi:10.1111/j.1365-2672.2006.03072.x PMID:17184325

Walstra, P., Wouters, J., & Geurts, T. (2008). Milk for liquid consumption. In Dairy Science and Technology (pp. 421-444). CRC, Taylor & Francis.

Wernery, R., & Yagil, R. (2012). Medicinal properties in camel milk for treatment of Epidemic Diseases. *Proceedings of the 3rd ISOCARD International Conference*, 225-227.

WHO. (2019). *Estimated incidence, mortality and prevalence worldwide in 2019*. Retrieved January 19, 2019, from http://globocan.iarc.fr/Pages/fact_sheets_cancer.aspx

Wu, H., Guang, X., Al-Fageeh, M., Cao, J., Pan, S., Zhou, H., . . . Alshanqeeti, A. (2014). Camelid genomes reveal evolution and adaptation to desert environments. *Nature Communications, 5*. Retrieved from https://www.nature.com/articles/ncomms6188

Yagil, R. (1987). Camel milk - A review. *Farm Animals*, *2*, 81–99.

Yahya, M., Alhaj, O. & Al-Khalifah, A. (2017). Antihypertensive effect of fermented skim camel (*Camelus dromedarius*) milk on spontaneously hypertensive rats. *Nutricion hospitalaria: organo oficial de la Sociedad Espanola de Nutricion Parenteral y Enteral*, *34*, 416-421.

Yamamoto, N., Akino, A., & Takano, T. (1994). Antihypertensive effect of the peptides derived from casein by an extracellular proteinase from Lactobacillus helveticus CP790. *Journal of Dairy Science*, *77*(4), 917–922. doi:10.3168/jds.S0022-0302(94)77026-0 PMID:8201050

Yassin, M. H., Soliman, M. M., Mostafa, S. A., & Ali, H. A. (2015). Antimicrobial effects of camel milk against some bacterial pathogens. *Journal of Food and Nutrition Research*, *3*(3), 162–168. doi:10.12691/jfnr-3-3-6

Yateem, A., Balba, M. T., Al-Surrayai, T., Al-Mutairi, B., & Al-Daher, R. (2008). Isolation of Lactic Acid Bacteria with Probiotic Potential from Camel Milk. *International Journal of Dairy Science*, *3*(4), 194–199. doi:10.3923/ijds.2008.194.199

Zagorski, O., Maman, A., Yaffe, A., & Meisler, A., Van creveld, C., & Yagil, R. (1998). Insulin in milk-a comparative study. *International Journal of Animal Sciences*, *13*, 241–244.

Zahedi, M., Salami, M., & Moslehishad, M. (2016). Fermented Camel Milk (Chal): Chemical, Microbial and Functional Properties. *Journal of Pharmaceutical and Health Sciences*, *4*(3), 193–204.

Chapter 8
Health-Improving and Disease-Preventing Potential of Camel Milk Against Chronic Diseases and Autism:
Camel Milk and Chronic Diseases

Mo'ez Al-Islam Ezzat Faris
University of Sharjah, UAE

Hadeel Ghazzawi
https://orcid.org/0000-0003-3045-4153
University of Jordan, Jordan

ABSTRACT

Camel milk has been used as part of the human diet since ancient times. This chapter tries to elaborate the different aspects of nutraceutical functional properties of camel milk, focusing on the nutritional composition, presence of bioactive zoochemicals and peptides, antioxidant nutrients (vitamin C), and health rendering properties of this unique milk. Recent research has identified camel milk as a prophylactic and therapeutic functional food due to its noticeable content of essential macronutrients, namely bioactive functional proteins and peptides, along with its considerable content of essential micronutrients. Indeed, the presence of this unique mixture has shown to be promising contributors to the management and prevention of chronic diseases, such as cancer, diabetes, liver and kidney, metabolic syndrome, inflammatory bowel diseases in adults, and autism. In vivo, in vitro, and epidemiological and experimental studies were reviewed, and molecular mechanisms were highlighted for better understanding of the health-promoting, disease-preventing potential of camel milk.

DOI: 10.4018/978-1-7998-1604-1.ch008

INTRODUCTION

Few past studies unraveled that camel milk (CM) treasures a plethora of considerable amounts of zoochemicals (compounds in animals that are believed to provide health benefits beyond the traditional nutrients that foods contain) and antioxidant vitamins such as C and E (Farah, 1993; Farah, Rettenmaier, & Atkins, 1992; Konuspayeva, Faye, & Loiseau, 2011), lactoferrins and lysosomes (El Sayed, Ruppanner, Ismail, Champagne, & Assaf, 1992; Konuspayeva, Faye, Loiseau, & Levieux, 2007), and immunoglobulins (Ebaid, Salem, Sayed, & Metwalli, 2011; El Sayed et al., 1992; Konuspayeva et al., 2007; Miniero et al., 2014) that may entail therapeutic potential. Several studies extensively reviewed and critically revised the significant therapeutic and prophylactic properties of CM, as a commonly and traditionally practiced medical intervention, and recently evident by modern research, with emphasis on anti-diabetic, antimicrobial and anti-inflammatory effects (Abdel Gader & Alhaider, 2016; Dubey, Lal, Mittal, & Kapur, 2015; Gizachew, Teha, Birhanu, & Nekemte, 2014; Hammam, 2019; Kalla, Manthani, & Keerthi, 2017; Khatoon & Najam, 2017; Mati et al., 2016; Mihic, Rainkie, Wilby, & Pawluk, 2016; Mirmiran, Ejtahed, Angoorani, Eslami, & Azizi, 2017; Mullaicharam, 2014; Niasari-Naslaji, Arabha, Atakpour, Salami, & Moosavi-Movahedi, 2012; C. Sharma & Singh, 2014; Shori, 2015; Yadav, Kumar, Priyadarshini, & Singh, 2015). Reports affirmed that the unique constitutes of CM in terms of the presence of a plethora of antioxidants, antiviral, antibacterial, antifungal, hypoglycemic, anti-tumor activity and anticancer properties, along with its ability to prevent aging and to affect autoimmune diseases (Al-Juboori, Mohammed, Rashid, Kurian, & El Refaey, 2013; Kula & Tegegne, 2016; Refaey, 2013; Sharma & Singh, 2014); all make camel milk a candidate functional and therapeutic food that deserves greater attention.

However, to the best of our knowledge, there is scarcity in the published research that gives explicit, comprehensive revision on the anti-cancer anti-inflammatory and anti-diabetic potentials of CM. Therefore, the current chapter tried to fill this gap and provide a comprehensive revision on the major research findings related to the effect of CM on the prevention, mitigation, and management of inflammation-related chronic diseases, namely cancer, diabetes, metabolic syndrome, and inflammatory bowel diseases.

CANCER

As part of the traditional medicine in the Middle East, CM has long been used in the prevention and treatment of numerous types of cancers (Korashy, Maayah, Abd-Allah, El-Kadi, & Alhaider, 2012), and people consume CM regularly as part of the common belief that it improves immunity against diseases and decreases the risk for cancer (Badawy, El-Magd, & Alsadrah, 2018). Some reports indicated that camel products, including both urine and milk, acquire anticancer effects (Al-Harbi et al., 1996; Al-Yousef et al., 2012; Mushref, 2006). This traditional application of CM could be found in ancient medicinal books that provide many quotes about the camel's benefits and nutraceutical values. Avicenna (980-1037 AD), the father of early modern medicine, stated the therapeutic uses for CM in treating diseases of the liver, spleen, kidney, cancer, and childhood diseases (Ibn-e-Sina, 2005; Zibaee et al., 2015).

Further, in traditional medicine for Arabs and Muslims, CM has long been used for remedial purposes, based on the fact that CM is mentioned in a praise context in the Holy Quran and Prophetic *Sunnah* (Saad, 2015). This belief in CM is reflected in the common conventional practice repeatedly reported among Arab cancer patients, who incorporate CM as part of complementary and alternative medicinal practices they follow to alleviate or treat cancers (Abuelgasim et al., 2018; Akhu-Zaheya & Alkhasawneh, 2012; Al-Amoudi, Cañas, Hohl, Distelhorst, & Thompson, 2015; Alrowais & Alyousefi, 2017; Jazieh et al., 2012; Mihic et al., 2016).

According to the Persian traditional, complementary medicine, CM has long been ethno-pharmacologically used for the treatment and prevention of uterine and gastrointestinal cancers. Moreover, examining the classic Persian medicine revealed that CM was the most functional natural liquid that may play an integral role in many chronic physiological and mental ailments including cancers (Hosseini, Zibaee, Yousefi, Taghipour, & Noras, 2015). Currently, acknowledging the nutraceutical and nutritional value of CM, and as a result of the prophylactic and therapeutic potential for human's health, the use of CM has been increased worldwide (Alavi, Salami, Emam-Djomeh, & Mohammadian, 2017).

In Vivo Studies

Indeed, there is a scarcity in the *in vivo* studies tackling the anti-tumor or chemo-preventive effect of CM against chemically induced colorectal cancer (CRC). In one of these prominent studies, Amr and colleagues examined the effect of fermented and unfermented camel and bovine milk on CRC in rodents after being injected with azoxymethane (AOM) chemical carcinogen. Colons were harvested, and the precarious lesions called aberrant crypt foci (ACF) were counted and determined for all tested groups (Amr et al., 2018). Significant reductions were observed in the total count of ACF of the colons (ranging from about 48% to about 62%) of the rats fed both CM and bovine milk diets in comparison to fed on positive control (standard diet without milk). However, no obvious changes were observed in the total ACF between unfermented and fermented diets or between the bovine milk and CM diets. Researchers concluded that CM displayed a chemo-preventive effect against colorectal carcinogenesis indicated by ACF, without an obvious impact for milk fermentation on the chemo-preventive potential (Amr et al., 2018).

Another recent *in vivo* study tried to investigate the impact of CM protein on AOM/dextran sodium sulfate-induced colitis in Balb/c mouse model of CRC during disease development. Tumor development and colitis-associated symptoms were observed during and at the end day of the experiment and included anti-inflammatory and pro-inflammatory cytokine gene expressions. Researchers found a noticeable reduction in colon inflammation symptoms and in the early stage development of CRC by the provision of CM whey protein, as revealed by reduced bloody stool and diarrhea, enhanced weight gain concurrent, with a diminution in gene expression of the inflammatory cytokine IL-6 evident in colon tissue.

Further, genetic expressions of both interleukin (IL)-8 and interferon (IFN)-γ were noticeably decreased in treated rodents. On the other hand, expression of the genes of the anti-inflammatory cytokines IL-10 was up-regulated in mice colons, whereas inducible nitric oxide synthase, a marker for inflamed mucosa, was down-regulated in mice treated with the CM whey. Similar genetic changes were observed in control mice treated with bovine milk except for IFN-γ, which was elevated. Researchers concluded that CM whey has the potential activity in retarding the progression of CRC in rodents principally through mitigating chemically-induced colonic inflammation (Al-Omari, Al-Ghariebeh, Alhaija, Al-Zoubi, & Al-Qaoud, 2019).

The reports of anti-cancer or chemo-preventive effect of CM could be ascribed to the presence of a group of bioactive zoo-chemicals along with essential nutrients that work synergistically in suppressing tumorigenesis and triggering normal cell division. Among these, bioactive peptides and proteins that have been gaining growing attention in the biomedical research. Variable types of bioactive peptides have been identified in CM protein including casein, α-lactalbumin, serum albumin, acidic whey protein, camel whey basic protein, lactoferrin, lysozymes, lactoperoxidase, peptidoglycan recognition protein (PGRP)-1 and immunoglobulins (Mati et al., 2016). Similar to bovine milk's proteins and bioactive peptides, CM bioactive peptides have been reported to display variable potential activities (Chapter 7) displayed from *in vitro* assays and include anti-inflammatory, anti-hypertensive, antimicrobial, anti-oxidative, and immunomodulatory activities (Mati et al., 2016), in addition to blood pressure-lowering effect, growth stimulation, mineral binding, opioid activities, and antimicrobial activities (Meisel, 2004). These bioactive peptides and proteins are liberated from CM either by enzyme hydrolysis with specific proteolytic enzymes, simulated gastrointestinal digestion, or during milk fermentation using bacterial proteolytic types (Mati et al., 2016). Among these bioactive peptides derived from CM; β-casein and whole casein exhibited high antioxidant activity, suggesting that ingesting and digesting CM protein can produce bioactive components that act as natural antioxidants, thus may entail a protective effect for the human body against cancer (Salami et al., 2011).

Peptidoglycan recognition protein (PGRP) is peptidoglycan that was first found in CM, with CM has the highest concentration (range of 105-130 mg/L, average 115.3 mg/L) of this protein in comparison to other animal milk sources (Kappeler, Heuberger, Farah, & Puhan, 2004; Mullaicharam, 2014). This protein has an obvious effect on breast cancer by controlling metastasis. It stimulates host immune response, and it has broad antimicrobial activity (Gizachew et al., 2014; Gul, Farooq, Anees, Khan, & Rehan, 2015; Stefan Kappeler, 1998; Yadav et al., 2015). Several reports indicated that PGRP was first discovered in CM and has an apparent suppressive effect on breast cancer by controlling metastasis (El-Hatmi, Girardet, Gaillard, Yahyaoui, & Attia, 2007; Sharma et al., 2011; Pradeep Sharma et al., 2012; Wernery, 2006; Yadav et al., 2015).

The reactive oxygen species work as free radicals attack cellular components, leading to the oxidation of proteins, lipids, and DNA; thus causing functional and structural changes to these molecules that may end with the development of cancer (Valko, Rhodes, Moncol, Izakovic, & Mazur, 2006). The reported anti-cancer potential of CM could be ascribed, in part, by virtue of its oligosaccharides, peptides and proteins which exhibit an ability to activate antioxidant enzyme systems such as catalase and superoxide dismutase (SOD), and to suppress the production of the highly reactive compound malondialdehyde (MDA) which is a strong oxidative stress marker (Roy & Deepak, 2014). Comparative study on whey protein from bovine and from camel milk unraveled that CM whey protein and its hydrolysates showed higher antioxidant potential when compared with bovine milk whey protein and its hydrolysates. Researchers ascribed such superiority in the antioxidant potential of whey protein and hydrolysates to the variations in the accessibilities and extents of antioxidant amino acids available in their primary structures (Chapter 2 and 7) and from the prevalence of α-lactalbumin as proteolytic substrates in camel whey (Ibrahim, Isono, & Miyata, 2018; Salami et al., 2010).

In Vitro Studies

A comparative study has been conducted to evaluate the anticancer activity of different mammalians' milk: with their whey and casein proteins tested against MCF7 cell line at different concentrations (0.5, 1 and 2 mg/ml) and using MTT assay. Results showed that CM casein showed the second highest cytotoxic activity, next to mare milk casein, and followed by donkey and cow milk caseins. Further, whey proteins demonstrated that CM whey protein showed more potent anticancer activity than showed by bovine and donkey milk, which presented weak anticancer activity (Shariatikia, Behbahani, & Mohabatkar, 2017). Hydrolysis of CM protein revealed that these hydrolyzed proteins could be used as a natural source of protein hydrolysates that possess antioxidant potentials and can be used as pharmaceutical and nutraceutical ingredient for human (Kumar, Chatli, Singh, Mehta, & Kumar, 2016). Another *in vitro* study done by Korashy and colleagues (Korashy et al., 2012) showed that CM was superior on cow's milk in profoundly suppressing human breast cancer cell line and MCF7 human hepatoma HepG2 cell line by induction of death receptors in both cell lines and suppressing cell proliferation, and by triggering anti-oxidative stress mechanisms. Authors concluded that CM activates both intrinsic and extrinsic apoptotic mechanisms (Korashy et al., 2012).

More recent study using camel milk exosomes (extracellular nanovesicles of 30 to 100 nm diameter that are produced by nearly all cell types) against MCF7 breast cancer cells (both *in vitro* and *in vivo*) showed that oral administration of CM and its exosomes (both orally and by local injection for the latter) hindered breast tumor progression as evident by triggering apoptosis (as indicated by higher caspase-3 activity, DNA fragmentation, *Bax* gene expression, and lower *Bcl2* gene expression), noticeable inhibition of oxidative stress (as expressed by decrease in MDA levels and *iNOS* gene expression); induction of antioxidant status as expressed by increased activities of superoxide dismutase (SOD), catalase (CAT), and glutathione peroxidase (GPX), along with noticeable reduction in expression angiogenesis-(VEGF), inflammation-(IL1β, NFκB), and metastasis-(MMP9, ICAM1) related genes; and higher immune response (high number of NK1.1 T cells in spleen, CD+8, CD+4). However, these anticancer effects were found to be superior for CM-derived exosomes, thought with less and immunomodulatory effect, than treatment by CM. These findings suggest that CM and its exosomes entail anticancer potential that presumably affects via induction of apoptosis and inhibition of inflammation, oxidative stress, metastasis and angiogenesis in the tumor microenvironment, making CM and its exosomes candidate to be used as an anticancer agent for cancer treatment (Badawy et al., 2018).

Studies indicated that the anticancer activity of fermented milk is triggered by inhibiting the angiotensin-converting enzyme (ICE)(Ayyash, Al-Dhaheri, Al Mahadin, Kizhakkayil, & Abushelaibi, 2018). Moreover, inhibition of proliferative cells of MCF7, Caco-2, and Hella was observed in CM treated cases. CM positively controlled all other health-promoting parameters like α-amylase, antioxidant, α-glucosidase inhibition, and proteolytic activity. Level of ascorbic acid, lysozyme, and lactoferrins are higher in CM. The higher contents of ascorbic acid make it free from being coagulated (Kappeler, Ackermann, Farah, & Puhan, 1999).

Camel milk contains a protein called alpha-lactalbumin (α-LA). A study showed that this protein demonstrated anticancer and pro-apoptotic activities against four types of human cancer cell lines: HepG-2 hepatoma, Caco-2 colon cancer, PC-3 prostate cancer, and MCF7 breast cancer as targets using MTT test, cell cycle analysis, annexin/PI staining, inhibition of tyrosine kinase and nuclear staining methods (Uversky, El-Fakharany, Abu-Serie, Almehdar, & Redwan, 2017). In another relevant study, casein with α-lactalbumin triggered a cytotoxic effect in HepG2 and HeLa cell lines. Further, casein with α-lactalbumin triggered apoptosis in both non-infected and infected HepG2 cells (Almahdy, EL-Fakharany, Ehab, Ng, & Redwan, 2011).

In a more recent and more comprehensive study investigating the anticancer, antihypertensive, antidiabetic, and antioxidant activities of CM fermented with CM probiotics revealed that CM demonstrated antiproliferative effect against Caco-2, MCF7, and HELA cancer cell lines, which were more inhibited when treated with water-soluble extracts of fermented CM (Ayyash et al., 2018). The most recent study using two cell lines: breast cancer MCF7 and colorectal cancer HCT 116 were cultured with different doses of CM. The effects of CM on cell death were tested using migration by *in vitro* scratch assay, viability by trypan blue exclusion assay and MTT assay, in addition to confocal microscopy and western blotting to confirm autophagy. Significant reductions were observed in cell viability, proliferation, as well as the migration of both the cells. Other tests revealed that CM treatment led to induction of autophagy. Researchers concluded that CM possess antiproliferative effects against human breast MCF7 and colorectal HCT 116 cancer cells by inducing autophagy (Krishnankutty et al., 2018).

Lactoferrin, a glycoprotein, is among the protective proteins in CM (Konuspayeva, Faye, & Loiseau, 2009; Konuspayeva et al., 2007) in higher quantities than bovine milk (Kappeler, Ackermann, Farah, & Puhan, 1999). Lactoferrin has been examined for its ability to repair DNA damage and to suppress *in vitro* colon cancer cell proliferation by virtue of its antioxidant properties (Habib, Ibrahim, Schneider-Stock, & Hassan, 2013). The anti-metastasis effect of lactoferrin might be related to the induction of apoptosis of these transformed cells, triggered by the activation of the *Fas* signaling pathway, suppressing cell proliferation due to its ability to transport iron into cells, acting as growth factor activator. Lactoferrin has potential in tumor treatment by blocking tumor cell proliferation (Fujita, Matsuda, Sekine, Iigo, & Tsuda, 2004; Tung et al., 2013; Zhang, Lima, & Rodrigues, 2014). In their work, Habib and colleagues examined the ability of CM lactoferrin to suppress colon cancer cell proliferation using *in vitro* cell line HCT-116 and DNA damage. The antioxidant capacity of lactoferrin was evaluated by free radical-scavenging activity (DPPH), ferric-reducing/antioxidant power assay (FRAP), total antioxidant activity, nitric oxide (NO) radical-scavenging assay, and DNA damage, compared with rutin and vitamin C (Habib et al., 2013). The study showed that CM lactoferrin exerts profound antioxidant potential in FRAP, DPPH assays, NO scavenging, and total antioxidant equivalents assays. Further, their study examined the ability of CM lactoferrin to block cancer cell growth and reported that high concentrations (3–5 mg/ ml) of CM lactoferrin inhibits the proliferation of HCT-116 colon cancer cells by as much as 56% (Habib et al., 2013). Cellular redox state and oxidative stress have been linked to cell death via apoptosis, DNA damage and a wide variety of chronic diseases, providing further therapeutic potential for CM lactoferrin (Tsuda & Sekine, 2000; Tsuda et al., 2000). Further, human and murine recombinant lactoferrin has shown an inhibitory effect against the development of experimental neoplasms in rodents (Wolf, Li, Taylor, & O'Malley Jr, 2003).

Camel milk fat (particularly polar lipids) also plays a role in augmenting the anti-cancer potential of CM (Maswadeh, Aljarbou, Alorainy, Alsharidah, & Khan, 2015). Further, one of the specific features of CM is the presence of conjugated linoleic acid (CLA), which has various functional properties, including the anticancer effect (Rodr,´omez, Pimentel, & Fontecha, 2017). Conjugated linoleic acid is reported to inhibit the initiation and progression of different types of cancers including colon, skin, breast, and stomach cancers (Ip, Singh, Thompson, & Scimeca, 1994; Pariza, 1999; Wangoh, Farah, & Puhan, 1998).

Alhaider and colleagues provided sufficiently *in vivo* evidence regarding the ability of CM to suppress carcinogenesis process by halting inflammatory angiogenesis via downregulating the proinflammatory and proangiogenic cytokines in an animal model (Alhaider, Abdel Gader, Almeshaal, & Saraswati, 2014). Researchers showed that CM treatment attenuated the main components of the macrophage recruitment, fibrovascular tissue, vascularization, collagen deposition and the levels of interleukin (IL)-1 β, IL-6, IL-17, vascular endothelial growth factor (VEGF), transforming growth factor-β and tumor necrosis factor-α. A regulatory function of CM on various parameters of the major components of inflammatory angiogenesis indicated the potential therapeutic benefit underlying the anti-tumor activities of CM observed in many cases.

Liver cancer is one of the most prevalent types of cancers throughout the world (Stewart & Kleihues, 2003). *In vivo* study revealed that CM suppressed murine hepatic carcinogenesis initiated by diethylnitrosamine and promoted by phenobarbitone (El Miniawy, Ahmed, Tony, Mansour, & Salah Khattab, 2014). A study on CM and cancer is not restricted on the chemo-preventive or the anti-tumor effect against different cancer *in vivo* or *in vitro* models. Cancer research extended to other aspects such as the anticytotoxic and antigenotoxic effect of CM in mice treated with cisplatin (a cancer chemotherapeutic drug) (Salwa & Lina, 2010). Results of this investigation revealed that CM has some antioxidant, anticytotoxic, and antigenotoxic effects, and suggested using CM as an adjuvant therapy with cancer therapeutics. This is supported by common practice in Kazakhstan where CM is used as an adjunct therapy to classical chemotherapy for some types of cancers, especially those related to the alimentary tract (Yadav et al., 2015).

Korashy and coworkers, in their attempt to examine the anti-tumor effect of CM against murine hepatoma Hepa-1c1c7 cells, showed for the first mechanistic evidence of the ability of CM to profoundly induce *Nqo1* and *Gsta1*, cancer protecting genes in Hepa 1c1c7 cells and halting the induction of *Cyp1a1*, a cancer-activating gene, at the transcriptional and posttranscriptional levels (Korashy, El Gendy, Alhaider, & El-Kadi, 2012). Authors concluded that CM entail a protective effect against or decrease the deleterious effects of various environmental carcinogens and toxicants such as a polycyclic aromatic hydrocarbon.

Using lyophilized CM (LCM), a study indicated that LCM fundamentally hindered proliferation and growth of human breast cancer BT-474 cells when compared with HEp-2 and HCC1937 BL cell lines through the induction of apoptotic pathways as indicated by both induction of death receptors in BT-474 and caspase-3 mRNA and its activity level (Hasson et al., 2015).

Using advanced techniques of transcriptomics and proteomics, results found by Yang and colleagues revealed that Xinjiang Bactrian CM contains an antitumor active fraction called TR35 which has the ability to efficiently inhibit Eca109 cell proliferation and induce its apoptosis (Yang et al., 2018). Furthermore, researchers found that this protein fraction has the ability to halt the growth of xenografted tumor in nude mice without loss in body weight. Furthermore, using RNA-Seq and 2-DE combined mass spectrometry analysis, they identified differentially expressed RNA and protein markers of apoptosis and necrosis. Authors ended up with the conclusion that Bactrian CM has a therapeutic potential that supports the historical anti-cancer use of CM in Northwest China. This research on Bactrian CM has been recently supported by another work by Wali and colleagues (2019) who successfully isolated and identified three new antioxidant peptides from the Bactrian CM hydrolysates (Wali et al., 2019).

INFLAMMATORY BOWEL DISEASES (IBD)

Inflammatory bowel diseases are autoimmune diseases characterized by persistent inflammation of the colon and include both Crohn's disease and ulcerative colitis (Fakhoury, Negrulj, Mooranian, & Al-Salami, 2014). Several reports indicated that microbial infection could be the underlying basic cause of Crohn's disease in humans, which resembles Johne's disease in cattle caused by an infection of Mycobacterium avium subspecies paratuberculosis (McNees, Markesich, Zayyani, & Graham, 2015; Naser, Sagramsingh, Naser, & Thanigachalam, 2014). Camel milk has powerful bactericidal properties and can rehabilitate the immune system. Thus, it may be useful in alleviating these inflammatory diseases affecting the human colon. It was observed that drinking non-pasteurized CM is beneficial to people with all the variety of symptoms associated with an infection of the alimentary tract (Shabo, Barzel, & Yagil, 2008).

Camel milk might represent a potential candidate for pharmacological efficacy on IBD with minimal adverse reactions (Arab et al., 2014). Due to its high content in major and trace minerals (magnesium, calcium, zinc, iron, and copper), vitamins (C, E, A, and B_2) and insulin, and lower content in sugar, fat, cholesterol, and protein (Darwish, Abd Raboh, & Mahdy, 2012); these factors of CM presumably may be helpful in alleviating or treating these inflammatory diseases (Moura, De Andrade, Dos Santos, Araújo, & Goulart, 2015). Dietary antioxidant vitamins (E and C) both act as exogenous antioxidant defenses which help in alleviating reactive oxygen species (ROS) which play crucial roles in normal response to growth factors, the immune response, and apoptotic elimination of damaged cells (Seifried, Anderson, Fisher, & Milner, 2007).

It also contains a relatively large amount of polyunsaturated fatty and linoleic acids, which are essential for human nutrition (Al Haj & Al Kanhal, 2010). With regard to the high risk of malnutrition in the course of IBD, nutritional support plays a crucial role in the management of these patients. CM has been consumed as an essential nutritional supplement with high energy and vitamin content to help immune-deficient patients (Arab et al., 2014). Malabsorption has been identified as a potential trigger for symptoms of IBD, such as bloating, abdominal pain, distension, malnutrition, and altered bowel habits (Barrett, Irving, Shepherd, Muir, & Gibson, 2009; Wiecek, Wos, Radziewicz-Winnicki, Komraus, & Grzybowska-Chlebowczyk, 2014). In addition to the presence of antioxidant nutrients, CM contains lactoferrin in higher concentration than cow milk. This protein is characterized by its substantial anti-inflammatory and antioxidant properties (Legrand, Elass, Carpentier, & Mazurier, 2005).

More studies are necessary to investigate if CM may be a valuable complementary approach for the management of IBD. The ability of CM and its peptides to suppress the inflammation in animals could entail a protective ability against inflammatory diseases such as those affecting the bowel (Abu-Qatouseh, Mallah, Issa, Sabri, & Shihab, 2019).

Camel milk is a potential candidate for pharmacological efficacy on inflammatory bowel diseases (IBD) with minimal adverse reactions (Arab et al., 2014). CM has been consumed as an essential nutritional supplement with high energy and vitamin content to help immune-deficient patients (Arab et al., 2014). Malabsorption syndrome has been identified as a potential trigger for symptoms of IBD, such as abdominal pain, bloating and distension, altered bowel habits, and malnutrition. Besides having antioxidant properties, CM lactoferrin presents marked antioxidant and anti-inflammatory properties, as explained deeply in the previous section. Given these properties, Arab et al. (2014) evaluated the effects of CM (10 mL/kg.bw/d) by gavage, one week before colitis induction and at the 4th-day post-induction against

2,4,6-trinitrobenzene sulfonic acid-induced colitis in rats. Attenuation of colon injury was observed through suppression of oxidative stress via reduction of lipid peroxides (malondialdehyde, MDA) activity and other oxidative stress products, along with boosting of the antioxidant defenses through the restoration of colonic reduced glutathione and total antioxidant capacity. More studies are necessary to investigate if CM may be a valuable complementary approach for the management of IBD (Arab et al., 2014).

DIABETES MELLITUS

The effect of camel milk consumption on diabetes mellitus (DM), one of main prevalent endocrinology disorders in the world is widely documented in the literature. Due to this specific importance, a special chapter (chapter 9) of the present book is dedicated to it.

METABOLIC SYNDROME (METS)

MetS have many terms, such as insulin resistance syndrome, deadly quartet, syndrome X, and syndrome X plus (Cameron, Shaw, & Zimmet, 2004). All of which have similar pathogenesis such abdominal obesity, hypertension, dyslipidemia, and impaired fasting glucose that contributes to increased cardiovascular morbidity and mortality (Cameron et al., 2004; Nagao & Yanagita, 2008). Insulin resistance with excessive fatty acids metabolic disorder mostly explicates metabolic disorder pathophysiology (Cameron et al., 2004). The syndrome is mainly contributing to a pro-inflammation state, which mainly contributes to increased risk for chronic diseases (Eckel, Grundy, & Zimmet, 2005). However; such oxidative stress state demands therapeutic attention for those at high risk. The fundamental approach is weight reduction and increased physical activity; however, drug treatment could be appropriate for diabetes and cardiovascular disease risk reduction (Cameron et al., 2004; Eckel et al., 2005; Nagao & Yanagita, 2008).

Different International Institutions diagnosed MetS by having 3 out of 5 of the following criteria: (1) waist circumference (WC >102 cm), (2) high-density lipoprotein cholesterol (HDL-C <40 mg/dL), (3) triglycerides (≥150 mg/dL), (4) blood pressure (≥130/≥85 mmHg) (5) fasting blood glucose (≥100 mg/d/L) (Espinosa-Marrón, Quiñones-Capistrán, Rubio-Blancas, del Pilar Milke-García, & Castillejos-Molina, 2019). Treatment with CM restores (Na^+/K^+)/ATPase as reported in animal studies. This may be due to insulin secretory effect along with decreasing peroxidative damage to membrane lipids (Al-Numair et al., 2010). Hyperglycemia can cause inhibition/ and reduction in the activities of (Na^+/K^+)- and Ca^{2+}/ ATPases; hence, alteration in the signal transduction pathways, and affect contractility, excitability, and cellular dysfunctions. This could be due to the restoration of insulin levels in diabetic rats administered with CM due to the presence of higher concentrations of insulin-like protein and zinc rich existence content in CM (Abdel Gader & Alhaider, 2016; Al-Numair et al., 2010; Aqib et al., 2019).

Recent reports in regards to CM health benefits included; hypotensive activity, hypoglycemic effect, oxidative stress reduction, hypocholesterolemic activity, and anti-carcinogenic and anti-inflammatory effects (Hamad, Abdel-Rahim, & Romeih, 2011), thus it could be a suitable food to tackle with MetS and its pathophysiological derangements. Lipid and glycemic profiles are the most major indexes among MetS patients. Abnormalities in these profiles are strongly correlated with increased oxidative damage (Espinosa-Marrón et al., 2019). Oxidative and inflammation could be refined and improved by the special anti-inflammatory effects of drinking CM consumption. CM rich antioxidant agents' composition such zinc, selenium, vitamins E, C, and glutathione peroxidase active system (Hamed, El Feki, & Gargouri, 2019; Mirmiran et al., 2017) could promote considering CM as a functional food for MetS patients.

Korish on 2014 launched promising results of the MetS treatment regarding DM due to CM consumption. CM is reported hypolipidemic, hypoglycemic, and anti-inflammatory effect in animals (Korish, 2014). In addition, the high content of magnesium, zinc, and trace element act as a strong defense against oxidative damage. Moreover, CM enhances the absorption and the metabolism of antioxidant vitamins such as vitamins C and E (Hamed et al., 2019; Sboui et al., 2010). Al-Ayadhi and Elamin in 2013 reported that glutathione GSH level after CM intake increased significantly. Moreover; CM content of zinc and vitamin E promotes GSH, GSHPx, and SOD levels. CM high contents of Mg and Zn and vitamin E boost GSH production (Al-Ayadhi & Elamin, 2013).

Besides, CM intake especially if combined with dates (common desert fruit) was found to increase the body immunity against free radical in a study on rats that were poisoned by lead acetate. This study showed (or proved) the powerful protective role of the mixture of CM with dates against damaging organs by lead peroxides toxic effect and free radicals (Al-Humaid, Mousa, El-Mergawi, & Abdel-Salam, 2010). Another study indicated the protective effect of CM against cadmium contamination among white Albino rats indicated by oxidative stress in the red blood cells (Mohammad, 2009).

CM and Obesity

Diet-induced obesity is recently a highlighted point of view. Visceral obesity is one the main cluster of the MetS, which majorly is caused by high fat- high cholesterol food intake combined with little physical activity (Cameron et al., 2004; Eckel et al., 2005), and, consequently, hyperlipidemia occurs. Alternative medicine recently is used widely and more often by 38% among the Americas and 80% among African and Asian countries (AlBedah et al., 2013; Korish & Arafah, 2013).

A significant reduction in body weight was reported in a study done on twenty male Wistar rats fed on high cholesterol diet for 6-8 weeks while compared with another group fed on high cholesterol diet plus CM (Korish & Arafah, 2013). Such finding would promote recommending CM intake among people who consume a regular high fat diet in order to prevent gaining weight. The low content of sugar and fat in CM composition (Abu-Lehia, 1989) would consider CM a convenience source to be included in the maintenance weight meal plan. Few reports highlighted the delaying in the gastric emptying effect of CM (Korish & Arafah, 2013); which mean higher satiety sensation leading to less desirable to eat.

CM and Blood Pressure

Angiotensin I-converting dipeptidyl carboxypeptidase enzyme (ACE) is associated with the regulation of blood pressure through increasing fluid retention (Smith & Vane, 2003) that is found in fermented dromedary CM protein. Factors that inhibit ACE reduce blood pressure (Quan, Tsuda, & Miyamoto, 2008); therefore; ACE inhibitors commonly are prescribed for MetS-related hypertension treatment (Kochi et al., 2014). Recent studies indicated the positive effect of CM intake as an antihypertensive agent (Korish & Arafah, 2013). Raw CM consumption due to its probiotic bacteria-fermented content has peptides with ACE inhibitory activity and hence could be effective in blood pressure control (Ejtahed et al., 2015). The Antihypertensive properties of camel milk has been discussed in details in Chapter 7.

CM and Lipid Profile

Recent studies indicated the positive effect of CM intake as a cholesterol-lowering agent (Al Haj & Al Kanhal, 2010). Excess reactive oxygen species enhance the oxidative stress, which inhibits antioxidant mechanisms hence boosting chronic inflammatory responses to hypercholesterolemia (Al Haj & Al Kanhal, 2010; Feldstein et al., 2005; Kojda & Harrison, 1999). Coronary heart disease (CHD) is one outcome of metabolic disorder, which is of the significant reasons for death in the industrialized nations. Raised pressure of blood in combination with high total blood cholesterol level are viewed as a noteworthy risk factor for CHD. Consumption of CM has been accounted to have a cholesterol-lowering impact *in vivo* (Al Haj & Al Kanhal, 2010; Elayan, Sulieman, & Saleh, 2008). The cholesterol-lowering component of CM is yet indistinct, yet various speculations have been proposed. Interaction between CM bioactive peptides proteins and cholesterol promote cholesterol reduction. In addition, the existence of orotic acid in CM is believed to decrease cholesterol level in both human and in rats (Al Haj & Al Kanhal, 2010).

Significant improvements were remarked by a significant reduction in total cholesterol, triglycerides, LDL-C, and VLDL-C levels as per Korish and Arafah's study on twenty male Wistar rats as described above in the CM and obesity section. Fortunately; the second group significantly decreased the atherogenic index (AI), which indicates the protective anti-atherosclerosis effect of CM intake among animals (Korish & Arafah, 2013). Intake of CM could have an anti-inflammatory effect against oxidative damage due to its content of antioxidants (Mirmiran et al., 2017) that is indicated to have a strong positive association with abnormal lipid profiles (Al-Aubaidy & Jelinek, 2014).

It is established that CM fatty acids profile is favorable in regard to human wellbeing (Al Haj & Al Kanhal, 2010). The more unsaturated fatty acids content, the wiser healthy diet choices (Vessby, 2003). CM fats are higher in long-chain PUFAs (Konuspayeva, Lemarie, Faye, Loiseau, & Montet, 2008), in unsaturated fats contents especially the essential fatty acids (Abu-Lehia, 1989; Haddadin, Gammoh, & Robinson, 2008; Sawaya, Khalil, Al-Shalhat, & Al-Mohammad, 1984) compared with bovine milk (Bracco, Hidalgo, & Bohren, 1972) while it is lower in cholesterol and saturated fat contents (Konuspayeva et al., 2008).

L-carnitine concentration is high in CM, which has a positive function regarding the lipid profile. Directly by reducing the absorption of exogenous cholesterol (Alhomida, 1996; Longo, Frigeni, & Pasquali, 2016), thus promotes hypolipidemic state and indirectly, by transferring of long-chain fatty acids to mitochondria for catabolic in β-oxidation (Bloomer, Butawan, Farney, & McAllister, 2019; Longo et al., 2016).

Camel milk is probably safe to be consumed by healthy people. This has been extrapolated from the results of Alabdulkarim (2012) who showed that CM, as well as cow milk consumption, reduced significantly total cholesterol level, triglyceride level, and liver enzymes (ALT and AST) of adult female Albino rats. Nonetheless, the effect of camel milk was the same as that of cow milk (Alabdulkarim, 2012).

The cholesterol-lowering efficacy of CM has been suggested in experimental animals (Elayan et al., 2008) as well as humans (Buonopane, Kilara, Smith, & McCarthy, 1992). Nonetheless, the exact related mechanisms are not clear. For instance, Li and Papadopoulos (1998) suggested that there might be an interaction between CM short peptides and blood cholesterol (Li & Papadopoulos, 1998). On the other hands, others (Buonopane et al., 1992; Rao, Chawan, & Pulusani, 1981) suggest that orotic acid might be involved. Elayan et al. (2008) suggested that CM probably inhibited hepatic cholesterol synthesis *in vivo* (Elayan et al., 2008). Recently, Hamed et al. (2018) showed that some cardio-preventive effects of fermented CM using *Lactococcus lactis* subsp *creemoris* might be attributed to the inhibition of CCl4-induced toxicity *in vivo* (Hamedet al., 2018).

Recently, Yahya et al. (2018) showed that administering adult male Wistar rats skim fermented CM (fermented by *Lactobacillus helvictus* and *Streptococcus thermophilus*) significantly reduced the levels of serum cholesterol and atherogenic index (LDL-cholesterol/HDL-cholesterol) (Yahya, Alhaj, AL-Khalifah, & Almnaizel, 2018). Interestingly, these results were accompanied by feeding high cholesterol diets. Moreover, the histopathological examination of the rat liver showed that tissue degeneration, stenosis, fibrosis, as well as inflammation were ameliorated by administering fermented CM compared to non-fermented. The researchers suggested that *Lactobacillus helvictus* and *Streptococcus thermophilus* reduction of endogenous cholesterol synthesis, intestinal cholesterol absorption, and inhibition of cholesterol synthesizing enzymes.

Within the same context, Elzhrani (2018) showed that CM reduced significantly total cholesterol and triglycerides. On the other hand, HDL-cholesterol reduced remarkably. The researcher showed that these cholesterol-lowering effects are related to the improvement of the body oxidative status indicated by the reduction of the enzyme's catalase, and peroxidase enzymes.

Moreover, most recent research showed the cholesterol-lowering effect of CM in rats but with an increase in HDL-cholesterol synthesis. The researchers highlighted that feeding CM to the rats increased fecal excretion of cholesterol, improved hepatic glutathione peroxidase, and attenuated hepatic thiobarbituric acid (Elzhrani, 2018).

CM and Blood Glucose

Communities who consume CM habitually showed a low prevalence of diabetes as it is reported in several reports (Agrawal et al., 2007). Such findings were assured by animal studies (Agrawal et al., 2007; Korish & Arafah, 2013; Mirmiran et al., 2017). High cholesterol diet is associated habitually with hyperglycemia. Surprisingly, in Korish and Arafah's study when CM was added to the high cholesterol diet group for eight weeks, this group showed a reduction in the HOMA-IR (insulin resistance assessment), a significant reduction in random blood glucose and in fasting insulin level (significant fasting hypoglycemia) (Korish & Arafah, 2013). The anti-diabetic effect of camel milk will be discussed in Chapter 9.

CM content of insulin-like protein and insulin is high almost 52 unit of insulin in each 1 liter of CM (Agarwal et al., 2003; Zagorski et al., 1998) as detected by radioimmunoassay analysis, which indicates considering CM as a natural product not only for glycemic control but also to preserve the normal lipid profile (Soleymanzadeh, Mirdamadi, Mirzaei, & Kianirad, 2019). As mentioned in the previous section (CM and diabetes mellitus), CM has small particles of insulin-like molecules, which have similar interaction with insulin receptors (Malik et al., 2012). In addition, the special features of CM protein (lysozyme, lactoferrin, and lactoperoxidase) are indigestible by the stomach enzyme (pepsin); hence, those proteins are not coagulated at low pH. Moreover, their capacity for buffering is better than other types of milk proteins (bovine) (Al haj & Al Kanhal, 2010).

The high content of antioxidant (zinc, selenium, vitamin C) in CM (Mirmiran et al., 2017) plays an important role as anti-inflammatory effects and immune modulatory functions on the pancreatic β-cells protection (Ebaid, 2014). However, CM's whey protein is assumed to increase glutathione and reduce reactive oxygen (Ebaid et al., 2011).

Twelve alloxan-treated dogs were entered an experimental study to compare between the CM (first group) vs. bovine milk (second group) intakes on the MetS parameters (blood glucose, total cholesterol, and total protein). After three weeks, hypoglycemic effects were observed among the first group. After five weeks, the first group showed a statistically significant reduction in blood glucose levels, in total cholesterol, and in total proteins. Oppositely, after feeding bovine milk to the second group significant rising in high blood glucose level, in cholesterol levels and in total proteins concentrations (Sboui et al., 2010). Most of the beneficial hypoglycemic effects of CM have been noticed on diabetic subjects (human or animal) but not on healthy cases (Sboui et al., 2010). This might be explained by CM normalizing impact on blood parameters (whether glycemia, lipids, and pressure).

More detail is given in chapter 9 "anti-diabetic effect of camel milk".

HEPATORENAL DISEASES AND CM

CM consumption is ordinarily used in the treatment of human diabetes, liver disease, respiratory disorders, gallstones, general fatigue, and gastric ulcers. Quite a few scientific studies have define the CM therapeutic possessions, due to its richness in antioxidant (Bouhaddaoui et al., 2019).

Fermented camel milk (FCM) showed favorable effects among oxidative damage in kidney diseases. In an animal study, pretreatment female mice with FCM, significant reduction in oxidative stress prevented the renal dysfunction. As well as the reduction in plasma uric acid, creatinine, lactate dehydrogenase (LDH), urea, and electrolytes levels which are the toxicity biomarker of kidney diseases. Hence, consumption of CM in general and FCM in specific would consider as anti-oxidative stress factors and supportive in the kidney damage prevention agents (Hamed et al., 2018).

Lactoferrin (LF) is a multifunctional protein (Åbrink, Larsson, Gobl, & Hellman, 2000). It was found to have an immunity function in the kidney against free iron availability in urine by recovering iron to be used in the metabolic process (Åbrink et al., 2000) and protecting body tissue from iron-induced lipid peroxidation (ferric reducing power), and cell growth regulation DNA and RNA binding (Soboleva, Sedykh, Alinovskaya, Buneva, & Nevinsky, 2019). LF has also been found to participate in protecting kidney from non-microbial oxidative injury and inflammation (Åbrink et al., 2000) and primary defense against microbial and viral infections (Soboleva et al., 2019). LF from CM showed superior potential against *E.coli* more than bovine and human LF (Almehdar, El-Baky, Alhaider, & Redwan, 2019).

In 2019 in Iran, among 44 adolescent chronic kidney disease CKD patients, a therapeutic protocol of 400 milliliters of camel milk with 10 milliliters of Tarangabin syrup orally for 3 months plus conventional therapy was applied. This study showed improving in renal function in patients with CKD through regulating glucose and anti-inflammatory, laxative, and immune-stimulatory function (Hosseini et al., 2019). Favorable effects were demonstrated from the fermented camel milk intake on liver enzymes aspartate aminotransferase (AST) and alanine aminotransferase (ALT) and their ratio (Fallah, Feizi, Hashemipour, & Kelishadi, 2018). Moreover, CM had shown biochemical and cellular features enhancing of experimental nonalcoholic fatty liver disease (NAFLD) (Korish et al.; 2013). It is well publicized that liver diseases pathogenesis is modified by improving lactic acid bacteria LAB intestinal balance properties (Xu, Xiu, Zhang, Du, & Wang, 2019).

Liver diseases are monitoring by many parameters (Ameen & Hameed, 2019). In 2019, an animal study tested the protective effect of feeding LAB isolated from Mongolian CM among mice suffered from acute liver injury induced by lipopolysaccharide (LPS)/D-galactosamine (D-GalN). A significant reduction in the expression of AST and ALT in serum and liver, and the expression of tumor necrosis factor (TNF)-α and interleukin (IL)-6 was presented. Finally, this study concluded using *Lactobacillus paracasei* subsp. *paracasei* from LAB CM as a probiotic potential for inhibiting the inflammation-based liver injury diseases (Xu et al., 2019). Other study presented significant increasing in glutathione (GSH) level and the enzymatic antioxidants activities superoxide dismutase, glutathione peroxidase, and catalase in liver due to an *in vitro* antioxidant activity of fermented camel milk with *Lactococcus lactis* subsp. *cremoris* (Hamed et al., 2019).

AUTISM SPECTRUM DISORDERS (ASD)

In 2019, the Centers for Disease Control and Prevention (CDC) released the recent autism prevalence (CDC, 2019). They established that in every 59 children about 1 child would be identified by ASD among all racial, ethnic and socioeconomic groups with boys being four times more vulnerable to ASD than girls (Baio et al., 2018; CDC, 2019).

ASDs are defined as a neurodevelopmental disorder with onset prior to 3 years of age. ASDs is combined with many chronic conditions characterized by shortage in social interaction, growth and mental retardation, stereotyped repeated restricted behavior (Cekici & Sanlier, 2019), impairments in language interaction, feeding problem with unusual eating patterns (Li, Ou, Li, & Xiang, 2017), high incidence of autoimmune disease, gastrointestinal disease (Al-Ayadhi & Elamin, 2015). Intestinal inflammation interfere the absorption of micronutrients (Adams, 2013; Adams & Holloway, 2004). Yet, the etiology of such disorder is not fully understood. Multifactorial pathophysiology such as genetic, neurologic, metabolic, oxidative stress, and immunologic all are involved in the ASDs (Al-Ayadhi & Elamin, 2015). ASDs are similar to other neurodevelopmental disorders that are related to increased endotoxins in plasma (Cekici & Sanlier, 2019).

The therapeutic interventions are complicated and are not yet effective due to the biological complexity aspects, especially that different brain areas are involved in these disorders (Zeina, Al-Ayadhi, & Bashir, 2014). At the point when the significance of nutrition is considered, one should take in account that the potential impacts of nutritional intake on people with ASD are conceivably crucial. Ongoing studies have investigated different dietary methodologies to figure out how to diminish the risk of ASD side effects (Golik, 2014).

Disputes influencing gastrointestinal tract GIT are extremely upsetting in ASD children such as steatorrhea, constipation, diarrhea, hypersensitivities, metabolic disorders, undernourished (especially mineral deficiency), eating disorder, and sustenance fixations (Cekici & Sanlier, 2019; Hamzawy, El-Ghandour, Abdel-Aziem, & Ali, 2018; Tas, 2018). They may also suffer from abnormal sensory, which may result in addition to the GIT problems, affects their nutritional intake (Tas, 2018).

The role of oxidative stress in numerous neurological diseases (Alzheimer's disease, Down syndrome, Parkinson's disease, schizophrenia, and ASDs) has been established by prevalent studies (Al-Ayadhi & Elamin, 2015). The reactive oxygen species ROS is the blamed mediator of damaging brain cells especially if exceed cells' antioxidant defense capacity leading to autism apoptosis and pathology (Hamzawy et al., 2018; Shohami, Beit-Yannai, Horowitz, & Kohen, 1997). Autistic children are found to experience irregularities in their behavioral, sleep disturbances, as well as disturbances in their GIT due to SOD cumulative (McGinnis, 2004). Alternating the antioxidant enzymes and non-enzymatic antioxidant molecules levels reduce oxidative stress hence improve autistic behavior (Yorbik, Sayal, Akay, Akbiyik, & Sohmen, 2002).

Due to CM unique composition of being high in important minerals (more of iron, calcium, zinc, magnesium, potassium, and copper) and vitamins (A, B_2, E, and C), lower in fat, cholesterol, and lactose with the absence of beta-casein and beta-lactoglobulin (Chapter 2). In addition, CM is considered richer than other milk types in inflammation-inhibiting contents (protective proteins) (immunoglobulins (Igs), lysozymes, lactoferrin, lactoperoxidase, N-acetyl-glucosaminidase, and peptidoglycan recognition protein (PGRP)(Al-Ayadhi & Elamin, 2015; Al-Ayadhi & Elamin, 2013; Cekici & Sanlier, 2019; Li et al., 2017). All of which would promote considering CM to decrease the oxidative stress biomarkers of ASD to rehabilitate the immune system (Al-Ayadhi & Elamin, 2015; Cekici & Sanlier, 2019). Camel milk unique constituents' size is only one-tenth of human antibodies and considered nanobodies (Yosef Shabo & Yagil, 2005), since CM Igs are more capable than human antibodies (which are unable) to enter the tissues, and the cells hence have therapeutic potencies in infection and immunity (Zafra et al., 2011). They are also able to neutralize the active enzyme belonging to an infectious agent such as bacteria or virus (Al-Ayadhi & Elamin, 2013). Therefore, CM owes its potential viability in ASDs treatment and improves their side effects with their hypoallergenic properties and antibodies (Al-Ayadhi & Elamin, 2013; Cekici & Sanlier, 2019). The nanobodies' small size of an important role in promoting the positive reaction against immunity diseased patients (Yosef Shabo & Yagil, 2005). The accumulative in superoxide dismutase SOD is assumed to increase the plasma myeloperoxidase one of the effectors of GI pathology among ASD patients (Al-Ayadhi, Halepoto, Al-Dress, Mitwali, & Zainah, 2015).

Due to its unique compositions, many papers considered CM as an ideal antioxidant food (Al-Ayadhi et al., 2015; Zeina et al., 2014). Recent studies showed that CM is the sole functional food tested on ASDs (Brondino et al., 2015) and intended to be considered as a substitute (food item) of the antioxidants supplement for its potential therapeutic characteristics to improve ASDs symptoms (Tas, 2018).

Irregular lipid profiles are a common feature of ASD (Meguid, Atta, Gouda, & Khalil, 2008). Discrepancies in dietary intake of lipids, fatty acids, and cholesterol may influence the development of autism-related behavioral outcomes (Bell et al., 2010). Recent papers considered that the alteration in essential fatty acids profile (Chapter 2) would be an indicator of autistic-like behaviors in the autistic patients (Meguid et al., 2008). Studies showed that autism children had higher AA verse DHA and EPA compared to healthy children (Bell et al., 2010; Meguid et al., 2008; Sliwinski, Croonenberghs, Christophe, Deboutte, & Maes, 2006). Imbalances in cholesterol levels have also been associated with ASD (Tierney et al., 2006). CM fatty acids' content is favorable to increase the healthy lipids' profile in consumers. CM is richer than bovine milk in long chain fatty acids, unsaturated fatty acids, especially EFA (AA, DH, and EPA), cholesterol (Al Haj & Al Kanhal, 2010). All of which represents a satisfactory dairy source to improve the lipid profile among ASD patients. Accumulation of heavy metals in the central nervous system is observed in ASD children. Those children are unable to detox their CNS from mercury, lead, aluminum, arsenic, and cadmium, which exaggeration neurotoxic effects (Gorini, Muratori, & Morales, 2014).

Restricted case studies, suggest recommending CM to treat disorders such as dairy food allergy, DM type 1 and 2, autism, fatty liver disease, Crohn's disease and diarrhea hepatitis B, and other autoimmune diseases (Cekici & Sanlier, 2019; Hamzawy et al., 2018; Mirmiran et al., 2017). Camel milk is still not used clinically in treating ASDs in many countries like Saudi Arabia, which put more effort on the researcher to approve CM participation in healing ASDs (Zeina et al., 2014).

Important progression in "The Childhood Autism Rating Scale" CARS scores and antioxidant activity amongst ASDs children treated for 2 weeks by consuming CM were recorded by controlled, double-blind, randomized trials RCT (Al-Ayadhi & Elamin, 2013; Bashir & Al-Ayadhi, 2014; Brondino et al., 2015). Raw CM was administered to 15 ASDs children and resulted in promising outcomes-recorded by CARs score-in comparison to boiled CM and bovine milk by Laila Al-Ayadhi and her colleagues. It was also noticed that significant increase in SOD level after CM administration would be explained by the remarkable content of zinc, copper, magnesium, and vitamin E in CM (Cekici & Sanlier, 2019). A similar finding was found previously in 2013, by a double-blind RCT to investigate the effect of raw CM on 24 ASDs patient verse boiled CM on 25 ASDs patients and altogether were compared to bovine milk as placebo (Al-Ayadhi et al., 2015).

In 2015, Al-Ayadhi and Elamin also tried to evaluate the behavioral differences two weeks before and two weeks after consuming CM (boiled and raw) by running RCT amongst 65 ASDs children. They recorded significant differences in CARS, (The Social Responsiveness Scale) SRS and (autism treatment evaluation checklist) ATEC scales, after daily consumption of CM for 2 weeks, which demonstrates the promising therapeutic intervention of CM by reducing the opioids effects which might explain these results (Al-Ayadhi et al., 2015; Cekici & Sanlier, 2019; Hamzawy et al., 2018). Camel milk works as a hunter for free radical and has antioxidant roles which innate immune response as conducted by earlier studies via regulating the inflammatory and apoptotic pathways (Hamzawy et al., 2018). Wernery in 2012 tested the effect of consuming 500 mL pasteurized CM for eight weeks on eight children with ASD. They documented a positive effect on behavioral and pathophysiological disorders (Wernery et al., 2012).

Dairy food allergy is recorded in ASD patients, which puts more hope to be prevented by recommending CM consumption. Again, it is important to retain that CM is deficient of beta-casein and beta-lactoglobulin, the most allergic compounds found in other milk sources (Al-Ayadhi et al., 2015). The hypoallergenic effect of camel milk has been discussed in Chapter 7.

This connection between ASD and malnourishment has been clarified through different systems, yet the perfect dietary methodology stays tricky. Bigger scale preliminaries concentrating on the portion of CM are expected to decide its impact on oxidative stress biomarkers and thusly as an ASD treatment. It is very important to take caution from promoting CM that is not well-controlled or contaminated due to considering ASDs as an immunity deficient disorder.

FUTURE RESEARCH DIRECTIONS

Future research should be directed toward conducting more controlled randomized controlled trials (Mihic; Rainkie, Wilby, & Pawluk, 2016) tackling variable diseases with emphasis on diabetes, cancer, and inflammatory bowel diseases, to investigate the variable metabolomics, lipidomic and transcriptomic impacts of CM consumption, to elaborate the impact of CM and fermented CM on gut microbiome and its related immunological and inflammatory aspects.

CONCLUSION

Camel milk could be easily described as a candidate functional food with variable health-promoting, disease-ameliorating potentials. Camel milk products have components-stimulated metabolic effects that have unique features due to the integration characteristic between functional foods components and their bioactive nutrients. Cumulative evidence showed that CM is helpful in suppressing the carcinogenesis process, in halting initiated carcinogens, and in stopping metastasis for different neoplasms. Further, CM has been repeatedly shown to help in normalizing blood sugar and blood lipids and normalizing metabolic syndrome components. Finally, recent reports indicated that CM could be an effective adjuvant therapy for inflammatory bowel diseases and cancers, with a plausible beneficial effect for patients with autism.

REFERENCES

Abdel Gader, A. G. M., & Alhaider, A. A. (2016). The unique medicinal properties of camel products: A review of the scientific evidence. *Journal of Taibah University Medical Sciences*, *11*(2), 98–103. doi:10.1016/j.jtumed.2015.12.007

Åbrink, M., Larsson, E., Gobl, A., & Hellman, L. (2000). Expression of lactoferrin in the kidney: Implications for innate immunity and iron metabolism. *Kidney International*, *57*(5), 2004–2010. doi:10.1046/j.1523-1755.2000.00050.x PMID:10792619

Abu-Lehia, I. H. (1989). Physical and chemical characteristics of camel milkfat and its fractions. *Food Chemistry*, *34*(4), 261–271. doi:10.1016/0308-8146(89)90103-9

Abu-Qatouseh, L., Mallah, E., Issa, H., Sabri, I., & Shihab, P. (2019). Antimicrobial And Anti-Inflammatory Activity Of Camel Milk Derived Immune Proteins And Peptides Against Propionibacterium Acnes. *International Journal of Biology. Pharmacy and Allied Sciences*, *8*, 163–173.

Abuelgasim, K. A., Alsharhan, Y., Alenzi, T., Alhazzani, A., Ali, Y. Z., & Jazieh, A. R. (2018). The use of complementary and alternative medicine by patients with cancer: A cross-sectional survey in Saudi Arabia. *BMC Complementary and Alternative Medicine*, *18*(1), 88. doi:10.118612906-018-2150-8 PMID:29530034

Adams, C. M. (2013). Patient report: Autism spectrum disorder treated with camel milk. *Global Advances in Health and Medicine: Improving Healthcare Outcomes Worldwide*, *2*(6), 78–80. doi:10.7453/gahmj.2013.094 PMID:24349886

Adams, J. B., & Holloway, C. (2004). Pilot study of a moderate dose multivitamin/mineral supplement for children with autistic spectrum disorder. *Journal of Alternative and Complementary Medicine (New York, N.Y.)*, *10*(6), 1033–1039. doi:10.1089/acm.2004.10.1033 PMID:15673999

Agarwal, R., Swami, S., Beniwal, R., Kochar, D., Sahani, M., Tuteja, F., & Ghouri, S. (2003). Effect of camel milk on glycemic control, risk factors and diabetes quality of life in type-1 diabetes: A randomized prospective controlled study. *Journal of Camel Practice and Research*, *10*(1), 45–50.

Agrawal, R., Budania, S., Sharma, P., Gupta, R., Kochar, D., Panwar, R., & Sahani, M. (2007). Zero prevalence of diabetes in camel milk consuming Raica community of north-west Rajasthan, India. *Diabetes Research and Clinical Practice*, *76*(2), 290–296. doi:10.1016/j.diabres.2006.09.036 PMID:17098321

Agrawal, R., Jain, S., Shah, S., Chopra, A., & Agarwal, V. (2011). Effect of camel milk on glycemic control and insulin requirement in patients with type 1 diabetes: 2-years randomized controlled trial. *European Journal of Clinical Nutrition*, *65*(9), 1048–1052. doi:10.1038/ejcn.2011.98 PMID:21629270

Agrawal, R., Singh, G., Nayak, K., Kochar, D., Sharma, R., Beniwal, R., ... Gupta, R. (2004). Prevalence of diabetes in camel milk consuming 'RAICA' Rural Community of North West Rajasthan. *International Journal of Diabetes in Developing Countries*, *24*, 109–114.

Agrawal, R., Swami, S., Beniwal, R., Kochar, D., Sahani, M., Tuteja, F., & Ghorui, S. (2003). Effect of camel milk on glycemic control, lipid profile and diabetes quality of life in type 1 diabetes: A randomised prospective controlled cross over study. *The Indian Journal of Animal Sciences*, *73*(10), 1105–1110.

Agrawal, R. P., Saran, S., Sharma, P., Gupta, R. P., Kochar, D. K., & Sahani, M. S. (2007). Effect of camel milk on residual β-cell function in recent onset type 1 diabetes. *Diabetes Research and Clinical Practice*, *77*(3), 494–495. doi:10.1016/j.diabres.2007.01.012 PMID:17320238

Agrawal, R. P., Sharma, P., & Gafoorunissa, S. J. (2011). Effect of camel milk on glucose metabolism in adults with normal glucose tolerance and type 2 diabetes in Raica community: A crossover study. *Acta Bio Medica Atenei Parmensis*, *82*(3), 181–186. PMID:22783713

Akhu-Zaheya, L. M., & Alkhasawneh, E. M. (2012). Complementary alternative medicine use among a sample of Muslim Jordanian oncology patients. *Complementary Therapies in Clinical Practice*, *18*(2), 121–126. doi:10.1016/j.ctcp.2011.10.003 PMID:22500850

Al-Amoudi, S., Cañas, J., Hohl, S. D., Distelhorst, S. R., & Thompson, B. (2015). Breaking the Silence: Breast Cancer Knowledge and Beliefs Among Somali Muslim Women in Seattle, Washington. *Health Care for Women International*, *36*(5), 608–616. doi:10.1080/07399332.2013.857323 PMID:24351062

Al-Aubaidy, H. A., & Jelinek, H. F. (2014). Oxidative stress and triglycerides as predictors of subclinical atherosclerosis in prediabetes. *Redox Report*, *19*(2), 87–91. doi:10.1179/1351000213Y.0000000080 PMID:24520969

Al-Ayadhi & Elamin. (2015). *Camel milk as a potential therapy as an antioxidant in autism spectrum disorder (ASD)*. Apple Academic Press.

Al-Ayadhi, Halepoto, Al-Dress, Mitwali, & Zainah. (2015). Behavioral benefits of camel milk in subjects with autism spectrum disorder. *Journal of the College of Physicians and Surgeons--Pakistan*, *25*(11), 819–823. PMID:26577969

Al-Ayadhi, L., & Elamin, N. (2013). Camel milk as a potential therapy as an antioxidant in autism spectrum disorder (ASD). *Evidence-Based Complementary and Alternative Medicine*. PMID:24069051

Al Haj, O. A., & Al Kanhal, H. A. (2010). *Compositional, technological and nutritional aspects of dromedary camel milk*. doi:10.1016/j.idairyj.2010.04.003

Al-Harbi, M. M., Qureshi, S., Ahmed, M. M., Raza, M., Baig, M. Z. A., & Shah, A. H. (1996). *Effect of camel urine on the cytological and biochemical changes induced by cyclophosphamide in mice*. doi:10.1016/0378-8741(96)01399-2

Al-Humaid, A., Mousa, H., El-Mergawi, R., & Abdel-Salam, A. (2010). Chemical composition and antioxidant activity of dates and dates-camel-milk mixtures as a protective meal against lipid peroxidation in rats. *American Journal of Food Technology*, *5*(1), 22–30. doi:10.3923/ajft.2010.22.30

Al-Juboori, A., Mohammed, M., Rashid, J., Kurian, J., & El Refaey, S. (2013). Nutritional and medicinal value of camel (Camelus dromedarius) milk. *WIT Transactions on Ecology and the Environment*, *170*, 221–232. doi:10.2495/FENV130201

Al-Numair, K. S., Chandramohan, G., Kamalakkannan, N., Alsaif, M. A., & Sundaraselvan, G. (2010). Effect of camel milk on the activities of ATPases in normal and streptozotocin-diabetic rats. *Polish Journal of Food and Nutrition Sciences*, *60*(4).

Al-Omari, M. M., Al-Ghariebeh, R. B., Alhaija, A. A. A., Al-Zoubi, H., & Al-Qaoud, K. M. (2019). Camel milk whey inhibits inflammatory colorectal cancer development via down regulation of pro-inflammatory cytokines in induced AOM/DSS mouse model. *Emirates Journal of Food and Agriculture*, *31*(4), 256–262. doi:10.9755/ejfa.2019.v31.i4.1935

Al-Yousef, N., Gaafar, A., Al-Otaibi, B., Al-Jammaz, I., Al-Hussein, K., & Aboussekhra, A. (2012). *Camel urine components display anti-cancer properties in vitro*. doi:10.1016/j.jep.2012.07.042

Alabdulkarim, B. (2012). Effect of camel milk on blood glucose, cholesterol, triglyceride and liver enzymes activities in female albino rats. *World Applied Sciences Journal*, *17*(11), 1394–1397.

Alavi, F., Salami, M., Emam-Djomeh, Z., & Mohammadian, M. (2017). Nutraceutical properties of camel milk. In *Nutrients in Dairy and their Implications on Health and Disease* (pp. 451–468). Elsevier. doi:10.1016/B978-0-12-809762-5.00036-X

AlBedah, A., Khalil, M., Elolemy, A. T., Al, A. M., Al, S. E., Al-Yahia, O. A., ... Henary, B. Y. (2013). The use of and out-of-pocket spending on complementary and alternative medicine in Qassim province, Saudi Arabia. *Annals of Saudi Medicine*, *33*(3), 282–289. doi:10.5144/0256-4947.2013.282 PMID:23793433

Alhaider, A. A., Abdel Gader, A. G. M., Almeshaal, N., & Saraswati, S. (2014). Camel milk inhibits inflammatory angiogenesis via downregulation of proangiogenic and proinflammatory cytokines in mice. *APMIS*, *122*(7), 599–607. doi:10.1111/apm.12199 PMID:24320686

Alhomida, A. (1996). Total, free, short-chain and long-chain acyl carnitine levels in Arabian camel milk (Camelus dromedarius). *Annals of Nutrition & Metabolism*, *40*(4), 221–226. doi:10.1159/000177925 PMID:8886250

Almahdy, O., EL-Fakharany, E. M., EL-Dabaa, E., Ng, T. B., & Redwan, E. M. (2011). Examination of the activity of camel milk casein against hepatitis C virus (genotype-4a) and its apoptotic potential in hepatoma and hela cell lines. *Hepatitis Monthly*, *11*(9), 724–730. doi:10.5812/kowsar.1735143X.1367 PMID:22235215

Almehdar, H. A., El-Baky, N. A., Alhaider, A. A., & Redwan, E. M. (2019). Immunogenicity comparison of lactoferrin purified from Saudi Arabia camel clans milk. *Human Antibodies*, 1–6. PMID:30372672

Alrowais, N. A., & Alyousefi, N. A. (2017). The prevalence extent of Complementary and Alternative Medicine (CAM) use among Saudis. *Saudi Pharmaceutical Journal*, *25*(3), 306–318. doi:10.1016/j.jsps.2016.09.009 PMID:28344484

Ameen, S. H., & Hameed, A. K. (2019). Therapy Role of Camel Milk for the Treatment of Hepatitis Mice Which Induces via Listeria Monocytogenes. *Indian Journal of Public Health Research & Development*, *10*(2), 537. doi:10.5958/0976-5506.2019.00347.4

Amr, A. M., Takruri, H. R., Shomaf, M. S., Alhaj, O. A., & Faris, M. E. A.-I., & Abdel-Rahm, W. M. (2018). Fermented Camel (Camelus dromedarius) and Bovine Milk Attenuate Azoxymethane-induced Colonic Aberrant Crypt Foci in Fischer 344 Rats. *Pakistan Journal of Nutrition*, *17*(4), 179–189. doi:10.3923/pjn.2018.179.189

Aqib, A. I., Kulyar, M. F.-A., Ashfaq, K., Bhutta, Z. A., Shoaib, M., & Ahmed, R. (2019). Camel milk Insuline: Pathophysiological and molecular Repository. *Trends in Food Science & Technology*, *88*, 497–504. doi:10.1016/j.tifs.2019.04.009

Arab, H. H., Salama, S. A., Eid, A. H., Omar, H. A., Arafa, E.-S. A., & Maghrabi, I. A. (2014). *Camel's milk ameliorates TNBS-induced colitis in rats via downregulation of inflammatory cytokines and oxidative stress*. doi:10.1016/j.fct.2014.04.032

Ayyash, M., Al-Dhaheri, A. S., Al Mahadin, S., Kizhakkayil, J., & Abushelaibi, A. (2018). In vitro investigation of anticancer, antihypertensive, antidiabetic, and antioxidant activities of camel milk fermented with camel milk probiotic: A comparative study with fermented bovine milk. *Journal of Dairy Science*, *101*(2), 900–911. doi:10.3168/jds.2017-13400 PMID:29224862

Badawy, A. A., El-Magd, M. A., & Alsadrah, S. A. (2018). Therapeutic Effect of Camel Milk and Its Exosomes on MCF7 Cells In Vitro and In Vivo. *Integrative Cancer Therapies*. doi:10.1177/1534735418786000 PMID:29986606

Baio, J., Wiggins, L., Christensen, D. L., Maenner, M. J., Daniels, J., Warren, Z., ... White, T. (2018). Prevalence of autism spectrum disorder among children aged 8 years—autism and developmental disabilities monitoring network, 11 sites, United States, 2014. *MMWR. Surveillance Summaries*, *67*(6), 1–23. doi:10.15585/mmwr.ss6706a1 PMID:29701730

Barrett, J. S., Irving, P., Shepherd, S. J., Muir, J. G., & Gibson, P. R. (2009). Comparison of the prevalence of fructose and lactose malabsorption across chronic intestinal disorders. *Alimentary Pharmacology & Therapeutics*, *30*(2), 165–174. doi:10.1111/j.1365-2036.2009.04018.x PMID:19392860

Bashir, S., & Al-Ayadhi, L. Y. (2014). Effect of camel milk on thymus and activation-regulated chemokine in autistic children: Double-blind study. *Pediatric Research*, *75*(4), 559–563. doi:10.1038/pr.2013.248 PMID:24375082

Bell, J. G., Miller, D., MacDonald, D. J., MacKinlay, E. E., Dick, J. R., Cheseldine, S., ... O'Hare, A. E. (2010). The fatty acid compositions of erythrocyte and plasma polar lipids in children with autism, developmental delay or typically developing controls and the effect of fish oil intake. *British Journal of Nutrition, 103*(8), 1160–1167. doi:10.1017/S0007114509992881 PMID:19995470

Bloomer, R. J., Butawan, M., Farney, T. M., & McAllister, M. J. (2019). An Overview of the Dietary Ingredient Carnitine. In *Nutrition and Enhanced Sports Performance* (pp. 605–617). Elsevier. doi:10.1016/B978-0-12-813922-6.00051-5

Bouhaddaoui, S., Chabir, R., Errachidi, F., El Ghadraoui, L., El Khalfi, B., Benjelloun, M., & Soukri, A. (2019). Study of the Biochemical Biodiversity of Camel Milk. *The Scientific World Journal.* PMID:31093015

Bracco, U., Hidalgo, J., & Bohren, H. (1972). Lipid composition of the fat globule membrane of human and bovine milk. *Journal of Dairy Science, 55*(2), 165–172. doi:10.3168/jds.S0022-0302(72)85454-7 PMID:4672739

Brondino, N., Fusar-Poli, L., Rocchetti, M., Provenzani, U., Barale, F., & Politi, P. (2015). Complementary and alternative therapies for autism spectrum disorder. *Evidence-Based Complementary and Alternative Medicine.* PMID:26064157

Buonopane, G. J., Kilara, A., Smith, J. S., & McCarthy, R. D. (1992). Effect of skim milk supplementation on blood cholesterol concentration, blood pressure, and triglycerides in a free-living human population. *Journal of the American College of Nutrition, 11*(1), 56–67. doi:10.1080/07315724.1992.10718197 PMID:1541797

Cameron, A. J., Shaw, J. E., & Zimmet, P. Z. (2004). The metabolic syndrome: Prevalence in worldwide populations. *Endocrinology and Metabolism Clinics, 33*(2), 351–375. doi:10.1016/j.ecl.2004.03.005 PMID:15158523

CDC. (2019). *Data & Statistics on Autism Spectrum Disorder.* Retrieved from https://www.cdc.gov/ncbddd/autism/data.html

Cekici, H., & Sanlier, N. (2019). Current nutritional approaches in managing autism spectrum disorder: A review. *Nutritional Neuroscience, 22*(3), 145–155. doi:10.1080/1028415X.2017.1358481 PMID:28762296

Darwish, H. A., Abd Raboh, N. R., & Mahdy, A. (2012). *Camel's milk alleviates alcohol-induced liver injury in rats.* doi:10.1016/j.fct.2012.01.016

Dubey, U., Lal, M., Mittal, A., & Kapur, S. (2015). *Therapeutic potential of Camel Milk.* doi:10.9755/ejfa.2015-04-122

Ebaid, H. (2014). Promotion of immune and glycaemic functions in streptozotocin-induced diabetic rats treated with un-denatured camel milk whey proteins. *Nutrition & metabolism, 11*(1), 31. doi:10.1186/1743-7075-11-31 PMID:25009576

Ebaid, H., Salem, A., Sayed, A., & Metwalli, A. (2011). Whey protein enhances normal inflammatory responses during cutaneous wound healing in diabetic rats. *Lipids in Health and Disease, 10*(1), 235. doi:10.1186/1476-511X-10-235 PMID:22168406

Eckel, R. H., Grundy, S. M., & Zimmet, P. Z. (2005). The metabolic syndrome. *Lancet*, *365*(9468), 1415–1428. doi:10.1016/S0140-6736(05)66378-7 PMID:15836891

Ejtahed, H. S., Naslaji, A. N., Mirmiran, P., Yeganeh, M. Z., Hedayati, M., Azizi, F., & Movahedi, A. M. (2015). Effect of camel milk on blood sugar and lipid profile of patients with type 2 diabetes: A pilot clinical trial. *International Journal of Endocrinology and Metabolism*, *13*(1). doi:10.5812/ijem.21160 PMID:25745496

El-Hatmi, H., Girardet, J.-M., Gaillard, J.-L., Yahyaoui, M. H., & Attia, H. (2007). *Characterisation of whey proteins of camel (Camelus dromedarius) milk and colostrum*. doi:10.1016/j.smallrumres.2006.04.001

El Miniawy, H. M. F., Ahmed, K. A., Tony, M. A., Mansour, S. A., & Salah Khattab, M. M. (2014). *Camel milk inhibits murine hepatic carcinogenesis, initiated by diethylnitrosamine and promoted by phenobarbitone*. doi:10.1016/j.ijvsm.2014.10.004

El Sayed, I., Ruppanner, R., Ismail, A., Champagne, C. P., & Assaf, R. (1992). Antibacterial and antiviral activity of camel milk protective proteins. *The Journal of Dairy Research*, *59*(2), 169–175. doi:10.1017/S0022029900030417 PMID:1319434

Elayan, A. A., Sulieman, A., & Saleh, F. (2008). The hypocholesterolemic effect of Gariss and Gariss containing bifidobacteria in rats fed on a cholesterol-enriched diet. *Asian J Biochem*, *3*, 43–47. doi:10.3923/ajb.2008.43.47

Elzhrani, M. S. (2018). Camel milk improvement of antioxidant and lipid profile in hypercholesterolemic rabbits. *Journal of Cell and Animal Biology*, *12*(1), 1–4. doi:10.5897/JCAB2017.0455

Espinosa-Marrón, A., Quiñones-Capistrán, C. A., Rubio-Blancas, A., del Pilar Milke-García, M., & Castillejos-Molina, R. A. (2019). *Hyperglycemia: The Metabolic Syndrome Component That Aggravates Erectile Dysfunction in Mexican Patients*. Academic Press.

Fakhoury, M., Negrulj, R., Mooranian, A., & Al-Salami, H. (2014). Inflammatory bowel disease: Clinical aspects and treatments. *Journal of Inflammation Research*, *7*, 113–120. doi:10.2147/JIR.S65979 PMID:25075198

Fallah, Z., Feizi, A., Hashemipour, M., & Kelishadi, R. (2018). Positive Effect of Fermented Camel Milk on Liver Enzymes of Adolescents with Metabolic Syndrome: A Double Blind, Randomized, Cross-over Trial. *Materia Socio-Medica*, *30*(1), 20. doi:10.5455/msm.2018.30.20-25 PMID:29670474

Farah, Z. (1993). Composition and characteristics of camel milk. *The Journal of Dairy Research*, *60*(4), 603–626. doi:10.1017/S0022029900027953 PMID:8294611

Farah, Z., Rettenmaier, R., & Atkins, D. (1992). Vitamin content of camel milk. *International Journal for Vitamin and Nutrition Research*, *62*(1), 30–33. PMID:1587705

Feldstein, A. E., Papouchado, B. G., Angulo, P., Sanderson, S., Adams, L., & Gores, G. J. (2005). Hepatic stellate cells and fibrosis progression in patients with nonalcoholic fatty liver disease. *Clinical Gastroenterology and Hepatology*, *3*(4), 384–389. doi:10.1016/S1542-3565(04)00616-0 PMID:15822044

Fujita, K.-i., Matsuda, E., Sekine, K., Iigo, M., & Tsuda, H. (2004). Lactoferrin enhances Fas expression and apoptosis in the colon mucosa of azoxymethane-treated rats. *Carcinogenesis*, *25*(10), 1961–1966. doi:10.1093/carcin/bgh205 PMID:15192017

Gizachew, A., Teha, J., Birhanu, T., & Nekemte, E. (2014). Review on medicinal and nutritional values of camel milk. *Nature and Science*, *12*(12), 35–41.

Golik, F. (2014). Case study: The effects of excess fructose in a patient with autism spectrum disorder infections. *Journal of the Australasian College of Nutritional and Environmental Medicine*, *33*(3), 13.

Gorini, F., Muratori, F., & Morales, M. A. (2014). The Role of Heavy Metal Pollution in Neurobehavioral Disorders: A Focus on Autism. *Review Journal of Autism and Developmental Disorders*, *1*(4), 354–372. doi:10.100740489-014-0028-3

Gul, W., Farooq, N., Anees, D., Khan, U., & Rehan, F. (2015). Camel milk: A boon to mankind. *Int J Res Stud Biosci*, *3*, 23–29.

Habib, H. M., Ibrahim, W. H., Schneider-Stock, R., & Hassan, H. M. (2013). *Camel milk lactoferrin reduces the proliferation of colorectal cancer cells and exerts antioxidant and DNA damage inhibitory activities*. doi:10.1016/j.foodchem.2013.03.039

Haddadin, M. S., Gammoh, S. I., & Robinson, R. K. (2008). Seasonal variations in the chemical composition of camel milk in Jordan. *The Journal of Dairy Research*, *75*(1), 8–12. doi:10.1017/S0022029907002750 PMID:17971263

Hamad, E., Abdel-Rahim, E., & Romeih, E. (2011). Beneficial effect of camel milk on liver and kidneys function in diabetic Sprague-Dawley rats. *Int J Dairy Sci*, *6*(3), 190–197. doi:10.3923/ijds.2011.190.197

Hamed, H., Chaari, F., Ghannoudi, Z., ElFeki, A., Ellouz, S. C., & Gargouri, A. (2018). Beneficial effects of fermented camel milk by lactococcus lactis subsp cremoris on cardiotoxicity induced by carbon tetrachloride in mice. *Biomedicine and Pharmacotherapy*, *97*, 107–114. doi:10.1016/j.biopha.2017.10.057 PMID:29080450

Hamed, H., El Feki, A., & Gargouri, A. (2019). Evaluation of the hepatoprotective effect of combination between fermented camel milk and Rosmarinus officinalis leaves extract against CCl 4 induced liver toxicity in mice. *Journal of Food Science and Technology*, *56*(2), 824–834. doi:10.100713197-018-3542-y PMID:30906040

Hamed, H., Gargouri, M., Boulila, S., Chaari, F., Ghrab, F., Kallel, R., ... El Feki, A. (2018). Fermented camel milk prevents carbon tetrachloride induced acute injury in kidney of mice. *The Journal of Dairy Research*, *85*(2), 251–256. doi:10.1017/S0022029918000250 PMID:29785914

Hamzawy, M. A., El-Ghandour, Y. B., Abdel-Aziem, S. H., & Ali, Z. H. (2018). Leptin and camel milk abate oxidative stress status, genotoxicity induced in valproic acid rat model of autism. *International Journal of Immunopathology and Pharmacology*, *32*. doi:10.1177/2058738418785514 PMID:30004275

Hasson, S., Al-Busaidi, J. Z., Al-Qarni, Z. A., Rajapakse, S., Al-Bahlani, S., Idris, M. A., & Sallam, T. A. (2015). In vitro apoptosis triggering in the BT-474 human breast cancer cell line by lyophilised camel's milk. *Asian Pacific Journal of Cancer Prevention, 16*(15), 6651–6661. doi:10.7314/APJCP.2015.16.15.6651 PMID:26434890

Hosseini, S. M. A., Anushiravani, M., Mojahedi, M. J., Hami, M., Zibaee, S., Rakhshandeh, H., ... Tavassoli, A. P. (2019). The efficacy of camel milk and Tarangabin (manna of Alhagi maurorum (combination therapy on glomerular filtration rate in patients with chronic kidney disease: A randomized controlled trial. *Avicenna Journal of Phytomedicine*.

Hosseini, S. M. a.-R., Zibaee, S., Yousefi, M., Taghipour, A., & Noras, M. (2015). Camels Milk: Nutrition and Health Perspectives Iranian Traditional Medicine. *International Journal of Pediatrics, 3*(5.1), 915-920.

Ibn-e-Sina, A. (2005). *Al-Qanun fit-tib, volume three* [The Canon of Medicine]. Beirut: Alaalami Beirut library Press (research of ebrahim shamsedine).

Ibrahim, H. R., Isono, H., & Miyata, T. (2018). Potential antioxidant bioactive peptides from camel milk proteins. *Animal Nutrition, 4*(3), 273–280. doi:10.1016/j.aninu.2018.05.004 PMID:30175255

Ip, C., Singh, M., Thompson, H. J., & Scimeca, J. A. (1994). Conjugated linoleic acid suppresses mammary carcinogenesis and proliferative activity of the mammary gland in the rat. *Cancer Research, 54*(5), 1212–1215. PMID:8118808

Jazieh, A. R., Al Sudairy, R., Abulkhair, O., Alaskar, A., Al Safi, F., Sheblaq, N., ... Tamim, H. (2012). Use of complementary and alternative medicine by patients with cancer in Saudi Arabia. *Journal of Alternative and Complementary Medicine (New York, N.Y.), 18*(11), 1045–1049. doi:10.1089/acm.2011.0266 PMID:22906212

Kalla, K., Manthani, V., & Keerthi, S. (2017). Camel Milk An White Gold Of Dessert-A Review. *International Archive of Applied Sciences and Technology*, *8*(3), 74–83.

Kappeler, S., Heuberger, C., Farah, Z., & Puhan, Z. (1998). *Compositional and structural analysis of camel milk proteins with emphasis on protective proteins*. ETH Zurich.

Kappeler, S., Heuberger, C., Farah, Z., & Puhan, Z. (2004). Expression of the peptidoglycan recognition protein, PGRP, in the lactating mammary gland. *Journal of Dairy Science, 87*(8), 2660–2668. doi:10.3168/jds.S0022-0302(04)73392-5 PubMed

Kappeler, S. R., Ackermann, M., Farah, Z., & Puhan, Z. (1999). Sequence analysis of camel (Camelus dromedarius) lactoferrin. *International Dairy Journal, 9*(7), 481–486. doi:10.1016/S0958-6946(99)00117-X

Khatoon, H., & Najam, R. (2017). Bioactive Components in Camel Milk: Their Nutritive Value and Therapeutic Application. In Nutrients in Dairy and their Implications on Health and Disease (pp. 377-387). Elsevier.

Kojda, G., & Harrison, D. (1999). Interactions between NO and reactive oxygen species: Pathophysiological importance in atherosclerosis, hypertension, diabetes and heart failure. *Cardiovascular Research, 43*(3), 652–671. doi:10.1016/S0008-6363(99)00169-8 PMID:10690328

Konuspayeva, G., Faye, B., & Loiseau, G. (2009). *The composition of camel milk: A meta-analysis of the literature data.* doi:10.1016/j.jfca.2008.09.008

Konuspayeva, G., Faye, B., & Loiseau, G. (2011). Variability of vitamin C content in camel milk from Kazakhstan. *Journal of Camelid Science*, *4*, 63–69.

Konuspayeva, G., Faye, B., Loiseau, G., & Levieux, D. (2007). *Lactoferrin and Immunoglobulin Contents in Camel's Milk (Camelus bactrianus, Camelus dromedarius, and Hybrids) from Kazakhstan.* doi:10.3168/jds.s0022-0302(07)72606-1

Konuspayeva, G., Lemarie, É., Faye, B., Loiseau, G., & Montet, D. (2008). Fatty acid and cholesterol composition of camel's (Camelus bactrianus, Camelus dromedarius and hybrids) milk in Kazakhstan. *Dairy Science & Technology*, *88*(3), 327–340. doi:10.1051/dst:2008005

Korashy, H. M., El Gendy, M. A., Alhaider, A. A., & El-Kadi, A. O. (2012). Camel milk modulates the expression of aryl hydrocarbon receptor-regulated genes, Cyp1a1, Nqo1, and Gsta1, in murine hepatoma Hepa 1c1c7 cells. *BioMed Research International*. PMID:22570534

Korashy, H. M., Maayah, Z. H., Abd-Allah, A. R., El-Kadi, A. O., & Alhaider, A. A. (2012). Camel milk triggers apoptotic signaling pathways in human hepatoma HepG2 and breast cancer MCF7 cell lines through transcriptional mechanism. *BioMed Research International*. PMID:22654482

Korish, A. (2014). The antidiabetic action of camel milk in experimental type 2 diabetes mellitus: An overview on the changes in incretin hormones, insulin resistance, and inflammatory cytokines. *Hormone and Metabolic Research. Hormon- und Stoffwechselforschung. Hormones et Metabolisme*, *46*(06), 404–411. doi:10.1055-0034-1368711 PMID:24627103

Korish, A. A., & Arafah, M. M. (2013). Camel milk ameliorates steatohepatitis, insulin resistance and lipid peroxidation in experimental non-alcoholic fatty liver disease. *BMC Complementary and Alternative Medicine*, *13*(1), 264. doi:10.1186/1472-6882-13-264 PMID:24119413

Krishnankutty, R., Iskandarani, A., Therachiyil, L., Uddin, S., Azizi, F., Kulinski, M., ... Mohammad, R. M. (2018). Anticancer Activity of Camel Milk via Induction of Autophagic Death in Human Colorectal and Breast Cancer Cells. *Asian Pacific journal of cancer prevention. APJCP*, *19*(12), 3501. PMID:30583676

Kula, J. T., & Tegegne, D. (2016). Chemical composition and medicinal values of camel milk. *Int J Res Stud Biosci*, *4*(4), 13–25.

Kumar, D., Chatli, M. K., Singh, R., Mehta, N., & Kumar, P. (2016). Enzymatic hydrolysis of camel milk proteins and its antioxidant properties. *Journal of Camel Practice and Research*, *23*(1), 33–40. doi:10.5958/2277-8934.2016.00005.9

Legrand, D., Elass, E., Carpentier, M., & Mazurier, J. (2005). Lactoferrin. *Cellular and Molecular Life Sciences*, *62*(22), 2549–2559. doi:10.100700018-005-5370-2 PMID:16261255

Li, H., & Papadopoulos, V. (1998). Peripheral-type benzodiazepine receptor function in cholesterol transport. Identification of a putative cholesterol recognition/interaction amino acid sequence and consensus pattern. *Endocrinology*, *139*(12), 4991–4997. doi:10.1210/endo.139.12.6390 PMID:9832438

Li, Y.-J., Ou, J.-J., Li, Y.-M., & Xiang, D.-X. (2017). Dietary supplement for core symptoms of autism spectrum disorder: Where are we now and where should we go? *Frontiers in Psychiatry*, *8*, 155. doi:10.3389/fpsyt.2017.00155 PMID:28878697

Longo, N., Frigeni, M., & Pasquali, M. (2016). Carnitine transport and fatty acid oxidation. *Biochimica et Biophysica Acta (BBA)-. Molecular Cell Research*, *1863*(10), 2422–2435.

Malik, A., Al-Senaidy, A., Skrzypczak-Jankun, E., & Jankun, J. (2012). A study of the anti-diabetic agents of camel milk. *International Journal of Molecular Medicine*, *30*(3), 585–592. doi:10.3892/ijmm.2012.1051 PMID:22751901

Maswadeh, H. M., Aljarbou, A. N., Alorainy, M. S., Alsharidah, M. S., & Khan, M. A. (2015). *Etoposide Incorporated into Camel Milk Phospholipids Liposomes Shows Increased Activity against Fibrosarcoma in a Mouse Model*. doi:10.1155/2015/743051

Mati, A., Senoussi-Ghezali, C., Ahmed Zennia, S. S., Almi-Sebbane, D., El-Hatmi, H., & Girardet, J.-M. (2016). Dromedary camel milk proteins, a source of peptides having biological activities –. *RE:view*. doi:10.1016/j.idairyj.2016.12.001

McGinnis, W. R. (2004). Oxidative stress in autism. *Alternative Therapies in Health and Medicine*, *10*(6), 22–36. PMID:15624347

McNees, A. L., Markesich, D., Zayyani, N. R., & Graham, D. Y. (2015). Mycobacterium paratuberculosis as a cause of Crohn's disease. *Expert Review of Gastroenterology & Hepatology*, *9*(12), 1523–1534. doi:10.1586/17474124.2015.1093931 PMID:26474349

Meguid, N. A., Atta, H. M., Gouda, A. S., & Khalil, R. O. (2008). Role of polyunsaturated fatty acids in the management of Egyptian children with autism. *Clinical Biochemistry*, *41*(13), 1044–1048. doi:10.1016/j.clinbiochem.2008.05.013 PMID:18582451

Meisel, H. (2004). Multifunctional peptides encrypted in milk proteins. *BioFactors (Oxford, England)*, *21*(1-4), 55–61. doi:10.1002/biof.552210111 PMID:15630170

Mihic, T., Rainkie, D., Wilby, K. J., & Pawluk, S. A. (2016). *The Therapeutic Effects of Camel Milk: A Systematic Review of Animal and Human Trials*. doi:10.1177/2156587216658846

Miniero, R., Mazza, G., Pasqua, A., Dolceamore, T., Zurlo, F., Mahdi, A., & Britti, D. (2014). Composition and therapeutic use of camel milk. *Large Animal Review*, *20*(3), 125–132.

Mirmiran, P., Ejtahed, H.-S., Angoorani, P., Eslami, F., & Azizi, F. (2017). Camel Milk Has Beneficial Effects on Diabetes Mellitus: A Systematic Review. *International Journal of Endocrinology and Metabolism*, *15*(2), e42150–e42150. doi:10.5812/ijem.42150 PMID:29026408

Mohammad, D. (2009). Camel's milk protects against cadmium chloride-induced hypochromic microcytic anemia and oxidative stress in red blood cells of white albino rats. *American Journal of Pharmacology and Toxicology*, *4*(4), 136–143. doi:10.3844/ajptsp.2009.136.143

Moura, F. A., De Andrade, K. Q., Dos Santos, J. C. F., Araújo, O. R. P., & Goulart, M. O. F. (2015). *Antioxidant therapy for treatment of inflammatory bowel disease: Does it work?* doi:10.1016/j.redox.2015.10.006

Mullaicharam, A. (2014). A review on medicinal properties of camel milk. *World J Pharm Sci*, *2*(3), 237–242.

Mushref, F. (2006). In vitro anticancer agent I-Tissue culture study of human lung cancer cells A549 II-Tissue culture study of mice leukemia cells L1210. *Int J Cancer Res*, *2*(4), 330–344. doi:10.3923/ijcr.2006.330.344

Nagao, K., & Yanagita, T. (2008). Bioactive lipids in metabolic syndrome. *Progress in Lipid Research*, *47*(2), 127–146. doi:10.1016/j.plipres.2007.12.002 PMID:18177744

Naser, S. A., Sagramsingh, S. R., Naser, A. S., & Thanigachalam, S. (2014). Mycobacterium avium subspecies paratuberculosis causes Crohn's disease in some inflammatory bowel disease patients. *World Journal of Gastroenterology*, *20*(23), 7403–7415. doi:10.3748/wjg.v20.i23.7403 PMID:24966610

Niasari-Naslaji, A., Arabha, H., Atakpour, A., Salami, M., & Moosavi-Movahedi, A. (2012). Camel Milk and its Bioactive Molecules in Medical Treatments. *Science Cultivation*, *2*(1), 20–24.

Pariza, M. (1999). *Conjugated linoleic acid and the control of cancer and obesity*. doi:10.1093/toxsci/52.suppl_1.107

Rao, D. R., Chawan, C., & Pulusani, S. (1981). Influence of milk and thermophilus milk on plasma cholesterol levels and hepatic cholesterogenesis in rats. *Journal of Food Science*, *46*(5), 1339–1341. doi:10.1111/j.1365-2621.1981.tb04168.x

Refaey, A. T. A.-J. S. E. (2013). *Nutritional and medicinal value of camel (Camelus dromedarius) milk*. Food and Environment. doi:10.2495/fenv130201

Rodr, L. M., Gomez, M. P.-G., Pimentel, L. L., & Fontecha, J. (2017). Milk fat components with potential anticancer activity—a review. *Bioscience Reports*, *37*. doi:10.1042/BSR20170705 PMID:29026007

Roy, T., & Deepak, D. (2014). Antioxidant properties of milk oligosaccharides from various ruminants. *International Journal of Pharma and Bio Sciences*, *5*(2), 400–408.

Saad, B. (2015). Greco-Arab and Islamic diet therapy: Tradition, research and practice. *Surge*, *1*(1).

Salami, M., Moosavi-Movahedi, A. A., Ehsani, M. R., Yousefi, R., Haertle, T., Chobert, J.-M., ... Ebadi, S. A. (2010). Improvement of the antimicrobial and antioxidant activities of camel and bovine whey proteins by limited proteolysis. *Journal of Agricultural and Food Chemistry*, *58*(6), 3297–3302. doi:10.1021/jf9033283 PMID:20175528

Salami, M., Moosavi-Movahedi, A. A., Moosavi-Movahedi, F., Ehsani, M. R., Yousefi, R., Farhadi, M., ... Haertlé, T. (2011). Biological activity of camel milk casein following enzymatic digestion. *The Journal of Dairy Research*, *78*(4), 471–478. doi:10.1017/S0022029911000628 PMID:21910944

Salwa, M. Q., & Lina, A. F. K. (2010). *Antigenotoxic and anticytotoxic effect of camel milk in mice treated with cisplatin*. doi:10.1016/j.sjbs.2010.02.010

Sawaya, W., Khalil, J., Al-Shalhat, A., & Al-Mohammad, H. (1984). Chemical composition and nutritional quality of camel milk. *Journal of Food Science*, *49*(3), 744–747. doi:10.1111/j.1365-2621.1984.tb13200.x

Sboui, A., Djegham, M., Khorchani, T., Hammadi, M., Barhoumi, K., & Belhadj, O. (2010). Effect of camel milk on blood glucose, cholesterol and total proteins variations in alloxan-induced diabetic dogs. *International Journal of Diabetes and Metabolism*, *18*(1), 5–11. doi:10.1159/000497686

Seifried, H. E., Anderson, D. E., Fisher, E. I., & Milner, J. A. (2007). A review of the interaction among dietary antioxidants and reactive oxygen species. *The Journal of Nutritional Biochemistry*, *18*(9), 567–579. doi:10.1016/j.jnutbio.2006.10.007 PMID:17360173

Shabo, Y., Barzel, R., & Yagil, R. (2008). Etiology of Crohn's disease and camel milk treatment. *Journal of Camel Practice and Research*, *15*(1), 55–59.

Shabo, Y., & Yagil, R. (2005). Etiology of autism and camel milk as therapy. *International Journal on Disability and Human Development: IJDHD*, *4*(2), 67–70. doi:10.1515/IJDHD.2005.4.2.67

Shariatikia, M., Behbahani, M., & Mohabatkar, H. (2017). Anticancer activity of cow, sheep, goat, mare, donkey and camel milks and their caseins and whey proteins and in silico comparison of the caseins. *Molecular Biology Research Communications*, *6*(2), 57. PMID:28775991

Sharma, C., & Singh, C. (2014). Therapeutic value of camel milk–a review. *Advanced Journal of Pharmacie and Life Science Research*, *2*(3), 7–13.

Sharma, P., Dube, D., Singh, A., Mishra, B., Singh, N., Sinha, M., ... Singh, T. P. (2011). *Structural Basis of Recognition of Pathogen-associated Molecular Patterns and Inhibition of Proinflammatory Cytokines by Camel Peptidoglycan Recognition Protein*. doi:10.1074/jbc.m111.228163

Sharma, P., Dube, D., Sinha, M., Dey, S., Kaur, P., Sharma, S., & Singh, T. P. (2012). Structural basis of heparin binding to camel peptidoglycan recognition protein-S. *International Journal of Biochemistry and Molecular Biology*, *3*(1), 86. PMID:22509483

Shohami, E., Beit-Yannai, E., Horowitz, M., & Kohen, R. (1997). Oxidative stress in closed-head injury: Brain antioxidant capacity as an indicator of functional outcome. *Journal of Cerebral Blood Flow and Metabolism*, *17*(10), 1007–1019. doi:10.1097/00004647-199710000-00002 PMID:9346425

Shori, A. B. (2015). Camel milk as a potential therapy for controlling diabetes and its complications: A review of in vivo studies. *Journal of Food and Drug Analysis*, *23*(4), 609–618. doi:10.1016/j.jfda.2015.02.007 PMID:28911476

Sliwinski, S., Croonenberghs, J., Christophe, A., Deboutte, D., & Maes, M. (2006). Polyunsaturated fatty acids: Do they have a role in the pathophysiology of autism? *Neuroendocrinology Letters*, *27*(4), 465–472. PMID:16891996

Soboleva, S. E., Sedykh, S. E., Alinovskaya, L. I., Buneva, V. N., & Nevinsky, G. A. (2019). Cow Milk Lactoferrin Possesses Several Catalytic Activities. *Biomolecules*, *9*(6), 208. doi:10.3390/biom9060208 PMID:31146486

Soleymanzadeh, N., Mirdamadi, S., Mirzaei, M., & Kianirad, M. (2019). Novel β-casein derived antioxidant and ACE-inhibitory active peptide from camel milk fermented by Leuconostoc lactis PTCC1899: Identification and molecular docking. *International Dairy Journal*.

Stewart, B. W., & Kleihues, P. (2003). *World cancer report*. Academic Press.

Tas, A. A. (2018). Dietary strategies in autism spectrum disorder (ASD). *Progress in Nutrition*, *20*(4), 554–562.

Tierney, E., Bukelis, I., Thompson, R. E., Ahmed, K., Aneja, A., Kratz, L., & Kelley, R. I. (2006). Abnormalities of cholesterol metabolism in autism spectrum disorders. *American Journal of Medical Genetics. Part B, Neuropsychiatric Genetics*, *141*(6), 666–668. doi:10.1002/ajmg.b.30368 PMID:16874769

Tsuda, H., & Sekine, K. (2000). Milk components as cancer chemopreventive agents. *Asian Pacific Journal of Cancer Prevention*, *1*(4), 277–282. PMID:12716300

Tsuda, H., Sekine, K., Ushida, Y., Kuhara, T., Takasuka, N., Iigo, M., . . . Moore, M. A. (2000). *Milk and dairy products in cancer prevention: focus on bovine lactoferrin*. doi:10.10161383-5742(00)00040-5

Tung, Y.-T., Chen, H.-L., Yen, C.-C., Lee, P.-Y., Tsai, H.-C., Lin, M.-F., & Chen, C.-M. (2013). Bovine lactoferrin inhibits lung cancer growth through suppression of both inflammation and expression of vascular endothelial growth factor. *Journal of Dairy Science*, *96*(4), 2095–2106. doi:10.3168/jds.2012-6153 PMID:23462173

Uversky, V. N., El-Fakharany, E. M., Abu-Serie, M. M., Almehdar, H. A., & Redwan, E. M. (2017). Divergent anticancer activity of free and formulated camel milk α-lactalbumin. *Cancer Investigation*, *35*(9), 610–623. doi:10.1080/07357907.2017.1373783 PMID:28949782

Valko, M., Rhodes, C., Moncol, J., Izakovic, M., & Mazur, M. (2006). Free radicals, metals and antioxidants in oxidative stress-induced cancer. *Chemico-Biological Interactions*, *160*(1), 1–40. doi:10.1016/j.cbi.2005.12.009 PMID:16430879

Vessby, B. (2003). Dietary fat, fatty acid composition in plasma and the metabolic syndrome. *Current Opinion in Lipidology*, *14*(1), 15–19. doi:10.1097/00041433-200302000-00004 PMID:12544656

Wali, A., Yanhua, G., Ishimov, U., Yili, A., Aisa, H. A., & Salikhov, S. (2019). Isolation and Identification of Three Novel Antioxidant Peptides from the Bactrian Camel Milk Hydrolysates. *International Journal of Peptide Research and Therapeutics*, 1–10.

Wangoh, J., Farah, Z., & Puhan, Z. (1998). Composition of milk from three camel (camelus dromedarius) breeds in Kenya during lactation. *Milchwissenschaft. Milk Science International*, *53*(3), 136–139.

Wernery, R., Joseph, S., Johnson, B., Jose, S., Tesfamariam, M., Ridao-Alonso, M., & Wernery, U. (2012). Camel milk against Autism–A preliminary report. *Journal of Camel Practice and Research*, *19*(2), 143–147.

Wernery, U. (2006). Camel milk, the white gold of the desert. *Journal of Camel Practice and Research*, *13*(1), 15.

WHO. (2006). *Definition and diagnosis of diabetes mellitus and intermediate hyperglycaemia: report of a WHO/IDF consultation*. WHO.

Wiecek, S., Wos, H., Radziewicz-Winnicki, I., Komraus, M., & Grzybowska-Chlebowczyk, U. (2014). Disaccharidase activity in children with inflammatory bowel. *The Turkish Journal of Gastroenterology*, *25*(2), 185–191. doi:10.5152/tjg.2014.3994 PMID:25003680

Wolf, J. S., Li, D., Taylor, R. J., & O'Malley, B. W. Jr. (2003). Lactoferrin inhibits growth of malignant tumors of the head and neck. *ORL, 65*(5), 245–249. doi:10.1159/000075220 PMID:14730178

Xu, R., Xiu, L., Zhang, Y., Du, R., & Wang, X. (2019). Probiotic and hepatoprotective activity of lactobacillus isolated from Mongolian camel milk products. *Beneficial Microbes*, 1–12. PMID:31122041

Yadav, A. K., Kumar, R., Priyadarshini, L., & Singh, J. (2015). Composition and medicinal properties of camel milk: A Review. *Asian Journal of Dairy and Food Research, 34*(2), 83–91. doi:10.5958/0976-0563.2015.00018.4

Yahya, M. A., Alhaj, O. A., AL-Khalifah, A. S., & Almnaizel, A. T. (2018). Hypocholesterolemic effect of camel milk on rats fed a high-cholesterol diet. *Emirates Journal of Food and Agriculture, 30*(4), 288–294. doi:10.9755/ejfa.2018.v30.i4.1664

Yang, J., Dou, Z., Peng, X., Wang, H., Shen, T., Liu, J., & Lia, G. Y. G. (2018). Transcriptomics and proteomics analyses of anti-cancer mechanismsof TR35eAn active fraction from Xinjiang Bactrian camel milk inesophageal carcinoma cell. *Clinical Nutrition (Edinburgh, Lothian)*. doi:10.1016/j.clnu.2018.10.013

Yorbik, O., Sayal, A., Akay, C., Akbiyik, D., & Sohmen, T. (2002). Investigation of antioxidant enzymes in children with autistic disorder. *Prostaglandins, Leukotrienes, and Essential Fatty Acids, 67*(5), 341–343. doi:10.1054/plef.2002.0439 PMID:12445495

Zafra, O., Fraile, S., Gutiérrez, C., Haro, A., Páez-Espino, A. D., Jiménez, J. I., & De Lorenzo, V. (2011). Monitoring biodegradative enzymes with nanobodies raised in Camelus dromedarius with mixtures of catabolic proteins. *Environmental Microbiology, 13*(4), 960–974. doi:10.1111/j.1462-2920.2010.02401.x PMID:21219561

Zagorski, O., Maman, A., Yaffe, A., Meisler, A., Van Creveld, C., & Yagil, R. (1998). Insulin in milk-a comparative study. *International Journal of Animal Sciences, 13*, 241–244.

Zeina, R. M., Al-Ayadhi, L., & Bashir, S. (2014). Autism spectrum disorder: Main problem waiting for solution in Kingdom of Saudi Arabia. *Autism, 8*(8), 487–490.

Zhang, Y., Lima, C. F., & Rodrigues, L. R. (2014). Anticancer effects of lactoferrin: Underlying mechanisms and future trends in cancer therapy. *Nutrition Reviews, 72*(12), 763–773. doi:10.1111/nure.12155 PMID:25406879

Ziistics of Camel Milk in Children: A Systematic Review. (n.d.). *Electronic Physician, 7*(7), 1523-1528. doi:10.19082/1523

Chapter 9
Potential Anti-Diabetic Effect of Camel Milk

Rajendra Prasad Agrawal
https://orcid.org/0000-0002-3214-7264
S. P. Medical College, India

Ritvik Agrawal
S. P. Medical College, India

Mo'ez Al-Islam Ezzat Faris
University of Sharjah, UAE

Hadeel Ali Ghazzawi
https://orcid.org/0000-0003-3045-4153
University of Jordan, Jordan

ABSTRACT

Based on empirical observations regarding the low prevalence of diabetes mellitus in population drinking regularly camel milk, camel scientists have investigated and assessed the effect of regular camel milk consumption on glycaemic status of diabetic patients and animal models. All the experiments' results concluded to the reduction of blood glucose and glycosylated haemoglobin. The hypothesis of high quantity of natural insulin in camel milk was proposed, but the quantities reported in the literature could not explain by itself the beneficial effect of camel milk consumption. It is stated that the lack of coagulum formation of camel milk the stomach was supposed to act as an effective vehicle (under internal nanoparticles) to take the milk insulin unchanged throughout the digestive tract and absorbed in the intestine. Other proteins in higher concentrations in camel milk than in other milk could interact with insulin receptor and contribute by their antioxidant and inti-inflammatory effect to regeneration of beta-cells in pancreas.

DOI: 10.4018/978-1-7998-1604-1.ch009

INTRODUCTION

Camel milk presents some specificities in its composition as emphasized in the chapter 2 (Camel milk composition and nutritional value) of the present book. Indeed, its fine composition could differ from other ruminant milks regarding minerals (Gorban & Izzeldin, 1997), vitamins, especially vitamin-C (Konuspayeva, Faye & Loiseau, 2011; Yadav et al., 2015), and some proteins as lactoferrin known for their anti-viral and anti-bacterial properties (Habib, Ibrahim, Scheider-Stock & Hassan,. 2013), present in higher quantity in camel milk (Konuspayeva, Faye, Loiseau & Levieux, 2007) and with higher bioactivity (Conesa et al., 2008). Other bioactive proteins as immunoglobulins and lysozyme are also expected in higher quantity in camel milk (El-Agamy, 2009). The health effect of camel milk is in relationship with its different components, especially those having antioxidant activity which contribute to remove free radicals, or those having protective effect which may have possible role for enhancing immune defence mechanism. Those aspects are widely described in the chapter 7 (Exploring potential therapeutic properties of camel milk) of the present book. Therefore, the present chapter is focused on the role of camel milk in the regulation of glycaemia in diabetic patients giving to this product a reputation of anti-diabetic adjuvant (Agrawal, Kochar, Sahani, Tuteja & Ghouri, 2007a).

BACKGROUND

Diabetes mellitus (DM) is the world's prevalent endocrine disorder caused by several aetiologies, implicating dysfunction of macronutrients metabolism. Usually, two forms of DM called DM type 1 (T1DM) resulting autoimmune destruction of insulin-producing Langerhans β-cells of the pancreas, and DM type 2 (T2DM), a metabolic disorder due to insulin resistance and relative insulin deficiency leading to high glycaemia. The global prevalence of DM is dramatically growing worldwide expected to reach 4.4% of the total human population in 2030, mainly in the third world countries (Wild, Roglic, Green, Sicree & King, 2004). The beneficial effect of regular consumption of camel milk (CM) on diabetic patients is described for long time empirically, notably in the Middle East (Mohamad et al., 2009; Malik, Al-Senaidy, Skrzypczak-Jankun & Jankun, 2012) and Ethiopia (Alema & Yusuf, 2014). In tribal population living with camel and consuming regularly its milk, low prevalence of diabetes was observed, notably in Raika pastoralist population (Agrawal et al., 2004a).

In a further study focused on the Raika community, it has been reported that the diabetes prevalence was negligible among the Raika population consuming camel milk while it was 0.7% in Raika community not consuming camel milk (Agrawal, Budania, Sharma, Gupta & Kochar, 2007b). These prevalences were 0.4% and 5.5% in non-Raika community consuming and not consuming camel milk, respectively (Agrawal et al., 2007b). It was concluded that the protective effect of regular camel milk consumption to DM is a reality, but the mechanisms of this beneficial effect requires to be investigated.

Figure 1. Weekly variations of blood glucose levels in diabetic dogs receiving 500 ml CM/day (T1), diabetic dogs receiving 500ml cow milk/day (T2), and healthy dogs (T3) from week1 to week5 (from after Sboui et al., 2010b)

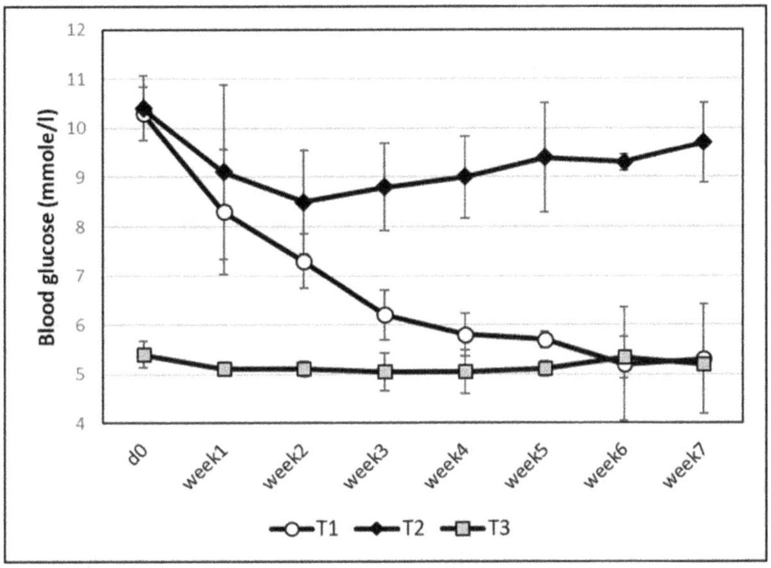

EFFECT OF CAMEL MILK CONSUMPTION ON DM

Several studies on laboratory animals like rats (Kebir, Aichouni & Zahzeh, 2017) or dogs (Sboui, Djegham, Khorchani, Hammadi, Barhoumi, & Belhadj, 2010) and human (Agrawal et al., 2005) were achieved and all of them concluded to the reduction of blood glucose and glycosylated haemoglobin (HbA1c) as well as the body mass index (BMI), c-peptide and other parameters related to type-1 diabetes (Table 1).

Animal Studies

Camel milk intake gives successful beneficial effect for patients with T1DM as demonstrated successfully in animal studies (Al Haj & Al Kanhal, 2010; Mirmiran., Ejtahed, Angoorani, Eslami & Azizi, 2017; Hammam, 2019). Among diabetic rats, many studies had ended up with a conclusion that feeding camel milk for a time longer than 30 days had an anti-hyperglycaemic effect and consequently may prevent the medical health consequences that accompany with T1DM diseases. Indeed, feeding of CM to diabetic rats reduced not only the levels of blood glucose, but also urea, uric acid and creatinine, and increased albumin, albumin/globulin ratio and contributed to alleviate liver and renal damage associated with streptozotocin-induced diabetic rats (Khan, Alzohairy, & Mohieldein, 2013). A study had been done on chemically triggered diabetic dogs ended up with the result that feeding fresh CM can be used to treat alloxan-treated dogs (Sboui, Djegham, Korchani, Hammadi, Barhoumi & Belhadj, 2010a), but the effect depended on the quantity of camel milk used to treat diabetic dogs, starting from 250 ml CM/day, no effect being observed with 100 ml/day (Sboui, Khorchani, Djegham, Agrebi, Elhatmi & Belhadj, 2010b). After 5 weeks of camel milk distribution to diabetic dogs, the blood glucose concentration reached normal level and was maintained still for 2 weeks after the end of CM treatment. Reversely, no

Table 1. Effect of camel milk on glycaemic control and insulin requirement in type 1 diabetic patients (from after Agrawal et al., 2005)

	Group 2: Camel milk group		
Variables	Before Treatment	After Treatment	p value
BMI (Kg/m^2)	17±4.4	19.7±2.97	0.001
HbA$_1$c (%)	7.8±1.38	6±0.96	0.001
Dose of Insulin (units/day)	32±12	17.83±12.40	0.005
Mean Blood Sugar (mg/dl)	119±19	95.42±15.70	0.001
Plasma Insulin (μIU/ml)	6.91±2.13	18.17±7.12	0.03
C-Peptide (ng/ml)	0.18±0.04	0.24±0.07	NS
Anti Insulin Antibody (%)	22.92±5.45	21.84±7.34	NS

* NS = Not Significant

hypoglycaemic effect was observed in diabetic dogs receiving cow milk (figure 1). Another study was conducted to evaluate the effect of raw, pasteurized and boiled camel milk on Alloxan- induced diabetic dogs. If raw camel milk appeared as solution to treat alloxan-induced diabetic dogs, this hypoglycaemic effect disappeared after boiling at 100°C (Mullaicharam, 2014) but is maintained with pasteurized milk (Sboui, Khorchani, Djegham, Agrebi, Dalleli & Belhadj, 2012).

Similar findings were shown in an experimental study for assessing camel milk whey proteins affection on lymphocytes sensitivity in rats after four months of streptozotocin (STZ)-induced T1DM. The data provided evidence of a protective role of camel milk whey in decreasing the tendency of the offspring of diabetic mothers to develop diabetes and related complications (Mahmoud, Badr & El-Shinnawy, 2016).

Human Studies

Several studies in adult diabetic patients were achieved. Seven randomized controlled trials to assess the beneficial effect of consuming camel milk, along with insulin therapy in T1DM patients were implemented in India. Their conclusion ended up with similar results in that the effect of camel milk on glucose homeostasis parameters was positively demonstrated in improving the treatment routine by a significant declension in fasting blood glucose, HbA1c, and the mean doses of insulin infusion. Fortunately, some patients stopped receiving insulin therapy after 8 months of camel milk consumption (Agarwal et al., 2003; Agrawal, Beniwal, Kochar, et al., 2005; Agrawal et al., 2004a; Mirmiran et al., 2017).

In a 2-years trial achieved on diabetic children, it was observed a significant decrease in all parameters: the mean blood glucose decreased from 118.58±19 to 93.16±17.06mg/dl, HbA1c levels from 7.81±1.39 to 5.44±0.81% and insulin doses from 32.50±9.99 to 17.50±12.09U/day. Out of 12 subjects receiving camel milk, insulin requirement in 3 subjects reduced to zero, that is remarkable (Agrawal, Jain, Shah, Chopra & Agarwal, 2011).

Weight loss is one of the most noticeable effects in T1DM patients. It was not significantly shown and rather weight gaining observed in a protocol therapy done in treating T1DM patients by mixing insulin infusion therapy with camel milk intake. Moreover, this mixing therapy protocol showed a well-nourished impact and relatively lowered fat and cholesterol level with the anabolic effect of CM (El-Sayed, Al-Shoeibi, El-Ghany, & Atef, 2011). The unique combination of CM has considered CM insulin to be more effective than insulin injection in the management of T1DM patients (El-Sayed et al., 2011).

Breitling (2002) supposed that CM not only possesses an anti-diabetic activity but also performs as an insulin-like activity with affection on the immune regulation and modulation on β-cells (Breitling, 2002).

In a comprehensive systematic review for the data collection on the effect of camel milk intake on DM markers among all animal and clinical studies, the advantageous effects were demonstrated by lowering blood sugar, decreasing insulin resistance (indicated by homeostatic model assessment for insulin resistance, HOMA-IR) and improving lipid profiles (Mirmiran et al., 2017). The recommended dose of camel milk in most clinical trials was 500 mL/day for three months to achieve the enhancement of DM markers in diabetic patients (Mirmiran et al., 2017).

Camel milk also showed good tolerating effects, and importantly it didn't show any enhancement in hypoglycemic events especially that the T1DM therapeutic medical drugs either can't be affordable or have unfavorable contraindications or side effects (Aqib et al., 2019; Pari & Satheesh, 2004). Exploring a non-invasive insulin delivery have been persistently attempting endeavors to normalize insulin through various frameworks, including oral intake (Agarwal et al., 2003; Aqib et al., 2019). Hence, it is important to find more applicable and safer hypoglycemic agents (Aqib et al., 2019; Lemhadri, Zeggwagh, Maghrani, Jouad, & Eddouks, 2004). The objective of oral insulin treatment is to minimize the impacts of pancreas-secreted insulin to control hyperglycemia postprandial and to avoid hypoglycemia between food intake to control glycemic and enhance life quality (Agarwal et al., 2003; Aqib et al., 2019; Bussa et al., 2017). It was recommended by a recent study to include CM in the diabetic medical, nutritional therapy routine plan to achieve favorable reductions in blood glucose levels by as much as 20% (Bussa et al., 2017).

However, in their critical assessment of experiments regarding effect of camel milk on DM, Mihic et al., (Mihic, Rainkie & Wilby, 2016) concluded that if the studies of camel milk in animals with artificially induced diabetes have shown a trend toward improved plasma glucose and decreased insulin requirements, improvement in dyslipidemia, liver function, and diabetic nephropathy, "*these experiments support the need for human trials of sound methodological quality in order to determine any potential clinical benefits of camel milk in diabetic patients*". Especially, the expression "antidiabetic" used by most of the authors (for example, Kula & Tegegne, 2016) to evoke health effect of camel milk should be avoided to speak rather about "glycaemia' regulation effect".

INSULIN AND INSULIN-LIKE PROTEIN IN CAMEL MILK

The main hypothesis regarding the effect of camel milk as a food supplement comprising medicinal values for diabetic subjects, was the presence of high quantity of insulin or "insulin-like" protein able to be preserved in the digestive tract. The lack of coagulum formation of camel milk was supposed to act as an effective vehicle to take the milk insulin unchanged to the intestine, and consequently absorbed at least partly (Agrawal et al., 2005). The camel milk insulin would be encapsulated in internal nanoparticles in the form of lipid vesicles (Hammam, 2019). Nonetheless, it rather passes rapidly through the stomach to the intestine to be readily absorbed (Agrawal et al., 2005; Hammam, 2019) and to be safeguarded from proteolysis during the transference via the stomach and absorbed in the intestine (Malik et al., 2012). This action is not applied to insulin protein from other sources, which form coagulation in the stomach and, thus, cannot be utilized by the diabetic patient who takes insulin orally. Besides, drugs taken orally are not able to overcome the mucosal barriers and are consequently destroyed by gastric juices before reaching the bloodstream (Malik et al., 2012).

The primary treatment of type 1 diabetes being insulin replacement, camel milk could contribute as substitution of insulin deficiency, notably because at present entire physiological insulin replacement cannot be achieved in clinical cases, and metabolic disturbances cannot be normalized. Several authors stated that camel milk is enriched with insulin (Hammam, 2019; Niasari-Naslaji et al., 2012) but in fact the hypoglycaemic agent in camel milk is still unclear (Korish, 2014) even if the mechanism is better understanding. Analysis by radioimmunoassay indicated that CM contains a large concentration of insulin, almost 52 units insulin per litre of camel milk (Agarwal et al., 2003) which is higher than in cow milk (Zagorski et al., 1998). In the study of Wernery et al., (Wernery, Nagy, Bhai, Schiele & Johnson, 2006), the mean insulin value of fresh camel milk was 41.9 ± 7.38 U/L with a significant reduction after pasteurization, freeze drying or storage of camel milk at 4°C for 4 days as well as freezing at -20°C. However, the lack of coagulation of camel milk in acid environment was considered the main factor for its therapeutic effect on insulin-dependent diabetes mellitus patients (Wernery et al., 2006). For other authors, insulin concentration is considerably higher in human milk than camel milk (60.23 ± 41.05 U/L) whereas it is lower in bovine milk (16.32 ± 5.98 U/L) (Shehadeh et al., 2001).

The hypothesis of protein insulin-like was proposed by several authors also. It is stated for example that lactoperoxidase, lysozyme, lactoferrin, secretory immunoglobulin A, immunoglobulin G could have been approved to act like-insulin (Abdel Gader & Alhaider, 2016; Aqib et al., 2019). Indeed, these proteins could have immuno-modulatory effect on β-cell function and degradable of coagulum in acidic medium (Abdel Gader & Alhaider, 2016; Agrawal et al., 2007a). Camel milk could contain small molecule substances, which have 'insulin-like' function that minimizes insulin interaction with its receptor (Hammam, 2019; Malik et al., 2012). Camel Milk also has a good buffering capability and has different amounts of caseins and fatty acids that make larger lipid than observed in the milk of another mammal (Malik et al., 2012). A comparative study on insulin-like protein content in various milks revealed that camel milk contains three times more insulin like proteins than cow milk (Mehaia et al., 1995).

Some whey proteins of camel milk have a special amino acid sequence, which comprises 50% cysteine, henceforth has very close characteristics of the peptides from insulin family (Beg, von Bahr-Lindström, Zaidi, & Jörnvall, 1986). The morphology of the CM immunoglobulin could be also the secret of its "anti-diabetic" effect. The heavy chain of amino acids in the immunoglobulin counteracts autoimmunity and prevents damage of β-cells that are responsible for insulin secretion, and hence improves the glucose utilization and inhibits the hyperglycaemia (Korish, 2014). The existence of such insulin-like proteins was supported by the fact that amino acid sequence of some of the camel milk proteins is found to be rich in half cystine like some insulin family peptides (Beg et al. 1986b).

Moreover, camels eat desert plants such as salty plants, bushes, and herbs including neem hence some of the phytochemicals are secreted in their milk which, in turn, might have anti-diabetic action (Agrawal et al., 2007b). Although camel milk protein and other active zoo-chemicals are sensitive to high temperature (see Chapter 10) particularly after boiling temperature (100°C); this degradation is less on CM α-lactalbumin and immunoglobulin (IgG) in contrast to lactoferrin from bovine milk which is denatured totally (Sboui et al., 2010a). Moreover; CM contains a higher amount of zinc than bovine milk acting a key role in islets of β-cells secretory activity (Sboui et al., 2010a).

MECHANISM OF HYPOGLYCAEMIC EFFECT OF CAMEL MILK

The anti-diabetic properties of camel milk may be very complex involving many molecular and cellular mechanisms and aspects of glucose metabolism and transport as well as insulin synthesis and secretion (Alavi, Salami & Emam-Djomeh, 2018; Shori, 2015; Abdulrahman, Ismail & Al-Hosaini, 2016; Malik et al., 2012). Camel milk insulin inhibits hormones raising glucose-dependent insulinotropic peptide (GIP) and glucagon-like peptide-1 (GLP) (Korish, 2014) and TNF-α and TGF-β1 levels which are produced upon the pathogenesis of DM (Aqib et al., 2019).

From the molecular and cellular points of view, camel milk may act at different levels (Ayoub, Palakkott, Ashraf & Iratni, 2018) including: (i) direct effects on insulin receptor function and glucose transport in the insulin-sensitive tissues, (ii) direct and/or indirect effects on insulin secretion by the pancreatic β-cells, and (iii) effects on the survival, growth, and the overall activity of the pancreatic cells.

The link between the anti-diabetic properties of camel milk and its putative effects on insulin receptor activity appears obvious with the pivotal role of insulin receptor in glucose homeostasis (Haeusler, McGraw & Accili, 2018). This is also based on the assumption that camel milk contains insulin and/or insulin-like proteins that act directly on the insulin sensitive tissues and that may have specific properties in terms of stability, proteolysis, and absorption in the stomach, and their entry into the circulation before reaching their target tissues (Mihic et al., 2016; Shori et al., 2015; Malik et al., 2012). Those insulin-like proteins could act directly on the insulin receptor and potentiating it activity (Abdulrahman et al., 2016).

The improvement caused due to hypoglycaemic effect of camel milk or whey camel milk (Ebaid, 2014) through β-cell functions may be due to: (a) Euglycemia possibly reduces β-cell work, leading to β-cell rest, and thereby preserving β-cell function. (b) tolerance induction in the body due to high concentration of circulating insulin (antigen) leading to preservation of β-cell function. (c) camel milk immunoglobulins which are of relatively small size and weight due to only Y shaped main chain which might offer an interplay with host cell protein thereby leading to an induction or activation of regulatory cells and finally leading to a downward regulation of immune system and β-cell salvage, (d) protective effect of β-Cell function may be due to presence of half-cystine, lactoferrin or insulin like factor in camel milk (Agrawal et al. 2007a).

The other hypothesis consists of the direct or indirect action of camel milk on insulin synthesis and secretion by the pancreatic β–cells. Camel milk proteins may restore and increase insulin secretion by either (i) stimulating glucose-mediated insulin secretion, (ii) inhibiting the secretion of glucagon by the pancreatic α-cells and its function in liver, and/or (iii) inhibiting the key enzymes that indirectly control the secretion of insulin such as the dipeptidyl peptidase IV (DPP-IV) (Mudgil, Kamal, Yuen & Maqsood, 2018).

Many studies suggested that the implication of the immunomodulatory, the anti-inflammatory, and the anti-oxidative actions of camel milk components restore the function of the immune cells as well as the secretory function of the pancreatic β-cells (Tantawy, El-Sayed & El-Said, 2010). Indeed, the treatment of type 1-diabetic rats with camel milk whey proteins has shown to reduce the proinflammatory (IL-1b, IL-6), and tumor necrosis factor (TNFa) and to increase the anti-inflammatory (IL-2 and IL-4) cytokines (Badr, Sayed, Omar, Adel-Rahim, Ahmed & Mahmoud, 2017; Mahmoud, Badr & El-Shinnawy, 2016).

In addition of hypoglycaemic effect, camel milk and especially the whey proteins could contribute to the alleviation of wound healing due to DM. For example, a study demonstrated a replenishment of anti-oxidant enzymes as SOD (superoxide dismutase), CAT (catalase), and GSH (glutathione) on diabetic rats supplemented by camel milk peptides (Ebaid et al., 2015). By increasing the synthesis of those enzymes and improving the function of the cellular system of antioxidant protection, the camel milk improves the healing process. The beneficial effects of camel whey proteins on wound healing were also attributed to their anti-oxidative activity that enhances the proliferation of immune cells and accelerates the healing process. The mechanism includes the attenuation of the oxidative and the inflammatory processes through the reduction of the levels of pro-inflammatory cytokines (TNF-a and IL-6), the restoration of the anti-inflammatory IL-10 levels and the expression of b-defensins 2 and 3 (Badr, 2013; Ebaid et al., 2015). Moreover, the supplementation of diabetic mice with camel milk whey proteins modulated the expression of different chemokines as well as TGF-b in wound tissue (Veliogu Ögunc et al., 2008).

CONCLUSION

The "anti-diabetic" or at least the hypoglycaemic properties continue to be one of the fascinating hallmarks of camel milk. However, an important gap still occurs between all the convincing *in vivo* data using patients with diabetes or animal models, and cellular and molecular mechanisms of action.

REFERENCES

Abdel Gader, A. G. M., & Alhaider, A. A. (2016). The unique medicinal properties of camel products: A review of the scientific evidence. *Journal of Taibah University Medical Sciences*, *11*(2), 98–103. doi:10.1016/j.jtumed.2015.12.007

Abdulrahman, A. O., Ismael, M. A., Al-Hosaini, K., Rame, C., Al-Senaidy, A. M., Dupont, J., & Ayoub, M. A. (2016). Differential effects of camel milk on insulin receptor signalling – towards understanding the insulin-like properties of camel milk. *Frontiers in Endocrinology*, *7*, 4. doi:10.3389/fendo.2016.00004

Agarwal, R., Swami, S., Beniwal, R., Kochar, D., Sahani, M., Tuteja, F., & Ghouri, S. (2003). Effect of camel milk on glycemic control, risk factors and diabetes quality of life in type-1 diabetes: A randomized prospective controlled study. *Journal of Camel Practice and Research*, *10*(1), 45–50.

Agrawal, R. P., Beniwal, R., Sharma, S., Kochar, D. K., Tuteja, F. C., Ghorui, S. K., & Sahani, M. S. (2005). Effect of raw camel milk in type 1 diabetic patients: 1year randomised study. *Journal of Camel Practice and Research*, *12*(1), 27–31.

Agrawal, R. P., Budania, S., Sharma, P., Gupta, R., & Kochar, D. K. (2007b). Zero prevalence of diabetes in camel milk consuming Raica community of northwest Rajasthan, India. *Diabetes Research and Clinical Practice*, *76*, 290-296.

Agrawal, R. P., Jain, S., Shah, S., Chopra, A., & Agarwal, V. (2011). Effect of camel milk on glycemic control and insulin requirement in patients with type 1 diabetes: 2-years randomized controlled trial. *European Journal of Clinical Nutrition*, *65*(9), 1048–1052. doi:10.1038/ejcn.2011.98

Agrawal, R. P., Kochar, D. K., Sahani, M. S., Tuteja, F. C., & Ghouri, S. K. (2004b). Hypoglycemic activity of camel milk in streptozotocin induced diabetic rats. *International Journal of Diabetes in Developing Countries*, *24*, 47–49.

Agrawal, R. P., Saran, S., Sharma, P., Gupta, R., Kochar, D. K., & Sahani, M. S. (2007a). Effect of camel milk on residual β-cell function in recent onset type 1 diabetes. *Diabetes Research and Clinical Practice*, *77*, 494-495.

Agrawal, R. P., Sharma, P., Jain, S., Gafoorunissa, S. A., Ibrahim, B., Shah, D., ... Kaur, T. (2011). Effect of camel milk on glucose metabolism in adults with normal glucose tolerance and type 2 diabetes in Raica community: A crossover study. *Acta Biomedica*, *82*(3), 181–186.

Agrawal, R. P., Singh, G., Nayak, K. C., Kochar, D. K., Sharma, R. C., Beniwal, R., ... Gupta, R. (2004a). Prevalence of diabetes in camel milk consuming 'RAICA' Rural Community of North West Rajasthan. *International Journal of Diabetes in Developing Countries*, *24*, 109–114.

Al Haj, O. A., & Al Kanhal, H. A. (2010). Compositional, technological and nutritional aspects of dromedary camel milk. *International Dairy Journal*, *20*(12), 811–821. doi:10.1016/j.idairyj.2010.04.003

Alavi, F., Salami, M., & Emam-Djomeh, Z. (2018). Nutraceutical properties of camel milk. In *Nutrients in Dairy and Their Implications for Health and Disease* (pp. 451–468). Academic Press.

Aleme, A., & Yusuf, M. (2014). Traditional consumption, therapeutic value and its derived dairy products of dromedary camel (*Camelus dromedaries*) milk in Somali regional state, eastern Ethiopia: A review. *Global Journal of Animal Scientific Research*, *3*(1), 240–246.

Aqib, A. I., Kulyar, M. F.-A., Ashfaq, K., Bhutta, Z. A., Shoaib, M., & Ahmed, R. (2019). Camel milk Insuline: Pathophysiological and molecular Repository. *Trends in Food Science & Technology*, *88*, 497–504. doi:10.1016/j.tifs.2019.04.009

Ayoub, M. A., Palakkott, A. R., Ashraf, A., & Iratni, R. (2018). The molecular basis of the anti-diabetic properties of camel milk. *Diabetes Research and Clinical Practice*, *146*, 305–312. doi:10.1016/j.diabres.2018.11.006

Badr, G. (2013). Camel whey protein enhances diabetic wound healing in a streptozotocin-induced diabetic mouse model: The critical role of b-Defensin-1, -2 and -3. *Lipids in Health and Disease*, *12*(1), 46. doi:10.1186/1476-511X-12-46

Badr, G., Sayed, L. H., Omar, H. E.-D. M., Abd El-Rahim, A. M., Ahmed, E. A., & Mahmoud, M. H. (2017). Camel whey protein protects B and T cells from apoptosis, by suppressing activating transcription factor-3 (ATF-3)-mediated oxidative stress and enhancing phosphorylation of AKT and IjB-a in type I diabetic mice. *Cellular Physiology and Biochemistry*, *41*(1), 41–54. doi:10.1159/000455935

Beg, O. U., von Bahr-Lindström, H., Zaidi, Z. H., & Jörnvall, H. (1986). A camel milk whey protein rich in half-cystine: Primary structure, assessment of variations, internal repeat patterns, and relationships with neurophysin and other active polypeptides. *European Journal of Biochemistry*, *159*(1), 195–201. doi:10.1111/j.1432-1033.1986.tb09852.x

Breitling, L. (2002). Insulin and anti-diabetes activity of camel milk. *Journal of Camel Practice and Research*, *9*(1), 43–45.

Bussa, N., Belayneh, A., & Deressa, M. (2017). The Potential of Camel Milk and Extracts of Major Plants Browsed by the Animal for Diabetes Treatment. *East African Journal of Sciences*, *11*(2), 129–138.

Conesa, C., Sanchez, L., Rota, C., Pérez, M. D., Calvo, M., Farnaud, S., & Ewans, R. W. (2008). Isolation of lactoferrin from milk of different species: Calorimetric and antimicrobial studies. *Comparative Biochemistry & Physiology, Part B., 150*(1), 131–139. doi:10.1016/j.cbpb.2008.02.005

Ebaid, H. (2014). Promotion of immune and glycaemic functions in streptozotocin-induced diabetic rats treated with un-denatured camel milk whey proteins. *Nutrition & metabolism, 11*(1), 31. doi:10.1186/1743-7075-11-31

Ebaid, H., Abdel-salam, B., Hassan, I., Al-Tamimi, J., Metwalli, A., & Alhazza, I. (2015). Camel milk peptide improves wound healing in diabetic rats by orchestrating the redox status and immune response. *Lipids in Health and Disease, 14*(1), 132. doi:10.118612944-015-0136-9

El-Agamy, E. I. (2009). Bioactive components in camel milk. In Y. W. Park (Ed.), *Bioactive components in milk and dairy products* (pp. 159–194). Ames, IA: Wiley-Blackwell Publ. doi:10.1002/9780813821504.ch6

El Sayed, I., Ruppanner, R., Ismail, A., Champagne, C. P., & Assaf, R. (1992). Antibacterial and antiviral activity of camel milk protective proteins. *The Journal of Dairy Research, 59*(2), 169–175. doi:10.1017/S0022029900030417

Gorban, A. M. S., & Izzeldin, O. M. (1997). Mineral Content of Camel Milk and Colostrums. *The Journal of Dairy Research, 64*(3), 471–474. doi:10.1017/S0022029997002264

Habib, H. M., Ibrahim, W. H., Schneider-Stock, R., & Hassan, H. M. (2013). Camel milk lactoferrin reduces the proliferation of colorectal cancer cells and exerts antioxidant and DNA damage inhibitory activities. *Food Chemistry, 141*(1), 148–152. doi:10.1016/j.foodchem.2013.03.039

Haeusler, R. A., McGraw, T. E., & Accili, D. (2018). Biochemical and cellular properties of insulin receptor signalling. *Nature Reviews. Molecular Cell Biology, 19*(1), 31–44. doi:10.1038/nrm.2017.89

Hammam, A. R. (2019). Compositional and therapeutic properties of camel milk: A review. *Emirates Journal of Food and Agriculture, 31*(3), 148–152. doi:10.9755/ejfa.2019.v31.i3.1919

Kebir, N., Aichouli, A., & Zahzeh, T. (2017). Raw camel milk properties on alloxan-induced diabetic Wistar rats. *Romanian Journal of Diabetes Nutrition & Metabolic Diseases, 24*(1), 41–47. doi:10.1515/rjdnmd-2017-0005

Khan, A. A., Alzohairy, M. A., & Mohieldein, A. H. (2013). Antidiabetic effects of camel milk in streptozotocin-induced diabetic rats. *American Journal of Biochemistry and Molecular Biology, 3*(1), 151–158. doi:10.3923/ajbmb.2013.151.158

Konuspayeva, G., Faye, B., & Loiseau, G. (2011). Variability of vitamin C content in camel milk from Kazakhstan. *Journal of Camelid Science, 4*, 63–69.

Konuspayeva, G., Faye, B., Loiseau, G., & Levieux, D. (2007). Lactoferrin and Immunoglobin content in camel milk from Kazakhstan. *Journal of Dairy Science, 90*, 38–46. doi:10.3168/jds.S0022-0302(07)72606-1

Korish, A. A. (2014). The antidiabetic action of camel milk in experimental type 2 diabetes mellitus: An overview on the changes in incretin hormones, insulin. *Hormone and Metabolic Research. Hormon- und Stoffwechselforschung. Hormones et Metabolisme, 46*(6), 404–411. doi:10.1055-0034-1368711

Kula, J. T., & Tegegne, G. (2016). Chemical composition and medicinal values of camel milk. [IJRSB]. *International Journal of Research Studies in Biosciences*, *4*(4), 13–25.

Lemhadri, A., Zeggwagh, N.-A., Maghrani, M., Jouad, H., & Eddouks, M. (2004). Anti-hyperglycaemic activity of the aqueous extract of Origanum vulgare growing wild in Tafilalet region. *Journal of Ethnopharmacology*, *92*(2-3), 251–256. doi:10.1016/j.jep.2004.02.026

Mahmoud, M. H., Badr, G., & El Shinnawy, N. A. (2016). Camel whey protein improves lymphocyte function and protects against diabetes in the offspring of diabetic mouse dams. *International Journal of Immunopathology and Pharmacology*, *29*(4), 632–646. doi:10.1177/0394632016671729

Malik, A., Al-Senaidy, A., Skrzypczak-Jankun, E., & Jankun, J. (2012). A study of the anti-diabetic agents of camel milk. *International Journal of Molecular Medicine*, *30*(3), 585–592. doi:10.3892/ijmm.2012.1051

Mehaia, M. A., Hablas, M. A., Abdel-Rahman, K. M., & El-Mougy, S. A. (1995). Milk composition of Majaheim, Wadah and Hamra camels in Saudi Arabia. *Food Chemistry*, *52*(2), 115–122. doi:10.1016/0308-8146(94)P4189-M

Mihic, T., Rainkie, D., Wilby, K. J., & Pawluk, S. A. (2016). The therapeutic effects of camel milk: A systematic review of animal and human trials. *Journal of Evidence-Based Complementary & Alternative Medicine*, *21*(4), 110–126. doi:10.1177/2156587216658846

Mirmiran, P., Ejtahed, H. S., Angoorani, P., Eslami, F., & Azizi, F. (2017). Camel milk has beneficial effects on diabetes Mellitus: A systematic review. *International Journal of Endocrinology and Metabolism*, *15*(2), e42150.

Mohamad, R. H., Zekry, Z. K., Al-Mehdar, H. A., Salama, O., El-Shaieb, S. E., El-Basmy, A. A., ... Sharawy, S. M. (2009). Camel milk as an adjuvant therapy for the treatment of type 1 diabetes: Verification of a traditional ethnomedical practice. *Journal of Medicinal Food*, *12*(2), 561–465. doi:10.1089/jmf.2008.0009

Mudgil, P., Kamal, H., Yuen, G. C., & Maqsood, S. (2018). Characterization and identification of novel antidiabetic and anti-obesity peptides from camel milk protein hydrolysates. *Food Chemistry*, *259*, 46–54. doi:10.1016/j.foodchem.2018.03.082

Mullaicharam, A. (2014). A review on medicinal properties of Camel milk. *World Journal of Pharmaceutical Sciences*. Available online at: http://www.wjpsonline.com/

Niasari-Naslaji, A., Arabha, H., Atakpour, A., Salami, M., & Moosavi-Movahedi, A. (2012). Camel Milk and its Bioactive Molecules in Medical Treatments. *Science Cultivation*, *2*(1), 20–24.

Pari, L., & Satheesh, M. A. (2004). Antidiabetic activity of Boerhaavia diffusa L.: Effect on hepatic key enzymes in experimental diabetes. *Journal of Ethnopharmacology*, *91*(1), 109–113. doi:10.1016/j.jep.2003.12.013

Sboui, A., Djegham, M., Khorchani, T., Hammadi, M., Barhoumi, K., & Belhadj, M. (2010a). Effect of camel milk on blood glucose, cholesterol and total proteins variations in alloxan-induced diabetic dogs. *International Journal of Diabetes and Metabolism*, *18*(1), 5–11. doi:10.1159/000497686

Sboui, A., Khorchani, T., Djegham, M., Agrebi, A., Dalleli, A., & Belhadj, O. (2012). Camel Milk as Adjuvant to Treat Alloxan Diabetes: Effect of Heat Treatment on this Property. *Journal of Diabetes & Metabolism*, *3*(04), 190. doi:10.4172/2155-6156.1000190

Sboui, A., Khorchani, T., Djegham, M., Agrebi, A., Elhatmi, H., & Belhadj, O. (2010b). Anti-diabetic effect of camel milk in alloxan-induced diabetic dogs: A dose–response experiment. *Journal of Animal Physiology and Animal Nutrition*, *94*(4), 540–546. doi:10.1111/j.1439-0396.2009.00941.x

Shehadeh, N., Gelertner, L., Blazer, S., Perlman, R., Solovachik, L., & Etzioni, A. (2001). Importance of insulin content in infant diet: Suggestion for a new infant formula. *Acta Paediatrica (Oslo, Norway)*, *90*(1), 93–95. doi:10.1111/j.1651-2227.2001.tb00262.x

Shori, A. B. (2015). Camel milk as a potential therapy for controlling diabetes and its complications: A review of in vivo studies. *Journal of Food and Drug Analysis*, *23*(4), 609–618. doi:10.1016/j.jfda.2015.02.007

Tantawy, E., El-Sayed, G. R., & El-Said, E. S. (2010). Effect of Camel Milk on Oxidative Stresses in Experimentally Induced Diabetic Rabbits. *Veterinary Research Forum: An International Quarterly Journal*, *1*(1), 30–43.

Velioglu Ogunc¸, A., Manukyan, M., Cingi, A., Eksioglu-Demiralp, M., Özdemir Aktan, A. O., & Yalçın, A. S. (2008). Dietary whey supplementation in experimental models of wound healing. *International Journal for Vitamin and Nutrition Research*, *78*(2), 70–73. doi:10.1024/0300-9831.78.2.70

Wernery, U., Nagy, P., Bhai, I., Schiele, W., & Johnson, B. (2006). The effect of heat treatment, pasteurization and different storage temperatures on insulin concentrations in camel milk. *Milchwissenschaft. Milk Science International*, *61*(1), 25–28.

Wild, S., Roglic, G., Green, A., Sicree, R., & King, H. (2004). Global prevalence of diabetes—estimates for the year 2000 and projections for 2030. *Diabetes Care*, *27*(5), 1047–1053. doi:10.2337/diacare.27.5.1047

Yadav, A. K., Kumar, R., Priyadarshini, L., & Singh, R. (2015). Composition and medicinal properties of camel milk: A Review. *Asian Journal of Dairy and Food Research*, *34*(2), 83–91. doi:10.5958/0976-0563.2015.00018.4

Zagorski, O., Maman, A., Yaffe, A., Meisler, A., Van Creveld, C., & Yagil, R. (1998). Insulin in milk-a comparative study. *International Journal of Animal Sciences*, *13*, 241–244.

Chapter 10
Effects of Industrial Processing Methods on Camel Milk Composition, Nutritional Value, and Health Properties

Ali Ahmed Metwalli
University of Minia, Egypt

Yonas Hailu
Teagasc Food Research Centre, Ireland & Haramaya University, Ethiopia

ABSTRACT

Camel milk has a comparable gross composition with other milk sources including bovine milk with some minor differences in the molecular properties of proteins and fat. The limited amount of β-Lg and κ-Casein(CN) are involved in heat denaturation via formation of disulfide bridges in cow milk; their absence in camel milk result in different responses for heat treatment at different scale. Furthermore, differences between camel milk proteins compared to other milk resulted poor coagulation and reduce stability during processing of dairy products such as yogurt and cheese. The effect of different thermal processing methods on camel milk were discussed; however, high pressure processing (HPP) study on processing effect on camel milk is an area of research for more confirmation in-depth study. The industrial processing methods were found to effect important camel milk properties, nutritional values, and health properties compared to other animals including limiting bioactive proteins such as immunoglobulin, lactoferrin, lysozyme, and vitamins. This effect depends on the type of heat treatment applied.

INTRODUCTION

Camel milk has a comparable gross composition with other milk species including bovine milk. However, due to the unique molecular properties of these components (i.e. Fat and proteins) it is very challenging to implements the production process used for processing of other milk (Hailu et al., 2016a).

DOI: 10.4018/978-1-7998-1604-1.ch010

These differences include rennetability or coagulation properties, heat stability, curd formation (Hailu et al., 2016b; Farah, 1986; Ramet, 2001). Heat treatment of milk is an essential step to render milk safe for human consumption and extend its shelf life (Chapter 3). Moreover, heat treatment is an integral part of production process of different products i.e. cheese, yogurt, powders (see Chapter 5). There are varied heat treatment methods depending on applied time-temperature combination. This is including low temperature long time pasteurization (LTLT), high temperature short time pasteurization (HTST), sterilization, thermization and Ultra High Temperature (UHT). Among all, HTST pasteurization and UHT are the most commonly used methods in dairy industry (Benabdelkamel, et al., 2017).

The heat stability of camel milk is different compared to bovine milk (Farah, 1986; Ramet, 2001); whereas camel milk reported to have some different properties from bovine milk including poor stability at high temperatures. This is attributed to the casein micelle or deficiency of β-lactoglobulin and κ-casein in camel milk (Al Haj & Al Kanhal, 2010). The addition of neither urea nor formaldehyde alone has no effect on HCT of camel's milk heat stability (Alhaj, Metwalli, & Ismail, 2011), therefore, heat treatment should be carefully optimized. On the other hand, proteins sedimentation could be the main problem for camel milk preservation (Farah et al., 2004) due to their poor stability. Similarly, the overall purpose of heat treatment applied to other milk sources would have the same effect; however, the deleterious outcomes for production of a specific milk product type is not documented yet. The scientific reports made on effects of different factors on industrial processing of camel milk is not much, therefore other milk sources are used to show the possible implications and these types of milk are specified each time whenever referred. This chapter aims to provide an overview on industrial processing methods and their effect on camel milk composition, nutritional value and health properties.

Thermization

Thermization is a mild heat treatment of milk. It is used to extend the quality of raw milk at farms especially camel milk with poor hygienic quality (see Chapter 3); or could be used when raw camel milk is held chilled for some time, before further processing. Ramet (1984) reported that lag phase of raw camel milk (four to six hours) is greater than that of cow milk (two to three hours). The content of antimicrobial factors (Chapter 7) which would make growing of microbes harder are a unique features of camel milk (El-Agamy, 1998; 2000). The aim of this treatment is to control the growth of psychrophilic and psychrotrophic bacteria. The thermization temperature will not bring an irreversible change to the proteins and keep milk properties similar to fresh milk.

These psychrotrophic bacteria if not deactivated may release heat-resistant proteases and lipases into the milk. The bacterial enzymes (lipase and protease) will not be totally inactivated during thermization or even during pasteurization and result in increased off-flavors in case milk is used for cheese, milk powders and UHT treatment. Conditions used for thermization are 57–68oC for 15 s, followed by refrigeration. Thermized raw milk can be stored at a maximum temperature of 8°C for up to 3 days (IDF, 1984). This does not lead to full inactivation of all spoilage and pathogenic bacteria. Nowadays camel milk is produced and collected in small farms then sent directly to heat treatment without storage, hence thermization is not required. However, the increase in camel milk production and storage under cold temperature for few times at farms, lead to subjecting camel milk to thermization process as an essential stage. The bactericidal properties of camel milk might provide a substituting advantaged of thermization step; however, this may need further studies.

Pasteurization

Pasteurization is the process of heating a liquid milk to below the boiling point to destroy microorganisms and enzymes induced spoilage. Pasteurization conditions were adjusted to 143°F (61.7°C) for 30 minutes or 160°F (71.1°C) for 15 seconds to inactivate *Mycobacterium bovis* organism which is known to be responsible for tuberculosis. However, in 1957 these conditions were shown to be inadequate for the inactivation of *Coxiella burnetii* which causes Q fever in humans (Enright et al., 1957). New pasteurization conditions of 145°F (62.8°C) for 30 minutes using batch process, or at 161°F (71.7°C) for 15 sec by continuous process were adopted in order to inactivate *Coxiella burnetii*. These conditions are still in use today. The conditions required to inactivate *Mycobacterium tuberculosis* were just slightly less than those required to inactivate alkaline phosphatase. By this temperature-time combination, thermoduric bacteria were being recognized in pasteurized milk but not tuberculosis. Minimal conditions (temperature-time) for milk pasteurization are different from country to country. By early 1950s, HTST processing accounted for about 75% of all milk pasteurized in the UK, (Davis, 1955). A recent survey of the conditions used in Australian factories revealed a range from 72°C for 15 s to 78–80°C for 25 s (Juffs & Deeth, 2007). Recently, it has been reported that consumption of raw camel milk caused brucellosis disease in different countries especially in Mediterranean and gulf countries include, without limitation, Qatar, Saudi Arabia and Oman (Radwan, et al., 1995; Garcella, et al., 2016). Radwan, et al. (1995) reported that 34% of camel milk collected from Saudi Arabia contained *B. melitensis biovars* 1, 2 and 3. An outbreak of human brucellosis by *Brucella melitensis* in 14 persons in a rural area in Qatar was reported by Garcella, et al. (2016). *Brucella* among other pathogenic bacteria are destroyed by both batch (63°C for 30 minutes) and HTST (72°C for 15 seconds) pasteurization. The species that are killed by pasteurization are: *Brucella abortus; Campylobacter jejuni; Campylobacter coli; Coxiella burnetii; Pathogenic Escherichia coli (0157:H7); Listeria monocytogenes; Mycobacterium tuberculosis; Mycobacterium bovis; Salmonella enterica serotypes; Streptococcus pyogenes;* and *Yersinia enterocolitica* (Juffs, & Deeth (2007).

HEAT-INDUCED CHANGES IN PHYSICOCHEMICAL PROPERTIES OF PASTEURIZED MILK

Changes in the Color Values of Thermally Treated Milk

The values of the Hunter color attribute *L**, *a**, *b**, give insight about the effect of heat treatments on color differences of milk and milk products. Omar, Harbourne, and Oruna-Concha (2018) found that the HTST process caused an increase in *L* (whiteness) and* an increase in *a** (greenness) and *b** (yellowness) in both camel and bovine milk. However, the differences in lightness L* were significant in camel milk and insignificant in cow milk. Moreover, the overall color changes in camel milk after HTST treatment of ΔE was 1.48 compared to 0.61 in bovine milk. This reduction in lightness of camel milk during the HTST treatment may be the result of disintegration of casein micelles into smaller particles. This concept can be related to the poor heat stability of camel milk (Farah, 1989; Hailu, et al., 2016a) that upon heating casein stats to precipitate or aggregate. (Needs, Stenning, Gill, Ferragut, & Rich, 2000) reported that heat treatment of cow milk at 85°C for 20 min increased L* from 81.6 to 84.73 (ΔE was 3.13). Researchers also found that L* increase with decreasing pH value from pH 6.7 to 5.2. No further change in L* was noticed below pH 5.2. The same trend was also observed with *b**. While, a* continued to increase until the end of incubation at pH 4.4. Fig. 1 shows the effect of heat treatment at 100°C for 3 min on color of milk, the heated milk exhibiting whiter color than untreated milk. Heat treatments were reported to have a significant effect on the composition (Chapter 2) and properties (Chapter 7) of camel milk. El Hasan et al. (2017) reported that heat treatments (LTLT, HTST, and sterilization) caused a decrease of pH and increase in acidity.

Changes in pH

Fresh milk had a pH of 6.5–6.7, with average of 6.6 (see Chapter 2). Growth of microorganisms that ferment lactose to lactic acid or extensive lipolysis will lower pH values. However, higher pH values in milk may be encountered when the mineral balance of milk is altered by changes in the permeability of the blood milk barrier (e.g. in very late stages of the lactation cycle or during mastitis infection). Camel milk pH is decreased with increasing temperature (Alhaj et al. 2011), due to changes in dissociation of ionizable groups. Lowering camel milk pH, caused a delay effect on the micelle of camel milk. This effect was only observed at pH 5.5, while starts at the onset of acidification for bovine milk. During acidification of dromedary milk maximum of micelle and Pi (inorganic phosphate) solubilization took place at lower pH values of 4.9 and 4.8, respectively. Dromedary milk micelle seemed to maintain its integrity until pH 5.5 (Kherouatou et al., 2003). While, this phenomenon is observed tight after the acidification of fresh milk at a higher pH values compared to camel milk (Kherouatou et al., 2003). At pH 5.0 a state of transition characterized by deep biochemical modifications was observed in camel milk (Kherouatou et al., 2003; Hamadi et al., 2000). This fusion led to a real three-dimensional network, having some linear, continuous nodes and tightened to give a very reticulate network near pH 4.7. It reported that the reorganization of the dromedary milk casein micelle and of its sub-units below pH 5.0, would determine

Figure 1. Changes in appearance of untreated milk (A) and heated milk at 100°C for 3 min
Adopted from Considine et al. (2007)

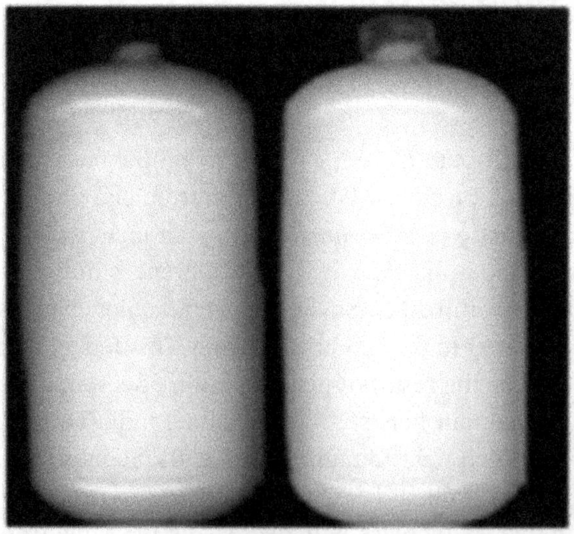

the rheological properties of the acid gel of dromedary milk. During the lowering of pH, these particularities marked the progress of the coagulation process that led to a pseudo curd (Kherouatou et al., 2003).

Milk pH decreases upon heating to temperatures <80°C in a linear fashion with increasing temperature (Ma & Barbano, 2003) as shown in Fig. 2. Heat-induced reductions in pH at this temperature range are primarily due to shifts in the mineral balance (Ca + Mg: cit + P) of milk, and are largely reversible on subsequent cooling (at temperature >100°C the reaction is mainly irreversible). The heat induced loss of CO_2 provides a counteracting increase in pH, but generally occur at lower extent. Severe heat treatment decreases the pH of milk further due to thermolytic breakdown of lactose to organic acids, especially formic acid (Berg, 1992). It has been demonstrated that the rate of pH decreasing of camel milk using commercial starter cultures is possible. The acidification rate in camel milk, however, was found to be lower than in bovine milk (Berhe et al., 2018). Moreover, Bekele, Hansen, Eshetu, Ipsen and Hailu (2019) demonstrated that the rate of pH decrease in camel milk depends on the type of used culture. Researchers found that the thermophilic culture resulted in faster acidification than mesophilic culture.

Rennet Clotting Time

Rennet coagulation time of camel milk significantly changes to an extent depending on the severity of heating applied (Al Haj & Al Kanhal, 2010). For example, a mild heat treatment, such as high-temperature short-time (HTST) or low temperature-long time (LTLT) pasteurization, has no negative impact on rennet coagulation properties of camel milk (Genene, Hansen, Eshetua, Hailu, & Ipsen, 2019). This is maybe preferable to restore the mineral equilibrium in milk which has been cold-stored, during which time solubilization of colloidal calcium phosphate occur. Manufacturing of cheese from camel milk using the existing traditional processing conditions used for milk of other livestock is difficult and has been considered as impossible (Brezovečki, et al., 2015; Berhe, Seifu, Ipsen, Kurtu, & Hansen, 2017). Difficulties including long coagulation time, weak curd, and low cheese yield were reported to be associated with the limitation of cheese production from camel milk (Bornaz et al., 2009). The large casein

Figure 2. Correlation between temperature and milk pH
Data adopted from Ma and Barbano (2003)

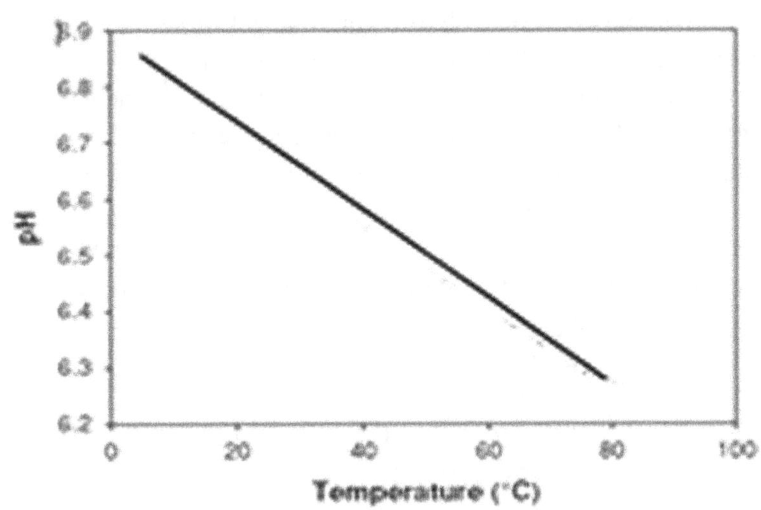

micelle size, low casein content and small amount of κ-CN in camel milk are also found to be responsible for these problems (Barłowska, Szwajkowska, Litwińczuk, & Król, 2011). Casein to whey protein ratio may also play an important role. Cow, sheep, goat and buffalo milk has casein to whey protein ratio of 80:20, while this ratio in camel milk is 72:28 (Rafiq et al. 2016). The manufacture and challenges of camel milk cheese was discussed in detail in Chapter 6.

Moreover, variation of casein ratios in camel milk is crucial factor (Brezovečki et al., 2015) as reported in Chapter 6. The lower κ-casein content and higher casein micellar size; as well as high mineral levels in camel milk lead to decrease the protein stability (heat coagulation time and rennet clotting time). The coagulum/curd obtained from camel milk using bovine rennet showed a fragile and heterogeneous structure. Camel milk after calf rennet addition was found to coagulate 2 - 3 times slower than cow's milk (Farah & Rüegg, 1989). The increase in the number of large casein micelles lead to prolong the coagulation time; this could be attributed to the reduced κ-CN content (Sagar, Mehta, Wadwani, Dargi, & Aparnthi, 2016). However, coagulation of camel milk through the action of both rennets (cow and camel) was due to the pepsin content in the rennet preparation used (Wangoh et al., 1993; Mal, & Pathak, 2009). The higher the pepsin content in rennet results in the faster coagulation time. Furthermore, long rennet clotting time of camel milk may be attributed to the different amino acid content of casein micelles. Hailu et al., (2016a) reported that κ-casein of camel milk has an additional proline residue at site 95 which plays an important role in protein stability against chymosin enzyme. The sensitive bond for hydrolysis by chymosin (Phe97-Ile98) in camel κ-casein was compared with (Phe105-Met 106) in bovine κ-casein (Kappeler, Farah, & Puhan, 1998; Hailu et al., 2016a). Several attempts were used to improve camel milk coagulation (see Chapter 6) including the addition of starter culture of lactic acid bacteria and calcium chloride to camel milk lead to reduce clotting time, improve curd firmness and increase cheese yield (Zubeir & Jabreel, 2008; Khan, Athar, & Aslam, 2004; Ahmed & Zubeir, 2011). However, Konuspayeva, Camier, Gaucheron, and Faye, (2014) used coagulant agent Chy-Max (camel chymosin produced by Hansen© Denmark) for coagulation of camel milk at 20 and 36°C with the addition of calcium chloride. Researchers reported that coagulation time was faster at 30°C with stronger curd firmness than at 20°C. Calcium chloride had no changes on clotting time at 20 or 30°C.

Mal and Pathak (2009) prepared cheese made from camel heated to 72°C for 15 sec after addition of 0.02% $CaCl_2$ or $CaSO_4$ 0.015% and 600 mg/L rennet or pepsin. Under these conditions, coagulation time was found to range between 1.5-2 hours for rennet and 10-15 minutes for pepsin. Genene et al. (2019) studied the effect of heat treatment on rennet clotting time and gel strength of camel milk in comparison with bovine milk. Their results revealed that rennet clotting time of unheated camel milk was higher than that of unheated cow milk (6.8 min against 4.2 min). The authors (Genene et al., 2019) attributed the shorter gelation times to the higher efficiency of camel rennet on camel and bovine milk. Moreover, gel formation for camel milk has been reported to occur after 95% of the κ-casein has been cleaved. Unlike bovine milk, this phenomenon occurred at a substantially lower level of 60–70% (Lomholt & Qvist, 1997) for varying casein hydrolysis or with 85% (Hailu et al., 2016b) in cow milk. On the other hand, subjecting milk to heat treatments of 65° for 30 min and 72 for 30 sec (almost similar to pasteurization conditions) lead the rennet-induced gelation times of camel and cow milk to significant increase and the camel milk did not coagulate at a temperature of 75 °C/5 min or above. While, the cow milk did not coagulate within the observation time (60 min) at 90 °C/5min. The time to attain maximum gel strength was significantly increased for both types of milk as the severity of the heat treatment increased (Genene et al., 2019). Increasing the concentration of camel milk 2 to 4 folds using ultra filtration improved rennet clotting time and gel strength (Hassl, Jorgensen, & Janhoj, 2011). Ramet, 2001 prepared semi-hard cheese from camel milk processed by thermization (low heat pasteurization) with adding mesophilic culture and 4.8 g rennet / 100 kg camel milk. Under these conditions clotting time takes between 10 to 30 min. Moreover, Vikas and Farah (1991) produced semi-hard cheese similar to blue or limburger cheese from camel milk heated at 65°C for 30 min in open fire then, cooled to 35°C. After addition of mesophilic culture (5%), 0.25 g / L citric acid (pH reached to 5.6-5.7) and rennet, camel milk clotted in 40 min. Although, Mohamed, Larsson-Raznikiewicz, and Mohamud (1990) prepared hard cheese from camel milk smoked with fired wood to prevent microbial growth. The results showed that the rennet clotting time for non-smoked milk was longer than smoked one; this could be due to the lower pH of smoked milk. Qadeer, Huma, Sameen & Iqbal (2015) conducted a study to optimize the processing conditions (temperature, pH, $CaCl_2$ and the addition of buffalo milk) to produce camel milk cheese. The researchers concluded that heating temperature of 65 °C for 30 min, pH 5.5, 0.06% $CaCl_2$ addition and incorporation of 10% buffalo milk were the optimum condition for production of camel cheese with good quality. Heat treatment process of 65 °C/30 min or 72 °C/30 sec is recommended for making cheese from camel milk (Genene et al., 2019). However, Kamal, Foukani, and Karoui, (2017) showed that preheating of camel milk at 50°C negatively affected its gelation properties, while rennet-induced gelation of camel milk was prevented with preheating at 70°C for 10 minutes. It is very important to note the variation in time of heating for the effect of heat treatment of proteins and functional properties.

Fermented Camel Milk

Traditionally, raw camel milk can ferment naturally at ambient temperature (26–29°C) for one or two days without heat treatment and without addition of starter cultures (Lore, Mbugua, & Wangoh, 2005). However, fermented camel milk manufactured by traditional methods (see Chapter 3) often shows a great variation in taste and flavor and is usually of poor hygienic quality that do not meet the acceptable quality requirements (Farah, Streiff, & Bachmann, 1990; Elmoslih et al., 2016). It has also been reported that the properties of fermented camel milk differ according to preparation methods (Shori, 2012). The manufacture of fermented camel milk products was discussed in detail in Chapter 5. Berhe et al., (2018) examined eight starter cultures for camel milk fermentation and reported that all investigated cultures were able to acidify camel milk and reached a final pH at a level similar to what was obtained in bovine milk, but the speed of acidification was generally lower in camel milk. This may be attributed to presence of inhibitory substances in camel milk (Al Haj & Al Kanhal, 2010) or due to reduced availability of nutrients (Chapter 7). When camel milk was mixed with cow milk or supplemented with cow casein hydrolysate before fermentation process, higher fermented rate was reported. This is attributed to the long fermentation time of camel milk and unavailability of micronutrient in camel milk for growth of starter culture. Alhaj, Al-Khalifa, Metwalli, Ismail and Ali (2017) prepared fermented dairy product from camel milk in which the camel milk was heated at 85° C for 30 minutes, then milk cooled to 60° C. Thereafter, κ-carrageenan added at a concentration of 0.02% to avoid whey off problems. Camel milk was then cooled before adding probiotic bacterial culture, and incubated at 40° C and 45° C for 4 to 12 hours depending on the type of starter culture used. This treatment lead to higher contents of antioxidant, antimicrobial and D- amino acid than raw camel milk. The sensory properties of fermented milk were also acceptable (Alhaj et al., 2017).

UHT Process

Ultra-high temperature processing uses continuous flow and subject's milk to 135 - 150°C for 3 to 5 seconds, then packaged, aseptically with an anticipated shelf life of 6 months stored/distributed under ambient conditions (Vazquez-Landaverde, Qian, & Torres, 2007). All microorganisms able to grow at ambient temperature are destroyed. Changes in chemical, physical and organoleptic of the product are kept to minimum under these conditions of very high temperature and short time. UHT treatment requires high quality raw milk that is heat stable with low microbial counts and acceptable flavor. It has been reported by Farah et al. (2004) that camel milk is stable after direct UHT process together with refrigeration to achieve five week of shelf life. Furthermore, proteins sedimentation is the main challenge of the preserved UHT camel milk, hence selected additives are required to achieve physical stability (Farah et al., 2004). The combinations of time-temperature used in UHT systems are determined by the time needed to inactivate heat-resistant bacterial endospores such as those of *Bacillus stearothermophilus* (Datta & Deeth, 2007) with minimum physico-chemical changes which decrease the sensory and nutritional qualities of the product. Figure 3 shows the relation between chemical changes and bactericidal effect at different temperature. Whereas, very high temperature cause very low chemical changes in relation to bactericidal effect (discussed later in this Chapter).

Temperatures ranging between 137-145°C with holding times of 8-2 s are commonly used for UHT treatment of milk and dairy products (Gedam, Prasad, & Vijay, 2007). It can be concluded from Figure 3 that temperatures lower than ~135°C, with a long holding times are required while at higher temperature (e.g. >150°C), very short holding periods (fraction in second), which are difficult to achieve in practice, are required to destroy most bacterial spores.

Types of Processing Systems

Steam, hot water, and electricity are heating media for UHT equipment. The sterilizers utilizing steam or hot water can be classified as direct or indirect heating systems. In direct heating systems, steam is

Figure 3. Relative chemical effect with change in temperature for the same bactericidal effect
Data adopted from Datta et al. (2002)

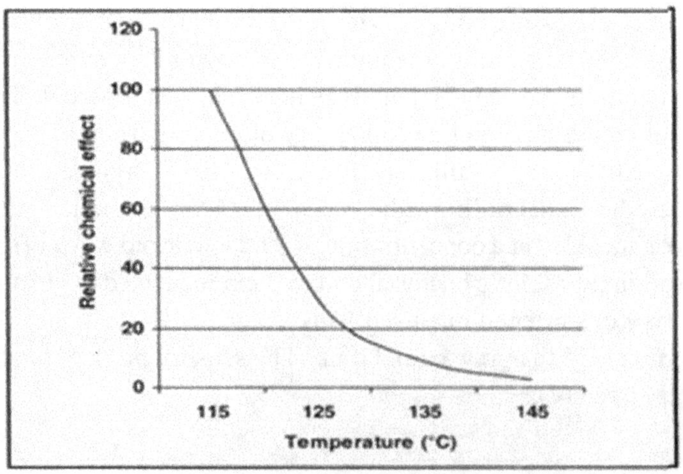

directly mixed with the product. The product temperature increases almost instantly due to the latent heat of vaporization. Direct heating systems include steam injection (steam into milk) and steam infusion (milk into steam). Figure 4 shows the profiles of UHT processing in direct and indirect mode.

The culinary steam must be high quality and impart no off-flavors to the product. By direct heating, the increase in volume of the liquid is approximately 11% (Lewis & Heppell, 2000). The condensed steam is removed later as the heated milk is cooled in a vacuum chamber. The preheating and final cooling steps are always performed using indirect heat exchangers.

On the other hand, the indirect system, the product and heating medium do not have contact, as a barrier (heat exchanger) is present. Indirect heating models include indirect spiral tubes, indirect tubes, indirect plate, and electricity are used (Bylund, 2003).

Effect of UHT Treatment on Physico-Chemical Properties of Milk

Effect on Appearance and Color

It is well known that milk becomes browner with increased severity of heating, the browning being consequence of Maillard reaction between the amino groups of milk lysine and the aldehyde groups of lactose. Omar et al. (2018) studied the changes in color of UHT treated camel milk with HTST and high-pressure processes. Authors reported that the lowest L^* value was observed in UHT-treated camel milk (from 67.77 to 61.83), which indicates increased darkness of the treated milk. The reduction in the lightness of camel milk during the UHT treatment may be the result of disintegration of casein micelles into smaller particles. While, L^* was the highest in UHT-treated bovine milk (increased from 66.81 to 68.94), which indicates an increase in the lightness of the milk. This increase in the lightness of UHT-treated bovine milk may be due to denaturation and association of whey proteins with casein micelles, in particular β-Lactoglobulin. Similar results for bovine milk have been reported by Rufian-Henares, Guerra-Hernandez, and Garcıa-Villanova, (2006). These researchers found that after UHT treatment of

Figure 4. Typical time-temperature profiles of UHT processing: direct, infusion or injection: indirect mode
Redrawn from Deeth and Datta (2011)

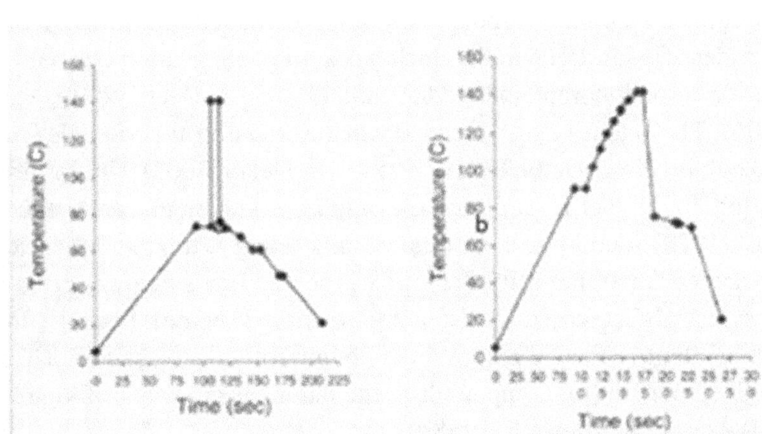

bovine milk the lightness of milk increase by 11 units compared with the untreated samples. Values a^* and b^* were also increased in both types of milk after UHT treatment. Moreover, the ΔE values (changes in L* values before and after UHT treatment) were markedly higher in camel milk than those in bovine milk after UHT treatment.

Rennet Coagulation Properties of UHT Treated Milk

The rennet clotting time of unheated camel milk was higher than that of unheated cow milk (6.8 min against 4.2 min) as reported by Genene et al., (2019). In contrast, Omar et al. (2018) reported that the RCT of the raw camel milk was much shorter than that of bovine milk (16.16 min for camel milk against 31.18 for bovine milk). The rennet coagulation time of camel milk affected by many factors including pH, type of enzyme, concentration of enzyme, mineral balance of the substrate and concentration of the substrate (casein). The heating temperature of 65 °C for 30 min, at pH 5.5, and addition of 0.06% $CaCl_2$ and incorporation of 10% buffalo milk were the optimum condition for production of camel cheese with good quality (Qadeer, Huma, Sameen & Iqbal, 2015). After UHT treatment both camel and cow milk could not form a curd (Ham *et al.* 2008; Omar et al. 2018). The heat-induced inhibition of rennet coagulation is mainly attributed to micelle aggregation, the decreased concentration of ionic calcium, and the association of denatured whey proteins with the casein micelles in heat-treated milk (Vasbinder, Rollema, & Kruif, 2003).

Effect on Milk Flavor (Cooked Flavor)

Immediately after processing, UHT milk has a very strong sulphurous or off-flavor which is commonly defined as 'cooked' flavor. The components responsible for this flavour are volatile sulphur compounds and free sulphydryl groups which are generated from the thermal denaturation of whey proteins, predominantly β-lactoglobulin (Al-Attabi, D'arcy, & Deeth, 2009). β-lactoglobulin is rich in cysteine in bovine milk, it contains 5 cysteine residues four of which form disulfide bonds leaving one free sulfhydryl group. While, camel milk is lacking β-lactoglobulin (Genene et al., 2019; Hailu et al., 2016a); but still have cooked flavor due to presence of other milk proteins containing sulfur amino acid either methionine or cysteine. Thermal denaturation allows these volatile sulphur-containing components to liberate from cysteine residues. Hydrogen sulphide, carbonyl sulphide, methanethiol, dimethyl sulphide and carbon disulphide have been identified in UHT milk which has a good correlation between 'cooked' flavor intensity and total volatile sulphur compounds (Al-Attabi, D'arcy, & Deeth, 2009; Vazquez-Landaverde, Torres, & Qian, 2006). The intensity of cooked flavor depends on type of UHT treatment (direct or indirect method) and holding time (Datta, Elliott, Perkins, & Deeth, 2002). Unlike direct heated milk, the indirect method has initially higher level of volatile sulphur components, and hence a stronger cooked flavor. Badings et al. (1978) found that heat treated milk using a tubular heat exchanger at 137.5°C for 5 s had a higher cooked flavor intensity than milk processed by steam injection at 141-145°C. The cysteine-HCL content sharply increased after heat treatment in raw milk from 4.1 mg / L to 10.07 mg / L. The cysteine-HCL content in treated recombined bovine milk decreased after UHT treatment. This is attributed to the reduction of sulfur compounds in the latter case to using of high heat powdered milk (Metwalli, Shalabi, Bayoumi, & Metwalli, 1988b).

Irreversible denaturation of protective proteins (β-lg, α-la, IgG and BSA) in skim milk occurred mainly during preheating causes the liberation of -SH group. The volatile sulphydryl compounds oxidize during storage, this may lead to decrease in cooked flavor intensity and improve flavor acceptability of milk (Oldfield, Taylor, & Singh, 2005). Dissolved oxygen level in UHT milk is crucial factor on oxidizing -SH groups during storage. In general, dissolved oxygen content in indirect type UHT treatment is higher than direct UHT treatment because of the flash-cooling step during direct UHT removes not only the excess water but also volatile compounds and dissolved oxygen (Datta, et al., 2002). Cysteine-HCL reduced during storage of UHT milk produced both from raw or recombined milk Metwalli et al. (1988b). The rate of -SH group decrease during storage depends on the concentration of residual oxygen in treated milk. The decline of reactive-SH during storage may attributed to volatilization or oxidation to disulfides or rebuilt in protein structure but not to sulphydryl oxidase where 40% of its activity remains after pasteurization and completely inactivated by UHT treatment (Farkey & Imifadon, 1995). Among all tested treatments (HTST, UHT, and HP), only two sulphurs compounds (dimethyl disulphide and dimethyl trisulphide) were detected at low levels of heat treatment. Compared to cow milk, sulphurs concentrations in camel milk after UHT were more than double (Omar et al., 2018). α-lactalbumin contains no free-SH group therefore, no participation occurred during formation of cooked flavor in UHT milk. It is noteworthy to mention that camel milk contains high contents of serum albumin and immunoglobulin than cow milk. These types of protein contain free-SH groups which may play role on UHT treated camel milk.

Effect of UHT Treatment on Whey Proteins Denaturation

It has been reported that camel milk proteins composition differs from bovine milk (see Chapter 2). The major identified whey proteins in camel milk was α-lactalbumin, followed by lactoferrin and serum albumin (Elagamy, 2000). In contrast, β-lactoglobulin is the primary whey protein in bovine milk, followed by α-lactalbumin and bovine serum albumin (Omar et al., 2018). α-Lactalbumin is the most heat-resistant whey protein. Serum proteins are denatured during heat treatment to a greater or lesser extent, depending on the severity of the heat treatment, and these changes have important consequences for some milk products.

Most studies on denaturation of whey proteins after heat treatments depend on measuring of whey protein nitrogen (WPN = non-casein nitrogen (NCN) - non-protein nitrogen (NPN) before and after heat treatment. Metwalli, Shalabi, Bayoumi, and Metwalli (1988a) found that Non-Casein Nitrogen (NCN) in bovine milk decreased after heat treatment as a result of whey protein denaturation lead to precipitation with casein at pH 4.6. The NCN also gradually increased during storage for 24 weeks. This phenomenon suggests a partial proteolysis of UHT milk proteins during storage as a result of heat resistant bacterial proteases. Heat treatment of cow and camel milk at range of 63 to 90°C decrease the NCN of both cow and camel milk depending on the heating temperature. The percentage of NCN decrease was higher in cow milk, for instance at 90°C the percentage of whey protein denaturation was 81% in cow treated milk while it was 50% for camel milk (Farah, 1986). So, it seems that the camel whey proteins are more heat resistant than those in cow milk. UHT treatment of whey proteins of camel and cow milk showed a high level of denaturation in camel whey proteins. Among camel whey proteins, α-lactalbumin underwent the highest level of denaturation (65.55 ± 0.29%), followed by serum albumin (12.58 ± 0.88%) and lactoferrin (3.65 ± 0.54%). Omar et al. (2018) showed that α-lactalbumin was the most sensitive whey protein to UHT treatment. Similarly, Felfoul et al. (2017) reported that α-lactalbumin was the most heat-sensitive whey protein in camel milk heated at 80 °C for 60 sec. While, camel serum albumin was the most resistant. In contrast, β-lactoglobulin was the primary whey protein in bovine milk, followed by α-lactalbumin and bovine serum albumin for heat denaturation. The levels of heat-induced denaturation of β-lactoglobulin, α-lactalbumin and bovine serum albumin after UHT treatment were 85.68, 51.06 and 5.37%, respectively. However, Elagamy (2000) reported that α-lactalbumin of camel milk was more heat resistant than those in cow and buffalo milk after heating up to 100°C. Furthermore, α-lactalbumin from camel milk exhibited less denaturation than in bovine milk after heat treatment for 90°C/5 min (Genene et al., 2019). Authors reported that 67% of α-lactalbumin was in native state (un-denatured) compared with raw milk, this value being only 5% in treated cow milk. Kamal and Karoui (2017) used the front-face fluorescence spectroscopy coupled with chemometric technique to characterize changes in camel milk following heat treatments in the range 55-75 °C from 0.5 min up to 30 min in comparison with cow milk. Researchers (Kamal & Karoui, 2017) followed the changes in the fluorescence intensities of Nicotinamide Adenine Dinucleotide (NADH), vitamin A and fluorescent Maillard reaction products as indicator for severity of heat treatments. The results exhibited that changes in the fluorescence intensity of the fluorescent Maillard reaction products spectra appeared to be the most sensitive probe to detect changes in camel milk as a function of heat treatment and holding time. Researchers also determined the activation energies of camel milk and cow milk under the same conditions. The results showed that average values of the activation energy for the camel milk heated in the 55-75 °C were between 47- 85 kJ.mol-1, while it was in the range of 22-73 kJ.mol-1 for cow milk. These findings explain the faster cow milk whey proteins denaturation compared to camel milk whey proteins.

Protein Sedimentation

Heat treatment of milk often cause aggregates of denatured whey proteins and other milk components. These aggregates either precipitate or clump together on the surface of milk. The rate of sedimentation can be measured by the distribution of nitrogenous compounds in milk (CN, NCN and NPN).

Protein nitrogen is distributed in milk between casein, whey proteins and non-protein nitrogen. Metwalli et al. (1988a) found that non-casein nitrogen (NCN) decrease after UHT treatment and this may be attributed to partial denaturation of whey proteins and its precipitation with casein at pH 4.6 or/and formation complex between casein and whey protein as a result of heat treatment. During storage at 20°C, the NCN increased gradually from 100.61 mg/100 mL to 140.63 mg/ 100 mL after 20 weeks. This suggests that a partial proteolytic decomposition of UHT-milk protein occur during storage because of thermostable bacterial enzymes. UHT treated milk exhibits sedimentation during storage. Farah (1986) studied the effect of heat treatment (63°C - 90°C) on distribution of NCN in camel milk. He found that the NCN decreased on heating depending on the temperature used. Guthy et al., (1983) found slight increase in sediment value of indirect heated UHT milk during storage at 35°C with a sharp increase before gelation. Metwalli et al. (1988b) also found an increase in sediment values during storage for 24 weeks at 20°C. Most UHT milk develops a slight sediment during storage, but this is not usually a major problem. Generally, direct UHT processing produces more sedimentation than indirect processing. (Datta, et al., 2002). This is attributed to the fact that there is insufficient hot surface area available during direct processing to allow deposition of the sediment and consequently sediments occur during storage.

The larger casein micelles size are more render to precipitate after heat treatment and camel milk contains a great number of large micelles with average diameter of 380 nm, whereas the smallest micelles are found in bovine (150 nm), sheep (180 nm), and goat milk (260 nm) (Barłowska et al., 2011). Sedimentation of camel milk after UHT treatment is clear phenomenon and depend on type of heat treatment (direct or indirect). Figure 5 shows the amount of camel milk sedimentation after UHT treatment in indirect or direct way. The sediment values are significantly lower in indirect processing than those in direct system. Most of denatured whey proteins in indirect system precipitate on heat surface exchanger while no surface exchanger in direct method and consequently sediments occur during storage.

Farah, et al. (2004) studied sedimentation phenomenon in UHT treated camel milk. Researchers found that camel milk treated in indirect or direct method exhibited excessive sediment after 5 weeks storage at room temperature and results were not satisfactory. Malmgren (2015) reported that adding phosphate or citrate salts and increasing pH values decreased sediment formation in UHT-treated camel milk. It seems that alcohol stability of milk plays the measure role in heat stability of different types of milk. Sagar, et al. (2016) suggested alcohol stability test of 74% alcohol for UHT treatment for cow milk. On the other hand, this concentration of alcohol is not enough to stabilize camel milk against precipitation of UHT camel milk. Malmgren (2015) showed that increasing alcohol concentration to 80% overcome this problem in camel milk. The effect of ethanol stability on precipitation of camel milk after UHT treatment is shown in Figure 6.

Moreover, the effect of adding phosphate and citrate salts on the changes in pH, ionic ion activity, ethanol stability and formation of sedimentation after UHT treatment of goat milk were studied by Boumpa, Tsioulpas, Grandison & Lewis (2008) and Chen, Grandison, & Lewis (2012). Authors found that addition of stabilizer salts decreased the activity of calcium ion and increased the heat stability (decreased formation of precipitation). Researchers also found that sediment formation was markedly decreased, when temperature reduced from 140°C to 125 and 114°C. Furthermore, ethanol stability of 74% exhibited remarkable decrease in the formation of precipitation. However, ethanol stability of buffalo milk is lower than that of cow milk but is still stable for UHT treatments (Kaushik, 2015).

Figure 5. Shows the amount of camel milk sedimentation after UHT treatment in indirect or direct system
Adopted from Malmgren (2015)

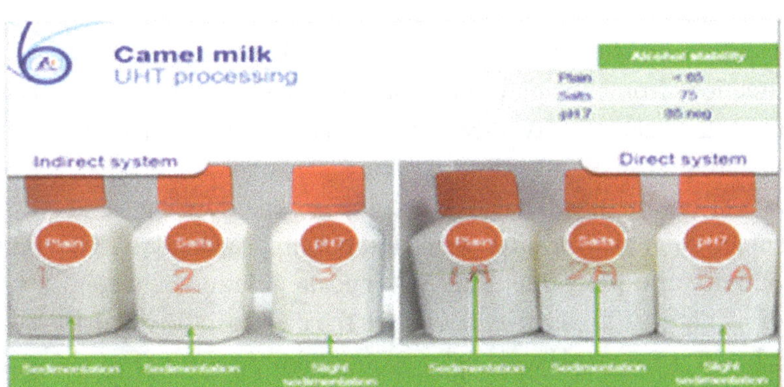

Figure 6. Correlation between ethanol stability and precipitation of camel milk after UHT treatment
Adopted from Malmgren (2015)

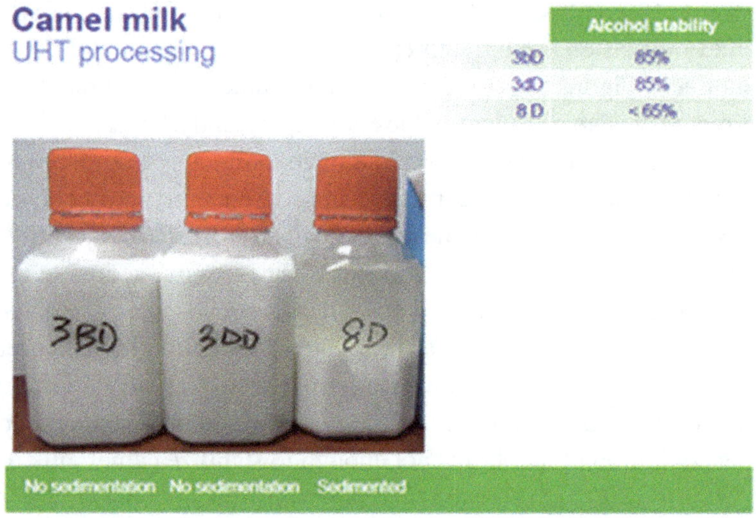
Camel milk
UHT processing
Alcohol stability
3BD 85%
3DD 85%
8D <65%
3BD
3DD
8D
No sedimentation No sedimentation Sedimented

Heat Coagulation Time of Milk (HCT)

The heat stability of milk has been the subject of many studies. The number of papers about the subject has become so large that it is difficult to grasp all the aspects studied. Despite of the fact that many of heat induced changes in milk have been extensively studied. Many phenomena are not fully understood particularly for some types of milk like camel milk.

Heat stability is defined as a coagulation time, which means the time from immersion of milk sample in a thermostatically controlled oil bath at a certain temperature until the appearance of visible coagulation (Fox, 1982). However, there are many other methods which can be used to detect HCT such as: heat coagulation temperature, viscosity measurement, heat exchanger fouling, sediment formation and changes in casein micelle size.

Basically, heat stability is the stability of casein particles to irreversible coagulation at high temperature. Metwalli (1992) reported that the stability of casein micelles upon heating depends on:

1. **Casein composition and their fraction ratios**, especially κ-casein content. This type of casein protects other fractions from precipitation in the presence of calcium and adds steric repulsion into micelles increasing the heat stability. κ-casein may also affect casein micelles size, a larger κ-casein content corresponding to small micelles.
2. **Volume fraction of casein micelles**, if the volume occupied by the same mass of casein micelles is large, the van der Waals attraction is weak and possibly stronger steric repulsion.
3. **Calcium ion activity and pH value**. There is opposite relation between Ca^{2+} activity and the pH of milk samples. A higher Ca^{2+} activity decreases the electrostatic repulsion consequently the heat stability. The relation between pH and heat coagulation time at 140°C is shown in Figure 7 for type A and B milk.

Figure 7. Schematic pH-heat coagulation time profile for type A (O) and type B (X) milk at 140°C

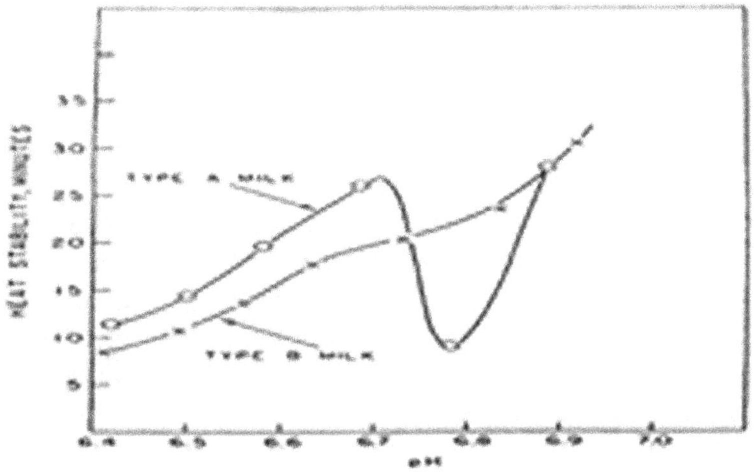

4. **The micellar colloidal calcium phosphate content (MCCP)**, the micelles are generally exhibit less heat stable with higher MCCP content. The casein of buffalo and camel milk contain higher MCCP and have less heat stability.
5. Heat stability of serum protein free-casein micelles (SPFCM) was lower than that of skimmed milk. The addition of 6 mM urea increased HCT at pH higher than pH 6.8. Figure 8 shows the HCT of SPFCM at 140°C.

Heat Coagulation time at higher temperature depends on the type of milk. Cow milk is more heat stable than buffalo, goat and camel milk. Sagar et al. (2016) found that the average heat stability of cow, buffalo and camel milk samples analyzed were 30 min, 26 min and 2.2 min, respectively at 140 °C. This indicates that heat stability of camel milk is very poor at high temperature. Moreover, camel milk was found (Metwalli et al., 2013) to coagulate at 140°C within 2 min (heating up time); while maximum

Figure 8. Effect of pH and urea addition on the heat stability of type A milk (open square), serum protein free casein micelles (open circle) and serum protein-free casein micelles + 6 mM urea (open triangle)
Ddata adopted from Metwalli (1992)

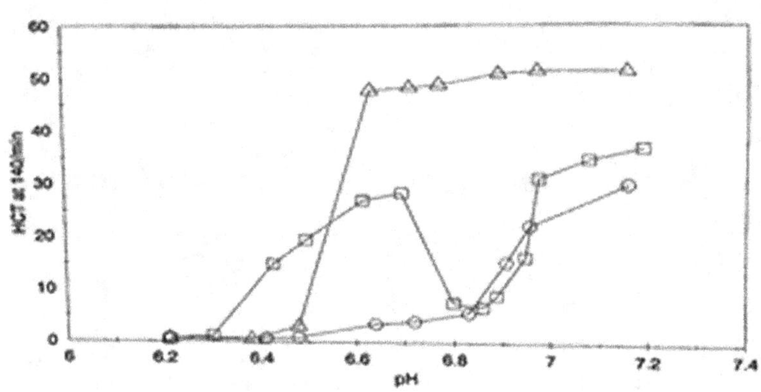

heat stability was observed at 120°C and pH higher than 6.8 (about 7 min), while the required time-temperature for commercial sterilizing process is 121°C for 15 min. The addition of urea to camel milk at a concentration of 10 and 30 mM urea did not improve the heat stability. However, dialysis of camel milk against Jennes and Koops buffer (1962) markedly increased the HCT of camel milk. It seems therefore that the composition of serum camel milk plays a role in heat stability. Alhaj et al. (2011) reported the precipitation of camel milk proteins during sterilization (121°C for 15 min) at pH 6.5 to 6.8, while, no precipitation was observed at pH > 7.0.

The effect of initial pH on precipitation of camel milk during sterilization at 121°C for 15 min is elucidated in Figure 9. At higher pH values (> pH 7.0) no precipitations have been observed. Alhaj et al. (2011) also reported that the addition of sodium phosphate salt in concentration of 1 mM/L prevent formation of protein precipitate at pH values 6.8 – 7.3 as shown in Figure 10. The authors concluded that addition of κ-casein at a concentration of 2 mg/mL or EDTA at a concentration of 6 mM/L could convert the camel milk from type A to type B.

High Pressure

The application of high pressure (HP) to milk dates to the end of the 19th century (Hite, 1899). High level of food safety can be done by traditional treatments but they lead to degradation of various food quality and nutritious attributes. The scientists make a great effort to minimize the undesirable effects on food quality. They used a number of non-thermal processing technologies including, but not limited, high pressure (HP), pulsed electric field, power ultrasonic, ionizing radiation, ultra violet decontamination, pulsed white light. Among these, high pressure processing (HPP) is the most promising technology for food applications and considered as high-hydrostatic pressure processing (HHPP) or ultrahigh-pressure processing (UHPP). Nevertheless, of its nomenclature, the technology has been cited as one of the best innovations in food processing during the past 50 years (Dunne, 2005). Camel milk was found to have some different properties from cow milk including poor heat stability at high temperature. This milk was reported not to be sterilized at natural pH due to instability of protein (Alhaj et al., 2011); therefore HHP

Figure 9. Sterilized whole camel milk at natural pH 6.5 or after adding NaOH to adjust the pH up to 8.0
Adopted from Alhaj et al. (2011).

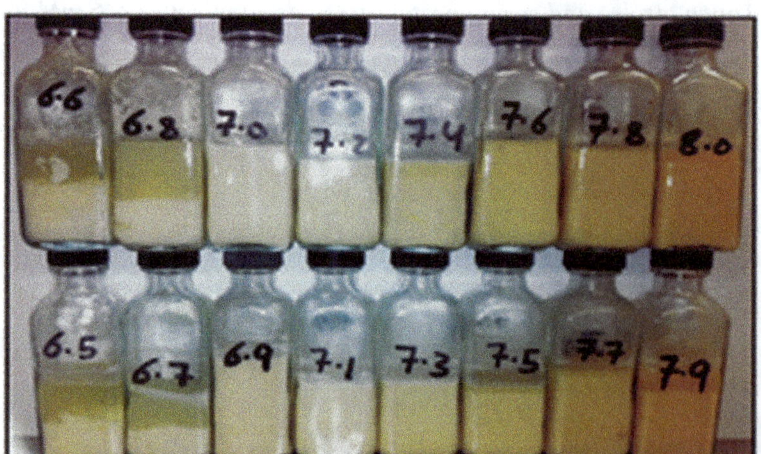

Figure 10. Heat stability of whole camel milk containing 1 mM sodium phosphate after adjustment the pH in the range 6.8-7.3
Adopted from Alhaj et al. (2011).

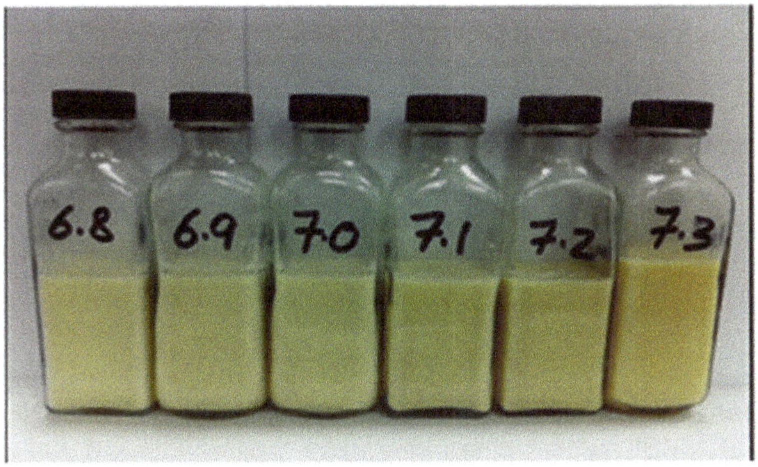

technology could alternate UHT treatment and extend its shelf life. In HPP, food is subjected to vary HP in the range of 100 to 1000 MPa at processing temperature ranged from 0°C to 100°C with exposure time of few seconds to 20 minutes. The pressure used in food technology increases the temperature of foods approximately 2–3°C / 100 MPa. Pressures used in the HP treatment of foods may have great effect on the ionic, hydrogen and hydrophobic bonds whereas may have no effect on covalent bonds.

Mechanism of High-Pressure Processing

Pressure vessel and pressure-generating device are the main components in HPP unit. It operates by placing the food on the top of the vessel and tightly closing it, then from the bottom of the vessel a water contain a small amount of soluble oil will be pumped as a source of pressure medium. However, the compressibility of the water need to be checked and a pressure higher than higher than 600 MPa water volume is compressed by up to 15%. After reaching the target pressure, in order to save further energy and maintain the pressure inputs to the system the pump or piston is stopped, the valves are closed. Finlay, a uniform pressure is conveyed throughout the very minimal or no heating of the product. Figure 11 shows a uniform transmitted pressure in the pressure vessel.

High pressure treatment applied in industries for food and dairy product development is currently either a batch or semi-continuous process. Application of pressure over the food system results in various physical and chemical changes. During pressure treatment, physical compression of the system occurs which results in a volume reduction and an increase in temperature and energy. At HP treatment i.e. >200 MPa and with a combination of 0–40°C temperature range a covalent bonds are almost unaffected and as a result of hydrophobic and ionic interactions are alteration the tertiary and quaternary structures of molecules are maintained (Hendrickx, Van Den, & Weemaes, 1998). Molecules with α-helices structure are less stable against pressure than with β-sheets (Goyal, Sharma, Upadhyay, Sihag, & Kaushik, 2013). HPP is usually carried out with water or water containing a small amount of soluble oil as a hydraulic fluid to facilitate the operation and compatibility with food materials (Earnshaw, 1996).

Figure 11. Schematic batch type of pressure processing system. (Pressure is exerted equally from all sides during holding time.)

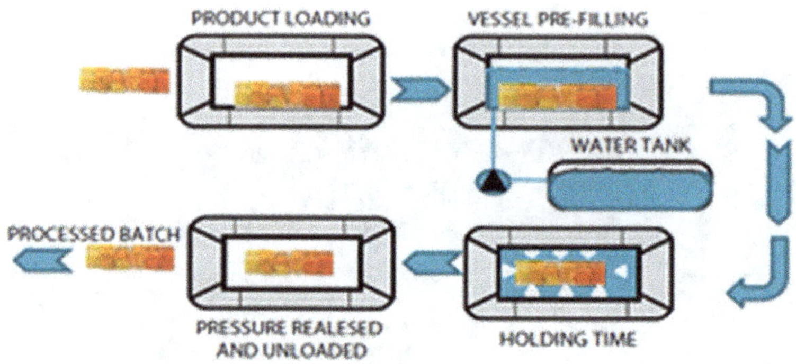

Inhibition and Destruction of Microorganisms in Milk Using HPP

Milk is a perishable commodity and spoils very easily. Its low acidity, high water activity and high nutrient content make it the perfect media for both vegetative and spore forming bacteria, including those which cause food poisoning (pathogens). Spore forming bacteria are thermo-resistant and important for milk deterioration. Heat treatments such as pasteurization, sterilization and ultra-high temperature (UHT) are the main heat treatments applied to microbial stabilization of milk, since they are simple.

Studies indicated that by applying the HPP both the pathogenic and spoilage microorganisms can be inactivated and it is possible to obtain 'raw' milk with treatment of pressure about 400 to 600 MPa of a microbiological quality comparable to that of pasteurized (72°C, 15 s) milk depending on the microbiological quality of milk (Buffa, Trujillo, & Guamis, 2001a; Goyal et al. 2013). A shelf-life of thermally pasteurized milk of 10 days at 10 °C can be obtained using a pressure treatment of at least 400 MPa for 15 min or 500 MPa for 3 min (Goyal et al. 2013).

Bacterial cells in the stationary phase being more resistant than those in the growth phase and HP at 600 MPa for 15 min at 20–30oC can destroy most of the vegetative cells of microorganisms (Thimson & Short, 1965). The bacterial spores are always more resistant than vegetative cells and they can survive at pressure of 1000 MPa. However, pressures between 50–300 MPa can stimulate the germination of bacterial spores. Heating or mild pressure treatments can be applied for inactivation of germinated spores.

Gram-positive bacteria are more resistant to pressure process than gram-negative bacteria. Gram-positive microorganisms can be inactivated at a high pressure (500–600 MPa) at 25°C for 10 min, while gram-negative microorganisms requires lower pressure treatments (300 - 400 MPa) at 25°C for 10 min. The thickness of cell wall of gram positive bacteria might be responsible for this variation. Vegetative cells of yeasts and molds are the most pressure sensitive. Pressures between 300 and 600 MPa inactivate molds, yeasts, and most of the vegetative bacterial cells (Smelt, 1998; Goyal et al. 2013). Studies on the effect of variation in pressure resistance on growth stage (exponential and stationary phase) with respect to growth temperature (8° and 30°C) between two strains of *Listeria monocytogenes*, *Bacillus cereus*, and *Pseudomonas fluorescens*. Results showed that stationary-phase cells were significantly more resistant than exponential-phase cells to pressure for all three species studied. Growth temperature had a significant effect at the two growth stages studied. Pressure treatment at 8°C induced significantly less spore germination than at 30°C (McClements et al., 2001).

On the other hand, studies on Ewe's milk containing 6% fat inoculated with *Listeria innocua* 910 CECT at a concentration of 10^7 CFU/ml showed that pressurizations at low-temperature (2°C) produced higher *Listeria innocua* inactivation than treatments at room temperatures (25°C). The kinetics of destruction of *L. innocua* were first order with *D*-values of 3.12 min at 2°C and 400 MPa, while it raised to 4 min at 25°C (Gervilla et al., 1997). In general, the descending order of inactivation is *P. fluorescens* >*E. coli* > *L. innocua* > *L. helveticus* > *S. aureus*. Moreover, *P. fluorescens*, *L. innocua,* and *L. helveticus* showed more resistance to HP at room temperature (25°C) than at low temperature (4°C), while, *E. coli,* and *S. aureus* showed lower resistance to HP at room temperature than at low temperature. However, *L. monocytogenes* and *E. coli* were the most pressure-resistant species at room temperature for HP treatment Patterson (2005). HP treatment at 400 MPa for 15 min and 550 MPa for 3 min completely inactivated *E. coli* in milk samples (Liepa, Zagorska, Galoburda, & Kostascuka, 2017). Hamad, et al. (2013) studied the effect of different levels of pressure (200, 250, 300 and 350 MPa) on mesophilic aerobic and psychrotrophic bacteria. They found that the bacterial loads reduced by up to 0.12, 0.44, 1.23 and 1.45, log cycles. When pressures increased to 400 to 600 MPa the reduction were up to 3.0 log cycles, which was the non-detectable level of these bacteria. They although concluded that treatment of 400 MPa seem to be enough to reduce microbial contamination of camel's milk to safe levels. Fitria, Buckow, Singh, Hemar, & Kasapis, (2015) claimed that high pressure treatment (1000 MPa) combined with heat treatment (above 60°C) considered equal to sterilization process due to its ability to inactivate bacterial spores at lower heat treatments.

MODIFICATION OF PHYSICO-CHEMICAL PROPERTIES OF MILK USING HPP

Effects of HPP on Appearance and Color

The most prominent difference between heat and pressure treatment of skim milk is the appearance of the milk directly after treatment. On heating, skim milk becomes whiter while pressure treated skim milk appears translucent or semi-translucent with slightly yellowish. The heated milk after storage remains white regardless of storage temperature. Pressure treated milk retains semi-transparent appearances if stored at 5°C, while storage at room temperature makes it more turbid (Cheftel, 1995). HP treated ewe's milk showed decrease in lightness (L^*) and an increase in greenness ($-a^*$) and yellowness ($+b^*$). This decrease in L^* value is due to disintegration of casein micelle (Farkas & Hoover, 2000). HPP of skim milk at 600 MPa for 15 min resulted in significant changes in the L^*, b^* and a^* values, that could be also perceived visually (Krebbers et al., 2003). The appearance of milk treated at 600 MPa is shown in Figure 12.

Increasing the sample's temperature from 4° to 43°C derived back color values of HP milk towards the values of untreated milk, but not to the same initial point. Treatment at 200 MPa at 20°C had only a slight effect on the L^* values, but treatment at 250–450 MPa significantly decreased the L^* value of pasteurized or reconstituted skim milk. Treatment at > 450 MPa had little further effect on the L^* values (Hayakawa et al., 1994). Cow's milk showed less sensitivity to pressure with respect to color change (Kolakowski, Reps, Dajnowiec, Szczepek, & Porowski, 1997). Kim, Kim, Choi, Min & Kwak (2008) studied the effect of high pressure treatment (200 MPa) and low temperature (-4°C) for 10, 20 and 30 min on physicochemical properties in milk they reported that the L^* values decreased in all treated

Figure 12. Untreated milk; D: high-pressure treated milk at 600 Mpa for 30 min
Data from Considine et al. (2007)

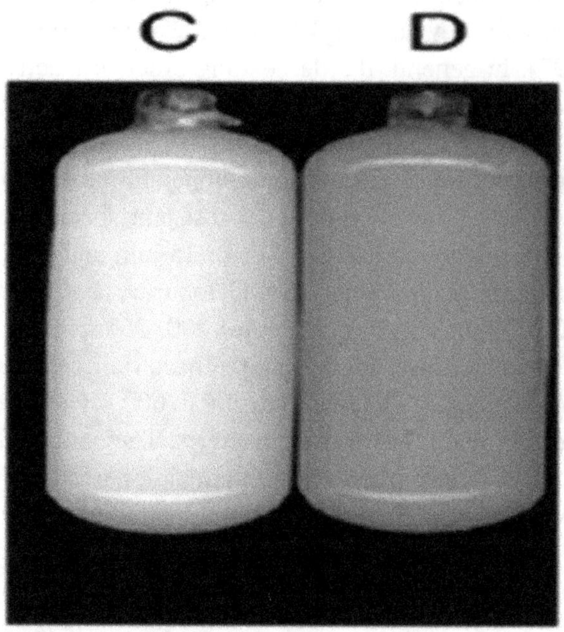

samples with increasing holding time whereas $-a^*$ and b^* -values were increased. However, the increase in treated samples at 10 min did not show significantly different values from that of raw milk sample.

Devi, Buckow, Singh, Hemar, and Kasapis (2015) and Omar et al. (2018) found that high-pressure treatment of bovine milk at 200 MPa caused a significant decrease in L^* with an accompanying increase in a* (greenness) and b* (yellowness) values. Increasing the pressure up to 800 MPa caused a further decrease in L^* and an increase in a* and b*. They attributed the reduction in L^* of bovine milk mainly to the dissociation of casein micelles by pressure into smaller particles, which increases the translucence of the milk. In contrast, a small reduction in L^* (1.88 units from 67.77 to 65.89) in HP-treated camel milk was observed after treatment at 200 MPa. Treatment at higher pressures ($\geq$400 up to 800 MPa) resulted in a further decrease in L^* in camel milk by up to 3.35 units (from 67.77 to 64.42). This slight reduction in L^* in camel milk compared with bovine milk during HP treatments is possibly the result of lower casein micelles disruption of camel milk (Omar et al. 2018). Treatments of buffalo milk at 250 or 400 MPa reduced L^* of buffalo milk slightly and that treatment at 600 or 800 MPa reduced L^* significantly, by up to 17 units after treatment (Huppertz et al. 2005).

Effects of HPP on Particle Size Changes

The physico-chemical and technological functionality of milk is affected by HP treatment. The casein micelles are disintegrated into smaller particles when milk is subjected to HP, (Cadesky, Walkling-Ribeiro, Kriner, Karwe, &. Moraru, 2017). This disintegration is accompanied by an increase of casein micelles number and calcium phosphate levels in serum phase of milk and by a decrease in the both non-casein nitrogen and serum nitrogen fractions, suggesting that the precipitation of whey proteins on casein micelles at pH 4.6 by centrifugation (Johnston et al., 1992; Law et al., 1998).

HPP of skim milk may increase or decrease casein micelles size depending on HP used. At about 300 MPa, it substantially decreases the size of the particles. The average decrease in size is from about 200 to 100 nm regardless of temperature at pressurization. However, pressure treatments in the range of 200 to <300 MPa causes the increase of particle size which is affected by pH of milk, temperature, pressure and duration of pressure processing (Huppertz et al., 2004).

Many reports suggested that the precipitation of denatured whey proteins may be responsible for this aggregation phenomenon, but successive studies carried on casein-free whey protein systems revealed that the aggregation is attributed to the casein micelles (Anema et al., 2005b). Changes in particle size of preheat milk at 90°C for 10 min was similar to those in unheated milk over the pressure range (100-300 MPa), demonstrating that the pre-denaturation of the whey proteins has little effect on the aggregation or disaggregation phenomenon in pressure-treated milk (Huppertz et al. 2004). The changes in particle size of HP treated milk was accompanied by a considerable increase in the level of serum casein, (Anema et al., 2005a). The aggregation of the casein micelles increases as the temperature and the duration of pressure treatment were increased. Pressure treatment of about 250 MPa and at temperatures above 20°C resulted in the formation two distinct populations: one with the particle size larger than the original casein micelles and other with smaller than original size of casein micelle (Gaucheron et al., 1997). Pothakamary et al. (1995) reported that the denaturation, coagulation, or gelation of proteins by HHP treatments is correlated with the extent of hydrophilicity or hydrophobicity of the protein. Moreover, the denaturation of whey proteins may be reversible (in the range of 101–304 MPa), or irreversible at >304 MPa depending on HHP treatment (Jaenicke, 1981; Goyal, et al. 2013). Reactions of denatured whey proteins with sulfur containing casein (K-casein and αs_2 casein) on HHP treatment may be responsible for casein micelle increase. The particle size of casein micelles decreased when the pH of the milk was reduced from the natural pH (6.7) to 6.5, with the increase in pressure, with a marked decrease in size above 200 MPa. A few studies have been carried out on HHP treatment of camel milk unlike the intensive research on the effect of high-pressure processing on cow milk proteins. It is important to study the effects of HHP on proteins and other constituents of different kinds of milk such as camel milk, which has been not much investigated. Recently, Omar et al. (2018) studied the effect of HP treatment on casein micelles in camel and cow milk. The results showed that the treatment of camel milk at 200 MPa caused a significant decrease in the size of casein micelles (from 171.23 nm to 135.23 nm) by 21% compared with untreated milk. Moreover, the casein micelle size of camel milk decreased by 25% (from 171.23 to 129.40 nm) with increasing the pressure from 400 to 800 MPa. Casein micelles in bovine milk behaved differently after HP treatment. A HP treatment of 200 MPa caused a small reduction in micelle size by 6% compared to untreated milk (from 143.45 to 134.90 nm) of bovine milk. However, increasing pressure (400–800 MPa) resulted a disintegration of bovine milk casein micelles from 143.45 to 71.52 nm than casein micelles in camel milk. This reduction in casein micelle size into smaller particles at higher pressure is likely to be due to disruption of the intra-micellar van der Waals, hydrophobic and electrostatic interactions and changes in the solubilization of micellar calcium phosphate (Needs, Stenning, Gill, Ferragut, & Rich, 2000; Huppertz, Smiddy, Upadhyay, & Kelly, 2006). The decrease in the size of casein micelles in camel milk was considerably smaller than in bovine milk after HP treatments, which might be due to the differences in the primary structure of micelles between the two kinds of milk and to the large casein micelle size of camel milk. The absence of β-lactoglobulin, lack of K-casein high mineral content such as magnesium, inorganic phosphorus, sodium and potassium may be involved.

Effects of HPP on Rennet Coagulation Time (RCT)

Rennet coagulation time (RCT) of milk is an index of the gelation and proper time for curd manipulation during cheese process. Application of high pressure may affect the RCT depending on the applied pressure (López-Fandiño, 2006). HP treatment at <150 MPa had no effect on the RCT, while a HP of 200 to 600 MPa significantly reduced the RCT (Desorby-Banon et al., 1994; Liepa, Zagorska, & Galoburda 2017). Moreover, RCT was reduced markedly after the treatment of 600 MPa. In general, rennet coagulation properties were increased for milk subjected to 200 MPa for 30 min (Lopez Fandino et al., 1996). The pressure-induced disintegration of the casein micelles appears to reduce the rennet coagulation time and cutting time; while denaturation of the whey proteins increases the RCT and eventually the curd cutting time, in a similar fashion to that for the heated milk. Rennet coagulation time decreases with increasing pressure and heat treatment time (Huppertz et al., 2005). RCT of HP treated milk is also dependent on temperature and pH of the milk. Treatment at 50–60°C (200 MPa) delayed the rennet coagulation of milk (Lopez Fandino, De La Fuente, Ramos, & Olano, 1998). Acidification of milk (pH-5.5) before HP treatment decreased its RCT, whereas alkalization (pH 7.0) had the opposite effect (Arias et al., 2000).

In general, rennet coagulation properties are found to enhance (Lopez Fandino 2006; Buffa, et al., 2001a) when milk subjected to 100–500 MPa pressures for 30 min, although higher pressures of 300 MPa are found in the same study to increase the rennet coagulation time of milk. The drop-in particle size produced by high pressure treatment is accompanied by conformational changes of spherical particles into chains. The RCT of the raw camel milk was much shorter than that of bovine milk (Omar et al., 2018). The reduction in the RCT of bovine milk after HP treatment at 200 MPa is believed to be the result of the dissociation of micellar κ-casein and the disruption of casein micelles, which led to an increase in the surface area for inter-micellar interactions with less κ-casein available to provide steric stabilization (Huppertz et al., 2006; Needs et al., 2000). In contrast, the RCT properties of camel milk differed from that of bovine milk for HP treatments responses. The HP treatment of 200 and 400 MPa significantly increased the RCT of camel milk by 55.90 and 109.39%, (from 16.16 to 25.20 and 33.84 min) respectively, compared to untreated milk. HP-treated camel milk at 200 MPa had lower rate of rennet induced gel formation than that of untreated milk during the first 30 min (Omar et al. 2018). This increase in the RCT and strength of the rennet-induced coagulum from camel milk treated at 200 MPa might be due to restricted effect of HP on disruption of casein micelles and whey protein denaturation in camel milk.

Cheese Production from HP-Treated Milk

Milk pasteurization (heating at 72–74 °C for 15 s or 63°C for 30 min) destroys pathogenic and most of spoilage microorganisms, and it is the most important heat treatment applied to cheese milk to ensure the safety and quality of the final products. However, milk pasteurization is known to undesirably affect the development of many sensory characteristics of cheese by decreasing the number of small peptides and free amino acids formed which leads to alterations in cheese texture and delayed ripening process

(Grappin & Beuvier, 1997). In general, pasteurized milk cheeses have received lower flavor intensity scores than raw milk cheeses (Lacotte, et al. 2015). High pressure technology can be used to increase the microbiological safety and quality of cheese milk to produce high quality cheeses. The protein modifications, i.e. whey protein denaturation and micelle disintegration, and alters mineral equilibrium by HP treatment affect the technological properties of milk, improving the rennet coagulation, accelerating cheese ripening and yield properties of cheese milk (Costabel, et al 2016; Trujillo, 1999; Buffa et al., 2001b). About 90% of β-lactoglobulin denatured at 800 MPa at low temperature; while 100% denaturation were observed at pressure 300 MPa at 60°C or at 400 MPa at 40°C (Lopez-Fandino 1998; Ye, et al. 2004). In addition, microbiological quality of cheeses from HP-treated milk (500 MPa for 15 min at 20 °C) was comparable to pasteurized milk (72 °C for 15 s) cheeses (Buffa et al., 2001b). However, the application of HP technology to cheese milk causes differences in cheese composition and ripening in comparison to pasteurized milk cheese. The HP-treated milk cheeses have higher moisture, salt and total free amino acids contents than raw or pasteurized milk cheeses (Costabel, et al. 2016; Trujillo et al., 1999). The activity of plasmin enzyme in pasteurized and pressurized milk is higher than in untreated milk (Costabel, et al 2016). On the other hand, cheeses made from HP-treated milk showed a similar level of lipolysis to cheeses made from raw milk; whereas the level of lipolysis in cheese made from pasteurized milk was lower (Buffa et al., 2001b). This behavior was explained by heat-sensitive but partial pressure-resistant characteristics of the indigenous milk lipase. The cheeses made from raw or HP treated milk were firmer and less fracturable than cheeses made from pasteurized milk, but differences became less notable at the end of ripening (Buffa et al. (2001b).

The report made on acceleration of cheese ripening using HP indicated as cheese exposed to HP at 50 MPa for 3 d at 25°C had characteristics typical of a 6-month-old commercial cheddar cheese (Yokoyama et al., 1992). Moreover, further studies on ripening of cheddar cheese shows an improved Cheddar cheese obtained at 50 MPa among the ranges of HP examined i.e. from 0.1 to 300 MPa for 3 days at 25°C after cheese making. A cheddar cheese (O'Reilly, O'Connor, Murphy, Kelly & Beresford, 2000b) and other cheese varieties (Kolakowski, et al., 1998; Saldo et al., 1999) report shows a different level of proteolysis; however, the method of cheese production by these authors is not the same which might be one of the reasons for the observed variation. Acceleration of cheese ripening have been tested under another HP conditions that involved 'high' HP treatments (400–600 MPa) short times (5–15 min) or an initial 'high' HP treatment (400–600) short times (5–15 min) followed by a 'low' HP treatment (50 MPa) long times (72 h) and different cheese varieties. The results showed that long treatments at moderate pressure produce an increase in proteolysis in comparison with short and intense treatments (Costabel, et al 2016). The enhancement effect is assumed to be caused by the release of starter enzymes and higher plasmin activity in treated samples than the others untreated samples (Costabel, et al 2016) .αS_1- and β-CN. Break-down and nitrogen content in soluble fractions was significantly higher in cheeses treated at 400 MPa, as well as soluble peptides and free amino acid amount increased. They reported also that the peptide profiles and content of total free amino acids in 60-day old treated cheese were similar to the fully ripened control cheeses for 90 day. Costabel, et al. 2016; Saldo et al., 2002). To date, no studies have been done on the production and acceleration of ripening of hard cheese from HP treated camel milk. Because camel milk contains no β-lactoglobulin, it will be expected that the properties of hard cheese prepared from camel milk at HP will be better than other types of milk containing β-lactoglobulin. However, further research is required to evaluate the full applicability of HP in accelerating the cheese ripening in different types of milk. The manufacture and challenges of camel milk cheese was discussed in details in Chapter 6.

Effects of HP-Processing on Yogurt and Fermented Dairy Products

Yogurt, is a custard-like food with a tart flavor, prepared from milk curdled by bacteria, especially *Lactobacillus delbrueckii subsp. bulgaricus* and *Streptococcus thermophilus,* and can be found in three states: set yogurt, stirred yogurt and fluid or drinking yogurt. The manufacture of yogurt from camel milk was discussed in details in Chapter 5. Among the processes involved in fermented milk and yogurt processing, the most important are homogenization, pasteurization and fermentation. Two strategies have been used to improve fermented milk and yogurt quality and preservation by means of HP, i.e. making fermented milk and yogurt from HP treated milk and pressurization to inactivate microbiota. The properties of acid set gels prepared from HP treated milk showed improved texture (rigidity and resistance to breaking) and syneresis resistance (Johnston et al., 1994). Most of the viscosity improvement is achieved after pressurization for 15 min at 400 MPa and for 5 min at 600 MPa with slight further increase up to 60 min. Yogurt firmness increases as pressure increases, and treatments of 350 MPa at 25°C and 500 MPa at 55°C showed no differences in whey syneresis compared with pasteurized milk (Ferragut et al., 2000). During storage at 4°C for 20 days, yogurts made from HP treated milk showed a good stability in terms of firmness and water retention compared with yogurt made from the untreated milk. Milk treatment with pressures of only 10% of pressure-treated milk (400–600 MPa for 10 min at 25°C) resulted in a creamy product that maintained the taste of the conventional yogurt, which would be advantageous since only a small proportion of the milk has to be pressurized and the improvement in texture is clearly perceived (Capellas et al., 2001; Trujillo et al., 2002). Research studies have described the disintegration of the casein micelles into smaller particles and the simultaneous increase in the amount of caseins and calcium phosphate in the serum phase which improved the water holding capacity of yogurt (Johnston et al. 1992). Further, the combination of HP and thermal treatment increased the yogurt viscosity and lowered gelation time compared to HP treated samples (Ferragut et al., 2000). The study conducted on ewe's milk yoghurt at different HP (200, 350 and 500 MPa) for 15 min and temperature of 10, 25 and 55 °C compared with milk pasteurized at 70 °C, 10 milk showed that the yogurt firmness increased with increase in pressure, and a 350 MPa pressure treatments at - 25°C and 500 MPa at 55 °C showed no differences in whey syneresis compared with pasteurized milk (Ferragut et al., 2000) In same study, *Lactobacillus delbrueki* activity was inactivated in yogurt was treated by HP (400 MPa, 15 min), while *Streptococcus thermophilus* was more resistant to the pressurization, and it was found that the degree of inactivation was dependent on the strain and varied from 35.3 to 99.9%. The shelflife of yogurt treated by HP processing can be increased via complete inactivation of lactic acid bacteria (Reps et al., 1999 & 2001). To date, no reports made on HP- treatment of camel milk for yogurt making from camel milk. Yogurt making effort from camel milk is challenged by the poor texture development (Berhe et al., 2017) and the probable application of HP-treatment might have a positive effect on camel yogurt texture; this need a further confirmation. The manufacture of yogurt from camel milk was discussed in details in Chapter 5.

Effects of HP-Processing on Fat Globule

The size of fat globules in camel milk are the smallest among all ruminants (Khalesi, Salami, Moslehishad, Winterburn, & Moosavi-Movahedi, 2017). Fat globules in camel milk (2.99 μm) are smaller than those of cow milk (3.44 - 4.53 μ m) (Couvreur , Hurtaud , Marnet , Faverdin , & Peyraud, 2007) and buffalo milk (8.7 μ m), ewe (3.30 μ m) but similar to those of goat milk (3.19 μm) (El-Zeini, 2006). So, the creaming rate in raw camel milk is lower than other types of milk because smaller fat globule size and absence of agglutinin (Farah & Ruegg, 1991). The effect of high pressure used in homogenization of milk on fat globules is different than HP technique. The effect of HP technique will be discussed here. A 450 MPa pressure at 10 or 25 °C did not change the fat globule size distribution, or the flow behavior. However, increasing the hydrostatic pressure up to 500 MPa resulted some modifications on size and distribution of milk fat globules of ewe's milk (Dumay, 1996). HP treatments at 25 and 50 °C showed a tendency to increase the number of small globules in the range 1–2 μm, whereas at 4 °C the tendency was the reverse and there was no damage on the milk fat globule membrane occurred (Gervilla et al., 2001). These modifications on distribution of milk fat globules could be due to phenomenon of aggregation and disaggregation of fat globules. This provides some advantages for HP-treated milk, that HP treatment at 25 and 50 °C increases the stabilit, whereas at 4 °C (low temperatures) it increases the creaming-off (Gervilla et al., 2001). Buchheim and Abou El Nour (1992) found that the crystallization of fat globule increased with prolong of pressure treatment and was maximal after processing at 300–500 MPa. Moreover, the crystallization proceeded during further storage at 23 °C after pressure release. Whipping properties of HP treated cream improved when cream was treated at pressures up to 600 MPa for up to 2 min (Eberhard et al., 1999) probably due to better crystallization of milk fat. The denaturation of whey protein increased and resulted in longer whipping time and destabilization of whipped cream by increasing the pressure and time HP treatment. Below 400 MPa no noticeable effects on whipping properties of cream were found. The oleic acid was not affected but autoxidation of linoleic acid was increased by pressures from 350 MPa though the effects were small and no new oxidation products, compared with thermal treatment, were formed (Butz, et al., 1999). The authors advise the need for complementary studies in milk and milk products.

EFFECT OF HEAT TREATMENTS ON BIOLOGICAL VALUE OF CAMEL MILK

Insulin-Like Peptide

It is well stablished that camel milk has revealed high concentration of insulin like peptide caused in prevention and control of diabetes (Chapter 7 and 9). These peptides in camel milk possess a special characteristic. These features include resistant to proteolytic enzymes, encapsulated in lipid vesicles that makes passage through the stomach and entry into the blood stream, absorption into circulation easier than those from other sources (Abrhaley & Leta, 2018). Camel milk contains large concentrations of insulin ranging from 58.67 - 150 U/L compared to17.01 U/L in cow milk (Abrhaley & Leta, 2018, Hamad et al., 2011; Mullaicharam, 2014). Human, goat and cow milk contain also insulin-like peptides which degraded easily by proteolytic enzymes and stomach acidity. Unlike to other milks, the coagulum of camel milk is soft and it passes through stomach fast. The concentration of insulin-like peptide in human, camel, and bovine milk was found to be 2.7 μg/ml, 1.7 μg/ml and 0.5 μg/ml, respectively. These results were confirmed by Agrawal et al. (2005). The potential anti-diabetic effect of camel milk is discussed in details in Chapter 9.

Biological activity of insulin-like peptide in camel milk were extensively studied on animal (Agrawal, 2005; Romeih, Hamad, & Abdel-Rahim, 2011), on human (Agrawal et al. 2003, 2009). Romeih, et al. (2011) and different types of milk (bovine, camel and buffalo) on the blood glucose level of 30 diabetic rats. The results showed that a reduction in blood glucose level in camel milk treated diabetic rats by about 49% while 11.6% and 11.1% for the bovine and buffalo groups, respectively were recorded. Other experiments revealed that a significant reduction in mean blood glucose was reported and the dose of insulin requirement decreased and confirmed that camel milk is safe and efficacious in improving long-term glycemic control, with a significant reduction in the doses of insulin in type 1 and 2 diabetic patients (Badr, 2013; Sboui et al., 2009; Agrawal et al., 2003 & 2011). Insulin-like peptides may lose their biological effect on heat treatments. The blood glucose levels in raw treated camel milk decreased from 169.68 ± 28.7 mg/dL to 81.54 ± 11.4 mg/dL ($p < 0.02$) after 4 weeks of treatment, whereas diabetic rats treated with pasteurized camel milk showed a slight decrease in blood glucose levels (from 135.45 ± 20.91 mg/dL to 113 ± 29.09 mg/dL) (Agrawal et al., 2005). The concentration of insulin in raw camel milk, whey and casein were 3.7 ± 0.47, 4.69 ± 0.45 and 0.85 ± 0.85 respectively, the corresponding valued in pasteurized forms were 0.7± 0.67, 0.91 ± 0.83 and 0.3 ± 0.39 (Hamoud, 2015). These observations proof that insulin-like peptides are thermolabile and loss their biological effect on heat treatments. However, the glucose blood levels significantly decreased in dogs treated with raw camel milk (from 10.16 ± 1.16 to 5.22 ± 1.06 mmol/l) and pasteurized milk (the same results as in raw milk) Whereas, the animals receiving boiled camel milk demonstrated high blood glucose (10.5 ± 0.52 mmol/l) (Sboui, et al., 2012)

Immunoglobulin

Immunoglobulins are classified into five i.e. Immunoglobulin A (IgA), Immunoglobulin G (IgG), Immunoglobulin M (IgM), Immunoglobulin D (IgD) and Immunoglobulin E (IgE). Camel milk contains IgA, IgG and IgM. Camel milk had three different subclasses i.e. IgG_1, IgG_2 and IgG_3 (El-Agamy 1989). Camel milk contains the highest percentage of serum albumin, immunoglobulins and glycosylated whey proteins in the proportion of 26, 18 and 11% respectively, from total whey proteins in camel milk (El-Hatmi et al. 2006); while cow milk contains 6.2, 3.5 and 5.3 of serum albumin, immunoglobulins and glycosylated whey proteins (Fox, 2003). In human milk these proteins i.e. serum albumin, immunoglobulins and glycosylated whey proteins were found 7.5, 18 and negligible (Malacarne et al 2002). These proteins have high biological and nutritional values that may be affected with heat treatments. There are some available studies that examine the use of native camel whey proteins (undenatured) and denatured whey proteins on B and T cells of diabetic mice improving the residual of β cell function in the pancreas (Badr, Mohany, & Metwalli 2011); inflammatory responses of wound healing in diabetic rats (Ebaid, Salem, Sayed & Metwalli 2011) and wound healing in streptozotocin diabetic rats (Metwalli, Mahmoud, Ebaid, Ahmed & Ahmed; 2015; Ebaid, et al. 2015; Moustafa, et al. 2016; Ebaid, Abdel-Salam, Hassan, Al-Tamimi, Metwalli & Alhazza, 2017). Endurance of neurosystem (Ajarem et al. 2017). El-Agamy, (2000) found that the protective proteins for microbial factors such as immunoglobulins lost their activities on heating of camel, cow and buffalo milk at 65°C for 30 min, whereas the lysozyme and lactoferrin not losing their activity. However, Griffiths (2010) and Uniacke-lowe, et al. (2010) reported that the effect of heat treatments on the activity of immunoglobulin depend on its type (i.e. IgG in cow and buffalo milk completely lost its activity on heating at 75°C for 30 min compared to 68.7% in camel milk). The two-dimensional differential gel electrophoresis mass spectrometry of camel milk revealed high degree of similarity (isoelectric point, molecular weight and protein fluorescence intensity) between raw milk and those heated at 65°C for 1h while the similarity was low between raw milk and milk heated at 98°C for 1h (Benabdelkamel, et al. (2017). It has been reported that IgG is the most heat stable while IgM is the least thermostable.The antigen binding region of Ig is more thermolabile than the rest of molecule regions (Uniacke-Lowe, 2010; Zagorska & Ciprovica, 2012). However, during pasteurization (72°C/15 sec) only 10 -30% of bovine milk Ig activity is lost, whereas (UHT) treatment (138_C/4 s) destroys the majority of Ig of milk (Claeys, et al. 2013).

Lactoferrin

Camel milk contains slightly higher content of lactoferrin than cow and buffalo milk but lower than human milk (see Chapter 7). The lactoferrin concentration in raw camel milk varied between 2.3 mg/mL (Niaz et al. 2017) and 0.229 ± 0.135 mg/ (Konuspayeva et al. 2007). Lactoferrin concentration in camel milk represents more than 2-3 times lactoferrin in other types of milk except human milk (El-Agamy, 2009). Although, camel lactoferrin contains the highest value of N – acetylglucosamine compared to other ruminant milk types. Heating milk at 85°C for 30 min caused complete inactivation of lactoferrin in camel, cow and buffalo milk while the residual activity of lactoferrin of human milk were 91, 59 and 27% on heating at 56°C for 15 min, 62.5 for 5 and 30 min respectively (Abd-Elsalam & El-shibiny, 2011). However, heat treatment of camel milk at 63 and 98°C for 1h completely denatured the protective proteins such as lactoferrin, lactoperoxidase, and peptidoglycan recognition protein (PGRP) after 98 °C of heating 1h, while this effect is very minimal after heating at 63 °C for 1h (Benabdelkamel et al., 2017). The antimicrobial activity of Lactoferrin has been attributed mainly to direct binding of LF to the microbial membrane, especially to lipopolysaccharide in Gram - negative bacteria, causing the cell wall of bacteria permeable, binding of iron from medium leading to inhibition of iron-need bacteria and prevention attachment of microorganisms to epithelial cells or enterocytes (Korhonen, 2009). Lactoferrin revealed antimicrobial effect against wide range of pathogenic microbes such as *E. coli; Staphylococcus aureus; Streptoccccus mutans; Listeria monocytogenes; Clostridium perfringens; Candida albicans; Helicobacter pylori; Pseudomonas aeruginosa; Salmonella typhimurium; S. enteriditis; Vibrio cholerae;* and against hepatitis viruses (B, C and G), HIV virus, and rotavirus (Pan, Rowney, Guo & Hobman, 2007). Food and Drug Administration (FDA) qualified the lactoferrin as "Generally Recognized as Safe (GRAS)". The potential antimicrobial effect of camel milk was discussed in details in Chapter 7.

Lysozyme

The concentration of lysozyme in camel milk is higher (i.e. ranged between 228, and 500 μ g/100 mL) (El-Agamy et al. 1998) than those in other ruminant milk (cow, buffalo, goat and sheep) but lower than those in non-ruminant milk (human, mare and donkey) (El-Agamy & Nawar, 2000). Cow milk contains 0.24 mg to 0. 89 mg/mL; while lysozyme in human milk is 7 - 37 μ g/100 mL (El-Agamy et al. 1998). The equivalent concentration of lysozyme in camel milk was, 8, 10, 11, and 18 times that of goat, sheep, cow and buffalo milk respectively (El-Agamy & Nawar 2000). Heating of camel milk at 65 ° C for 30 min has no effect on lysozymes. However, at 85°C for 30 min, the activity lysozymes were 56, 74, and 81.7% for the unheated milk of camel, cow, and buffalo milk, respectively. Hence camel milk lysozyme is more heat resistant than those of cow and buffalo milk. However, in human milk it loses activity very quickly at 72 °C (Chandan, Shahani, & Holly, 1964). The activity of lysozyme was measured before and after pasteurization against *Clostridium tyrobutyricum, Bacillus megaterium, Bacillus mojavensis, Clavibacter michiganensis, Xanthomonas campestris,* and *Escherichia coli.* The pasteurization did not affect the activity of lysozyme in jenny milk except for *B. mojaventis*, which showed resistance to lysozyme in milk samples subjected to heat treatments (Cosentino et al., 2016).

Vitamins

Water soluble vitamins (i.e. B-Complex and Vitamin C) and fat-soluble vitamins (A, E, D and K) are essential nutrients found in foods (see Chapter 2). They perform a specific function in the body system which is crucial for maintaining optimal health (see Chapter 8). Milk and milk products have different levels of both types of vitamins. It has been demonstrated that camel milk is the richest milk in vitamin C (Mehaia, 1992; El- Agamy, & Nawar 2000; Kamal & Karoui 2017) and niacin (Farah et al 1992). Camel milk has more 4 – 6 times vitamin C than cow milk (Konuspayeva, Faye & Loiseau, 2011). Consumption of two cups of camel milk can supply 160% of the recommended daily intake of vitamin D and riboflavin (Farah, 1996). Camel milk contains comparable levels of thiamin, vitamin B_6 and vitamin B_{12} with cow milk but lower than cow milk in riboflavin (B_2), Pantothenic acid and folate. However, higher contents of water-soluble vitamins are found in camel milk than human milk except pantothenic acid (Jelliffe, & Jelliffe, 1978; El-Agamy, 2009). In general, ruminant milk has higher vitamin content than non-ruminant milk types (human, donkey, and mare milk). Very little information is available about the effect of heat treatments on camel milk vitamins. Vitamin C is the most sensitive vitamins for heat treatments but its heat sensitivity in camel milk is higher than in cow milk (Medhammar et al., 2012). Vitamin loss during heating depends on severity of heat treatment. Renner, (1983) studied the effect of pasteurization, UHT and conventional sterilization on loss of vitamins B1, B2, folic acid and vitamin C. Pasteurization caused loss <10, 0 - 8, <10 and 10 – 25% compared to respectively, 0 – 20, <10, 5 – 20 and 5 – 30% in UHT treatment and 20 – 50, 20 – 50, 30 – 50 and 30 -100% in sterilized milk. Thiamin (B_1) loss during UHT treatment and storage for 60 days were studied by Metwalli, et al. (1988a). The average loss during UHT treatment was in the range 10.03 - 12.46% and the loss increased to 16.07 – 20.29% during storage at room temperature. Mehaia, (1992) studied the effect of heat treatments at different temperature (63, 73, 80, 90 and 100°C for 10, 15 and 30 min), on the loss of vitamin C and riboflavin in camel milk. The results revealed that heating of camel milk at 63, 80, 90 and 100°C for 30 min results in a loss of vitamin C content of about 27, 41, 53 and 67%, respectively. While the losses in cow milk were 18, 26, 36 and 48% in order. No significant loss (0 – 7%) was observed in riboflavin on heating camel and cow milk at different used temperatures. Vitamins A, E, D_3, B_1, B_2, B_6, B_{12} and C were not affected by pasteurization (Wernery, Hanke, Braun & Johnson, 2003). Moreover, only small or no losses have been reported for vitamins B_6, niacin, panthothenic acid, biotin, A, D and E, even during conventional sterilization (Wernery, et al 2003; MacDonald et al. 2011; Claeys, et al. 2013). Losses in fat soluble vitamins (A, E, D and K) are more likely to be caused by sun light and oxygen rather than heat treatments. Vitamins C, folate (B9) and riboflavin (vitamin B2) may completely disappear within a few days in the presence of O2 and exposure to light.

Minerals

Major and trace minerals are bioactive in physiology and metabolism of the human body. There is strong relationship between minerals and the occurrence of some diseases such as osteoporosis, hypertension, cancer, and cardiovascular disease and help body to use carbohydrate, proteins and fat. The contribution of milk minerals to the diet is significant for calcium, phosphorus sodium, potassium, chloride, zinc, and iodine. Mineral content of different types of milk illustrated in Table 1. The mineral content of ruminant milk is much higher than in non-ruminant milk (Table 1). Although there are major differences in the mineral content of milk from different species. Camel milk has a greater amount of Na, K,

Table 1. Mineral content (mg/100 mL) of different species of milk

minerals	Human	Camel	Cow	Buffalo	Goat	Ewe
Ca mg %	28-34	106 - 190	117	184	134	198
Na mg %	10 - 18	69	48 - 58	44.75 - 51	41	27 – 81
K mg %	53-62	156 -170	143	101.6	181	120
Mg mg%	3 - 4	7.4 - 12	11	18 -29	16	18 - 22
P mg %	14-43	72 104	89 -117	85-293	79-153	124-175
Cit mg %	77-80	128	160	177.6	70 - 180	104 – 205
Cl mg %	60	132	110	63.82	150	150
Zn ppm	1.6 – 3.8	4 - 5	3.8 – 4.0	0.2 – 2.4	3.2 – 56	4.0 – 9.0
Fe ppm	0.2 - 0.5	1.3 – 4.4	0.3 – 0.8	0.42 – 2.0	0.5 – 1.0	0.8 – 1.4
Cu mg/L	0.2- 0. 6	1.3 – 1.8	0.1 – 0.8	0.07 – 0.4	0.2 0.5	0.3 -0.5
Ash	0.23	0.6 – 0.9	0.7	0.8	0.8	0.9

Data adopted from: Jilo, & Tegegne, (2016); Medhammar et al., (2012); Abd; El-Salam & El-Shibiny, (2011); El-Agamy, (2009); Pandya & Haenlein, 2009; Shamsia, (2009); Sheng & Fang, (2009); Arthur, Smith,. & Hartmann, (1989)

Zn, Fe, Cu and Mn than bovine milk (Chapter 2). Camel milk contains 1.3 – 4.4 mg/L (Fe), 4 - 5 mg/L (Zn), 1.3 1.8 mg/ L (Cu), (Jilo, & Tegegne, 2016). Medhammar et al., 2012; El-Agamy, 2009; Abd El-Salam & El-Shibiny, 2011; Pandya & Haenlein, 2009; Shamsia, 2009; Sheng & Fang, 2009); while the corresponding values cow milk were 0.3 – 0.8 mg/L, 3.8 – 4.0mg/ L and 0.1 – 0.8 mg/L, respectively. The concentration of Mg and Fe in camels' milk was higher (i.e. 7–20-fold and 4–10-fold, respectively) than in human milk, cows 'milk respectively (Farida & Srikumar, 2001). The concentration of citrate in camel milk is lower than in cow milk, this may give advantage to camel milk in medicinal properties where, lactoferrin activity is enhanced with low levels of citrate. The ratio of Ca: P in camel milk is 1.68 versus 1.13 and 1.08 (Table 1) for cow and human milk respectively.

The heat treatments of milk may have influence on mineral composition in the way that concentration of dietary minerals in heat treated milk is different than concentration in raw milk (Malbe et al., 2010. The pasteurized camel milk at 72°C for 5 min had the same calcium, zinc, copper and iron content with the raw camel milk (Wernery et al. 2003).

CONCLUSION

Camel milk was consumed mainly in fresh form, however due to the technological advancement and currently due to the increased demand for a variety of dairy products a number of camel milk-based products are available on the market. However, the industrial production process of camel milk products is in a very initial stage compared to cow milk-based products. This book chapter assessed the existing study on the effect of industrial production process on camel milk composition, nutritional value and health properties. Camel milk qualitative and quantitative compositions are the vital points that contribute for the variation observed in terms of heat treatment response from camel milk. The absence of β-lactoglobulin in camel milk, presence scarce amount of κ-casein and higher proportion of β-casein are the major contributor. As β-lactoglobulin and κ-casein are known to be involved in heat denaturation due to formation of disulfide bridges in cow milk, their absence in camel milk resulted different response for heat treatment applied at different scale. Application of high-pressure process on camel milk appears as a possible option for production of improved products from camel milk. The presence of bioactive component such as immunoglobulins, lactoferrins, and lysozymes along with promising health functionality may furnish opportunity for product application. However, due to scattered scientific reports existing a confirmation study on some of the effect of heat treatments and health benefits is strategic.

REFERENCES

Abd El-Salam, M. H., & El-Shibiny, S. (2011). A comprehensive review on the composition and properties of buffalo milk. *Dairy Science & Technology*, *91*(6), 663–699. doi:10.100713594-011-0029-2

Abrhaley, A., & Leta, S. (2018). Medicinal value of camel milk and meat. *Journal of Applied Animal Research*, *46*(1), 552–558. doi:10.1080/09712119.2017.1357562

Agrawal, R., Sahani, M., Tuteja, F., Ghouri, S., Sena, D., Gupta, R., & Kochar, D. K. (2005). Hypoglycemic activity of camel milk in chemically pancreatectomized rats-an experimental study. *International Journal of Diabetes in Developing Countries*, *25*(3), 75–79. doi:10.4103/0973-3930.22776

Agrawal, R., Swami, S., Beniwal, R., Kochar, D., Sahani, M., Tuteja, F., & Ghouri, S. (2003). Effect of raw camel milk on glycemic control, risk factors and diabetes quality of life in type-1 diabetes: A randomized prospective controlled study. *Journal of Camel Practice and Research*, *10*, 45–50.

Ahmed, N., & Zubeir, I. E. (2011). Effect of Salt Level on Some Physical and Chemical Properties and Acceptability of Camel Milk Cheese. *Journal of Camelid Science*, *4*, 40–48.

Ajarem, J., Allam, A., Ebaid, H., Maodaa, S., AL-Sobeai, S. M., Rady, A. M., ... Sabri, M. I. (2015). AL-Sobeai S, Rady A, Metwalli A, Altoom N, Ibrahim, & Sabri M (2015) Neurochemical, structural and neurobehavioral evidence of neuronal protection by whey proteins in diabetic albino mice. *Behavioral and Brain Functions*, *11*(1), 7. doi:10.118612993-015-0053-0 PMID:25888881

Al-Attabi, Z., D'arcy, B. R., & Deeth, H. C. (2009). Volatile sulphur compounds in UHT milk. *Critical Reviews in Food Science and Nutrition*, *49*(1), 28–47. doi:10.1080/10408390701764187 PMID:18949597

Al Haj, O. A., & Al Kanhal, H. A. (2010). Compositional, Technological and Nutritional aspects of Dromedary Camel Milk - a Review. *International Dairy Journal*, *20*(12), 811–821. doi:10.1016/j.idairyj.2010.04.003

Al-Juboori, A. T., Mohammed, M., Rashid, J., Kurian, J., & El Refaey, S. (2013). Nutritional and medicinal value of camel (*Camelus dromedarius*) milk. *WIT Transactions on Ecology and The Environment*, *170*, 221–232. doi:10.2495/FENV130201

Alhaj, O. A., Al-Khalifa, A. S., Metwalli, A. A., Ismail, E. & Ali, H. S. (2017). *Method of making a fermented dairy product from camel milk.* Patent Number: 9623057.

Alhaj, O. A., Metwalli, A. A. M., & Ismail El, A. (2011). Heat Stability of Camel Milk Proteins after Sterilisation Process. *Journal of Camel Practice and Research*, *18*(2), 277–282.

Anema, S. G., Lowe, E. K., & Stockman, R. (2005a). Particle size changes and casein solubilization in high-pressure-treated skim milk. *Food Hydrocolloids*, *19*(2), 257–267. doi:10.1016/j.foodhyd.2004.04.025

Anema, S. G., Stockman, R., & Lowe, E. K. (2005b). Denaturation Of Β-Lactoglobulin In Pressure Treated Skim Milk. *Journal of Agricultural and Food Chemistry*, *53*(20), 7783–7791. doi:10.1021/jf050326x PMID:16190631

Arias, M., Lopez-Fandino, R., & Olano, A. (2000). Influence of PH on the Effects of High Pressure on Milk. *Milchwissenchaft*, *55*(4), 191–194.

Arthur, P. G., Smith, M., & Hartmann, P. (1989). Milk lactose, citrate and glucose as markers of lactogenesis in normal and diabetic women. *Journal of Pediatric Gastroenterology and Nutrition*, *90*(4), 488–496. doi:10.1097/00005176-198911000-00016 PMID:2621526

Badr, G. (2013). Camel whey protein enhances diabetic wound-healing in a streptozotocin-induced diabetic mouse model: The critical role of β-defensin-1, -2 and -3. *Lipids in Health and Disease*, *12*(1), 46. doi:10.1186/1476-511X-12-46 PMID:23547923

Badr, G., Mohany, M., & Metwalli, A. (2011). Effects of undenatured whey protein supplementation on CXCL12- and CCL21-mediated B and T cell chemotaxis in diabetic mice. *Lipids in Health and Disease*, *9*(10), 203. doi:10.1186/1476-511X-10-203 PMID:22070978

Balny, C., & Masson, P. (1993). Effects of High Pressure on Proteins. *Food Reviews International*, *9*(4), 611–628. doi:10.1080/87559129309540980

Barłowska, J., Szwajkowska, M., Litwińczuk, Z., & Król, J. (2011). Nutritional Value and Technological Suitability of Milk from Various Animal Species Used for Dairy Production. *Comprehensive Reviews in Food Science and Food Safety*, *10*(6), 291–302. doi:10.1111/j.1541-4337.2011.00163.x

Bekele, B., Hansen, E. B., Eshetu, M., Ipsen, R., & Hailu, Y. (2019). Effect of starter cultures on properties of soft white cheese made from camel (*Camelus dromedarius*) milk. *Journal of Dairy Science*, *102*(2), 1108–1115. doi:10.3168/jds.2018-15084 PMID:30591338

Benabdelkamel, H., Masood, A., Alanazi, I. O., Alzahrani, D. A., Alrabiah, D. K., AlYahya, S. A., & Alfadda, A. A. (2017). Proteomic profiling comparing the effects of different 121 heat treatments on camel (*Camelus dromedarius*) milk whey proteins. *International Journal of Molecular Sciences*, *18*(4), 2–15. doi:10.3390/ijms18040721 PMID:28350354

Berg, E. H. (1992). *Reaction of lactose during heat treatment of milk: A quantitative study* (Ph.D Thesis). Wageningen Agricultural University, The Netherlands.

Berhe, T., Ipsen, R., Seifu, E., Kurtu, M. Y., Eshetu, M., & Hansen, E. B. (2018). Comparison of the Acidification Activities of Commercial Starter Cultures in Camel and Bovine Milk. *Lebensmittel-Wissenschaft + Technologie*, *89*, 123–127. doi:10.1016/j.lwt.2017.10.041

Berhe, T., Seifu, E., Ipsen, R., Kurtu, M. Y., & Hansen, E. B. (2017). Processing Challenges and Opportunities of Camel Dairy Products. *International Journal of Food Sciences*, *2*, 1–8. doi:10.1155/2017/9061757 PMID:29109953

Bornaz, S., Sahli, A., Attalah, A., & Attia, H. (2009). Physicochemical Characteristics and Renneting Properties of Camels' Milk: A Comparison with Goats', Ewes' and Cows' Milks. *International Journal of Dairy Technology*, *62*(4), 505–513. doi:10.1111/j.1471-0307.2009.00535.x

Boumpa, T., Tsioulpas, A., Grandison, A. S., & Lewis, M. J. (2008). Effects of phosphates and citrates on sediment formation in UHT goats' milk. *The Journal of Dairy Research*, *75*(2), 160–166. doi:10.1017/S0022029908003166 PMID:18474132

Brezovečki, A., Čagalj, M., Dermit, Z. F., Mikulec, N., Ljoljić, D. B., & Antunac, N. (2015). Camel Milk and Milk Products. *Camel Milk. Mljekarstvo*, *65*, 81–90.

Buchheim, W., & Abou El Nour, A. M. (1992). Induction of Milkfat Crystallisation In the Emulsified State by High Hydrostatic Pressure. *Fett Wissenschaft Technologie*, *94*(10), 369–373. doi:10.1002/lipi.19920941003

Buffa, M., Trujillo, A. J., & Guamis, B. (2001a). Rennet Coagulation Properties of Raw, Pasteurised And High Pressure-Treated Goat Milk. *Milchwissenschaft. Milk Science International*, *56*(5), 243–246.

Buffa, M., Trujillo, A. J., & Guamis, B. (2001b). Changes in Textural, Microstructure, And Colour Characteristics During Ripening of Cheeses Made from Raw, Pasteurised Or High-Pressure-Treated Goats' Milk. *International Dairy Journal*, *11*(11–12), 927–934. doi:10.1016/S0958-6946(01)00141-8

Butz, P., Zielinski, B., Ludwig, H., & Tauscher, B. (1999). The Influence of High Pressure on The Autoxidation of Major Unsaturated Fatty Acid Constituents of Milk. In H. Ludwig (Ed.), *Advances in High Pressure Bioscience and Biotechnology* (pp. 453–456). Heidelberg, Germany: Springer. doi:10.1007/978-3-642-60196-5_82

Bylund, G. (2003). *Dairy processing handbook*. Tetra Pak Processing Systems AB.

Cadesky, L., Walkling-Ribeiro, M., Kriner, K. T., Karwe, M. V., & Moraru, C. I. (2017). Structural changes induced by high-pressure processing in micellar casein and milk protein concentrates. *Journal of Dairy Science*, *100*(9), 7055–7070. doi:10.3168/jds.2016-12072 PMID:28647329

Capellas, M., Mor-Mur, M., & Needs, E. C. (2001). *Physical Properties of Yoghurt from Pressurised Concentrated and Fortified Milks*. In Eurocaft Meeting, Berlin, Germany.

Chandan, R. C., Shahani, K. M., & Holly, R. G. (1964). Lysozyme Content of Human Milk. *Nature*, *204*(4953), 76–77. doi:10.1038/204076a0 PMID:14240122

Chaplin, L. C., & Lyster, R. L. J. (1988). Effect of Temperature on The Ph Of Skim Milk. *The Journal of Dairy Research*, *55*(2), 280. doi:10.1017/S0022029900026108

Cheftel, J. C. (1995). Review: High-Pressure, Microbial Inactivation and Food Preservation. *Food Science & Technology International*, *1*(2–3), 75–90. doi:10.1177/108201329500100203

Chen, B. Y., Grandison, A. S., & Lewis, M. J. (2012). Comparison of Heat Stability of Goat Milk Subjected to Ultra-High Temperature and In-Container Sterilization. *Journal of Dairy Science*, *95*(3), 1057–1063. doi:10.3168/jds.2011-4367 PMID:22365189

Claeys, W. L., Cardoen, S., Daube, G., De Block, J., Dewettinck, K., Dierick, K., ... Herman, L. (2013). Raw or heated cow milk consumption: Review of risks and benefits. *Food Control*, *31*(1), 251–262. doi:10.1016/j.foodcont.2012.09.035

Considine, T., Patel, H. A., Anema, S. G., Singh, H., & Creamer, L. K. (2007). Interactions of milk proteins during heat and high hydrostatic pressure treatments— A Review. *Innovative Food Science & Emerging Technologies*, *8*(1), 1–23. doi:10.1016/j.ifset.2006.08.003

Cosentino, C., Labell, C., & Elshafie, H. S. (2016). Effects of different heat treatments on lysozyme quantity and antimicrobial activity of jenny milk. *Journal of Dairy Science*, *99*(7), 5173–5179. doi:10.3168/jds.2015-10702 PMID:27157571

Costabel, L. M., Bergamini, C., Vaudagna, S. R., Cuatrin, A. L., Audero, G., & Hynes, E. (2016). Effect of high-pressure treatment on hard cheese proteolysis. *Journal of Dairy Science*, *99*(6), 4220–4232. doi:10.3168/jds.2015-9907 PMID:27016833

Cronshaw, H. B. (1947). *Dairy Information*. London: Dairy Industries Ltd.

Datta, N., & Deeth, H. C. (2007). *Advances in Thermal and Non-Thermal Food Preservation*. Ames, IA: Blackwell Publishing. doi:10.1002/9780470277898.ch4

Datta, N., Elliott, A. J., Perkins, M. L., & Deeth, H. C. (2002). Ultra-high-temperature (UHT) treatment of milk: Comparison of direct and indirect mods of heating. *Australian Journal of Dairy Technology*, *57*(3), 211–227.

Davis, J. G. (1955). *A Dictionary of Dairying (2nd ed.)*. London: Leonard Hill.

Deeth, H. C. (2002). Lipolysis in Milk and Dairy Products – A Research Journey. *Food Australia*, *54*, 433–436.

Deeth, H. C., & Datta, N. (2011). Heat Treatment of Milk; Ultra-High Temperature Treatment (UHT): Heating Systems. In Encyclopedia of Dairy Sciences (2nd ed.; pp. 699-707). San Diego, CA: Academic Press.

Desorby-Banon, S., Richard, F., & Hardy, J. (1994). Study of Acid and Rennet Coagulation of High Pressurized Milk. *Journal of Dairy Science*, *77*(11), 3267–3274. doi:10.3168/jds.S0022-0302(94)77267-2

Devi, A. F., Buckow, R., Singh, T., Hemar, Y., & Kasapis, S. (2015). Colour Change and Proteolysis of Skim Milk during High Pressure Thermal–Processing. *Journal of Food Engineering*, *147*, 102–110. doi:10.1016/j.jfoodeng.2014.09.017

Dunne, C. P. (2005). *High Pressure Keeps Food Fresher*. Available At http://www.Natick.Army.Mil/About/Pao/05/05-22.Htm

Earnshaw, R. (1996). High Pressure Food Processing. *Nutrition & Food Science*, *2*(2), 8–11. doi:10.1108/00346659610108966

Ebaid, H., Abdel-Salam, B., Hassan, I., Al-Tamimi, J., Metwalli, A., & Alhazza, I. (2017). Erratum to: Camel milk peptide improves wound healing in diabetic rats by orchestrating the redox status and immune response. *Lipids in Health and Disease*, *16*(1), 43. doi:10.118612944-017-0421-x PMID:28219371

Ebaid, H., Salem, A., Sayed, A., & Metwalli, A. (2011). Whey protein enhances normal inflammatory responses during cutaneous wound healing in diabetic rats. *Lipids in Health and Disease*, *10*(1), 235. doi:10.1186/1476-511X-10-235 PMID:22168406

Eberhard, P., Strahm, W., & Eyer, H. (1999). High Pressure Treatment of Whipped Cream. *Agrarforschung*, *6*(9), 352–354.

Ejtahed, H., Niasari Naslaji, A., Mirmiran, P., Zraif Yeganeh, M., Hedayati, M., Azizi, F., & Moosavi Movahedi, A. (2014). Effect of Camel Milk on Blood Sugar and Lipid Profile of Patients with Type 2 Diabetes: A Pilot Clinical Trial. *International Journal of Endocrinology and Metabolism, 13*(1). doi:10.5812/ijem.21160 PMID:25745496

Eksterend, B., Larsson, M., & Perlmann, C. (1980). Casein micelle size and composition related to the enzymatic coagulation process. *Biochimica et Biophysica Acta*, *660*(3), 361–366. doi:10.1016/0304-4165(80)90284-6 PMID:6772232

El-Agamy, E. I. (1989). *Biological activity of protective proteins of camel milk against pathogenic and nonpathogenic bacteria and viruses* (Ph.D. Thesis). Alexandria University, Alexandria, Egypt.

El-Agamy, E. I. (1998). Antimicrobial factors and nutritive value of human milk and other species. Journal of Agricultural Science. *Mansoura University.*, *23*, 245–254.

El-Agamy, E. I. (2000). Effect of heat treatment on camel milk proteins with respect to antimicrobial factors: A comparison with cows' and buffalo milk proteins. *Food Chemistry*, *68*(2), 227–232. doi:10.1016/S0308-8146(99)00199-5

El-Agamy, E. I. (2009). Chapter 6: bioactive components in camel milk. In Y.W. Park (Ed.), Bioactive components in milk and dairy products (pp. 159-194). Wiley-Blackwell.

El-Hatmi, H., Levieux, A., & Levieux, D. (2006). Camel (Camelus dromedarius) immunoglobulin G, α-lactalbumin, serum albumin and lactoferrin in colostrum and milk during the early postpartum period. *The Journal of Dairy Research*, *73*(3), 288–293. doi:10.1017/S0022029906001713 PMID:16566855

El-Zeini, H. M. (2006). Microstructure, rheological and geometrical properties of fat globules of milk from different animal species. *Polish Journal of Food and Nutrition Sciences*, *15*, 147–154.

Elhasan, S. M., Bushara, A. M., Abdelhakam, K. E., Elfaki, H. A., Eibaid, A. I., Farahat, F. H., & Sukrab, A. M. (2017). Effect of heat treatments on physico-chemical properties of milk samples. [JAIR]. *Journal of Academia and Industrial Research*, *6*, 40–46.

Enright, J. B., Sadler, W. W., & Thomas, R. C. (1957). Thermal Inactivation of *Coxiella Burnetii* and Its Relation to Pasteurization of Milk. *American Journal of Public Health*, *47*, 695–700. doi:10.2105/AJPH.47.6.695 PMID:13424814

Fantuz, F., Salimei, E., & Papademas, P. (2016). Macro-and micronutrients in non-cow milk and products and their impact on human health. In *Non-Bovine Milk and Milk Products* (pp. 209–261). Cambridge, UK: Academic Press. doi:10.1016/B978-0-12-803361-6.00009-0

FAO. (2013). Milk and Dairy Products in Human Nutrition. Rome: Wiley-Blackwell. doi:10.1186/1471-2458-11-95

Farah, Z. (1986). Effect of Heat Treatment on Whey Proteins of Camel Milk. *Milchwissenschaft. Milk Science International, 41*(12), 763–765.

Farah, Z. (1996). *Camel milk properties and products*. St. Gallen, Switzerland: SKAT.

Farah, Z., Eberhard, P., Meyer, J., Rehberger, B., Thomet, A., & Gallmann, P. U. (2004). *UHT processing of camel milk*. Retrieved from http://www.agroscope.admin.ch/publikationen/einzelpublikation/index.html?lang=en&aid=11827&pid=19150

Farah, Z., Rettenmayer, R., & Atkins, D. (1992). Vitamin content of camel milk. *International Journal for Vitamin and Nutrition Research, 62*, 30–33. PMID:1587705

Farah, Z., & Rüegg, M. W. (1989). The size distribution of casein micelles in camel milk. *Food Microstructure, 8*, 211–216.

Farah, Z., & Ruegg, M. W. (1991). The creaming properties and size distribution of fat globules in camel milk. *Journal of Dairy Science, 74*(9), 2901–2904. doi:10.3168/jds.S0022-0302(91)78472-5

Farah, Z., Streiff, T., & Bachmann, M. R. (1990). Preparation and Consumer Acceptability Tests of Fermented Camel Milk in Kenya. *The Journal of Dairy Research, 57*(2), 281–283. doi:10.1017/S002202990002690X

Farida, M., & Srikumar, T. (2001). Trace elements and their distribution in protein fractions of camel milk in comparison to other commonly milks. *The Journal of Dairy Research, 68*(3), 463–469. doi:10.1017/S0022029901005003 PMID:11694048

Farkas, D. F., & Hoover, D. G. (2000). High Pressure Processing: Kinetics of Microbial Inactivation for Alternative Food Processing Technologies. *Journal of Food Science, 65*, 47–64. doi:10.1111/j.1750-3841.2000.tb00618.x

Felfoul, I., Jardin, J., Gaucheron, F., Attia, H., & Ayadi, M. A. (2017). Proteomic Profiling of Camel and Cow Milk Proteins under Heat Treatment. *Food Chemistry, 216*, 161–169. doi:10.1016/j.foodchem.2016.08.007 PMID:27596405

Feligini, M., Bonizzi, I., Buffoni, J. N., Cosenza, G., & Ramunno, L. (2009). Identification and Quantification of α_{S1}, α_{S2}, β, and κ-Caseins in Water Buffalo Milk by Reverse Phase-High Performance Liquid Chromatography and Mass Spectrometry. *Journal of Agricultural and Food Chemistry, 57*(7), 2988–2992. doi:10.1021/jf803653v PMID:19256489

Ferragut, V., Martinez, V. M., Trujillo, A. J., & Guamis, B. (2000). Properties of Yogurts Made from Whole Ewe's Milk Treated by High Hydrostatic Pressure. *Milchwissenschaft. Milk Science International, 55*(5), 267–269.

Fitria, A., Buckow, R., Singh, T., Hemar, Y., & Kasapis, S. (2015). Colour change and proteolysis of skim milk during high pressure thermal-processing. *Journal of Food Engineering, 147*, 102–110. doi:10.1016/j.jfoodeng.2014.09.017

Fox, P. F. (2003). The major constituents of milk. In G. Smit (Ed.), *Dairy Processing, Improving Quality* (pp. 5–38). Cambridge, UK: Woodhead Publishing Limited. doi:10.1533/9781855737075.1.5

Fuente, M. A., Olano, A., Casal, V., & Juárez, M. (1999). Effects of high pressure and heat treatment on the mineral balance of goats' milk. *The Journal of Dairy Research*, *66*(1), 65–72. doi:10.1017/S0022029998003264 PMID:10191474

Garcella, H. G., Garciab, E. G., Pueyob, P. V., Martínb, I. R., Arias, A. V., & Serranoa, R. N. A. (2016). Outbreaks of brucellosis related to the consumption of unpasteurized camel milk. *Journal of Infection and Public Health*, *9*(4), 523–527. doi:10.1016/j.jiph.2015.12.006 PMID:26796768

Gaucheron, F., Famelart, M. H., Mariette, F., Raulot, K., & Michel, F. (1997). Combined Effects of Temperature and High-Pressure Treatments on Physicochemical Characteristics of Skim Milk. *Food Chemistry*, *59*(3), 439–447. doi:10.1016/S0308-8146(96)00301-9

Gedam, K., Prasad, R., & Vijay, V. K. (2007). The Study on UHT Processing of Milk: A Versatile Option for Rural Sector. *World Journal of Dairy & Food Sciences*, *2*(2), 49–53.

Genene, A., Hansen, E. B., Eshetua, M., Hailu, Y., & Ipsen, R. (2019). Effect of Heat Treatment on Denaturation of Whey Protein and Resultant Rennetability of Camel Milk. *Lebensmittel-Wissenschaft + Technologie*, *101*, 404–409. doi:10.1016/j.lwt.2018.11.047

Gervilla, R., Capellas, M., Ferragut, V., & Guamis, B. (1997). Effect of High Hydrostatic Pressure on Listeria Innocua 910 CECT. *Journal of Food Protection*, *60*(1), 33–37. doi:10.4315/0362-028X-60.1.33 PMID:10465037

Gervilla, R., Ferragut, V., & Guamis, B. (2001). High Hydrostatic Pressure Effects on Color and Milk-Fat Globule of Ewe's Milk. *Journal of Food Science*, *66*(6), 880–885. doi:10.1111/j.1365-2621.2001.tb15190.x

Gervilla, R., Ferragut, V., & Guamis, B. (2001). High Hydrostatic Pressure Effects on Colour and Milk-Fat Globule of Ewe's Milk. *Journal of Food Science*, *66*(6), 880–885. doi:10.1111/j.1365-2621.2001.tb15190.x

Goyal, A., Sharma, V., Upadhyay, N., Sihag, M., & Kaushik, R. (2013). High Pressure Processing and Its Impact on Milk Proteins: A Review. *Journal of Dairy Science and Technology*, *2*, 1–9.

Griffiths, M. W. (2010). Improving the safety and quality of milk. In *Milk production and processing* (Vol. 1). Guelph, Canada: Woodhead Publishing Limited, University of Guelph.

Hailu, Y., Hansen, E. B., Seifu, E., Eshetu, M., Ipsen, R., & Kappeler, S. (2016a). Functional and Technological Properties of Camel Milk Proteins: A Review. *The Journal of Dairy Research*, *83*(4), 422–429. doi:10.1017/S0022029916000686 PMID:27845026

Ham, J. S., Shin, J. H., Noh, Y. B., Jeong, S. G., Han, G. S., Chae, H. S., ... Jo, C. (2008). Chemical and Microbiological Quality, Capillary Electrophoresis Pattern, and Rennet Coagulation of UHT-Treated and Irradiated Milk. *Food Science and Biotechnology*, *17*, 58–65.

Hamad, E. M., Abdel-Rahim, E. A., & Romeih, E. A. (2011). Beneficial effect of camel milk on liver and kidney function in diabetic Sprague-Dawley rats. *International Dairy Science*, *6*(3), 190–197. doi:10.3923/ijds.2011.190.197

Hamad, S. H., Al Eid, S. M., Al Jassas, F. M., & Abu Tarboush, H. (2013). *Use of High Hydrostatic Pressure for The Preservation of Camel's Milk*. International Conference Animal & Dairy Sciences, Las Vegas, NV.

Hamoud, A. M. (2015). *Characterisation of proteins in camel milk, the effect of heat treatment on physicochemical and functional properties related to yogurt* (PhD thesis). School of Life Sciences, Heriot-Watt University.

Hassl, M., Jorgensen, B. D., & Janhoj, T. (2011). Rennet gelation properties of ultrafiltration retentates from camel milk. *Milchwissenschaft. Milk Science International*, *66*, 80–84.

Hayakawa, I., Kanno, T., Yoshiyama, K., & Fujio, Y. (1994). Oscillatory Compared with Continuous High-Pressure Sterilization on *Bacillus Stearothermophilus* Spores. *Journal of Food Science*, *59*(1), 164–167. doi:10.1111/j.1365-2621.1994.tb06924.x

Hendrickx, M. L., Van Den, B. I., & Weemaes, C. (1998). Effects of High Pressure on Enzymes Related to Food Quality. *Trends in Food Science & Technology*, *9*(5), 197–203. doi:10.1016/S0924-2244(98)00039-9

Hite, B. H. (1899). The Effect of Pressure in the Preservation of Milk. *West Virginia Agricultural Experimental Station Bulletin*, *58*, 15–35.

Huppertz, T., Fox, P. F., & Kelly, A. L. (2004). High Pressure Treatment of Bovine Milk: Effects on Casein Micelles and Whey Proteins. *The Journal of Dairy Research*, *71*(1), 97–106. doi:10.1017/S002202990300640X PMID:15068072

Huppertz, T., Hinza, K., Zobrista, M. R., Uniacke, T., Kellya, A. L., & Fox, P. F. (2005). Effects of High-Pressure Treatment on The Rennet Coagulation and Cheesemaking Properties of Heated Milk. *Innovative Food Science & Emerging Technologies*, *6*(3), 279–285. doi:10.1016/j.ifset.2005.03.005

Huppertz, T., Smiddy, M. A., Upadhyay, V., & Kelly, A. L. (2006). High-Pressure-Induced Changes in Bovine Milk: A Review. *International Journal of Dairy Technology*, *59*(2), 58–66. doi:10.1111/j.1471-0307.2006.00246.x PMID:16410058

Ibrahim, A. H. (2015). Effects of exopolysaccharide-producing starter cultures on physicochemical, rheological and sensory properties of fermented camel's milk. *Emirates Journal of Food and Agriculture*, *27*(4), 373–384. doi:10.9755/ejfa.v27i4.19911

IDF. (1984). *The Thermization Of Milk, Document No. 182*. Brussels: International Dairy Federation.

Jelliffe, D. B., & Jelliffe, E. F. (1978). *Human milk in the modern world: Psychosocial, nutritional and economic significance*. Oxford, UK: Oxford University Press. doi:10.1136/bmj.2.6151.1573

Jilo, K., & Tegegne, D. (2016). Chemical composition and medicinal values of camel milk. *International Journal of Research Studies in Biosciences*, *4*, 13–25.

Johnston, D. E., Austin, B. A., & Murphy, P. M. (1992). Effects of High Hydrostatic Pressure on Milk. *Milchwissenchaft*, *47*, 760–763.

Johnston, D. E., Austin, B. A., & Murphy, R. J. (1992). Effects of High Hydrostatic Pressure on Milk. *Milchwissenschaft. Milk Science International*, *47*(12), 760–763.

Johnston, D. E., Murphy, R. J., & Birks, A. W. (1994). Stirred-Style Yogurt-Type Product Prepared from Pressure Treated Skim-Milk. *High Pressure Research*, *12*(4-6), 215–219. doi:10.1080/08957959408201660

Juffs, H., & Deeth, H. C. (2007). *Scientific Evaluation of Pasteurisation For Pathogen Reduction in Milk and Milk Products*. Canberra: Food Standards Australia and New Zealand.

Kamal, M., Foukani, M., & Karoui, R. (2017). Effects of heating and calcium and phosphate mineral supplementation on the physical properties of rennet-induced coagulation of camel and cow milk gels. *The Journal of Dairy Research*, *84*(2), 220–228. doi:10.1017/S0022029917000152 PMID:28524011

Kamal, M., & Karoui, R. (2017). Monitoring of mild heat treatment of camel milk by front-face fluorescence spectroscopy. *Lebensmittel-Wissenschaft + Technologie*, *79*, 586–593. doi:10.1016/j.lwt.2016.11.013

Kappeler, S., Farah, Z., & Puhan, Z. (1998). Sequence Analysis of *Camelus Dromedarius* Milk Caseins. *The Journal of Dairy Research*, *65*(2), 209–222. doi:10.1017/S0022029997002847 PMID:9627840

Kaushik, R., Sachdeva, B., Arora, S., & Gupta, C. (2015). Effect of content on sensory and physico-chemical properties of laboratory-pasteurized calcium and vitamin D-fortified mixture of cow and buffalo milk. *International Journal of Dairy Technology*, *68*(1), 135–143. doi:10.1111/1471-0307.12166

Khalesi, M., Salami, M., Moslehishad, M., Winterburn, J., & Moosavi-Movahedi, A. A. (2017). Biomolecular content of camel milk: A traditional superfood t owards future healthcare industry. *Trends in Food Science & Technology*, *62*, 49–58. doi:10.1016/j.tifs.2017.02.004

Khan, H., Athar, I. H., & Aslam, M. (2004). Evaluation of Cheese Prepared by Processing Camel Milk. *Pakistan Journal of Zoology*, *36*, 323–326.

Kim, H. Y., Kim, S. H., Choi, M. J., Min, S. G., & Kwak, H. S. (2008). The Effect of High Pressure–Low Temperature Treatment on Physicochemical Properties in Milk. *Journal of Dairy Science*, *91*(11), 4176–4282. doi:10.3168/jds.2007-0883 PMID:18946121

Kolakowski, P., Reps, A., Dajnowiec, F., Szczepek, J., & Porowski, S. (1997). Effect of High Pressures on The Microflora of Raw Cow's Milk. In Proceedings of Process Optimization and Minimal Processing of Foods. Leuven, Belgium: Leuven University Press.

Konuspayeva, G., Camier, B., Gaucheron, F., & Faye, B. (2014). Some parameters to process camel milk into cheese. *Emirates Journal of Food and Agriculture*, *26*(4), 354–358. doi:10.9755/ejfa.v26i4.17277

Konuspayeva, G., Faye, B., & Loiseau, G. (2011). Variability of vitamin C content in camel milk from Kazakhstan. *Journal of Camelid Science*, *4*, 63–69.

Konuspayeva, G., Faye, B., Loiseau, G., & Levieux, D. (2007). Lactoferrin and mmunoglobulin Contents in Camel's Milk (*Camelus bactrianus, Camelus dromedarius,* and Hybrids) from Kazakhstan. *Journal of Dairy Science*, *90*(1), 38–46. doi:10.3168/jds.S0022-0302(07)72606-1 PMID:17183073

Korhonen, H. J. (2009). Bioactive Components in Bovine Milk. In Bioactive Components in Milk and Dairy Products (pp. 15-42). Wiley-Blackwell. doi:10.1002/9780813821504.ch2

Krebbers, B., Matser, A., Hoogerwerf, S., Moezelaar, R., Tomassen, M., & Berg, R. (2003). Combined High-Pressure and Thermal Treatments for Processing of Tomato Puree: Evaluation of Microbial Inactivation and Quality Parameters. *Innovative Food Science & Emerging Technologies*, *4*(4), 377–385. doi:10.1016/S1466-8564(03)00045-6

Lacotte, P., Gomez, F., Bardeau, F., Muller, S., Acharid, A., Quervel, X., ... Birlouez-Aragon, I. (2015). A fluorescence-based analyzer to assess cheese milk denatured whey proteins. *Journal of Dairy Science*, *98*(10), 1–10. doi:10.3168/jds.2015-9412 PMID:26210276

Law, A. J. R., Leaver, J., Felipe, X., Ferragut, V., Pla, R., & Guamis, B. (1998). Comparison of The Effects of High Pressure and Thermal Treatments on The Casein Micelles in Goat's Milk. *Journal of Agricultural and Food Chemistry*, *46*(7), 2523–2530. doi:10.1021/jf970904c

Lewis, M. J., & Heppell, N. (2000). *Continuous Thermal Processing of Foods: Pasteurization and UHT Sterilization*. Gaithersburg, MD: Aspen Publishers.

Liepa, M., Zagorska, J., & Galoburda, R. (2017). Effect of High Pressure Processing on Milk Coagulation Properties. *Research for Rural Development*, *1*, 223–229. doi:10.22616/rrd.23.2017.033

Liepa, M., Zagorska, J., Galoburda, R., & Kostascuka, S. (2018). Effect of High-Pressure Processing on Microbial Quality of Skimmed Milk. Proc. Latvian Acad. *Sci., Section B*, *72*, 118–122.

Lomholt, S. B., & Qvist, K. B. (1997). Relationship between Rheological Properties and Degree of K-Casein Proteolysis During Renneting Of Milk. *The Journal of Dairy Research*, *64*(4), 541–549. doi:10.1017/S002202999700246X

López-Fandiño, R. (2006). High pressure-induced changes in milk proteins and possible applications in dairy technology. *International Dairy Journal*, *16*(10), 1119–1131. doi:10.1016/j.idairyj.2005.11.007

Lopez Fandino, R., Carrascosa, A. V., & Olano, A. (1996). The Effects of High Pressure on Whey Protein Denaturation and Cheese-Making Properties of Raw Milk. *Journal of Dairy Science*, *79*(6), 929–1126. doi:10.3168/jds.S0022-0302(96)76443-3

Lopez Fandino, R., De La Fuente, M. A., Ramos, M., & Olano, A. (1998). Distribution of Minerals and Proteins between the Soluble and Colloidal Phases of Pressurized Milks from Different Species. *The Journal of Dairy Research*, *65*(1), 69–78. doi:10.1017/S0022029997002653

Lore, T. A., Mbugua, S. K., & Wangoh, J. (2005). Enumeration and Identification of Microflora In Suusac, A Kenyan Traditional Fermented Camel Milk Product. *Lebensmittel-Wissenschaft + Technologie*, *38*(2), 125–130. doi:10.1016/j.lwt.2004.05.008

Ma, Y., & Barbano, D. M. (2003). Milk pH As A Function Of co2 Concentration, Temperature, And Pressure in A Heat Exchanger. *Journal of Dairy Science*, *86*(12), 3822–3830. doi:10.3168/jds.S0022-0302(03)73989-7 PMID:14740816

MacDonald, L. E., Brett, J., Kelton, D., Majowicz, S. E., Snedeker, K., & Sargeant, J. M. (2011). A systematic review and meta-analysis of the effects of pasteurization on milk vitamins, and evidence for raw milk consumption and other health related outcomes. *Journal of Food Protection*, *74*(11), 1814–1832. doi:10.4315/0362-028X.JFP-10-269 PMID:22054181

Mal, G., & Pathak, K. M. L. (2009). *Camel Milk- properties and its products*. 2nd conference of ISO-CARD-2009, Djerba, Tunisia.

Malacarne, M., Martuzzi, F., Summer, A., & Mariani, P. (2002). Protein and fat composition of mare's milk: Some nutritional remarks with reference to human and cow's milk. *International Dairy Journal, 12*(11), 869–877. doi:10.1016/S0958-6946(02)00120-6

Malbe, M., Otstavel, T., Kodis, I. & Viitak, A. (2010). Content of selected micro and macro elements in dairy cows. *Agronomy Research, 8*(S2), 323-26.

Malmgren, B. (2015). *Challenges in processing of goat, buffalo and camel milk for longer shelf life*. Presentation to 7th international symposium on Sheep, Goat and other non-cow milk, Limossol, Cyprus.

McClements, J. M. J., Patterson, M. F., & Linton, M. (2001). The effect of growth stage and growth temperature in high hydrostatic pressure inactivation of some psychotropic bacteria in milk. *Journal of Food Protection, 64*(4), 514–522. doi:10.4315/0362-028X-64.4.514 PMID:11307889

Medhammar, E., Wijesinha-Bettoni, R., Stadlmayr, B., Nilsson, E., Charrondiere, U. R., & Burlingame, B. (2012). Composition of milk from minor dairy animals and buffalo breeds: a biodiversity perspective. *Journal of the Science of Food and Agriculture, 92*, 445-474.

Metwalli, A., Mahmoud, A., Ebaid, H., Ahmed, O. M., & Ahmed, R. R. (2015). Up-regulation of Hsp72 and keratin16 mediates wound healing in streptozotocin diabetic rats. *Biological Research, 48*(1), 54. doi:10.118640659-015-0044-5 PMID:26428860

Metwalli, A. A. M. (1992). *Changes in casein micellar structure during heating in the presence and absence of whey proteins* (Thesis). Minia University, Egypt.

Metwalli, A. A. M., Ismail, E. A., Alhaj, O. A., Saleh, K. A., & Ibrahim, F. S. (2013). The Effect of Urea and Formaldehyde on Heat Coagulation Time (HCT) Of Camel Milk. *Life Science Journal, 10*(3), 2113–2119.

Metwalli, N. H., Shalabi, S. I., Bayoumi, S. E., & Metwalli, A. A. M. (1988a). Effect of Ultra-High Temperature and Subsequent Storage on the Constituent of Recombined Milk: 1- Selected Chemical Characteristics and Nitrogen Distribution. *Minia Journal of Agricultural. Research for Development, 10*(3), 1225-1240.

Mohamed, M. A., Larsson-Raznikiewicz, M., & Mohamud, M. A. (1990). Hard cheese making from camel milk. *Milchwissenschaft. Milk Science International, 45*, 716–718.

Moustafa, M. G. F., Abdel-Mohsen, A. M., Ebaid, H., Hassan, I., & Al-Tamimi, J. (2016). Wound healing of different molecular weight of hyaluronan; in-vivo study. *International Journal of Biological Macromolecules, 89*, 582–591. doi:10.1016/j.ijbiomac.2016.05.021 PMID:27174907

Mullaicharam, A. R. (2014). A review on medicinal properties of camel milk. *World Journal of pharmaceutic. Science, 2*, 237–242.

Needs, E. C., Stenning, R. A., Gill, A., Ferragut, V., & Rich, G. T. (2000). High-Pressure Treatment of Milk: Effects on Casein Micelle Structure and On Enzymic Coagulation. *The Journal of Dairy Research, 67*(1), 31–42. doi:10.1017/S0022029999004021 PMID:10717841

Niaz, B., Zahoor, T., Randhawa, M. A., & Jamil, I. A. (2017). Solation of Lactoferrin from Camel Milk through Fast Protein Liquid Chromatography and its Antagonistic Activity against *Escherichia coli* and *Staphylococcus aureus*. *Pakistan Journal of Zoology*, *49*(4), 1307–1313. doi:10.17582/journal.pjz/2017.49.4.1307.1313

Oldfield, D. J., Taylor, M. W., & Singh, H. (2005). Effect of preheating and other process parameters on whey protein reactions during skim milk powder manufacture. *International Dairy Journal*, *15*(5), 501–511. doi:10.1016/j.idairyj.2004.09.004

Omar, A., Harbourne, N., & Oruna-Concha, M. J. (2018). Effects of industrial processing methods on camel skimmed milk properties. *International Dairy Journal*, *84*, 15–22. doi:10.1016/j.idairyj.2018.03.011

Pan, Y., Rowney, M., Guo, P., & Hobman, P. (2007). Biological properties of lactoferrin: An overview. *Australian Journal of Dairy Technology*, *62*, 31–42.

Pandya, A. J., & Haenlein, G. F. W. (2009). Chapter 5: bioactive components in buffalo milk. In Y. W. Park (Ed.), Bioactive components in milk and dairy products (pp. 105-158). Wiley-Blackwell.

Patterson, M. F. (2005). Microbiology of pressure-treated foods. *Journal of Applied Microbiology*, *98*(6), 1400–1409. doi:10.1111/j.1365-2672.2005.02564.x PMID:15916652

Perkins, M. L., & Deeth, H. C. (2002). Ultra-High-Temperature (UHT) Treatment of Milk: Comparison of Direct and Indirect Modes of Heating. *Australian Journal of Dairy Technology*, *57*, 211–227.

Qadeer, Z., Huma, N., Sameen, A., & Iqbal, T. (2015). Camel milk cheese: Optimization of processing conditions. *Journal of Camelid Science*, *8*, 18–25.

Radwan, A. I., Bekairl, S. I., Mukayel, A. A., AL-Bokmy, A. M., Prasad, P.V.S., Azar, F.N., & Coloyan, E. R. (1995). Control of *Brucella melitensis* infection in a large camel herd in Saudi Arabia using antibiotherapy and vaccination with Rev. 1 vaccine. *Revue Scientifique et Technique de.l'Office International des Epizooties, 14*, 719-732.

Rafiq, S., Huma, N., Pasha, I., Sameen, A., Mukhtar, O., & Khan, M. I. (2016). Chemical Composition, Nitrogen Fractions and Amino Acids Profile of Milk from Different Animal Species. *Asian-Australasian Journal of Animal Sciences*, *29*(7), 1022–1028. doi:10.5713/ajas.15.0452 PMID:26954163

Ramet, J. P. (1984). Les enzymes coagulantes en fromagerie. In *Le fromage*. Paris: Ed. Sepaic.

Ramet, J. P. (2001). The Technology of Making Cheese from Camel Milk (*Camelus Dromedarius*). *FAO Animal Production and Health Paper*, *113*, 31–33.

Reps, A., Warminska Radyko, I., & Dajnowiec, F. (1999). Effect of High Pressure on Yoghurt. In H. Ludwig (Ed.), *Advances in High Pressure Bioscience and Biotechnology* (pp. 453–456). Heidelberg, Germany: Springer. doi:10.1007/978-3-642-60196-5_102

Reps, A., Warminska Radyko, I., Krzyzewska, A., & Tomasik, J. (2001). Effect of High Pressures on *Streptococcus Salivarius* Subsp. *Thermophilus*. *Milchwissenschaft. Milk Science International*, *56*(3), 131–133.

Romeih, E., Hamad, E., & Abdel-Rahi, E. (2011). Beneficial Effect of Camel Milk on Liver and Kidneys Function in Diabetic Sprague-Dawley Rats. *International Journal of Dairy Science*, *6*(3), 190–197. doi:10.3923/ijds.2011.190.197

Rufian-Henares, J. A., Guerra-Hernandez, E., & Garcıa-Villanova, B. (2006). Colour measurement as indicator for controlling the manufacture and storage of enteral formulas. *Food Control*, *17*(6), 489–493. doi:10.1016/j.foodcont.2005.02.011

Sagar, S. P., Mehta, B. M., Wadwani, K. N., Dargi, V. B., & Aparnthi, K. D. (2016). Evaluation of Camel Milk for Selected Processing Related Parameters and Composition with Cow and Buffalo Milk. *Int. J. Of Health. Animal Science and Food Safety*, *3*, 27–37.

Saldo, J., Mcsweeney, P. L. H., Sendra, E., Kelly, A. L., & Guamis, B. (2002). Proteolysis in Caprine Milk Cheese Treated by High Pressure to Accelerate Cheese Ripening. *International Dairy Journal*, *12*(1), 35–44. doi:10.1016/S0958-6946(01)00169-8

Sboui, A., Khorchani, T., Djegham, M., Agrebi, A., Elhatmi, H., & Belhadj, O. (2009). Anti-diabetic effect of camel milk in alloxan-induced diabetic dogs: A dose response experiment. *Journal of Animal Physiology and Animal Nutrition*. PMID:19906135

Sboui, A., Khorchani, T., Djegham, M., Aroua Agrebi, A., Dalleli, A., & Belhadj, O. (2012). Camel Milk as Adjuvant to Treat Alloxan Diabetes: Effect of Heat Treatment on this Property. *Journal of Diabetes & Metabolism*, *3*(04), 1–5. doi:10.4172/2155-6156.1000190

Schreiber, R., & Hinrichs, J. (2000). Rennet coagulation of heated milk concentrates. *Le Lait*, *80*(1), 33–42. doi:10.1051/lait:2000105

Shamsia, S. M. (2009). Nutritional and therapeutic properties of camel and human milks. *International Journal of Genetics and Molecular Biology*, *1*, 52–58.

Sheng, Q., & Fang, X. (2009). Bioactive components in mare milk. In Y. W. Park (Ed.), Bioactive components in milk and dairy products (pp. 195-213). Wiley-Blackwell.

Shori, A. B. (2012). Comparative Study of Chemical Composition, Isolation and Identification of Micro-Flora in Traditional Fermented Camel Milk Products: Gariss, Suusac, and Shubat. *Journal of the Saudi Society of Agricultural Sciences*, *11*(2), 79–88. doi:10.1016/j.jssas.2011.12.001

Sing, R. R. B., & Patil, G. R. (1989). Storage stability of UHT buffalo milk. 1. Change in physico-chemical properties. *Indian Journal of Dairy Science*, *42*, 150–154.

Singh, H., Shalabi, S. I., Fox, P. F., Flynn, A., & Berry, A. (1988). Rennet coagulation of heated milk-influnce of pH adjustment before or after heating. *The Journal of Dairy Research*, *55*(2), 205–215. doi:10.1017/S0022029900026030

Smelt, J. M. (1998). Recent Advances in the Microbiology of High-Pressure Processing. *Trends in Food Science & Technology*, *9*(4), 152–158. doi:10.1016/S0924-2244(98)00030-2

Stage and Growth Temperature in High Hydrostatic Pressure Inactivation of Some Psychrotrophic Bacteria in Milk. (n.d.). *Journal of Food Protection*, *64*, 514–522. doi:10.4315/0362-028X-64.4.514

Suliman, S. O., Abdelrahman, S. H., & Khojali, S. M. E. (2013). Effect of Heat Treatment on Some Mineral Status of Camel Milk. *Journal of Animal Science*, *2*, 4–5.

Thimson, W. J., & Short, A. J. (1965). Resistance of Microorganisms to Hydrostatic Pressure. *Biotechnology and Bioengineering*, *7*(1), 139–159. doi:10.1002/bit.260070124

Trujillo, A. J., Capellas, M., Saldo, J., Gervilla, R., & Guamis, B. (2002). Applications of High-Hydrostatic Pressure on Milk and Dairy Products: A Review. *Innovative Food Science & Emerging Technologies*, *4*(4), 295–307. doi:10.1016/S1466-8564(02)00049-8

Trujillo, A. J., Royo, C., Guamis, B., & Ferragut, V. (1999). Influence of Pressurisation on Goat Milk and Cheese Composition and Yield. *Milchwissenschaft. Milk Science International*, *54*, 197–199.

Uniacke-Lowea, T., Huppertz, T., & Fox, P. F. (2010). Equine milk proteins: Chemistry, structure and nutritional significance. *International Dairy Journal*, *20*(9), 609–629. doi:10.1016/j.idairyj.2010.02.007

Vasbinder, A. J., Rollema, H. S., & Kruif, C. G. D. (2003). Impaired Rennetability of Heated Milk; Study of Enzymatic Hydrolysis and Gelation Kinetics. *Journal of Dairy Science*, *86*(5), 1548–1555. doi:10.3168/jds.S0022-0302(03)73740-0 PMID:12778565

Vazquez-Landaverde, P. A., Qian, M. C., & Torres, J. A. (2007). Kinetic Analysis of Volatile Formation in Milk Subjected to Pressure-Assisted Thermal Treatments. *Journal of Food Science*, *72*(7), 389–398. doi:10.1111/j.1750-3841.2007.00469.x PMID:17995641

Vazquez-Landaverde, P. A., Torres, J. A., & Qian, M. C. (2006). Quantification of trace volatile sulfur compounds in milk by solid-phase microextraction and gas chromatography-pulsed flame photometric detection. *Journal of Dairy Science*, *89*(8), 2919–2927. doi:10.3168/jds.S0022-0302(06)72564-4 PMID:16840607

Vikas, M., & Farah, Z. (1991). *Manufacture of cheese from camel milk. Report on field studies in Kenya*. ETH Zürich.

Wangoh, J., Farah, Z., & Puhan, Z. (1993). Extraction of camel rennet and its comparison with calf rennet extract. *Milchwissenschaft. Milk Science International*, *48*, 322–325.

Wernery, U., Hanke, B., Braun, F., & Johnson, B. (2003). The effect of heat treatment on som constituents. Preliminary report. *Milchwissenschaft. Milk Science International*, *58*, 277–279.

Ye, A., Anema, S. G., & Singh, H. (2004). High-Pressure–Induced Interactions between Milk Fat Globule Membrane Proteins and Skim Milk Proteins in Whole Milk. *Journal of Dairy Science*, *7*(12), 4013–4022. doi:10.3168/jds.S0022-0302(04)73542-0 PMID:15545361

Yokoyama, H., Sawamura, N., & Motobayashi, N. (1992). *Method for accelerating cheese ripening*. European Patent application EP 469 857 (0) A1.

Zagorska, J., & Ciprovica, I. (2012). The influence of heat treatment on antimicrobial proteins in milk. *World Academy of Science, Engineering and Technology*, *64*, 832–836.

Zubeir, I. E. M. E., & Jabreel, S. O. (2008). Fresh Cheese from Camel Milk Coagulated with Camiflo. *International Journal of Dairy Technology*, *61*(1), 90–95. doi:10.1111/j.1471-0307.2008.00360.x

Chapter 11
Camel Colostrum Composition, Nutritional Value, and Nutraceuticals

Zeineb Jrad
https://orcid.org/0000-0003-0463-4353
Arid Land Institute, Tunisia

Olfa Oussaief
https://orcid.org/0000-0003-3785-6083
Arid Lands Institute of Medenine, Tunisia

Touhami Khorchani
Arid Land Institute, Tunisia

Halima El-Hatmi
Arid Land Institute, Tunisia

ABSTRACT

Colostrum is an important source of nutrients and immune factors for the newborn. The nutrient profile and immunological composition of colostrum vary from species to species. The composition and characteristics of the colostrum of human, cows, and goats have been the subject of several studies. The study of the characteristics of camel colostrum is more recent. In this chapter, the current understanding of the composition of camel colostrum (i.e., carbohydrates, proteins, oligosaccharides, fats, vitamins, and minerals) is reviewed. A complete comparison with other animal colostrum in whole composition and nutritional value of camel colostrum will be investigated in the current chapter. Consequently, the aim of this chapter is to provide an overview of the vast research, underlining the significance of camel colostrum in feeding of human beings and to predict the potential possible role of camel colostrum that can play in the functional products market in the future.

INTRODUCTION

DOI: 10.4018/978-1-7998-1604-1.ch011

Data regarding camel colostrum are still limited compared to advanced camel milk. Indeed, there is only 33 references appeared between 1979 and 2019, 18 of them reported the physical and chemical composition of camel colostrum. Abu-Lehia, Al-Mohizea, and El-Beheri, (1989) conducted the first study on camel colostrum composition. Then, many works assessed the immunological quality and whey protein profile of camel colostrum. Finally, the recent references in relation with camel colostrum reported the physiological activity (Muslim, 2018; Towfik, 2018) and biological activities of camel colostrum proteins and/or their hydrolysates (Jrad et al., 2015; Jrad et al., 2019). In this chapter, the authors will investigate in depth, the physico-chemical properties of camel colostrum of both camel species (dromedary and bactrian). Then, the authors will describe in details the composition of camel colostrum, one by one (c.a. fat fraction, lactose, oligosaccharides, minerals, enzymes and whey proteins) as well as its role in human nutrition, compared to those of other animal colostrum including human, cow, goat, sheep, and buffalo. In this chapter, the authors will emphasize the biological and therapeutic values of camel colostrum.

BACKGROUND

The *Camelidae* subfamily is divided into two species: the dromedary with one-humped (*Camelus dromedarius*) and the bactrian with two-humped (*Camelus bactrianus*). The dromedary is more abundant in Africa, Middle-East and Asia than bactrian. On the other hand, the latter is mostly distributed in the arid regions of central Asia, Kazakhstan, Russia and China (FAO, 2016). This animal adapts well to the extremely harsh arid land environments (lack of water, solar radiation, high temperature, rare vegetation). Under such conditions, the camel can produce milk with\ potential health beneficial effects. In fact, recent studies indicate that camel milk contributes to the prevention and treatment of a multitude of intestinal (e.g., ulcers and inflammatory bowel) and systemic (e.g., obesity, hepatic steatosis, and diabetes) diseases that are associated with aging and nutrition. For these virtues, the use of camel milk and its products in human nutrition is gaining popularity. However, less is known about the camel colostrum use in human food products, despite been used in traditional medicine to treat edema in pregnant women and as an anti-scorbutic agent for the elderly. Camel colostrum is an "early" milk produced by milking glands of she-camel in the first five days after parturition. In subsequent two other days, it changes in mature milk (El-Hatmi, Girardet, Gaillard, Yahyaoui, & Attia, 2007). Obviously, breastfeeding of colostrum has various benefits for newly born of different species, however, the composition and nutritional value of different animal colostrum are highly varied depending on the needs of the newly born. The chemical composition of camel colostrum has been studied (Zhang et al., 2005, El-Hatmi et al., 2007, Konuspayeva et al., 2010) and there is a clear difference in the chemical composition (protein, lactose, fat, ash and total solids) of camel and other animal colostrum (cow, goat and sheep). In general, camel colostrum contains less lactose and fat, more protein, peptides, non-protein nitrogen, ash, vitamins and minerals, than other animal colostra.

Proteins are key components of colostrum, in particular the immunoglobulins G (IgG). The IgG content must be high enough to ensure a sufficient passive immunization. In addition, consumption of a sufficient amount of colostrum is crucial to meet the high energy demand of newly born small ruminants to support their thermoregulation. In camel colostrum, immunoglobulins consist of three main sub-classes, namely IgG1, IgG2, and IgG3 (Azwai Carter, & Woldehiwet, 1996). As reported by Hamers-Casterman et al. (1993), the two immunoglobulins sub-classes –IgG2 and IgG3- are devoid of light chains and have a molecular mass of 42 and 45 kDa, respectively. This feature in the protein composition of camel colostrum reflects a particular biological activity such as antimicrobial, anti-oxidant and anti-hypertensive properties (Jrad et al., 2014).

PHYSICAL PROPERTIES

The appearance of camel colostrum differs from that of other bovine species. Camel colostrum is translucent, thick, very dense, sticky and cream-colored (El Khasmi et al., 2005).

pH and Acidity

The pH and titrable acidity of bactrian camel colostrum ranges from 6.31 to 6.53 and 18-24°D, respectively (Bai, Zhao, & Zhang, 2009). Those of dromedary camel colostrum varies between 6.28-6.39 for pH and 31-34 °D (Jrad et al., 2015; Gorban & Izzeldin, 1997). The camel colostrum is slightly more acidic than the mature milk, although the richness of colostrum in proteins, this is due to the buffering capacity of colostrum.

The buffering capacity is defined as the resistance to change in pH upon addition of acid or base; the principal buffering components of milk are soluble phosphate, colloidal calcium phosphate, citrate, carbonate and proteins (Lucey, Hauth, & Gorry, 1993). McIntyre, Parrish, and Fountaine (1952) reported that the buffering capacity of bovine colostrum was greater than that of advanced cow milk and decreased rapidly during the first four milking.

Density and Specific Gravity

The density of bactrian camel colostrum is 1.055 for the first milking, which is in accordance with that of dromedary camel colostrum (1.05) as reported by El-Agamy (1994). The camel density decreases as lactation stage progressed and ranges from 1.034 to 1.037, in mature dromedary camel milk (Konuspayeva et al., 2010). The density of cow colostrum of the first day of parturition (1.055) is similar to that of camel colostrum and decrease thereafter, the viscosity of bactrian camel colostrum obtained from the first milking was 24.66 mPas, and demine progressively during lactation period (Zhao et al., 2015). Similar finding is reported in dromedary camel colostrum (Jrad et al., 2015).

CHEMICAL CONSTITUENTS

The chemical composition of camel colostrum is very variable from one study to another (Table 1).

There is a clear difference in the chemical composition (protein, lactose, fat, ash and total solids) of colostrum of both species (dromedary and bactrian). This variability is due to a number of factors, such as individuality, breed, parity, nutrition, and time *post-partum*. Camel colostrum is produced during the first week and lasts 5 days according to El-Hatmi et al. (2006), taken up to 2 days of transition, then from the 7th day, the secretion is considered as mature milk (Gorban & Izzeldin, 1997).

Table 1. Colostrum composition of the different mammalian species in (%) during 24 h after parturition

Species	Protein	Fat	Lactose	IgG	Reference
Dromedary	14.34–20.20	0.01 – 0.17	2.56–4.4	4.72–10.18	EL Hatmi, Levieux, & Levieux. (2006) ; Jrad et al. (2015) ; Omer and Eltinay (2008)
Bactrian	14.23-18.93	0.27 – 0.35	4.3-4.59	4.75–13.256	Ji, Zhang, & So. (2007) ; Zhang et al. (2005) ; Zhao, Bai, & Niu, (2015)
Cow	10–13.90	6.70– 8.00	1.80–2.50	1.6–3.4	Kehoe and Prescott (2007) ; Madesn, Rasmussen, Nielsen, Wiking, & Larsen, (2004)
Sheep	17.55–22.49	6.47–13.64	2.59–3.19	2.88–4.42	Moreno-Indias et al. (2012)
Goat	10.54 –17.13	43.8-80.3	31.9 –43.5	2.66–6.10	Kessler, Bruckmaier, & Gross. (2019) Moreno-Indias et al. (2012)
Buffalo	9.1–13.46	9.59–10	2.7–3.3	1.45–3.3	Abd El-Fattah, Ragab Abd Rabo, El-Dieb, & El-Kashef, (2012)

Proteins

Proteins are organic molecules composed of carbon atoms (C), hydrogen (H) and oxygen (O). However, their chemical structure is distinguished by the presence of nitrogen (N), a chemical element essential for their synthesis and which constitutes about 16% of their molecular weight. A large number of substances other than proteins also contain nitrogen, but protein remains the main source of nitrogen in the body and in food. The physiological energy value of the proteins is evaluated at 4 kcal (17 kJ) per gram. A person's protein needs depends not only on the extent of protein synthesis required for tissue renewal and growth within the body, but also on the quality of the protein that the person consumes. Indeed, the amino acid mixtures contained in dietary proteins are not all used in the same way by the body; depending on their composition, they meet the body's needs for amino acids, particularly for essential amino acids, to varying degrees (Dubost, 2006).

The proteins found in colostrum are an important source of peptides and amino acids that can modulate various physiological functions for the neonate. The protein content of dromedary camel colostrum ranged from 14.34 to 20.20% (El-Hatmi et al., 2006; Konuspayeva et al., 2007), which were similar to that of bactrian camel colostrum (Ji et al., 2007; Zhang et al., 2005). Moreover, there is no large differences in the protein content between camel and sheep colostrum, although their amounts are higher than those of cow, goat and buffalo colostra (Table 1). Protein content decreases gradually as the transition period advanced in colostrum of different species. The richness of camel (both species) in proteins is in diversified nutritional value of camel colostrum. In fact, camel colostrum proteins are known for their high nutritional value attributed to the high digestibility (Jrad et al., 2014) and desirable amino acid profile with satisfactory balance of essential amino acids (Kamal, Omar, & El-Saied, 2007). The major amino acids in camel colostrum of the first day of lactation is glutamic acid, which plays an important role in fetal nitrogen and carbon metabolism. Proline, leucine and aspartic acid are also found with high levels in camel colostrum (Kamal et al., 2007). A large amount of amino acids is required for newborn to synthetize protein and adsorb immunoglobulins (Ontsouka, Bruckmaier, & Blum, 2003).

Camel colostrum contains far less casein than milk (Jrad et al., 2014). However, the concentration of casein is higher in colostrum of different ruminants than in milk (Madsen et al., 2004) and decreases at each milking *post-partum* (Parrish, Wise, Hughes, & Atkeson. 1948). Sobczuk-Szul, Wielgosz-Groth, Wronski, & Rzemieniewski, (2013) reported that early cow colostrum contains reduced proportions of αs-casein, which increase with time *post-partum*, and elevated proportions of κ-casein, which decrease with time *post-partum*, while the proportion of β-casein remained constant throughout the lactation period.

Whey proteins are predominant in the protein fraction of camel colostrum, mainly immunoglobulins (IgG). Bactrian and dromedary camel colostrum lacks β-lactoglobulin, a major serum protein found in other livestock ruminant colostrum, which is similar to human colostrum. Therefore, camel colostrum is a good alternative to infant formula when breastfeeding is not universal (El-Agamy et al., 2009). Infant formula based on bovine milk is widely used as alternative to breast milk. However, there are many differences between human and cow milk and colostrum constituents. Therefore, to produce a better infant formula, camel colostrum is the most similar to breast-milk, in addition to its wealth in different nutrients and bioactive components.

The major whey proteins of camel colostrum are immunoglobolins (IgG1, IgG2, IgG3), camel serum albumin (CSA), lactoferrin (LF), lactalbumin (LA) and protein-peptone component 3 (PP3). The most abundant proteins in camel colostrum are as follows:

Immunoglobulins (Ig)

Colostrum is essential for the health of the newly born, whose endocrine systems and the nutritional state (Guilloteau et al., 1997; Blum & Hammon 2000) and the development and function of the gastrointestinal tract (Bühler, Hammon, Rossi, & Blum, 1998; Blum & Hammon 2000).

Colostrum is characterized by its very high level of immunoglobulins, which immediately following parturition, passes from mother's colostrum to the suckling young as are born without blood immunoglobulins, thereby conferring passive immunity (Marnila & Korohnen 2002; Tsioulpas, Grandison, & Lewis, 2007; Stelwagen et al., 2009). The Ig G is the most abundant colostral immunoglobulins in the ruminants' colostrum. The level is found to be higher in camel (Bactrian and dromedary) colostrum than the other species studied (Table 1). This particularity reflects the good quality of camel colostrum, because colostrum quality has a strong relationship with the colostral immunoglobulin level. Therefore, camel colostrum can be a source for producers, which make provision to have a good colostrum available if the mother does not provide enough colostrum for the newly born.

Camel colostrum of the first three days, consists of high contents of three main sub-classes of IgG, namely IgG1, IgG2, and IgG3 (Azwai et al., 1996). The immunoglobulins of sub-class1 (IgG1), which consists of the heavy and light chains with molecular weights of 55 and 30 kDa, respectively (H55, L30). The two other sub-classes (IgG2 and IgG3) are devoid of light chains and have a molecular mass of 42 and 45 kDa, respectively (Hamers-Casterman et al., 1993). It has been reported that these heavy chain antibodies interfere with several biological processes and may make it a good candidate for human therapy (Holt, Herring, Jespers, Woolven, & Tomlinson, 2003).

The variable domains of the camel immunoglobulin heavy chain are the smallest antibody fragments that bind the known antigens, their molecular weights vary between 11 and 15 kDa (Holt et al., 2003). Indeed, their small size in addition to their high affinity and specificity could make them particularly suitable for targeting antigens in clogged areas such as tumors or penetration into poorly vascularized tissues. These domains are also strongly expressed in yeasts and fungal species, for example, the VHH domains of camel antibody have been expressed in the *Saccharomyces cerevisiae* strain at levels exceeding 100 mg / L in a single culture and more than 1 g/L during batch fermentation (Frenken, Howell, Ledeboer, & van der Logt, 2000). The camel colostrum Ig G has already shown a great stability toward heat treatments (Ji, 2006). Given their specificities, camel immunoglobulins are good candidates for human therapy of rheumatoid arthritis or cancers diseases.

Camel Serum Albumin (CSA)

Similar to that of the human species, camel serum albumin (CSA) is the major protein of colostrum after immunoglobulins. It is the only whey protein that is not synthesized by the mammary gland but of blood origin. It passes into the milk by passive diffusion. This protein is involved in the transport of insoluble fatty acids in the blood and the metabolism and distribution of ligands (Carter & Ho, 1994).

Its average concentration in camel colostrum reported by El-Hatmi et al. (2007) decreased from 20.8 to 12.5 g / L during the first hour and 24 h *post-partum* respectively, and then stabilizes from the seven day of lactation to an average value of 10.8 g /L. The detailed information about the CSA content was not available regarding the bactrian camel colostrum. According to the literature, the serum albumin content in camel colostrum was higher than that of bovine (2.63 g/L), human (0.43 g/L) and goat colostrum (2.97 g/L) (Levieux & Ollier, 1999; Nagasawa, Kiyosawa & Takase, 1974; Levieux et al., 2002).

Colostrum of different species contains higher serum albumin than mature milk. In fact, the increased concentration of this whey protein in colostrum is an upshot of augmented leakage from the circulating blood, which may play a role in the transport of small molecules, such as free fatty acids released from adipocytes (Zhang et al., 2011; Evans 2002).

Lactoferrin (LF)

Several studies have shown that lactoferrin (LF) is very abundant in colostrum but is also found in other body fluids: tears, urine, saliva (Bennet & Kokocinski, 1973; Masson et al., 1971). Lactoferrin is a cationic iron-binding glycoprotein, part of the family of transferrins, and playing a key role in the defense of the organism. The concentration of LF in colostrum is higher than that in mature milk in most species; i.e., the average of LF in bactrian camel colostrum was more than 3 times higher than in advanced milk samples (Konuspayeva et al., 2007). The levels of LF in colostrum vary considerably between species. The mean LF content in colostrum of the dromedary camel from Tunisia was 1.21±0.28 g/L, with a maximum level of (2.3 g/l) was observed at 48 h after parturition, which was similar to that of bactrian camel colostrum (El-Hatmi et al., 2006, 2007; Konuspayeve et al., 2007). Moreover, Abd El-Gawad, El-Sayed, Mahfouz, & Abd El-Salam, (1996) and Zhang et al. (2005) have reported higher values of LF concentration in both dromedary (5.10 g/L) and bactrian (4.71% of total protein) in the colostrum of 2nd day of lactation. Human colostrum contains a high concentration of LF (2-7 g/L), whereas in other species the levels are relatively low including buffalo (0.123-1.085 g/L), cow (0.5-1 g/L), goat (0.072-0.088 g/L) and sheep (0.005 g/L) (Abd El-Fattah et al., 2012; Konuspayeva et al., 2007; Rachman, Maheswari, & Bachroem, 2015; Buchta, 1991). The amino acid sequences from milk of different species, namely the human (Rey, Woloshuk, de Boer, & Pieper, 1990), cow (Pierce et al., 1991), goat (Le Provest, Nocart, Guerin, & Martin, 1994), mare (Sharma & Singh, 1999), murine (Tian et al., 2008), buffalo (Paramasivam, 2008) and camel (Kappeler, Ackermann, Farah, & Puhan, 1999) were determined. The sequence identity between these LFs varies from 60 to 90% (Kappeler et al., 1999). The comparison of the sequence also reveals that the C-terminus of the different LFs are highly conserved, while the N-terminus show greater variations. In fact, the cationic N-terminus of LF is of special interest because to date, identified potent antimicrobial peptides obtained by enzymatic hydrolysis of LF were released from the N-terminal zone of the parent protein (Bellamy, Takase, Wakabayashi, Kawase, & Tomita, 1992). Despite the sequence similarities of the different LFs, they differ in functional details, including their relative affinities for iron, iron release, and receptor binding properties (Khan et al., 2001; Karthikeyan, Yadav, Paramasivam, Srinivasan, & Singh, 1999). The degree of saturation varied from15 to 20% in bovine, human and camel LF, thanks to two specific sites of iron chelation (Zhang et al., 2018; Jrad et al., 2019). Higher iron saturation values were observed in goat and sheep LF (Conesa et al., 2008). The LF protein, thus plays an important role during the early stages of life, and adult age in the assimilation of iron or its interest in human nutrition (Morr & Ha, 1993).

Besides its high nutritional value, the LF has a very important biological properties. Indeed, it has been demonstrated *in vitro* that camel LF has antimicrobial activities on a wide range of infectious agents such as bacteria, molds and viruses, anti-cancer and anti-oxidant, activities (Conesa et al., 2008; Ismael, El Hafez, Mahmoud, Elaraby, & Hassan 2013; Redwan et al., 2016, Habib, Ibrahim, Schneider-Stock, & Hassan, 2013). Moreover, the peptic hydrolysates of camel LF generated a potent antimicrobial peptides more active than the protein source against undesirable and spoilage bacteria (Jrad et al., 2019). Therefore, camel LF can be added in some foods to increase their safety and nutritional value. It has been demonstrated that high heat treatments didn't have a deleterious effect on bactrian and dromedary camel LF antibacterial activity as it observed in cow LF (Elagamy, 2000; Zhao, Bao, & Ha, 2007).

α-Lactalbumin (α-LA)

The α-Lactalbumin (α-LA) is a small protein with a molecular weight of 14,000 kDa and is the major whey protein in camel milk. Its average rate in dromedary camel colostrum is 2.2 g / L (El-Hatmi et al., 2007) and is similar to that of bactrian camel and bovine colostrum and advanced milk (2.04 g/l) as reported by Levieux and Ollier (1999). The α-LA has a strong analogy with lysozyme in molecular weight and amino acid sequences but they differ in their biological properties. It is known that α-LA does not exhibit a bactericidal effect such as lysozyme, this is probably due to the substitution of a molecule of glutamic acid of the active center of lysozyme by a molecule of histidine in the α-LA (Beg et al., 1986).

Various biological activities have been attributed to this protein. In fact, human α-LA is involved in the apoptosis of tumor cells and the trapping of free radicals. From a nutritional point of view, this protein contains all the essential amino acids. It represents an exceptional rate in Tryptophan, Cystine and Lysine.

Protein-peptone component 3 (PP3)

Lactophorin also known as proteose-peptones 3 (PP3) consisted of peptide fragments released by the trypsin hydrolysis of casein and belongs to the GlyCAM-1 family (Groenen, Dijkhof, & Van der Poel, 1995). It is a phosphorylated glycoprotein isolated and sequenced for the first time in camel milk by

Beg, von Bahr-Lindstrom, Zaidi, and Jornvall (1987). El Hatmi et al. (2007) detected PP3 only after the 48th hour after birth on the average amount of 2.7 g / L. The concentration of PP3 doubles when that of IgGs falls, which could confirm the idea that PP 3 may contribute to the immune function of IgGs when advanced milk replaces colostrum. No data are available concerning the detection and level of PP3 in the colostrum of different species.

LIPIDS AND FATTY ACIDS

Lipids are composed mainly of carbon atoms (C) and hydrogen (H); oxygen atoms (O) are also present, but they represent only a small proportion of the lipid mass. It is thanks to their rich carbon-hydrogen bonds that lipids are also a good sources of energy for the human body. In fact, the body draws 9 kcal (37 kJ) from each gram of lipid, which is more than twice the amount of energy it can extract from one gram of carbohydrate or protein. Therefore, fat content of colostrum serves as a source of energy, especially that colostrum is the first natural food taken with the newborn and that its content in nutrients is critical to his health and development (Kniazeva, Crawford, Seiber, Wang, & Han, 2004).

Fat is an important milk fraction, its synthesis is at the endoplasmic reticulum of mammary epithelial cells as droplets composed of a neutral triglyceride core surrounded by a tri-layered membrane. Milk fat is primarily composed of neutral lipids, cholesterol, and polar lipids, as well as a protein group from the cytoplasmic crescents and membrane. Certain fatty acids are known to be involved in many biological functions; and implicated health beneficial effects; however, their components and interspecies complexity have not yet been elucidated.

Dromedary camel colostrum is lower in fat content (0.1 g/L at 2 h postpartum) than mature milk (30 g/L) according to El Hatmi et al. (2006) and Merin et al. (2001). These authors reported that the fat content of colostrum is initially low, it will reach its highest level after about a week and then decrease. In the same manner, fat content in bactrian camel colostrum for the first milking were 0.27, 0.28 and 0.35% (Zhang et al., 2005; Ji et al., 2007; Zhao, Unelius, Bengtsson, Cannon, & Nedergaard, 1994), and progressively increased to its average levels during the first week (0.20%). This characteristic is found in the colostrum of the human and the mare, but not in that of the cow (8.04%; Alais, 1984), buffalo (11.31%, Coroian et al. 2013) and goat (9.4%, Marziali et al., 2018). In the colostrum of these ruminants, the fat content gradually decreased starting with first day *post-partum* until day seven.

Fatty acids

Nutritional aspects of milk fat have attracted public attention. The short and medium chain fatty acids (C4 - C14) are synthesized *de novo* in the mammary glands, whereas the long chain fatty acids (C15-C22) arise from both diet and *de novo* synthesis. Camel colostrum fat contains a relatively high content of polyunsaturated fatty acids, mainly $C_{18:1}$ (25.4– 26.05%) formatting and $C_{16:1}$ (8.1-13.9%) (8.1-13.9%), the rest being saturated fatty acids ($C_{12:0}$ – $C_{18:0}$) with a dominance of $C_{18:0}$ and $C_{16:0}$ fatty acids (Ayadi et al., 2019; Gorban & Izzeldin, 2001). The content of saturated fatty acids ($C_{12:0}$ - $C_{18:0}$) is lower in colostrum than in advanced milk, unlike polyunsaturated fatty acids (C18:1-C18:3), which have higher levels in camel colostrum than in mature milk (Zhang et al., 2005). Indeed, camel colostrum is rich in fatty acids linked with possible health benefits such as oleic acid (25.3 $\pm$ 1.58 g/100g), vaccenic acid (1.9 $\pm$ 0.04 g/100g) and rumenic acid (0.9 $\pm$ 0.06 g/100g) (Ayadi et al., 2019). Arachidonic (AA, 20:4

ω6) and docosahexaenoic (DHA, 22:6 ω3) acids, which are critical for neural and visual development, are also detected in camel milk at early stage of lactation at levels of 0.3±0.01% and 0.2±0.01% respectively (Ayadi et al., 2019; Gorban & Izzeldin, 2001). The abundance of long chain poly-unsaturated fatty acids in camel colostrum revealed its high nutritional value because those lipids are vital for normal growth and development of infants (Kniazeva, Crawford, Seiber, Wang, & Han, 2004). In the same manner, human colostrum fat constituted higher content in polyunsaturated fatty acids such as C18:1 ω-9 (36.21%) and C18:2 ω-6 (59.67%) than transitional and mature milk fat, with the corresponding lower content of saturated fatty acids (C16:0, 26.59% and C18:0, 8.13%) (Zou et al., 2012). Bioactive fatty acids DHA and AA are also present in human colostrum with a proportion of 1.01±0.37% and 0.48±0.26%, respectively (Fares et al., 2016), this may be regarded as the other common point between the human and camel colostrum.

In contrast, in goat and bovine colostrum, the saturated fatty acids (C16:0; C18:0 and C14:0) represent the main fatty acid compounds ranging from 47.7% to 58.4% of total fatty acids, whereas mono-unsaturated fatty acids (C18:1cis 9; 25.67%) are the second main fatty acid class (36.7–46.5%). On the other hand, polyunsaturated fatty acids do not change during lactation and ranged from 4.2% to 4.5% (Marziali et al., 2018).

Similar to goat colostrum, the buffalo counterpart, showed the highest titres of saturated fatty acids, i.e., butyric acid (C4:0), myristic acid (C14:0), palmitic acid (C16:0), oleic acid (C18:1) and the lowest values showed up in mono-unsaturated fatty acids (myristoleic acid (C14:1), pentadecanoic acid (C15:1)) (Coroian et al., 2013).

Many factors may affect the fatty acid composition in colostrum, including the species, the physiological state of mother, age and diet.

In conclusion, camel colostrum is the best nutritional diet compared to other species as it contains the highest level of healthy fatty acids such as oleic acid, vaccenic acid and rumenic acid. Its atherogenicity index was lower while overall-Δ^9-desaturase and health promoting indexes were higher than mature milk (Ayadi et al., 2019), which considered to have beneficial effects on human health.

Cholesterol and Triacyl-Glycerol

Cholesterol is present in a low amount in camel advanced milk and colostrum, but it is a very important compound for the development of cellular membranes. Cholesterol is the precursor of the hormones that are involved in the development of the nervous system and it has an effect on the sphingolipids content (Contarini et al., 2014).

Triacylglycerol (TAG) components are classified according to the number of carbon atoms in short-chain (C26-C40), medium-chain (C42-C46) and long-chain (C48-C54) (Castro-Gómez et al., 2014). TAG are considered as an excellent biologically inert source of energy. In fact, short and medium TAG has the ability to diffuse from the gastrointestinal tract to the portal system and, therefore, can aid in the process of excess energy burning and weight loss, whereas the long chain-TAG help in maintaining the fluid condition of the fat at physiological temperatures (Castro-Gómez et al., 2014).

The percentage of cholesteryl ester and free cholesterol in camel colostrum is 0.1 and 0.84%, respectively, as determined by laser densitometric scanner. The remaining lipids are triacylglycerols-the main lipid fraction (96.24%) with low amount of short–chain TAG, and high level of long-chain TAG, free fatty acids (0.65%), diacylglycerols (0.7%) and phospholipids (1.2%) (Gorban & Izzeldin, 2001). In the same manner, the major lipid fraction in human colostrum is the TAG (10.04 g/L), the rest contain in descending order cholesterol, cholesterol ester and phospholipids (Brabas & Herrrera, 1998). Buffalo colostrum cholesterol concentration is higher than that of camel colostrum. It varied between 12.93 and 12.68%, according to the summer and winter season, and decreased to 9.02 and 7.88% at the end of the colostral period (Coroian et al., 2013).

Goat colostrum contains 5.2 mg/g of cholesterol and 7 g/100g of total triacylglycerol with 22% of short chain-TAG, 18.3% of medium chain-TAG and 59.7% of long chain-TAG (Marziali et al. 2017).

Several authors reported the decrease of cholesterol content during the advancement of the lactation in mammals like cow, goat and buffalo (Contarini et al. 2014; Faye, Bengoumi, Al-Masaud, & Konuspayeva, 2015). For the camel species, it's quite the opposite (Gorban & Izzeldin, 2001).

CARBOHYDRATES

Lactose

Lactose is known as "milk sugar", a reducing sugar, is the main carbohydrate found in milk and is the main carbon source fermentable by lactic acid bacteria. It is a disaccharide made up of the monosaccharides - glucose and galactose - which are joined by a β 1-4 glycosidic bond. It is present in varying concentrations in the milk of virtually all mammals (Oftedal, 1995). The lactose content remains relatively stable over the period from the first to the eighth day after parturition according to El-Hatmi et al. (2006). Conversely, in ruminant colostrum, which is also rich in most of its components such as proteins, fats and ashes, lactose is the only component found to be low in the first day after parturition and increases as a result (Merin et al., 2001). Dromedary camel colostrum possesses 2.56% of lactose, this content doubles in bactrian colostrum (El-Hatmi et al., 2006; Zhang et al., 2005).

Figure 1. Mean and SD of cholesterol concentrations (mg/100ml) in colostrum and mature milk from different species (goat, camel, cow and buffalo)
From after Contarini et al. (2014); Zaharia et al. (2011); Gorban and Izzeldin (2001)

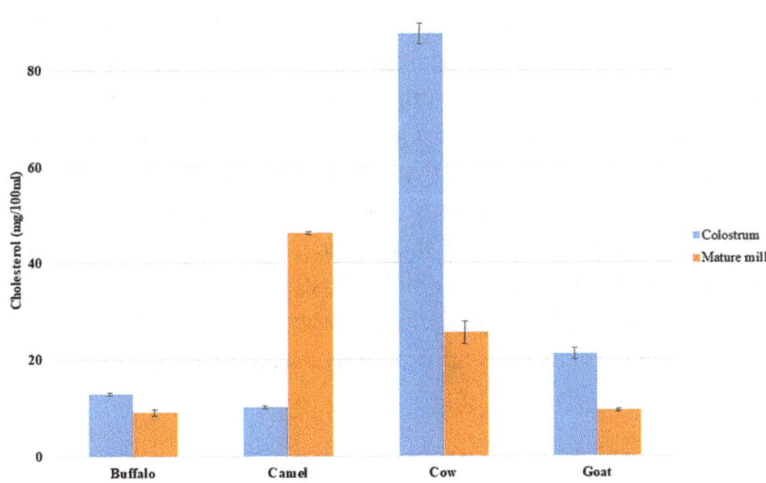

Oligosaccharides

In addition to lactose as the dominant saccharide, colostrum contains small amounts of other sugars, called oligosaccharides in which a lactose unit is usually located at the reducing end and defined as carbohydrates containing 3-10 monosaccharides covalently linked through glycosidic bonds. Oligosaccharides are biologically significant components of colostrum and milk, serving as soluble ligands for micro-organisms and that inhibit the attachment of pathogenic microorganisms and virus to the colonic mucosa, and as prebiotics, which stimulate the growth of *Bifidobacteria* within the newly born colon (Martín-Ortiz et al., 2016; Thum, Cookson, McNabb, Roy, & Otter 2015). Oligosaccharides are divided into two broad classes: neutral and acidic. Neutral oligosaccharides, or galacto-oligosaccharides (GOS), contain no charged carbohydrate residues and their structures are mainly based on lactose with the addition of neutral monosaccharides, whereas acidic oligosaccharides contain one or more negatively charged residues of N-acetylneuraminic acid or N-glycolylneuraminic acid and known as sialic acid (Gopal & Gill 2000). Camel colostrum contain at least 8 acidic oligosaccharides, which are with core units of lacto-N-neotetraose [LNnT; Gal(β1–4)GlcNAc(β1–3)Gal(β1–4)Glc], novoLNPI, and lacto-N-neohexaose [LNnH; Gal(β1–4)GlcNAc(β1–3)[Gal(β1–4)GlcNAc(β1–6)]Gal(β1–4)Glc], as well as 3′-SL and 6′-SL. In addition, there is a significant homology and heterogeneity were observed in oligosaccharides between camel and cow, as reported by Fukuda et al. (2010).

Fukuda et al. (2010) reported that bactrian camel colostrum contains a higher concentration of various sialyl oligosaccharides (0.20%) than bovine colostrum and mature camel milk (0.12%). This suggests that the bactrian camel mammary glands early in lactation similar to that observed with bovine colostrum only synthesize most of the sialyl oligosaccharides. Bactrian camel colostrum contains sialyl oligosaccharides with core units characterized as Gal(β1–3) Gal(β1–4)Glc (3′-GL) or Gal(β1–3)[Gal(β1–4)GlcNAc(β1–6)]Gal(β1–4)Glc (novoLNPI) (Fukuda et al., 2010). These oligosaccharides have not previously been characterized in any other colostrum or milk. This particularity can reflect a particular activity, as the biological activity of milk oligosaccharides is dependent on their individual structural characteristics. No information is available regarding dromedary camel colostrum oligosaccharides, but those of mature milk are studied by Alhaj et al. (2013) who detected two neutral and five acidic oligosaccharides in pasteurized dromedary milk. Afterwards Gangwar, Singh, & Deepak (2018), identified with the help of spectroscopic technique a novel oligosaccharides in camel milk named Medalose, which has never been elucidated from any type of milk or other natural source.

The concentration of oligosaccharides in bovine colostrum is approximately 0.7 to 1.2 g/mL (Nakamura et al., 2003). Higher average of oligosaccharides is reported in goat colostrum (2.4 g/L) and it changes during the lactation stage (0.7 g/L in mature milk) according to McGrath, Fox, Mcsweeney, & Kelly, (2016). Human colostrum contains high levels of oligosaccharides varied from 22 to 24 g/L, while mature milk encloses a lower amount ranged between 5 and 10 g/L (Kunz & Rudloff, 2002; Urashima, Fukuda, & Messer, 2012). Compared with human colostrum, the levels of oligosaccharides in colostrum and milk of domestic mammalian animals (cows, sheep, and goat) are much lower (Urashima et al., 2001).

Although the level of oligosaccharides in camel colostrum is lower than human milk, the higher content compared with other mammalian colostrum and the similarity of the structure of camel oligosaccharides compared with human milk could promote it as a source of oligosaccharides. In fact, camel colostrum is a good candidate as bio-functional ingredient for human infant formula due to the high content of oligosaccharides with healthy properties and as alternative formulas based on cow's milk poor in oligosaccharides, and especially that the addition of bovine milk oligosaccharides to infant formula has therefore been limited (Vandenplas, 2002).

MINERALS

Minerals and especially trace minerals are essential for the newborn because of their implications in various metabolic pathways. Milk is an important source of mineral substances, especially calcium, phosphorus, sodium, potassium, chloride, iodine, magnesium, and small amounts of iron. The main mineral compounds of milk are calcium and phosphorus, which are substantial for bone growth and the proper development of newly born. In addition, zinc is involved in the immune system and the synthesis of collagen. Copper is involved in the metabolism of phospholipids, lipids and glucose and calcium is involved in the formation of the skeleton. The mineral content of the dromedary and camel colostrum varies during the first week *post-partum* (Jrad et al., 2015). The greatest variation is recorded during the first two days of lactation (Abu-Lehia, 1991). The highest concentration ratio between colostrum and milk (ratio 19) is observed in iron. According to Zhang et al. (2005), calcium and phosphorus concentrations fell down after the parturition from 2.25 and 1.52 g/L, respectively, to 1.60 and 1.25 g/L after 2 h for bactrian camel colostrum. The contents of Na and K varies considerably during the lactation period, but, in general, Na content is higher and K content is lower in bactrian camel colostrum than in advanced milk. The concentration of Ca, Fe, Zn and Na in dromedary camel colostrum were 1464.9, 1.9, 18 and 437 mg/l, respectively. That of Mg is at the order of 174.3 µg/L. The values of trace minerals with the exception of Na and K, were higher in dromedary camel colostrum than mature milk (Gorban & Izzeldin, 1997; Konuspayeva et al., 2010). The goat colostrum contains a comparable level in Ca (1579 mg/kg), P (1400 mg/L) and Fe (1.46 mg/L) and very low concentrations of Zn (4.27 mg/L), Mg (85.77 mg/L), with camel colostrum (Yang, Chen, & Zhang, 2009).

At the first day of lactation, buffalo colostrum had higher concentrations of Mg, Na, K and Zn and lower concentration of P than cow colostrum. However, there were no differences between both colostra in Ca, Fe, Cu and Pb concentrations.

The high bioavailability of these minerals (i.e. Na, K, Ca, Fe, P and Mg) influences the unique nutritional value of camel colostrum. Therefore, camel colostrum can be incorporated in the gluten-free products for people with celiac disease, who are vulnerable in terms of proper dietary balance including an adequate supply of minerals. In fact, there is a mineral deficiency among people on a gluten-free diet and most of them refer to Mg, Fe, Zn, Cu (Vici, Belli, Biondi, & Polzonetti, 2016).

VITAMINS

Colostrum contains many vitamins whose concentrations are generally five to ten times higher than those of advanced milk (Levieux & Ollier, 1999). Camel colostrum concentrations of vitamin C vary from one study to another. Mohamed, Mousa, & Beynen, (2005) reported that the concentration is 49.1 ± 3.4 mg/L while Konuspayva, Faye, & Loiseau, (2011) noted that the vitamin content ranges from 79 to 204 mg/L. According to the same author, this rate is maintained at 34.0 ± 5.9 mg/ml during the first *post-partum* week and then drops to 22.2 ± 3.0 mg / L after 1 month. In addition to vitamin C, camel colostrum is rich in vitamins A (retinol), E (tocopherol) and vitamin B_1 (thiamine) with levels of 30.7 µg / 100 ml; 136.9 µg /100 ml and 72.7 mg / ml respectively (Stahl, Sallmann, Duehlmeier, & Wernery, 2006).

At calving, the concentration of vitamin A in buffalo colostrum are approximately 1.50 times lower than in cow colostrum. Vitamin E is higher in buffalo colostrum (342.00 UI/100mL) than cow colostrum (234.0 UI/100mL) (El-Fattah, Rabo, El-Dieb, & El-Kashef, 2012).

The availability of a relatively higher amount of vitamin C in camel colostrum is of significant relevance from the nutritional point as vitamin C has a powerful anti-oxidant action.

COLOSTRUM NUTRACEUTICALS

There is increasing evidence that colostrum is not solely a basic food of high nutritional value but that it also contains many bioactive compounds (lipids, vitamins, proteins, and derived hydrolytic peptides) of major interest for human health. *In vitro* analyses performed on purified proteins have revealed a great potential in camel colostrum proteins as they exhibit a diversity of biological activities. Various tools combining physicochemical, analytical, and in silico approaches can be used to identify hydrolytic peptides with potential bioactivities. It is remarkable that a lot of camel colostrum proteins have no identified physiological function described yet, besides providing essential amino-acids for humans. A few efforts have been made in the last years to further characterize biological activities of colostrum-derived hydrolytic peptides that may naturally occur during the digestive process.

It has been observed that dromedary camel colostrum has a potent antimicrobial activity against pathogenic bacteria like *Escherichia coli* and *Listeria monocytogenes* (Benkerroum, Makkaoui, Bennani, & Kamal, 2004). This could be explained by the richness of dromedary colostrum in lactoferrin. Besides their direct antimicrobial activity, which contributes to dromedary's colostrum preservation after milking, colostrum is the first food of newborn mammals; the question of the antimicrobial activity of lactoferrin after ingestion deserves thus also further study. Once ingested by mammals, proteins are first come in contact with chymosin (for newborn mammals) and/or pepsin (for mammals with a mature digestive system) for about 30 min at a low pH in the stomach (1 to 3 for mammals with a mature digestive system). Interestingly, the hydrolysis of bovine lactoferrin by pepsin results in the liberation of antimicrobial fragments with a higher antibacterial activity than the parent protein. Interestingly, Jrad et al. (2019) identified two potent antilisterial peptide analogs to lactoferrampin B and kaliocin-1 and 9 other different peptides presenting at least 50% similarity with 10 known antimicrobial peptides. Thanks to its biological functions, camel LF has potential for use as an ingredient in functional foods and nutraceuticals. Moreover, in Asia, LF has found applications in infant formulas, skim milk, facial cleansers, toothpaste, mouthwashes (Wakabayashi, Yamauchi, & Takase, 2006).

Besides the antimicrobial activity, dromedary camel colostrum exhibited a hypotensive and antioxidant activities. These activities improved after gastro-intestinal digestion (Jrad et al., 2014). In fact, there are very few studies in the field of bioactive peptides from colostrum of camels. The bioactive peptides derived from dromedary camel colostrum proteins display various bio-functionalities such as antioxidant activities, anticancer activities, reduction of blood pressure (angiotensin-converting enzyme (ACE)-inhibitory), opioid activities, mineral binding, growth stimulation, and ant-inflammatory activities. Jrad et al. (2014) identified 181 peptides in the dromedary colostrum hydrolysate, 25 of them presented strong sequence similarity with known bioactive peptides. At least 16 different biological activities were potentially carried by many peptides. Some of these peptides would also be precursors of small bioactive fragments released by gastrointestinal digestion and more easily absorbed by the intestinal barrier. The majority of these peptides are derived from β-casein. In fact, 6 peptides presented sequence homology with known ACE inhibitor peptides and 6 other are homologous to antioxidant peptides. Other bioactive peptides were derived from α_{S1} and α_{S2} casein, one of which is homologous to the *'Plasmodium falciparum* EBA-175 protein' peptide and four other peptides homologous to the preventive peptide of food allergies derived from bovine αs2 casein. Other peptides derived from κ-casein exhibited homology to Casoplatelin and Opioid antagonist peptides. Thus camel colostrum as source of bioactive peptides can be commercially process into capsules, tablets and powder by various nutraceutical manufacturing industries.

CONCLUSION

Milk from some minor dairy animals, such as camel, buffalo, yak and sheep, is of nutritional and economic importance in many countries. There is an increasing demand for natural milk from minor dairy animals, particularly from a camel, horse and yak. More importantly, many studies have investigated the specificity of milk from minor dairy animals and the possibility to use them as functional foods in the human diet, however information about colostrum of those species and their potential nutritional values are limited. Thus, this work investigated the principal composition of camel colostrum in comparison with cow, goat, buffalo and sheep colostra. The authors of this chapter note the high nutritional value of camel colostrum compared with the other studied species. In fact, it contains almost all the beneficial compounds found in other colostra, e.g., proteins, peptides, fatty acids, vitamins, and other bioactive compounds. Camel colostrum has higher levels of total protein, IgG, LF, long chain poly-unsaturated fatty acids, conjugated linoleic acid, and contents of vitamin C and oligosaccharides than those of cow, goat and buffalo colostra.

Consequently, camel colostrum preparations may contribute to human health care both as part of a health promoting diet and as an alternative or supplement to the medical treatment of specified human diseases

Consequently, it is interesting to create a colostrum bank for newborn that cannot be fed by its own mother immediately after birth and for preparation of immune colostrum products that can be used as feed supplements or colostrum substitutes for calves and human.

REFERENCES

Abd El-Fattah, A. M., Ragab Abd Rabo, F. H., El-Dieb, S. M., & El-Kashef, H. A. S. (2014). Preservation methods of buffalo and bovine colostrum as a source of bioactive components. *International Dairy Journal*, *39*(1), 24–27. doi:10.1016/j.idairyj.2014.04.008

Abd El-Gawad, I. A., El-Sayed, E. M., Mahfouz, M. B., & Abd El-Salam, A. M. (1996). Changes of lactoferrin concentration in colostrum and milk from different species. *Egyptian Journal of Dairy Science*, *24*, 297–308.

Abu-Lehia, H. (1991). Nitrogen distribution and mineral contents of camel colostrum. *Australian Journal of Dairy Technology*, *46*, 82–84.

Abu-Lehia, I. H., Al-Mohizea, I. S., & El-Beheri, M. (1989). Physical and chemical characteristics of camel colostrum. *Australian Journal of Dairy Technology (Australia)*, *44*(23), 34–36.

Alais, C. (1984). Les lipides. In Sciences du Lait. Principes des Techniques Laitidres, (pp. 61-106). Sepaic.

Alhaj, O. A., Taufik, E., Handa, Y., Fukuda, K., Saito, T., & Urashima, T. (2013). Chemical characterisation of oligosaccharides in commercially pasteurised dromedary camel (*Camelus dromedarius*) milk. *International Dairy Journal*, *28*(2), 70–75. doi:10.1016/j.idairyj.2012.08.008

Ayadi, M., Hammadi, M., Casals, R., Atigui, M., Khorchani, T., Samara, E. M., ... Caja, G. (2019). Influence of management type and stage of lactation on the performance and milk fatty acid profile of dairy camels (*Camelus dromedarius*). *The Journal of Agricultural Science*, *156*(9), 1111–1122. doi:10.1017/S0021859618001065

Azwai, S. M., Carter, S. D., & Woldehiwet, Z. (1996). Immunoglobulins of camel (*Camelus dromedarius*) colostrum. *Journal of Comparative Pathology*, *114*(3), 273–282. doi:10.1016/S0021-9975(96)80049-1 PMID:8762585

Bai, Y. H., Zhao, D. B., & Zhang, H. P. (2009). Physiochemical properties and amino acid composition of Alxa bactrian camel milk and shubat. *Journal of Camel Practice and Research*, *16*(2), 249–255.

Barbas, C., & Herrera, E. (1998). Lipid composition and vitamin E content in human colostrum and mature milk. *Journal of Physiology and Biochemistry*, *54*, 167–174. PMID:10217214

Beg, O. U., von Bahr-Lindstrom, H., Zaidi, Z. H., & Jornvall, H. (1986). A camel milk whey protein rich in half-cystine: Primary structure, assessment of variations, internal repeat patterns, and relationships with neurophysin and other active polypeptides. *European Journal of Biochemistry*, *159*(1), 195–201. doi:10.1111/j.1432-1033.1986.tb09852.x PMID:3743571

Bellamy, W., Takase, M., Wakabayashi, H., Kawase, K., & Tomita, M. (1992). Antibacterial spectrum of lactoferricin B, a potent bactericidal peptide derived from the N-terminal region of bovine lactoferrin. *The Journal of Applied Bacteriology*, *73*(6), 472–479. doi:10.1111/j.1365-2672.1992.tb05007.x PMID:1490908

Bennett, R. M., & Kokocinski, T. (1978). Lactoferrin content of peripheral blood cells. *British Journal of Haematology*, *39*(4), 509–521. doi:10.1111/j.1365-2141.1978.tb03620.x PMID:359033

Blum, J. W., & Hammon, H. (2000). Colostrum effects on the gastrointestinal tract, and on nutritional, endocrine and metabolic parameters in neonatal calves. *Livestock Production Science*, *66*(2), 151–159. doi:10.1016/S0301-6226(00)00222-0

Buchta, R. (1991). Ovine lactoferrin: Isolation from colostrum and characterization. *The Journal of Dairy Research*, *58*(2), 211–218. doi:10.1017/S0022029900029757 PMID:1856354

Bühler, C., Hammon, H., Rossi, G. L., & Blum, J. W. (1998). Small intestinal morphology in eight-day-old calves fed colostrum for different durations or only milk replacer and treated with long-R3-insulin-like growth factor I and growth hormone. *Journal of Animal Science*, *76*(3), 758–765. doi:10.2527/1998.763758x PMID:9535335

Carter, D. C., & Ho, J. X. (1994). Structure of serum albumin. In C. B. Anfinsen, J. T. Edsall, F. M. Richards, & D. S. Eisenberg (Eds.), *Advances in protein chemistry* (pp. 153–203). New York: Academic Press.

Castro-Gómez, M. P., Rodriguez-Alcalá, L. M., Calvo, M. V., Romero, J., Mendiola, J. A., Ibañez, E., & Fontecha, J. (2014). Total milk fat extraction and quantification of polar and neutral lipids of cow, goat, and ewe milk by using a pressurized liquid system and chromatographic techniques. *Journal of Dairy Science*, *97*(11), 6719–6728. doi:10.3168/jds.2014-8128 PMID:25200790

Conesa, C., Sánchez, L., Rota, C., Pérez, M. D., Calvo, M., Farnaud, S., & Evans, R. W. (2008). Isolation of lactoferrin from milk of different species: Calorimetric and antimicrobial studies. *Comparative Biochemistry and Physiology. Part B, Biochemistry & Molecular Biology*, *150*(1), 131–139. doi:10.1016/j.cbpb.2008.02.005 PMID:18387837

Contarini, G., Povolo, M., Pelizzola, V., Monti, L., Bruni, A., Passolungo, L., ... Degano, L. (2014). Bovine colostrum: Changes in lipid constituents in the first 5 days after parturition. *Journal of Dairy Science*, *97*(8), 5065–5072. doi:10.3168/jds.2013-7517 PMID:24931528

Coroian, A., Erler, S., Matea, C. T., Mireşan, V., Răducu, C., Bele, C., & Coroian, C. O. (2013). Seasonal changes of buffalo colostrum: Physicochemical parameters, fatty acids and cholesterol variation. *Chemistry Central Journal*, *7*(1), 40. doi:10.1186/1752-153X-7-40 PMID:23442377

Dubost, M. (2006). La nutrition. Chenelière.

El-Agamy, E. I. (1994, October). Camel colostrum. II. Antimicrobial factors. In *Proceedings of the Workshop on Camels and Dromedaries as Dairy Animal* (pp. 24-26). Academic Press.

El-Agamy, E. I., Nawar, M., Shamsia, S. M., Awad, S., & Haenlein, G. F. (2009). Are camel milk proteins convenient to the nutrition of cow milk allergic children? *Small Ruminant Research*, *82*(1), 1–6. doi:10.1016/j.smallrumres.2008.12.016

El-Agamy, E. I., Ruppanner, R., Ismail, A., Champagne, C. P., & Assaf, R. (1992). Antibacterial and antiviral activity of camel milk proteins. *The Journal of Dairy Research*, *59*(2), 169–175. doi:10.1017/S0022029900030417 PMID:1319434

El-Fattah, A. M. A., Rabo, F. H. A., El-Dieb, S. M., & El-Kashef, H. A. (2012). Changes in composition of colostrum of Egyptian buffaloes and Holstein cows. *BMC Veterinary Research*, *8*(1), 19. doi:10.1186/1746-6148-8-19 PMID:22390895

El-Hatmi, H., Girardet, J. M., Gaillard, J. L., Yahyaoui, M. H., & Attia, H. (2007). Characterisation of whey proteins of camel (*Camelus dromedarius*) milk and colostrum. *Small Ruminant Research*, *70*(2-3), 267–271. doi:10.1016/j.smallrumres.2006.04.001

El-Hatmi, H., Levieux, A., & Levieux, D. (2006). Camel (*Camelus dromedarius*) immunoglobulin G, α-lactalbumin, serum albumin and lactoferrin in colostrum and milk during the early post partum period. *The Journal of Dairy Research, 73*(3), 288–293. doi:10.1017/S0022029906001713 PMID:16566855

El Khasmi, M., Riad, F., Safwate, A., El Abbadi, N., Farh, M., Faye, B., & Coxam, V. (2005). La chamelle allaitante face au stress calcique: une fonction endocrine adaptée aux conditions désertiques. *Science et changements planétaires/Sécheresse, 16*(4), 261-267.

Elagamy, E. I. (2000). Effect of heat treatment on camel milk proteins with respect to antimicrobial factors: A comparison with cows' and buffalo milk proteins. *Journal of Food Chemistry, 68*(2), 227–232. doi:10.1016/S0308-8146(99)00199-5

Fares, S., Sethom, M. M., Feki, M., Cheour, M., Sanhaji, H., Kacem, S., & Kaabachi, N. (2016). Fatty acids profile in preterm Colostrum of Tunisian women. Association with selected maternal characteristics. *Prostaglandins, Leukotrienes, and Essential Fatty Acids, 112*, 32–36. doi:10.1016/j.plefa.2016.08.002 PMID:27637338

Faye, B., Bengoumi, M., Al-Masaud, A., & Konuspayeva, G. (2015). Comparative milk and serum cholesterol content in dairy cow and camel. *Journal of King Saud University-Science, 27*(2), 168–175. doi:10.1016/j.jksus.2014.11.003

Frenken, L. G., Howell, S., Ledeboer, A. M., & van der Logt, C. P. (2003). *U.S. Patent No. 6,670,453*. Washington, DC: U.S. Patent and Trademark Office.

Fukuda, K., Yamamoto, A., Ganzorig, K., Khuukhenbaatar, J., Senda, A., Saito, T., & Urashima, T. (2010). Chemical characterization of the oligosaccharides in Bactrian camel (*Camelus bactrianus*) milk and colostrum. *Journal of Dairy Science, 93*(12), 5572–5587. doi:10.3168/jds.2010-3151 PMID:21094729

Gangwar, L., Singh, R., & Deepak, D. (2018). Structure elucidation of a novel oligosaccharide (Medalose) from camel milk. *Journal of Molecular Structure, 1153*, 157–161. doi:10.1016/j.molstruc.2017.10.006

Gopal, P. K., & Gill, H. S. (2000). Oligosaccharides and glycoconjugates in bovine milk and colostrum. *British Journal of Nutrition, 84*(S1), 69–74. doi:10.1017/S0007114500002270 PMID:11242449

Gorban, A. M. S., & Izzeldin, O. M. (1997). Mineral content of camel milk and colostrum. *The Journal of Dairy Research, 64*(3), 471–474. doi:10.1017/S0022029997002264 PMID:9275262

Groenen, M. A. M., Dijkhof, R. J. M., & Van der Poel, J. J. (1995). Characterization of a GlyCAM1-like gene (glycosylation dependent cell adhesion molecule 1) which is highly and specifically expressed in the lactating bovine mammary gland. *Gene, 158*(2), 189–195. doi:10.1016/0378-1119(95)00138-V PMID:7607540

Guilloteau, P., Huërou-Luron, I. L., Chayvialle, J. A., Toullec, R., Zabielski, R., & Blum, J. W. (1997). Gut regulatory peptides in young cattle and sheep. *Journal of Veterinary Medicine Series A, 44*(1-10), 1-23.

Habib, H. M., Ibrahim, W. H., Schneider-Stock, R., & Hassan, H. M. (2013). Camel milk lactoferrin reduces the proliferation of colorectal cancer cells and exerts antioxidant and DNA damage inhibitory activities. *Food Chemistry, 141*(1), 148–152. doi:10.1016/j.foodchem.2013.03.039 PMID:23768340

Hamers-Casterman, C., Atahouch, T., Muyldermans, S., Robinson, G., Hamers, C., Songa, E. B., ... Hamers, R. (1993). Naturally-occuring antibodies devoid of light chains. *Nature*, *363*(6428), 446–448. doi:10.1038/363446a0 PMID:8502296

Holt, L. J., Herring, C., Jespers, L. S., Woolven, B. P., & Tomlinson, I. M. (2003). Domain antibodies: Proteins for therapy. *Trends in Biotechnology*, *21*(11), 484–490. doi:10.1016/j.tibtech.2003.08.007 PMID:14573361

Ismael, A. B., El Hafez, S. M. A., Mahmoud, M. B., Elaraby, A. K. A., & Hassan, H. M. (2013). Development of new strategy for non-antibiotic therapy: Dromedary camel lactoferrin has a potent antimicrobial and immunomodulator effects. *Advances in Infectious Diseases*, *3*(04), 231–237. doi:10.4236/aid.2013.34034

Ji, R. M. T. (2006). *Studies on molecular evolution of domestic and wild bac-trian and the physical–chemical properties of camel milk*. Diss. ETHNo. 219208.

Ji, R. M. T., Zhang, H. P., & So, Y. L. M. (2007). Chemical compositions and dynamic changes of Mongolian Gobi Red Bactrian camel milk. *Chinese Journal of Food Science*, *28*(8), 399–403.

Jrad, Z., El Hatmi, H., Adt, I., Girardet, J. M., Cakir-Kiefer, C., Jardin, J., ... Oulahal, N. (2014). Effect of digestive enzymes on antimicrobial, radical scavenging and angiotensin I converting enzyme inhibitory activities of camel colostrum and milk proteins. *Dairy Science & Technology*, *94*(3), 205–224. doi:10.100713594-013-0154-1

Jrad, Z., El-Hatmi, H., Adt, I., Gouin, S., Jardin, J., Oussaief, O., ... Oulahal, N. (2019). Antilisterial activity of dromedary lactoferrin peptic hydrolysates. *Journal of Dairy Science*, *102*(6), 4844–4856. doi:10.3168/jds.2018-15548 PMID:31005319

Jrad, Z., Oulahal, N., Adt, I., Khorchani, T., Degraeve, P., & El-Hatmi, H. (2015). Camel colostrum: Nutritional composition and improvement of the antimicrobial activity after enzymatic hydrolysis. *Emirates Journal of Food and Agriculture*, *27*(4), 384–389. doi:10.9755/ejfa.v27i4.19912

Kamal, A. M., Omar, A., & El-Saied, K. M. (2007). Changes in amino acids profile of camel milk protein during the early lactation. *International Journal of Dairy Science*, *2*(3), 226–234. doi:10.3923/ijds.2007.226.234

Kappeler, S. R., Ackermann, M., Farah, Z., & Puhan, Z. (1999). Sequence analysis of camel (*Camelus dromedarius*) lactoferrin. *International Dairy Journal*, *9*(7), 481–486. doi:10.1016/S0958-6946(99)00117-X

Karthikeyan, S., Yadav, S., Paramasivam, M., Srinivasan, A., & Singh, T. P. (2000). Structure of buffalo lactoferrin at 3.3 Å resolution at 277 K. *Acta Crystallographica. Section D, Biological Crystallography*, *56*(6), 684–689. doi:10.1107/S0907444900005151 PMID:10818344

Kehoe, T. J., & Prescott, E. C. (2007). *Great depressions of the twentieth century*. Research Department, Federal Reserve Bank of Minneapolis.

Kessler, E. C., Bruckmaier, R. M., & Gross, J. J. (2019). Immunoglobulin G content and colostrum composition of different goat and sheep breeds in Switzerland and Germany. *Journal of Dairy Science*, *102*(6), 5542–5549. doi:10.3168/jds.2018-16235 PMID:30904298

Khan, J. A., Kumar, P., Paramasivam, M., Yadav, R. S., Sahani, M. S., Sharma, S., ... Singh, T. P. (2001). Camel lactoferrin, a transferrin-cum-lactoferrin: Crystal structure of camel apo-lactoferrin at 2.6 Å resolution and structural basis of its dual role. *Journal of Molecular Biology*, *309*(3), 751–761. doi:10.1006/jmbi.2001.4692 PMID:11397094

Kniazeva, M., Crawford, Q. T., Seiber, M., Wang, C. Y., & Han, M. (2004). Monomethyl branched-chain fatty acids play an essential role in *Caenorhabditis elegans* development. *PLoS Biology*, *2*(9), e257. doi:10.1371/journal.pbio.0020257 PMID:15340492

Konuspayeva, G., Faye, B., & Loiseau, G. (2011). Variability of vitamin C content in camel milk from Kazakhstan. *Journal of Camelid Science*, *4*, 63–69.

Konuspayeva, G., Faye, B., Loiseau, G., & Levieux, D. (2007). Lactoferrin and Immunoglobulin contents in camel's milk (*Camelus bactrianus, Camelus dromedarius*, and *Hybrids*) from Kazakhstan. *Journal of Dairy Science*, *90*(1), 38–46. doi:10.3168/jds.S0022-0302(07)72606-1 PMID:17183073

Konuspayeva, G., Faye, B., Loiseau, G., Narmuratova, M., Ivashchenko, A., Meldebekova, A., & Davletov, S. (2010). Physiological change in camel milk composition (*Camelus dromedarius*) 2: Physico-chemical composition of colostrum. *Tropical Animal Health and Production*, *42*(3), 501–505. doi:10.100711250-009-9450-4 PMID:19763867

Kunz, C., & Rudloff, S. (2002). Health benefits of milk derived carbohydrates. *Bulletin of the International Dairy Federation*, *375*, 72–79.

Leprovost, F., Nocart, M., Guerin, G., & Martin, P. (1994). Characterization of the goat lactoferrin cDNA: Assignment of the relevant locus to bovine U12 synteny group. *Biochemical and Biophysical Research Communications*, *203*(2), 1324–1332. doi:10.1006/bbrc.1994.2327 PMID:8093048

Levieux, D., Morgan, F., Geneix, N., Masle, I., & Bouvier, F. (2002). Caprine immunoglobulin G, β-lactoglobulin, α-lactalbumin and serum albumin in colostrum and milk during the early *post-partum* period. *The Journal of Dairy Research*, *69*(3), 391–399. doi:10.1017/S0022029902005575 PMID:12369410

Levieux, D., & Ollier, A. (1999). Bovine immunoglobulin G, beta-lactoglobulin, alpha-lactalbumin and serum albumin in colostrum and milk during the early post-partum period. *The Journal of Dairy Research*, *66*(3), 421–430. doi:10.1017/S0022029999003581 PMID:10480080

Lucey, J. A., Hauth, B., Gorry, C., & Fox, P. F. (1993). Acid–base buffering of milk. *Milchwissenschaft. Milk Science International*, *48*, 268–272.

Madsen, B. D., Rasmussen, M. D., Nielsen, M. O., Wiking, L., & Larsen, L. B. (2004). Physical properties of mammary secretions in relation to chemical changes during transition from colostrum to milk. *The Journal of Dairy Research*, *71*(3), 263–272. doi:10.1017/S0022029904000263 PMID:15354571

Marnila, P., Korhonen, H., Roginski, H., Fuquay, J. W., & Fox, P. F. (2002). *Encyclopedia of Dairy Science*.

Martín-Ortiz, A., Salcedo, J., Barile, D., Bunyatratchata, A., Moreno, F. J., Martin-García, I., & Ruiz-Matute, A. I. (2016). Characterization of goat colostrum oligosaccharides by nano-liquid chromatography on chip quadrupole time-of-flight mass spectrometry and hydrophilic interaction liquid chromatography-quadrupole mass spectrometry. *Journal of Chromatography. A, 1428*, 143–153. doi:10.1016/j.chroma.2015.09.060 PMID:26427327

Marziali, S., Guerra, E., Cerdán-Garcia, C., Segura-Carretero, A., Caboni, M. F., & Verardo, V. (2018). Effect of early lactation stage on goat colostrum: Assessment of lipid and oligosaccharide compounds. *International Dairy Journal, 77*, 65–72. doi:10.1016/j.idairyj.2017.09.004

Mcgrath, B. A., Fox, P. F., Mcsweeney, P. L. H., & Kelly, A. L. (2016). Composition and properties of bovine colostrum: A review. *Dairy Science & Technology, 96*(2), 133–158. doi:10.100713594-015-0258-x

McIntyre, R. T., Parrish, D. B., & Fountaine, F. C. (1952). Properties of the colostrum of the dairy cow. VII. pH, buffering capacity and osmotic pressure. *Journal of Dairy Science, 23*, 405–422.

Merin, U., Bernstein, S., Bloch-Damti, A., Yagil, R., Van Creveld, C., Lindner, P., & Gollop, N. (2001). A comparative study of milk serum proteins in camel (*Camelus dromedarius*) and bovine colostrum. *Livestock Production Science, 67*(3), 297–301. doi:10.1016/S0301-6226(00)00198-6

Mohamed, H. E., Mousa, H. M., & Beynen, A. C. (2005). Ascorbic acid concentrations in milk from Sudanese camels. *Journal of Animal Physiology and Animal Nutrition, 89*(1-2), 35–37. doi:10.1111/j.1439-0396.2004.00507.x PMID:19112713

Moreno-Indias, I., Sánchez-Macías, D., Castro, N., Morales-delaNuez, A., Hernández-Castellano, L. E., Capote, J., & Argüello, A. (2012). Chemical composition and immune status of dairy goat colostrum fractions during the first 10 h after partum. *Small Ruminant Research, 103*(2-3), 220–224. doi:10.1016/j.smallrumres.2011.09.015

Morr, C. V., & Ha, E. Y. W. (1993). Whey protein concentrates and isolates: Processing and functional properties. *Critical Reviews in Food Science and Nutrition, 33*(6), 431–476. doi:10.1080/10408399309527643 PMID:8216810

Muslim, E. T. (2018). Effect of usage Iraqi camel colostrum extract on some blood parameters in albino rats. *Al-Qadisiyah Journal of Veterinary Medicine Sciences, 17*(1), 138–141. doi:10.29079/vol17iss1art489

Nagasawa, T., Kiyosawa, I., & Takase, M. (1974). Lactoferrin and serum albumin of human casein in colostrum and milk. *Journal of Dairy Science, 57*(10), 1159–1163. doi:10.3168/jds.S0022-0302(74)85030-7 PMID:4473469

Nakamura, T., Kawase, H., Kimura, K., Watanabe, Y., Ohtani, M., Arai, I., & Urashima, T. (2003). Concentrations of sialyloligosaccharides in bovine colostrum and milk during the prepartum and early lactation. *Journal of Dairy Science, 86*(4), 1315–1320. doi:10.3168/jds.S0022-0302(03)73715-1 PMID:12741556

Oftedal, O. T. (1995). Comparative analysis of nonhuman milks. In R. G. Jensen (Ed.), *Handbook of milk composition* (p. 749-788). San Diego, CA: Academic Press. doi:10.1016/B978-012384430-9/50035-4

Omer, R. H., & Eltinay, A. M. (2008). Chemical composition of camel's colostrum and milk in United Arab Emirates. *Arab Universities Journal of Agricultural Sciences*, *16*(1), 127–134. doi:10.21608/ajs.2008.14620

Ontsouka, C. E., Bruckmaier, R. M., & Blum, J. W. (2003). Fractionized milk composition during removal of colostrum and mature milk. *Journal of Dairy Science*, *86*(6), 2005–2011. doi:10.3168/jds.S0022-0302(03)73789-8 PMID:12836936

Ontsouka, C. E., Bruckmaier, R. M., & Blum, J. W. (2003). Fractionized milk composition during removal of colostrum and mature milk. *Journal of Dairy Science*, *86*(6), 2005–2011. doi:10.3168/jds.S0022-0302(03)73789-8 PMID:12836936

Parrish, D. B., Wise, G. H., Hughes, J. S., & Atkeson, F. W. (1948). Properties of the colostrum of the dairy cow. II. Effect of prepartal rations upon the nitrogenous constituents. *Journal of Dairy Science*, *31*(10), 889–895. doi:10.3168/jds.S0022-0302(48)92273-5

Pierce, A., Colavizza, D., Benaissa, M., Maes, P., Tartar, A., Montreuil, J., & Spik, G. (1991). Molecular cloning and sequence analysis of bovine lactotransferrin. *European Journal of Biochemistry*, *196*(1), 177–184. doi:10.1111/j.1432-1033.1991.tb15801.x PMID:2001696

Rachman, A. B., Maheswari, R. R. A., & Bachroem, M. S. (2015). Composition and isolation of lactoferrin from colostrum and milk of various goat breeds. *Procedia Food Science*, *3*, 200–210. doi:10.1016/j.profoo.2015.01.022

Redwan, E. M., El-Baky, N. A., Al-Hejin, A. M., Baeshen, M. N., Almehdar, H. A., Elsaway, A., & Uversky, V. N. (2016). Significant antibacterial activity and synergistic effects of camel lactoferrin with antibiotics against methicillin-resistant *Staphylococcus aureus* (MRSA). *Research in Microbiology*, *167*(6), 480–491. doi:10.1016/j.resmic.2016.04.006 PMID:27130281

Rey, M. W., Woloshuk, S. L., deBoer, H. A., & Pieper, F. R. (1990). Complete nucleotide sequence of human mammary gland lactoferrin. *Nucleic Acids Research*, *18*(17), 5288. doi:10.1093/nar/18.17.5288 PMID:2402455

Rybicka, I., & Gliszczyńska-Świgło, A. (2017). Minerals in grain gluten-free products. The content of calcium, potassium, magnesium, sodium, copper, iron, manganese, and zinc. *Journal of Food Composition and Analysis*, *59*, 61–67. doi:10.1016/j.jfca.2017.02.006

Sharma, A. K., & Singh, T. P. (1999). Lactoferrin–metal interactions: First crystal structure of a complex of lactoferrin with a lanthanide ion (Sm3+) at 3.4 Å resolution. *Acta Crystallographica. Section D, Biological Crystallography*, *55*(11), 1799–1804. doi:10.1107/S0907444999009865 PMID:10531475

Sobczuk-Szul, M., Wielgosz-Groth, Z., Wronski, M., & Rzemieniewski, A. (2013). Changes in the bioactive protein concentrations in the bovine colostrum of Jersey and Polish Holstein–Friesian cows. *Turkish Journal of Veterinary and Animal Sciences*, *37*(1), 43–49.

Stahl, T., Sallmann, H. P., Duehlmeier, R., & Wernery, U. (2006). Selected vitamins and fatty acid patterns in dromedary milk and colostrum. *Journal of Camel Practice and Research*, *13*(1), 53–57.

Stelwagen, K., Carpenter, E., Haigh, B., Hodgkinson, A., & Wheeler, T. T. (2009). Immune components of bovine colostrum and milk. *Journal of Animal Science*, *87*(suppl. 13), 3–9. doi:10.2527/jas.2008-1377 PMID:18952725

Thum, C., Cookson, A., McNabb, W. C., Roy, N. C., & Otter, D. (2015). Composition and enrichment of caprine milk oligosaccharides from New Zealand Saanen goat cheese whey. *Journal of Food Composition and Analysis*, *42*, 30–37. doi:10.1016/j.jfca.2015.01.022

Towfik, A. I. (2018). Histological evaluation of camel colostrum extracts effects as a new biological therapy on auricular cartilage defect healing. *Al-Qadisiyah Journal of Veterinary Medicine Sciences*, *17*(2), 17–22. doi:10.29079/vol17iss2art497

Tsioulpas, A., Grandison, A. S., & Lewis, M. J. (2007). Changes in physical properties of bovine milk from the colostrum period to early lactation. *Journal of Dairy Science*, *90*(11), 5012–5017. doi:10.3168/jds.2007-0192 PMID:17954740

Urashima, T., Fukuda, K., & Messer, M. (2012). Evolution of milk oligosaccharides and lactose: A hypothesis. *Animal*, *6*(3), 369–374. doi:10.1017/S1751731111001248 PMID:22436215

Urashima, T., Saito, T., Nakamura, T., & Messer, M. (2001). Oligosaccharides of milk and colostrum in non-human mammals [review]. *Glycoconjugate Journal*, *18*(5), 357–371. doi:10.1023/A:1014881913541 PMID:11925504

Vandenplas, Y. (2002). Oligosaccharides in infant formula. *British Journal of Nutrition*, *87*(S2), S293–S296. doi:10.1079/BJN/2002551 PMID:12088532

Vici, G., Belli, L., Biondi, M., & Polzonetti, V. (2016). Gluten free diet and nutrient deficiencies: A review. *Clinical Nutrition (Edinburgh, Lothian)*, *35*(6), 1236–1241. doi:10.1016/j.clnu.2016.05.002 PMID:27211234

Wakabayashi, H., Yamauchi, K., & Takase, M. (2006). Lactoferrin research, technology and applications. *International Dairy Journal*, *16*(11), 1241–1251. doi:10.1016/j.idairyj.2006.06.013

Yang, X.-Y., Chen, J.-P., & Zhang, F.-X. (2009). Research on the chemical composition of Saanen goat colostrum. *International Journal of Dairy Technology*, *62*(4), 500–504. doi:10.1111/j.1471-0307.2009.00515.x

Zaharia, N., Salamon, R., Pascal, C., Salamon, S., & Zaharia, R. (2011). Changes in fatty acid composition and cholesterol content of goat colostrum. *Biotechnology in Animal Husbandry*, *27*(3), 1201–1208. doi:10.2298/BAH1103201Z

Zhang, H., Yao, J., Zhao, D., Liu, H., Li, J., & Guo, M. (2005). Changes in chemical composition of Alxa Bactrian camel milk during lactation. *Journal of Dairy Science*, *88*(10), 3402–3410. doi:10.3168/jds.S0022-0302(05)73024-1 PMID:16162513

Zhang, J. L., Han, X., Shan, Y. J., Zhang, L. W., Du, M., Liu, M., ... Ma, Y. (2018). Effect of bovine lactoferrin and human lactoferrin on the proliferative activity of the osteoblast cell line MC3T3–E1 in vitro. *Journal of Dairy Science*, *101*(3), 1827–1833. doi:10.3168/jds.2017-13161 PMID:29290425

Zhang, L. Y., Wang, J. Q., Yang, Y. X., Bu, D. P., Li, S. S., & Zhou, L. Y. (2011). Comparative proteomic analysis of changes in the bovine whey proteome during the transition from colostrum to milk. *Asian-A Australian Journal Animal Science*, *24*(2), 272–278. doi:10.5713/ajas.2011.10122

Zhao, D. B., Bai, Y. H., & Niu, Y. W. (2015). Composition and characteristics of Chinese Bactrian camel milk. *Small Ruminant Research*, *127*, 58–67. doi:10.1016/j.smallrumres.2015.04.008

Zhao, J., Unelius, L., Bengtsson, T., Cannon, B., & Nedergaard, J. (1994). Coexisting beta-adrenoceptor subtypes: Significance for thermogenic process in brown fat cells. *American Journal of Physiology. Cell Physiology*, *267*(4), C969–C979. doi:10.1152/ajpcell.1994.267.4.C969 PMID:7943293

Zhao, R. G. T., Bao, H. J., & Ha, S. S. R. (2007). Study on antibacterial activity and its influential factor of lactoferrin in Bactrian camel milk *in vitro. Progress of Veterinary. Medecine in China*, *28*(10), 22–26.

Zhao, S., Zhang, C., Wang, J., Liu, G., Bu, D., Cheng, J., & Zhou, L. (2010). Variations of immunoglobulins in colostrum and immune milk as affected by antigen releasing devices. *Asian-Australasian Journal of Animal Sciences*, *23*(9), 1184–1189. doi:10.5713/ajas.2010.90521

Zou, X.-Q., Guo, Z., Huang, J.-H., Jin, Q.-Z., Cheong, L.-Z., Wang, X.-G., & Xu, X.-B. (2012). Human milk fat globules from different stages of lactation: A lipid composition analysis and microstructure characterization. *Journal of Agricultural and Food Chemistry*, *60*(29), 7158–7167. doi:10.1021/jf3013597 PMID:22747344

Chapter 12
Camel Meat Production, Structure, and Quality

Isam Tawfik Kadim
University of Nizwa, Oman

Msafiri Mbaga
Sultan Qaboos University, Oman

Ghada Ahmed Ibrahim
University of Bahri, Sudan

Ikhlas Ahmed Nour
University of Khartoum, Sudan

ABSTRACT

This chapter aimed to discuss population, meat production, and quality characteristics of camels. Camels are considered environmentally friendly and well adapted to the desert's harsh arid and semiarid environment due to their high movability, adequate fodder demand, and water regulation. Camels are most populous in the East Africa and Middle East. Although approximately 250,000 camels are annually slaughtered in many countries and camels as a producer of meat is becoming much more significant, camel meat market has not yet developed. In 2019, the global camel meat production in Africa was leading with 419,933 tonnes production, followed by Asia (210,000 tonnes) and Europe (179 Tonnes). An important feature that characterizes camelid meat products is the low level of intramuscular and subcutaneous fat compared to red meat sources. Pre- and post-mortem factors should be carefully considered to improve camel meat quality characteristics. According to the health aspects and quality of camel meat, it can be successfully marketed alongside cattle, dear, sheep, and goat.

DOI: 10.4018/978-1-7998-1604-1.ch012

INTRODUCTION

The Camelidae is divided into Camelinae (dromedary and Bactrian) and Laminae (guanaco and Ilama) and Vicugna (vicuna and alpaca) (Saadoun & Cabera, 2008). The dromedary camel is mainly found in the Middle East, Asia and Africa, and Bactrian is prevalent in China, Russia, Kazakhstan and in central Asia. Camels are generally found in remote areas, mostly arid lands or high mountains, and the most numerous camel species (90%) in the world are the dromedaries (Kadim, Mahgoub & Purchas, 2008). The historical background of camels has been discussed in details in chapter 1. According to FAOSTAT, (2019), between 2000 and 2017, approximately 35 million camels in the world have enlarged in number by 72%, while camel meat production increased by 81%. Camel meat is mainly exported from the Horn of Africa to the Arabian Peninsula and from Western Africa to countries of Northern Africa (Faye, 2013). For many countries, camels are significant to the markets by providing quality food products. Due to increase of the human population, camel meat can accomplish the growing demand for meat sources (Saparov & Annageldiyev, 2005).

Camels are considered environmentally-friendly and very well adapted to desert harsh arid and semi-arid environment (discussed in chapter 17) because of their high movability, adequate fodder demand and water regulation. Globally, in terms of population, camels are most populous in the East Africa (Horn of Africa) and Middle East (see chapter 1), with eight of the top ten leading camel producers are in Africa. These are Somalia, Sudan, Kenya, Niger, Chad, Mauritania, Ethiopia, Pakistan, Mali and Yemen.

Meat quality characteristics of camel are described as tough, watery, and coarse in taste compared to other red meats (Kadim et al. 2008). However, many studies revealed that at similar ages, quality parameters of camel meat are compatible to beef (Kadim et al. 2008). An important feature that characterizes most camelid meat products is the low level of intramuscular and subcutaneous fat compared with many other red meat sources (Kadim et al., 2008). Currently, camelid meat products are receiving increased interest, not only in countries raising camels but also on a worldwide scale, owing to the meat unique health beneficial features (Chapter 13). Therefore, many countries of Asia and Africa started to consume camels' meat. A thorough understanding and optimization of the production steps for camelid meat products, including conservation and processing, are essential for successful upgrading, industrial implementation and marketing of camelid meat. Marketing the nutritional values of camelid meat products are a promising future perspective that can be used as a tool to enhance the value of quality camel meat. The nature of the meat characteristics outlined here, along with the ability of camels to thrive under conditions that may be a challenge to many other meat-producing species, suggest that meat production from camels has a valuable role to play in helping to meet future demands for meat. Almost 250,000 camels are annually slaughtered in many countries. However, camel meat market has not yet developed. Future research is needed for using the prospects of the camel as a meat source by broad spectrum research into effective production system, and enhanced meat technology. Some features of dromedary camel meat with distinctive emphasis on number of camel, meat manufacture, meat value characteristics and health aspects have been summarized in this chapter.

WORLD CAMEL POPULATION

Camels are mainly owned by nomadic people and pastoralists who are constantly moving in pursuit of pasture, therefore, it is difficult to exactly determine the number of camels in the world (Faye, 2013).

Table 1. Number of Camels in the World from 2014 to 2017 in thousand heads (FAOSTAT, 2019)

Year	World Number	Regional Distribution		
		Africa	Asia	Europe
2000	20,251.00	16,495.80	3,745.20	10
2001	20,778.80	17,109.20	3,660.60	9
2002	21,060.20	17,558.60	3,493.60	8
2003	21,557.20	18,043.70	3,505.90	7.6
2004	22,363.30	18,818.70	3,537.20	7.4
2005	22,318.00	18,730.50	3,580.00	7.4
2006	22,481.60	18,674.60	3,800.00	7.1
2007	25,399.10	21,541.80	3,850.10	7.2
2008	26,327.90	22,471.50	3,849.20	7.2
2009	25,854.00	21,974.90	3,872.10	7.0
2010	26,518.80	22,656.90	3,854.60	7.2
2011	26,765.10	22,849.40	3,908.40	7.3
2012	22,032.80	18,065.10	3,960.30	7.5
2013	22,600.30	18,476.70	4,116.10	7.5
2014	27,891.70	23,462.10	4,422.20	7.4
2015	33,125.40	28,592.40	4,525.60	7.4
2016	33,832.10	29,337.70	4,487.10	7.3
2017	34,830.00	30,126.00	4,696.80	7.2
Percentage growth (2000–17)	72.0	82.6	25.4	-28.0

Note: The numbers reported in this table does not include the wild Australian (Feral) camel population

Camels are also not usually subjected to compulsory and regular vaccination programs, as a result, an exhaustive census for camels is quite difficult. However, between 2000 and 2017, growing numbers of camels in the world was a trend. (FAOSTAT, 2019). This increase might be attributed to camel's higher capacity of adaptation to various environments (chapter 17), which lead to development of camels' farming in several countries. This was due to improve ecological image of camel farming and products in many countries in the world. According to FAOSTAT (2019, the total large camelids population in the world in 2017 was estimated at 34.8envi30 (Table 1). However, there are different national estimations, which may estimate the camel world population at probably around 40 million head. Out of this number, 30.126 million (or 86.5% of the camels in the world) were found in Africa. In terms of growth, world camel population (Table 1) grew by 72% over the period from 2000 to 2017. Regionally camel population grew by 82.6, 25.4 in Africa, Asia and decreased by -28 in Europe (Table 1).

Globally, in terms of population, camels are most populous in the East Africa (Horn of Africa) and Middle East, with eight of the top ten leading camel producers (Table 2) are in Africa. These are: Somalia, Sudan, Kenya, Niger, Chad, Mauritania, Ethiopia, Pakistan, Mali and Yemen (Table 2). In 2017 Chad was estimated to have 20.9% of all camels in the world followed by Somalia (20.7%), Sudan (13.9%), Kenya (9.6%) and Niger (5.1%). Therefore, these five countries jointly accounted for 70.3% of the global

Table 2. World top ten countries in camel population (thousand heads) (FAOSTAT, 2019)

Year	Somalia	Sudan	Kenya	Niger	Chad	Mauritania	Ethiopia	Pakistan	Mali	Yemen
2000	7,002	3,108	718	1,468	827	1,356	400	775	397	253
2001	7,079	3,203	819	1,487	877	1,411	410	767	591	264
2002	7,156	3,342	847	1,506	927	1,467	420	758	665	267
2003	7,200	3,503	895	1,526	977	1,511	435	751	748	350
2004	7,210	3,724	1,194	1,545	1,027	1,556	445	743	841	353
2005	7,230	3,908	931	1,565	1,077	1,603	459	736	674	357
2006	7,000	4,078	1,058	1,586	1,127	1,494	437	921	578	359
2007	7,000	4,238	3,156	1,606	1,327	1,494	615	933	852	365
2008	7,000	4,406	3,552	1,627	1,358	1,341	1,009	945	887	373
2009	7,000	4,560	2,971	1,654	1,391	1,351	808	958	904	384
2010	7,000	4,623	3,031	1,634	1,400	1,355	1,102	970	923	403
2011	7,000	4,715	3,091	1,655	1,435	1,400	979	983	941	436
2012	7,100	NA	2,865	1,677	1,450	1,425	916	995	960	443
2013	7,100	NA	2,899	1,698	1,500	1,500	1,098	1,008	979	454
2014	7,150	4,792	2,784	1,720	1,631	1,525	1,164	1,022	979	460
2015	7,202	4,809	3,060	1,743	6,414	1,418	1,228	1,035	999	455
2016	7,226	4,826	3,223	1,765	6,836	1,471	1,209	1,000	1029	442
2017	7,222	4,849	3,339	1,788	7,285	1,480	1,211	1,100	1193	447
% growth (00-17)	3.1	56.0	365.0	21.8	780.9	9.1	202.8	41.9	200.5	76.7

camel population in 2017. With regard to camel population growth, among the top ten camel producing countries, Chad is leading with 309% growth rate between 2000 and 2017 (Table 2). This is followed by Kenya (365%), Ethiopia (202.8%), Mali (200.5%), Yemen (76.7), Sudan (56%), Pakistan (41.9%), Niger (21.8%), and Mauritania (9.1%). The country with the lowest camel population growth was Somalia at 3.1% for the same period between 2000 and 2017. This indicates that camel had probably moved from Somalia to neighbouring countries such as Kenya and Ethiopia due to violence (war/fighting).

WORLD CAMEL MEAT PRODUCTION

Camel's meat is the major commodity income under conventional camel production systems. As a source of meat, the values of camel are rising due to healthy reasons in many societies that have never been used to consume camel meat before. Some of the factors that make the camels promising meat-produces are their ability to graze and utilize poor forages; ability to walk long distances; beside their ability to survive under harsh environments, extraordinary income rates of reserves, greater remains which provide a good amount of high nutritive value meat. (Kadim et al., 2008). Due to its medicinal properties, camels' meat is used in many countries of Asia and Africa (Bin Saeed, Al-Hamdan & Fontaine, 2005; Kurtu, 2004; Bekhit & Farouk, 2013). Globally, available statistics on camel meat production are scarce due to

Table 3. World camel meat production and regional distribution in tonnes (FAOSTAT, 2019)

Year	World Quantity	Regional Distribution		
		Africa	Asia	Europe
2000	347,998	239,598	108,093	308
2001	376,647	264,140	112,257	250
2002	367,927	259,247	108,480	200
2003	365,440	262,719	102,504	216
2004	380,927	277,164	103,495	268
2005	345,714	243,781	101,739	194
2006	392,748	286,836	105,724	188
2007	450,424	338,896	111,372	157
2008	496,708	380,998	115,538	172
2009	485,614	364,139	121,386	89
2010	522,794	402,116	120,514	164
2011	532,363	411,554	120,706	103
2012	537,521	415,760	121,627	134
2013	525,859	389,676	135,983	200
2014	585,398	396,289	188,934	175
2015	600,219	404,495	195,532	193
2016	605,471	406,799	198,493	178
2017	630,210	419,933	210,098	179
Growth % (2000 – 17)	81.1	75.3	94.4	-41.9

limited information on number of animals slaughtered and hence estimated amount of meat produced (Faye 2013). Based on FAOSTAT (2019) database (Table 3), in 2017 global camel meat production reached 630,210 tonnes. Africa was leading with 419,933 tonnes produced, followed by Asia (210,092 tonnes) and Europe (179 tonnes).

Table 3 shows that camel meat production grew faster in Asia between 2000 and 2017 at about 94.4%, followed by Africa at 75.3%. Camel meat production slowed down in Europe by -41.9% may be due to most of European consumers are not familiar with camel meat and marketing of nutritional values is not developed. Globally however there was a 81.1% growth in camel meat production between 2000 and 2017 (Table 3). Share wise this regional camel meat production distribution translates to 72.4%, 27.6% and 0.0%, respectively for Africa, Asia and Europe.

In terms of top ten camel meat producers in the world, Sudan tops the list whereby in 2017 the country produced 146,000 tonnes, followed by Saudi Arabia (102,900 tonnes), Kenya (72,800), Somalia (46,900 tonnes), Egypt (39,600 tonnes), UAE (33,900 tonnes), Ethiopia (29,000 tonnes), Mauritania (24,300 tonnes), Mali (20,000 tonnes) and Niger (11,300 tonnes), (Table 4).

Table 4. World top ten camel meat producers in thousand tonnes (FAOSTAT, 2019)

Year	Sudan	Kenya	Egypt	Somalia	Saudia Arabia	UAE	Ethiopia	Niger	Mauritania	Mali
2000	81	15.1	39.7	39.1	39.8	13.1	11.1	11	19.9	6.3
2001	81.5	17.3	52	41.7	39.9	13.9	13.3	12	20.9	9.5
2002	80.5	17.8	46	40.8	40.5	14.6	13.4	12.2	22	10.7
2003	84	18.8	38.8	44.2	41.3	15.4	13.6	12.3	23	12
2004	88	25.1	39	44.5	42	17.5	13.9	12.5	23.5	13.5
2005	61	19.6	40	44.7	41.1	16.9	13.3	12.6	24	10.8
2006	101	22.2	43.8	44.2	39.6	21.5	12.8	12.8	22.5	9.2
2007	106	66	37.4	44.2	41.1	24.2	17.7	13	22.5	13.6
2008	119.4	74.6	45.3	44.2	41.1	23.8	28.9	13.2	21.6	14.2
2009	124.6	62.4	36.8	44.2	42	29.7	22.5	17.4	22	14.5
2010	128.5	64.5	48	44.2	43	30.1	31.5	27.4	23	14.8
2011	139	64.5	47.3	44.2	43.6	30.2	28.1	27.6	23.5	15
2012	140	64.5	47.3	45.9	44	30.2	28.1	28	23.5	15
2013	142	65.1	38.0	45.9	45.8	27.8	28.1	9.4	22.1	16.0
2014	143	59.8	40.0	46.0	95.1	30.6	28.1	10.7	24.6	16.3
2015	144	65.8	38.0	46.6	97.2	31.5	28.1	11.3	23.0	16.7
2016	145	70.3	39.0	46.7	100.1	32.8	28.1	10.3	24.0	17.2
2017	146	72.8	39.6	46.9	102.9	33.9	29.0	11.3	24.3	20.0
Growth% (00-17)	80.8	382.0	-0.2	20.0	158.5	158.5	161.3	2.6	21.9	217.7

CAMEL MEAT CONSUMPTION

It has been proven that compared to other red meats, camel meat is healthier (Kadim & Sahi, 2018, Kadim, Mahgoub, Al-Marzooqi, Khalaf, & Raiymbek, 2013b). Camel meat is much healthier (will be discussed in details in chapter 13) because it has less fat than all the other red meats for example beef and mutton. Camel meat has been consumed for many years, especially in the Middle East and Africa and it is said to be delicious, tasty and healthy. The popularity of camel meat is increasing fast with time because of its high quality and comparability with regular beef meat (Kadim et al., 2008). The camel brisket, ribs and loin are among the preferred parts, and the hump is considered a delicacy. To add value, camel meat has been processed into a variety of mouth-watering and sumptuous products such as: sausage (Kargozari et al., 2014), burgers, patties and shawarma (Farouk & Bekhit, 2013).

MUSCLE STRUCTURE

Camel skeletal muscle is composed of long fibres assured together by intramuscular connective tissue through (Figure 1). Skeletal muscle fibres are composed of thousands of myofibrils that are made up

Figure 1. Microstructure of camel muscles

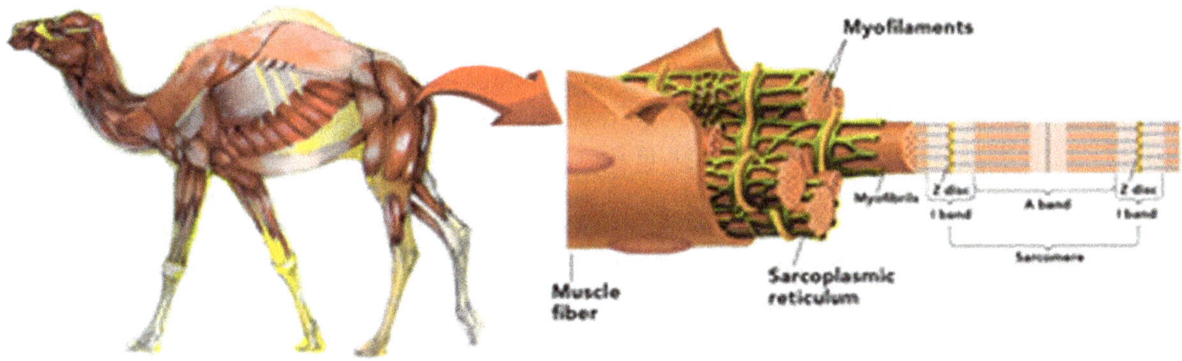

of thousands of protein filaments packed together (Colville & Bassert, 2002). Myofibrils are composed of myosin (thick filaments) and actin (thin filaments) filaments, which are prearranged in units called sarcomeres. According to Helliwell (1999), each sarcomere consists of one set of myosin and two sets of actin. Through structural changes, myosin has the ability to convert chemical energy into mechanical energy and is the utmost lavish skeletal-muscle protein in camels. Actin having the main structural role, while tropomyosin and troponin are calcium-activated complexes involved with controlling muscle contraction, actin, troponin and tropomyosin are the main proteins of the thin filament (Clark, McElhinny, Beckerle, & Gregorio, 2002). Skeletal muscles fibres have many nuclei located beneath the sarcolemma, which surrounds the sarcoplasm, or cytoplasm of the muscle fibre (Colville & Bassert, 2002). Collagen and elastin fibres make the connective tissue of skeletal muscle. A collagen membrane that is synthesized by muscle fibres, endomysial fibroblasts and endothelial cells (Abrahamson, 1986) surrounds each skeletal muscle fibre. The forces of the skeletal muscle contraction are conveyed to bones through the collagenous structures of tendons, and fasciae (Helliwell, 1999). A layer of thick epimysium connective tissue surrounds each muscle. The bundle of muscle fibres is covered by a thinner perimysium connective tissue, while individual muscle fibres are covered by delicate endomysium connective tissue (Leeson, Lesson, & Paparo, 1985). Epimysium is Type I collagen; perimysium consisted from Type I and III of collagen, while the endomysium contains Type III, IV and V collagens (Duance, Stephens, Dunn, Bailey, & Dubowitz, 1980). Arrangement of myofibres, myofibrils, and myofilaments influence the appearance of meat texture (Swatland, 1984). The morphology, composition and amount of intramuscular connective tissue vary within camel muscles. The large variation in tenderness between different camel muscles may be due to different intramuscular connective tissue content. However, the quantity, arrangement and dispersal of intramuscular connective tissue are probably the maximum mutable phenotypic alteration between camel muscles within an animal and signify a great dissimilarity in protein expression and revenue. Given the large influence of intramuscular connective tissue on meat tenderness, even minor-changes of its appearance and income may have major prospective for decreasing undesired changes in meat soreness.

ELECTRON MICROSCOPY STRUCTURE OF CAMEL MUSCLE

Skeletal muscle structure of camel was examined in details using scanning electron microscopy (Figures 2 and 3). Figure 2 shows fibres with well-defined sarcolemma, endomysium and perimysium. According to Pospiech et al. (2003), in general the proportions of myofibrillar proteins constitute between 50% and 55% of the total muscle protein, although in some cases the proportion can go up to 80% (Pearson & Greaser, 1999). The myofibrillar protein plays a significant role in the structural integrity and functioning of camel skeletal muscle. The major constituents in myofibrils are the myosin (C-protein) and actin (tropomyosin, troponin) filaments, which alternate regularly along the length of the fibre. These proteins are located in sarcomeres, within which actin and myosin seized in position by a host of supportive proteins such as desmin and α-actinin. A longitudinal arrangement of contractile proteins marks in alternating light and dark areas that extends from one myofibril to another across the fibre creating cross-striations, which are referred to as bands (Figure 3). The center of the A band is the M-line and the less dense are in the center of the A band which is called the H-Zone (Figure 3). Sarcomere is the basic contracting unit of the muscle fibre, while I band is shared with the adjacent fibre sarcomere (Colville & Bassert, 2002).

Each camel muscle consists of a highly complex arrangement of connective tissue, which provides hold and physical support to muscle fibres as well as being medium through which all the nutrients and waste passes between the muscle fibres and capillaries. Connective tissues consist of fixed and free cells embedded in a matrix of proteins and sulphated carbohydrates (Locker, 1989). Individual muscle fibres are surrounded by endomysium, containing the blood capillaries and nerve connections necessary for muscle function (Varnam & Sutherland, 1995). The structural stability provided by connective tissue is largely determined by the properties of collagen fibres, which are immensely strong, relatively inextensible and stable (Locker, 1989). The perimysium generally accounts for 80% of the total collagen content in skeletal muscles. Therefore, it is considered as a structural element in determining meat tenderness.

High amount of oxidative enzymes are present in camel muscles associated to other red meat (Saltin, Rose, & Henckel, 1994). The latter authors listed that by increasing ability of mitochondrial electron transport to rise in the capacity to produce ATP, in camel muscles, oxidative enzymes show a great rate of respiratory regulator and firmly united oxidative phosphorylation. However, little is known about the

Figure 2. Electron micrograph of a transverse section of the camel muscle. MB: muscle bundle; MF: myofibrils; E: enodmysium, P:perimysium, S: interperimysium space

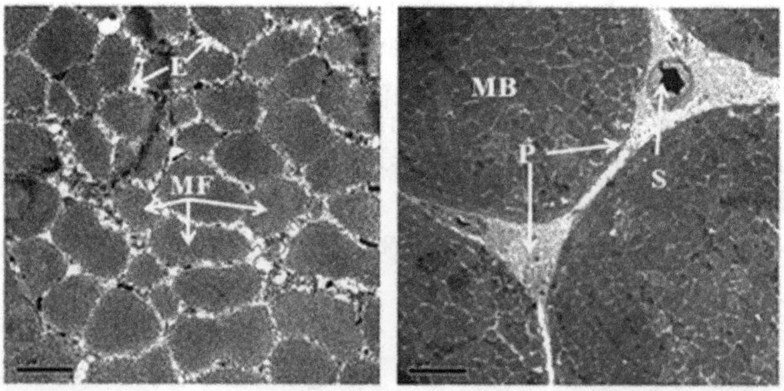

Figure 3. Electron micrograph of a longitudinal section of the camel muscle (Magnifications × 2500 (1) and 2000 (2). Z: Z-line, SL; sarcomere length, I: I-band, A: A-band, H: H-zone)

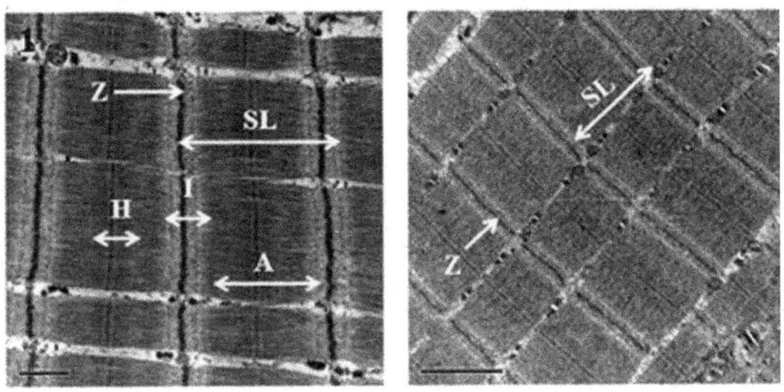

factors, which regulate the biogenesis of mitochondria and the biosynthesis of specific mitochondrial ingredients of camel muscles. It is stated that in both construction and number of mitochondria in animals, mitochondria in skeletal muscles are able to undergo adaptive changes (Lee & Lardy, 1965). The acclimatization of camels to different environmental conditions, therefore, may be because of rise in number and size of mitochondria and a change in the structure of the mitochondria in camel skeletal muscles.

MUSCLE FIBRE TYPES

Although, enzyme activities and substrate levels in skeletal camel muscles have not been investigated, camel's muscles are made up of three basic fibre categories divided by biochemical and physiological approaches (Kadim et al., 2013a). Similarly, Saltin et al. (1994), Baker & Santer (1990) and Rahelic & Puac (1981) stated that based on muscle oxidative capacity (succinate dehydrogenase (SDH), adenosine 5-triphosphate substrate (ATPase) and glycolytic capacity using NADH-tetrazoliumreductase enzyme) camel skeletal muscles can be classified into three muscle fibre types. Moreover, Brooke & Kaiser (1970) classified skeletal muscle fibre types as Types I, IIA and IIB, while Ashmore, Tompkins, and Doerr (1972) used Type βR (red), αR (intermediate) and αW (white). Types I R, II R and II W classification were used or Types I, IIA, IIX, IIB using antibody and mRNA staining.

Type I (slow oxidative fibre) has a moderate shrinking speed and a less myosin ATPase activity; therefore, they are focused for steady, constant motion and hardy to fatigue. Type I cells are tinny with a good vessel stock for effectual gas conversation and they are ironic in mitochondria and myoglobin that gives them a red colour. Type IIA (fast oxidative-glycolytic fibres) have a fast shrinkage speediness and a high myosin ATPase activity and resilient to tiredness. They have a good vessel supply for effective gas conversation and rich in mitochondria and myoglobin. Type IIB (fast glycolytic fibres) have a fast shrinkage speediness and a high myosin ATPase activity but easily fatigued.

Differences in the comparative incident of Type I, IIA and IIB fibres among camel muscles were stated by Kadim, Mahgoub, Al-Marzooqi & Khalaf (2009a); Kadim et al. 2009b, 2013a), Kassem, El-Sayed, & Ahmed (2004) and Saltin et al. (1994). Though, Kadim et al. (2009a, b; 2013a) did not report dominant fibre types in individual camel muscles. Camel GM muscle had a pronounced pre-

Table 5. In the racing camel, composition of muscle in different locomotors muscles (n=6, mean± standard error (Saltin et al., 1994)

	Muscle[1]							
Measurement	**D B**	**TB**	**BB**	**SI**	**GM**	**ST**	**BF**	**VL**
Proportion%								
Type I	49.3±5.0	35.9±3.7	66.6±16.6	93.6±3.2	73.6±2.9	19.4±2.6	50.8±3.6	27.6±2.6
Type IIA	41.2±5.0	44.9±4.4	32.4±17.6	4.9±2.9	25.6±2.6	63.0±6.6	41.4±2.7	50.8±3.1
Type IIB	9.5±6.0	19.2±3.7	1.1±1.10	1.2±0.9	0.8±0.8	17.6±5.1	7.8±4.0	21.5±2.1
Area (μm²)								
Type I	4806±241	5100±563	4108±44	7283±643	5817±140	4604±391	4287±339	4572±722
Type IIA	7179±933	6170±1112	3888±838	8099±1198	6061±585	9396±1082	4938±388	7232±803
Type IIB	8256±1333	7821±1006		5364±668		10708±1180	6379±504	7848±535

[1]Muscle: DB;*deltoid brach*ii, TB*: triceps brachii;* BB *biceps brachii;* SI: *supraspinatus* GM: *gluteus medius;* ST: *semitendinosus;* BF: *biceps femoris,* VL*: vastus lateralis*

Table 6. In dromedary camel, composition of muscle in six locomotors muscles (n=10 mean± standard error) (Kadim et al., 2013a)

	Muscle[1]					
Measurement	**SI**	**TB**	**LT**	**ST**	**SM**	**BF**
Proportion%						
Type I	33.9±2.29	32.3±1.99	32.2±2.01	37.0±3.15	30.1±1.76	33.4±2.33
Type IIA	31.2±1.8	32.4±2.21	32.6±2.54	30.5±2.91	36.4±3.31	35.5±2.65
Type IIB	34.9±2.17	35.3±3.10	35.2±3.31	32.5±2.54	33.5±2.21	31.1±2.22
Area (μm²)						
Type I	5393±437	6588±399	7487±410	6357±321	4451±334	6878±445
Type IIA	5892±460	7157±471	8165±411	7640±367	5502±291	7189±411
Type IIB	6392±317	7671±482	8649±448	8031±417	6455±357	7756±391

1 Muscle: DB; deltoid brachii, TB: triceps brachii; BB biceps brachii; SI: supraspinatus GM: gluteus medius; ST: semitendinosus; BF: biceps femoris, VL: vastus lateralis

dominance of muscle fibre Type I (73.6%), while the ST had only 19.4% (Saltin et al., 1994; Table 5). Camel SI muscle contained an average of 93.6% Type I fibres whereas the BB had 35.9% of Type I fibres. In contrast, Kadim et al. (2013a) found that camel *SI* had 34.4% Type I (Table 6). Saltin et al. (1994) reported that the proportion of muscle fibre Type IIB in the BB, ST and VL in the dromedary ranged between 10 to 21%. The amount of Type I was significantly higher in the ST muscle than the IS TB, LT or SM muscles, while the proportion of Type IIA was considerably advanced in SM and BF muscles than in IS and *ST* muscles (Kadim et al., 2013a). The same authors establish that the quantity of Type IIB fibre was considerably greater in the LT and TB muscles than in BF muscle (Table 6). In contrast, Kadim et al., (2009a, b) in similar camel breeds found that the proportion of Type IIB muscle fibres was significantly higher than Type I oxidative or Type IIA high-oxidative in camel LT muscles. In this respect, camels might have a large proportion of Type II fibres as it has an excellent ability sur-

Table 7. Coefficients of variation % for different measurements on gluteus medius (GM) (n=6, mean± standard error) (Saltin et al., 1994)

Type I Fibres	14.8+8.5
Type IIA Fibres	52.9+25.9
Type IIB Fibres	83.0+79.0
Area – Type I fibres	15.9+2.4
Area – Type IIA fibres	24.7+8.7

vive during starvation periods. However, high proportion of Type IIA was more than Type I and Type IIB fibre types in LT of two-year-old camel muscles (Kassem et al., 2004). In variance to the current research, Saltin et al., (1994) reported that GM muscles in racing camels had a clear pre-dominance of muscle fibre Type I (73.6%), while the ST muscle had only 19.4% (Type I fibres), and the SI muscle contained an average of 93.6% Type I fibres while the TB muscle had 35.9% Type I fibres. Saltin et al. (1994) reported a considerable difference among the eight muscles in the camel. Compared with horses and donkeys (Snow & Guy, 1981; Snow & Harris, 1985), the difference between muscles in the camel in different studies is quite substantial. Differences between the findings of various studies might be attributed to the heterogeneity of camels because there are no well-defined camel breeds as in other farm animals. Sampling techniques is another possible cause of variation. Inconsistency in dimensions may be shown in the study of Saltin et al. (1994), where muscle fibre composition was based on a small tissue sample (biopsy). In a homogeneous muscle type distribution, muscles of the various fibre types do not constitute a problem of sampling (Ariano, Armstrong, & Edgerton, 1973). In camel muscles, fibre types are heterogeneously mixed (Heneiksen-Larsen, Lexell, & Sjostrom, 1983; Saltin et al., 1994). The high coefficient of variation values for Type I, IIA and IIB fibres relate to a heterogeneous dissemination of muscle fibre types in camels (Table 7).

MUSCLE FIBRE AREA

The range of diverse muscle fibre types varied between muscles within the same breed of camels and between different muscle fibre types. In camel skeletal muscles, Type I fibres were the smallest in size with Type IIA in the middle and Type IIB the largest (Kadim et al., 2009a, b, 2013a). Saltin et al. (1994) established that the SI muscles had the smallest fibre Type IIA while fibre Type IIA was smaller than Type I in the BB. The largest fibre sizes of the fibre types were in the SI and ST muscles. Type IIB fibres were the biggest in the ST muscle, whereas the same fibre type was the smallest in the SI muscle (Table 5). Although, there is a distinct variation in camel Type IA fibre proportions, there are some modifications in fibre size when substrate and enzyme levels are alike (Saltin et al., 1994). This could result in minor alterations in metabolic profiles of the various muscle fibres in camels, which could be due to glycogen content rather than enzyme activities. Based on the staining of SDH, the difference in staining intensity is quite marked when comparing type I and II fibres.

Camels have larger mean muscle fibre areas than cattle, goats, sheep, dogs or horses (Snow & Harris, 1985; Essen-Gustavsson, 1986). The significantly larger size of muscle fibres in camels than in cows is most possibly related to animal size (141 kg and 304 kg carcass weight for cattle and camel, correspondingly) (Kadim et al., 2009a). This is mainly due to the considerable size in many muscle fibre types. Saltin et al. (1994) compared muscle fibre sizes between breeding camels and racing camels and found that the racing camel had a larger muscle fibre area. They concluded that the breeding camels may have smaller muscle fibre areas because they had been out of training for more than 1 year.

The diameter of diverse muscle fibre types varied between individual muscles and among different muscle fibre types (Table 6). Though no noteworthy alterations in muscle fibre type diameters within each muscle were noted, Type I fibres were arithmetically the lowest with Type IIA fibres in the middle and Type IIB fibres the biggest. Parallel results were stated by Kadim et al. (2009a, b; 2013a) in camel. Kadim et al. (2013a) reported that the IS and ST muscles had, considerably, the lowest muscle fibre types compared with others muscles. Kadim et al. (2013a) establish that the SM, IS muscles had the smallest muscle fibre types compared with other muscles. The largest Type I, Type IIA and Type IIB was in the BF muscle. Kadim et al. (2013a) found that the largest Type I was in BF muscle, while the largest Type IIA and Type IIB fibres were found in the LT muscle. However, Saltin et al. (1994) found that the SI muscle had the smallest Type IIA fibre while Type IIA fibre was smaller than the Type I fibre in the BB muscle. Saltin et al. (1994) reported that even when substrate and enzyme levels were similar, there were some differences in fibre size. This could be due to small variation in metabolic profiles of the different muscle fibres in camels, which, in turn, may be because of glycogen content instead of enzyme activities.

Skeletal muscle fibre characteristics is affected by neuromuscular junction activity, exercise, stress, hormones and aging (Pette & Staron, 1990). The quality characteristics of meat are determined by the muscle structure, fibre types, architecture, connective tissue and ageing. Interrelation exist among meat quality and muscle fibre type's fabric (Cassens & Cooper, 1971; Ashmore et al., 1972). Variations in fibre type proportions between muscles within the same camel and between camels in different studies were reported by Kadim et al. (2009a, b; 2013b), Kasseem et al. (2004) and Saltin et al. (1994). Muscle fibre type fabric, fibre areas and the capillary density of specific muscles are significant factors affecting different pre- and post-mortem biochemical reactions. A characteristic of skeletal muscles is its diversity of different kinds of fibres, which, differ among themselves (Pette & Staron, 1990). The larger the size of muscle fibre is the tougher the meat. Type II fibres with glycolytic metabolism are larger than Type I. Type I fibres are rich in lipids and red in colour. Therefore, they contribute to taste and colour, which are in turn related to metabolic differences. Camel meat quality parameters such as pH, water-holding capacity, colour, and tenderness are influenced by muscle fibre type. The relationship between meat quality and proportion of various muscle fibre types was reported by Calkin, Dutson, Smith, Carpenter, & Davis (1981). When the proportion of α-white fibre increases in muscles, there will be more connective tissue, less intramuscular fat, and the meat will be less tender than muscles with more β- red fibres. Dransfield (1981) reported that muscle fibre-type plays a major role in postmortem tenderization. Slow-twitch (β-red) muscles have the highest amount of calpain as well as the highest amount of calpastatin (calpain inhibitor), which prevents proteolysis (Koohmaraie, 1988). More amount of proteinase inhibitor decrease proteolysis, resulting in slow postmortem aging rates.

MEAT QUALITY CHARACTERISTICS

Compared to other red meat animals, camel meat is frequently regarded as inferior quality. This might be endorsed to slaughter older camels at the end of their productive life, which has a direct bearing on the magnitude of demand for meat outside the camel herding societies. However, numerous studies reported

Table 8. Effect of age on some meat quality characteristics of the dromedary camel longissimus thoraces (LT) muscle

	Kadim et al. (2006)			Kadim et al. (2009b)	
	Age group (year)			Age group (year)	
	1-3	3-5	5-8	1-2	8-10
Ultimate pH	5.91	5.84	5.71	5.68	5.65
WB- Shear force value (Newton)	68.4	79.5	131.9	6.74	8.90
Sarcomere length (μm)	1.85	1.24	1.06	1.66	1.60
Myofibrillar fragmentation Index%	80.99	73.3	60.4	72.2	67.3
Expressed juice (cm^2/g)	29.6	27.36	21.26	38.1	37.4
Cooking loss %	26.06	23.72	22.42	23.4	22.0
Colour parameters					
L^* (lightness)	37.74	34.03	31.69	39.1	38.1
a^* (redness)	13.37	13.82	16.18	16.5	15.6
b^* (yellowness)	6.09	6.78	7.26	5.58	6.29

that comparable to those of beef, meat quality characteristics from young dromedary camel are superior (Kadim et al., 2006, 2009b). Meat quality characteristics of 2-3 years-old beef and 2-4 years-old camel are similar (Kadim & Mahgoub, 2008). During cooking the camel meat loses more water than beef (48% vs. 37%) whereas between the two species no tenderness differences were observed, according to Kamoun (1995a, b). In order to optimize the best age for slaughtering camel for high quality meat, effect of age on meat quality is discussed. With increasing animal age, meat becomes less tender and of inferior quality. The effect of camel age on meat quality parameters are shown in Table 8 (Kadim et al., 2006). Whereas, Kamoun (1995a, b) reported that for meat quality, age is not a predominant factor, in the case of camels slaughtered between one and four years of age and fed the same diet. Kadim et al. (2006) and Dina & Klintegerg (1977) suggested that between one to three years of age the male camels should be slaughtered. This might be less than 3 year of age, camels were not yet fully-grown (60-70% of full live weight), and consequently, their meat is tender.

ULTIMATE MUSCLE pH

The final pH of muscles is a result of lactic acid addition through glycolysis that marks meat quality structures (Simek, Vorlova, Malota, Steinhauserova, & Steinhauser, 2003). Laack, Kauffman, & Greaser (2001) noted that 40-50% of variation in muscle ultimate pH is controlled by glycogen concentration. On the other hand, Warris (1990) stated that it requirements 0.81g/100g of glycogen to reduce the pH of one kg of muscle from 7.2 to 5.5. In general, the ultimate pH of camel muscles is the consequence of several aspects including pre-slaughter handling, post-mortem treatment, glycogen storage and muscle physiology. A high final pH in camel meat is a result of low muscle glycogen as a result of pre-slaughter stress, including, poor nutrition, rough handling and long transportation. The declining and ultimate pH can affect muscle colour, tenderness, expressed juice, cooking time, flavour, and drip loss. There is a variation in the final pH values among different camel muscles (Kadim et al., 2013a).

The final pH of camel meat varies between 5.5 and 6.6 (Kadim et al., 2006, 2009a, b; 2013a), with the young animals tend to have meat with a higher pH than older camels because of lower levels of glycogen. In this respect, Kadim et al. (2006) reported that three-year-old camel had 5.91 pH value while six-year-old one had 5.71 value. The final pH of camel muscles ranges between 5.53 and 5.75 and between 5.68 and 5.80 for electrically stimulated and non-stimulated camel carcasses, correspondingly (Kadim et al., 2009a). The breed of camels does not differ in terms of final muscle pH (Suliman, Sami, Alowaimer, & Koohmaraie, 2011).

TENDERNESS

One of the greatest significant organoleptic features of meat quality is tenderness (Koohmaraie, 1988). The most significant physiological parameters affecting meat tenderness are muscle structure, glycogen concentration, collagen content, solubility, and the actions of proteases and their inhibitors (Hocquette, Malek, Jailler, & Picard, 2005). The types of muscle structures and characteristics are depending on major variation in meat tenderness (Renand, Picard, Touraille, Berge, & Lepetit, 2001). Kamoun (1995b) identified that compare to the ST and TB muscles, LT muscle had more soluble collagen. The TB muscle had the highest shear force values, maximum connective tissue strength and lowest collagen solubility than LT, *ST*, SM, *PM* and VL in camel indicating that it is the toughest muscle in this group (Babiker & Youssif, 1990) The PM and LT muscles were the most tender and had less detectable connective tissue than other muscles. In another study, Kadim et al. (2013a) found that IS, *TB* and LT camel muscles had lower shear force values than ST, SM and BF muscles, which might be due to less connective tissue (Table 5).

Table 9. Meat quality characteristics of six muscles of the dromedary camel carcasses (1.5-2 year-old) (Kadim et al., 2013a)

	Muscle[1]					
	IS	TB	LT	ST	SM	BF
Ultimate pH	5.64	5.73	5.61	5.67	5.83	5.74
WB-Shear Force (kg)	6.31	6.72	6.51	9.02	12.9	10.3
Sarcomere Length (μm)	1.71	1.72	1.71	1.54	1.44	1.53
Myofibrillar Fragmentation Index%	75.8	74.0	74.2	70.3	65.3	70.5
Expressed juice (cm^2/g)	34.8	42.1	41.8	36.8	42.4	40.2
Cooking Loss %	31.6	29.2	33.5	28.5	30.6	29.5
Colour						
*L**	41.7	40.2	43.5	40.5	40.6	40.6
*a**	12.7	12.6	14.0	10.5	13.6	13.3
*b**	2.6	3.7	4.1	2.2	2.9	3.8

[1]Muscle: IS;*Infraspinatus*, TB; *Triceps brachii*, LT; *Longissimus thoracic*, ST; *Semitendinosus*, SM; *Semimembranosus*, BF; *Biceps femoris*

Tenderness is the most marked variation in meat quality characteristics between camel meat and other red meat animals (Mukasa-Mugerwa, 1981). At the end of their fruitful life (more than 10 year-old) camels are frequently slaughtered, which is classified as of low quality linked with other meat animals. Average shear force value of camel meat at 5-8 years was 48% and 40% higher than those of 1-3 and 3-5 year olds, respectively (Kadim et al., 2006). As animal matures, differences due to age may be associated to changes in muscle composition and structure, particularly in the nature and quantity of connective tissue (Asghar & Pearson, 1980). Important differences (P<0.05) were establish between the different ages (8, 16 and 26 months of age) and cuts for shear force values of camels (Dawood, 1995).

AGING

Archeologically, meat has been aged for a period of time at appropriate temperatures to improve its quality characteristics. Ageing is the process that causes an improvement in meat quality parameters over time and involves degradation of muscle structures by lysosomal enzymes (Hwang et al., 2003; Jaturasitha, Thirawong, Leangwunta, & Kreuzer, 2004). The improving ageing period of camel meat is depended on the type, size, breeds, and age of the animal. Moderate temperature storage may accelerate the ageing process by keeping carcasses at temperatures of 15°C or greater for few days (Petrovic, Grujic, & Petrovic, 1993). Kadim et al. (2009a) aged camel meat at 2-3°C for seven days to improve its quality characteristics and found that meat samples form the ageing group had more tender than the control samples (Table 10). This implies that ageing may be one of the post-mortem treatments to improve camel meat quality parameters.

Table 10. Effects of age and ageing on meat quality attributes of longissimus thoraces (LT) of dromedary camel (Kadim et al., 2009a)

	Age (year)							
	1-3		4-6		7-9		10-12	
	Ageing 7-day	Ageing 2-day	Ageing 7-day	Ageing 2-day	Ageing 7-day	Ageing 2-day	Ageing 7-day	Ageing 2-day
Ultimate pH	5.86	5.85	5.79	5.78	5.71	5.71	5.60	5.61
Expressed juice (cm2/g)	38.6	37.2	37.2	36.6	30.8	30.3	21.3	21.1
Cooking loss%	25.7	25.0	23.9	22.7	21.3	19.8	18.9	17.8
WB-shear force (kg)	7.28	8.10	8.41	8.97	9.14	9.76	11.29	12.79
Sarcomere length (μm)	1.73	14.71	1.65	1.67	1.48	1.47	1.39	1.37
Myofibrillar fragmentation index%	77.9	73.5	71.6	69.8	66.9	64.5	62.7	60.2
Lightness (L*)	40.5	39.80	38.71	36.86	35.31	33.72	30.15	28.47
Redness (a*)	15.6	15.7	16.9	16.1	18.2	19.0	19.9	19.5
Yellowness (b*)	5.40	5.51	6.04	6.03	7.03	7.05	7.93	7.98

EXPRESSED JUICE

Arrest of water inside the myofibrillar system is responsible for water holding capacity in meat. By giving density on meat can transfer water from the intercellar to the extracellular space and finally on the surface due to structural changes at sarcomeres level. It changes the holding capacity of water, minerals and vitamins (Beriain, Bass, Purroy, & Treacher, 2000). Moreover, Dyer & Dingle (1967) reported that meat water content is exaggerated by final pH, denaturation and arrangement of proteins by the ionic asset of the extracellular fluid and oxidation of lipids, which reduces proteins solubility. Kadim et al. (2006) found that camel's meat slaughtered at 1 to 3 years had more expressed juice compared to camels slaughtered at 5 to 8 years of age, possibly due to changes in fat content and the holding capacity of meat. Due to an intensification in the moisture to protein ratio, the expressed juice decreases as fat levels increase (Miller, Staffle, & Zirkle, 1968). Dawood (1995) mentioned that 8 month-old camel meats had expressively more water-holding capacities than meat from 26 month-old camels.

COLOUR (*L*, a*, b**)

The meat colour is linked to the chemical structure of myoglobin content. According to the age, species or muscle pH, myoglobin concentration (Gardner, Kennedy, Milton, & Pethick., 1999; Lawrie, 2006). There was a deleterious linear affiliation among muscle pH and its colour (Menzies & Hopkines, 1996). Protein degradation after slaughter is linked to the ultimate pH, which rises light sprinkle properties of meat and thus rises L*, a* and b* values. Small definitive pH and high meat temperature might lead to more protein deprivation resulting in higher colour values than the high ultimate pH meat samples. Postmortem glycolysis decreases muscle pH making muscle surfaces perkier and lightly wet. Camel LD muscles had higher lightness (L*), redness (a*) and yellowness (b*) values than ST and TB muscles (Babiker & Yousif, 1990). On the other hand, Suliman et al. (2011) reported that the colour of the BF muscle was not exaggerated by breed. A high redness (*a**) colour component in the camel meat was associated with a lower lightness (L*), while greater lightness connected with great fat content (Kadim et al., 2013a). The same authors found that ST muscle had the darkest colored lean compared to IS, LT, TB, SM, and BF muscles. The LT, SM and BF camel muscles had advanced redness (a*) values than ST muscle, while a* value for IS and TB muscles were in between. CIE a* values were similar among LT, SM and BF muscles (Kadim et al., 2013a). In camel, the highest average yellowness (b*) value was recorded in the LT muscle with comparable values to the TB and BF muscles. The camel age is directly related with colour of meat (Kadim et al., 2006).

ELECTRICAL STIMULATION

Electrical stimulation of freshly slaughtered animal's muscles is the elicitation of muscle contraction using electric impulses, which it mimic the action potential coming from the central nervous system, causing the muscles to contract. It should be in a series of short pulses, each of which causes the muscles to contract violently, but between pulses, the muscles return to their normal relaxed state (Hwang, Devine, & Hopkins, 2003). It can play a positive role in preventing cold shortening by accelerating the decline in pH and the onset of rigor mortis when the muscle temperature drops below 10°C, while the muscle still contains sufficient energy to cause contraction (Simmons et al., 2008). Carcasses must be chilled quickly following slaughter to minimize microbiological growth and to reduce weight loss. Electrical stimulation causes muscle contractions that convert muscle glycogen to lactic acid. In this state the muscles have no further energy to contract and will not cause cold shortening when chilled to 12°C. In camel, the electrical stimulation altered muscular morphology due to physical disturbance of the myofibrillar matrix (Kadim, et al., 2009a).

Histological images presented the presence of contracture bands encompassing mainly strained, vague and disturbed sarcomeres (Kadim et al., 2009 a,b). It could be interpreted that physical disruption per se lowers the resistance to mechanical shearing force. A change in camel muscle does not result from low stimulation unless there is markedly accelerated postmortem glycolysis (Kadim et al., 2009a). According to Kadim et al. (2009a, b), the positive effect of electrical stimulation on the rate of camel muscle pH decline is caused by accelerating muscle glycogen degradation and thus increasing the concentration of lactic acid, then the pH of stimulated muscle can reach a pH of 6.0 in several hrs instead of the 12 to 16 hrs that may be required for non-stimulated muscles. In dromedary camel, electrical stimulation consistently produced a more rapid glycolysis early post mortem in four age groups muscles (Kadim et al., 2009a). The greatest pH falls, 40 min post mortem, resulted from electrical stimulation applied 20 minutes after slaughter (Kadim et al., 2009a, b). At 40 min postmortem, the average pH decline in stimulated camel muscle were 0.12 below the non-stimulated group (Kadim et al., 2009a). After a relatively fast fall within the first 4 h, the mean pH values of camel muscles underwent a slow decline until the ultimate pH at 24 h postmortem (Kadim et al., 2009a, b).

CONCLUSION

In harsh environments, camels are a decent source of high nutritional meat. The camel has distinctive physiological characteristics, including a tolerance to low and high temperatures, water scarcity, poor vegetation, solar radiation and rough topography. Camels are commonly produced on poor nutrition under traditional systems and at old ages after completing a career in work are mostly slaughtered. When they are slaughtered at same ages, the quality characteristics of camel meat are similar to beef meat. The camel meat can be effectively marketed alongside that of dear, sheep, cattle, and goat, as per the quality parameters. To improve meat quality features, pre and postmortem factors should be carefully measured. Forthcoming research is necessary for developing the prospective of the camel as a basis of meat through multi-disciplinary research into effective manufacture systems, and better meat expertise and marketing.

REFERENCES

Abrahamson, D. R. (1986). Recent studies on the structure and pathology of basement membranes. *The Journal of Pathology*, *149*(4), 257–278. doi:10.1002/path.1711490402 PMID:2944999

Ariano, M. A., Armstrong, R. B., & Edgerton, V. R. (1973). Hind limb muscle fibre populations of five mammals. *The Journal of Histochemistry and Cytochemistry*, *21*(1), 51–55. doi:10.1177/21.1.51 PMID:4348494

Asghar, A., & Pearson, A. M. (1980). Influence of ante- and postmortem treatments upon muscle composition and meat quality. *Advances in Food Research*, *26*, 53–213. doi:10.1016/S0065-2628(08)60318-3

Ashmore, C. R., Tompkins, G., & Doerr, L. (1972). Postnatal development of muscle fibre types in domestic animals. *Journal of Animal Science*, *4*(1), 37–41. doi:10.2527/jas1972.34137x PMID:4258174

Babiker, S. A., & Yousif, O. K. (1990). Chemical composition and quality of camel meat. *Meat Science*, *27*(4), 283–287. doi:10.1016/0309-1740(90)90066-F PMID:22055364

Baker, D. M., & Santer, R. M. (1990). Development of a quantitative histochemical method for determination of succinate dehydrogenase activity in autonomic neurons and its application to the study of aging in the autonomic nervous system. *The Journal of Histochemistry and Cytochemistry*, *38*(4), 525–531. doi:10.1177/38.4.2319123 PMID:2319123

Bekhit, A. E., & Farouk, M. M. (2013). Nutritive and health value of camel meat. In I. T. Kadim, O. Mahgoub, B. Faye, & M. M. Farouk (Eds.), *Camel Meat and Meat Products* (pp. 205–223). CAB International. doi:10.1079/9781780641010.0205

Beriain, M.J., Bass, P., Purroy, A., & Treacher, T. (2000). Effect of animal and nutritional factors and nutrition on lamb meat quality. *Centre international de hautes études agronomiques méditerranéennes*, 75-86.

Bin Saeed, A. A., Al-Hamdan, N. A., & Fontaine, R. E. (2005). Plague from Eating Raw Camel Liver. *Advances in Food Research*, *26*, 53–213. PMID:16229781

Brooke, M. H., & Kaiser, K. K. (1970). Three myosin ATPase systems, the nature of their pH lability and sulfhydral dependence. *The Journal of Histochemistry and Cytochemistry*, *18*, 670–672. doi:10.1177/18.9.670 PMID:4249441

Calkin, C. R., Dutson, T. R., Smith, G. C., Carpenter, Z. I., & Davis, G. W. (1981). Relationship of fibre type composition to marbling and tenderness of bovine muscle. *Journal of Food Science*, *46*(3), 708–710. doi:10.1111/j.1365-2621.1981.tb15331.x

Cassens, R. G., & Cooper, C. (1971). Red and white muscle. *Advances in Food Research*, *19*, 1–45. doi:10.1016/S0065-2628(08)60030-0 PMID:5000245

Clark, K. A., McElhinny, A. S., Beckerle, M. C., & Gregorio, C. C. (2002). Striated muscle cytoarchitecture: An intricate web of form and function. *Annual Review of Cell and Developmental Biology*, *18*(1), 637–706. doi:10.1146/annurev.cellbio.18.012502.105840 PMID:12142273

Colville, T., & Bassert, J. M. (2002). *Clinical Anatomy and Physiology for Veterinary Technicians*. St Louis, MO: Mosby, Inc.

Dawood, A. (1995). Physical and Sensory characteristics of Najdi camel meat. *Meat Science*, *39*(1), 59–69. doi:10.1016/0309-1740(95)80007-7 PMID:22059763

Dina, D., & Klintegerg, R. (1977). *Proposal for a rural development training project and study concerned with camel utilization in arid lands in Ethiopia*. Academic Press.

Dransfield, E. (1981). Eating quality of DFD beef. *Veterinary Medicine and Animal Science*, *10*, 344–361.

Duance, V. C., Stephens, H. R., Dunn, M., Bailey, A. J., & Dubowitz, V. (1980). A role for collagen in the pathogenesis of muscular dystrophy. *Nature*, *284*(5755), 470–472. doi:10.1038/284470a0 PMID:7360283

Dyer, W. J., & Dingle, J. R. (1967). *Fish as Food* (G. Borgstrom, Ed.). Academic.

Essen-Gustavsson, B. (1986). Activity and inactivity-related muscle adaptation in the animal kingdom. In B. Saltin (Ed.), *Biochemistry of Exercise VI* (pp. 435–444). Champaign, IL: Human Kinetics Publishers.

FAOSTAT. (2015). *Food and Agricultural Organization, United Nations statistics*. Retrieved from http://faostat.fao.org/site/339/default.aspx

Farouk, M. M., & Bakhit, A. E. (2013). Processed Camel Meats. In I. T. Kadim, O. Mahgoub, B. Faye, & M. M. Farouk (Eds.), *Camel Meat and Meat Products* (pp. 186–204). CAB International. doi:10.1079/9781780641010.0186

Faye, B. (2013). Camel meat in the world. CAB International.

Gardner, G. E., Kennedy, L., Milton, J. T. B., & Pethick, D. W. (1999). Glycogen metabolism and ultimate pH of muscle merino, first-cross, and second-cross whether lambs as affected by stress before slaughter. *Australian Journal of Agricultural Research*, *50*(2), 175–181. doi:10.1071/A98093

Gheisari, H. R., Aminlari, M., & Shekarforoush, S. S. (2009). A comparative study of the biochemical and functional properties of camel and cattle meat during frozen storage. *Veterinarski Arhiv*, *79*, 51–68.

Helliwell, T. R. (1999). Muscle: Part 1- Normal structure and function. *Current Orthopaedics*, *13*(1), 33–41. doi:10.1016/S0268-0890(99)90083-X

Heneiksen-larsen, K. B., Lexell, J., & Sjostrom, M. (1983). Distribution of different fibre types in human skeletal muscles. I. Method for the preparation and analysis of cross-sections of whole tibialis anterior. *The Histochemical Journal*, *15*, 167–178. doi:10.1007/BF01042285 PMID:6343306

Hocquette, J. F., Malek, I. C., Jailler, R., & Picard, B. (2005). Recent advances in research on bovine muscle and meat sensory quality. II. Influence of rearing factors on muscle characteristics. *Cahiers Agricultures*, *14*, 365–372.

Hwang, I. H., Devine, C. E., & Hopkins, D. L. (2003). The biochemical and physical effects of electrical stimulation on beef and sheep meat tenderness. *Meat Science*, *65*(2), 677–691. doi:10.1016/S0309-1740(02)00271-1 PMID:22063428

Jaturasitha, S., Thirawong, P., Leangwunta, V., & Kreuzer, M. (2004). Reducing toughness of beef from BosIndicus draught steers by injection of calcium chloride: Effect of concentration and time postmortem. *Meat Science*, *68*(1), 61–69. doi:10.1016/j.meatsci.2004.02.004 PMID:22062008

Kadim, I. T., Al-Karousi, A., Mahgoub, O., Al-Marzooqi, W., Al-Maqbaly, R., Khalaf, S. K., & Raiymbek, G. (2013a). Physical, chemical, quality and histochemical characteristics of infraspinatus, triceps brachii, longissimus thoraces, biceps femoris, semitendinosus, and semimembranosus of dromedary camel (Camelus dromedaries) muscles. *Meat Science*, *93*, 564–571. doi:10.1016/j.meatsci.2012.11.028 PMID:23273465

Kadim, I. T., & Mahgoub, O. (2008). Effect of age on quality and composition of one-humped camel Longissimus thoracis muscle. *International Journal of Postharvest Technology and Innovation*, *1*(3), 327–336. doi:10.1504/IJPTI.2008.021467

Kadim, I. T., Mahgoub, O., Al-Marzooqi, W., Al-Zadgali, S., Annamali, K., & Mansour, M. H. (2006). Effects of age on composition and quality of muscle Longissimus thoracic of the Omani Arabian Camel (*Camelus dromedarius*). *Meat Science*, *73*(4), 619–625. doi:10.1016/j.meatsci.2006.03.002 PMID:22062561

Kadim, I. T., Mahgoub, O., Al-Marzooqi, W., & Khalaf, S. K. (2009a). Effect of low voltage electrical stimulation and splitting carcass on histochemical and meat quality characteristics of the one-humped camel (Camelus dromedaries) Longissimus thoracic muscle. *Journal of Camelid Science*, *2*, 30–40.

Kadim, I. T., Mahgoub, O., Al-Marzooqi, W., Khalaf, S. K., Mansour, M. H., Al-Sinani, S. S. H., & Al-Amri, I. S. (2009b). Effects of electrical stimulation on histochemical muscle fibre staining, quality, and composition of camel and cattle Longissimus thoracic muscles. *Journal of Food Science*, *74*(1), S44–S52. doi:10.1111/j.1750-3841.2008.00992.x PMID:19200120

Kadim, I. T., Mahgoub, O., Al-Marzooqi, W., Khalaf, S. K., & Raiymbek, G. (2013b). Nutritive Value, Quality and Health Aspects of the Dromedary (Camelus dromedaries) and Bactrian (Camelus bacterianus) Camel Meats: A Review. *Agricultural and Marine Sciences*, *18*, 7–24.

Kadim, I. T., Mahgoub, O., & Purchas, R. W. (2008). A review of the Growth, and of the Carcass and Meat Quality Characteristics of the One-humped Camel (Camelus dromedaries). *Meat Science*, *73*, 619–625. doi:10.1016/j.meatsci.2006.03.002 PMID:22063567

Kadim, I. T., & Sahi, A. B. A. (2018). Health aspects of camel meat: A review of literature. *Advances in Animal and Veterinary Sciences*, *6*(7), 271–272. doi:10.17582/journal.aavs/2018/6.7.271.272

Kamoun, M. (1995a). Dromedary meat: production, qualitative aspects and acpability for transformation. *Option Mediterraneennes.Serie B, Etudes Recherches,* (13), 105-130.

Kamoun, M. (1995b). *Evolution de la qualite de la carcasse et de la viande des dromadaires En function de la conduit zootechnique des animaux*. Rapport final relative a la bourse de recherché FIS no. 1372-2.

Kargozari, M., Moini, S., Basti, A. A., Emam-Djomeh, Z., Ghasemlou, M., Martin, I. R., ... Szumny, A. (2014). Development of Turkish dry-fermented sausage (sucuk) reformulated with camel meat and hump fat and evaluation of physicochemical, textural, fatty acid and volatile compound profiles during ripening. *Food Science and Technology (Campinas)*, *59*, 849–858.

Kassem, A., ElSayed, M. T., & Ahmed, A. (2004). Microstructural characteristics of Arabian camel meat. *Journal of Camelid Science*, *1*, 86–95.

Koohmaraie, M. (1988). The role of endogenous proteases in meat tenderness. *Reciprocal Meat Conference Proceedings*, *41*, 89-100.

Laack, R. V., Kauffman, R., & Greaser, M. (2001). Determinants of ultimate pH of meat. *Proceedings of 47th International Congress of Meat Science and Technology*, *1*, 22-26.

Lawrie, R. A. (2006). *Lawrie's Meat Science* (7th ed.). Cambridge, UK: Woodhead Publishing Limited. doi:10.1533/9781845691615

Lee, Y. P., & Lardy, H. A. (1965). Influence of thyroid hormones on 1-α-glycerophosphate dehydrogenases and other dehydrogenases in various organs of the rat. *The Journal of Biological Chemistry*, *240*, 1427–1436. PMID:14284758

Leeson, C. R., Lesson, T. S., & Paparo, A. A. (1985). Textbook of Histology (5th ed.). W. B. Saunders Company.

Locker, R. H. (1989). Muscle in to meat. In Meat Production and Processing. New Zealand Society of Animal Production.

Menzies, D. J., & Hopkins, D. L. (1996). Relationship between color and ph in lamb loins. *Proceedings of Australian Society of Animal Production*, *21*, 353.

Miller, W. O., Staffle, R. L., & Zirkle, S. B. (1968). Factors, which influence the water-holding capacity of various types of meat. *Food Technology*, *22*, 11390.

Mukasa-Mugerwa, E. (1981). The camel (Camelus dromedaries): A biographical review. International Livestock Centre for Africa.

Pearson, A. M., & Greaser, M. L. (1999). Flesh food and their analogues. In A. J. Rosenthal (Ed.), *Food texture: Measurement and Perception* (Vol. 1, pp. 228–255). Aspen Publishers, Inc.

Petrovic, L., Grujic, R., & Petrovic, M. (1993). Definition of the optimum freezing rate –2. Investigation of the physico-chemical properties of beef m. Longissimus dorsi frozen at different freezing rates. *Meat Science*, *33*(3), 319–331. doi:10.1016/0309-1740(93)90004-2 PMID:22060150

Pette, C., & Staron, S. (1990). Cellular and molecular diversities of mammalian skeletal muscle fibres. *Reviews of Physiology, Biochemistry and Pharmacology*, *116*, 1–76. PMID:2149884

Pospiech, E., Grzes, B., Lyczynski, A., Borzuta, K., Szalata, M., & Micolajczak, B. (2003). Muscle proteins and their changes in the process of meat tenderization. In Effect of genetic and non-genetic factors on carcass and meat quality of pigs. Poland Institute of Genetics and Animal Breeding.

Rahelic, S., & Puac, S. (1981). Fibre types in longissimus dorsi from wild and highly selected pig breeds. *Meat Science*, *5*(6), 451–455. doi:10.1016/0309-1740(81)90042-5 PMID:22054604

Renand, G., Picard, B., Touraille, C., Berge, P., & Lepetit, J. (2001). Relationships between muscle characteristics and meat quality traits of young Charolais bulls. *Meat Science*, *59*(1), 49–60. doi:10.1016/S0309-1740(01)00051-1 PMID:22062505

Saadoun, A., & Cabrera, M. C. (2008). A review of the nutritional content and technological parameters of indigenous sources of meat in South America. *Meat Science*, *80*(3), 570–581. doi:10.1016/j.meatsci.2008.03.027 PMID:22063568

Saltin, B., Rose, R. J., & Henckel, P. (1994). Skeletal muscle morphology and metabolic potential. *Acta Physiologica Scandinavica*, *150*(617), 24–32. PMID:8010123

Shehata, M. F. (2005). Carcass traits and meat quality of one-humped camels fed different halophytic forages: 2-Physical, chemical, and sensory characteristics of camel meat. *Journal of Agriculture Science*, *30*, 1943–1952.

Simek, J., Vorlova, L., Malota, L., Steinhauserova, I., & Steinhauser, L. (2003). Post-mortal changes of pH value and lactic acid content in the muscles of pigs and bulls. *Journal of Animal Science*, *7*, 295–299.

Simmons, N. J., Daley, C. C., Cummings, T. L., Morgan, S. K., Johnson, N. V., & Lombard, A. (2008). Reassessing the principles of electrical stimulation [Review]. *Meat Science*, *80*(1), 110–122. doi:10.1016/j.meatsci.2008.05.006 PMID:22063176

Snow, D. H., & Guy, P. S. (1981). Fibre type and enzyme activities of the gluteus medius in different breeds of horse. In J. Poortmans & G. Niset (Eds.), *Biochemistry of Exercise IV-B* (pp. 275–282). Baltimore, MD: University of Park Press.

Snow, D. H., & Harris, R. C. (1985). Thoroughbreds and greyhounds: biochemical adaptations in creatures of nature and of man. In Circulation, respiration and metabolism. Springer-Verlag. doi:10.1007/978-3-642-70610-3_17

Suliman, G., Sami, A., Alowaimer, A., & Koohmaraie, M. (2011). Effect of breed on the quality attributes of camel meat. *The Indian Journal of Animal Sciences*, *81*, 407–411.

Swatland, H. J. (1984). The structure and properties of meat. In *Structure and Development of Meat Animals* (pp. 153–200). Englewood Cliffs, NJ: INC.

Varnam, A. H., & Sutherland, J. P. (1995). *Meat and meat products: technology, chemistry and microbiology*. London: Chapman and Hall.

Warris, P. (1990). The handling of cattle pre-slaughter and its effects on carcass and meat quality. *Applied Animal Behaviour Science*, *28*(1-2), 171–186. doi:10.1016/0168-1591(90)90052-F

Chapter 13
Camel Meat Nutrient Content and Potential Health Benefits

Isam Tawfik Kadim
University of Nizwa, Oman

Roger Purchas
Massey University, New Zealand

Issa Al-Amri
University of Nizwa, Oman

Abdulaziz Alkindi
University of Nizwa, Oman

Ghulam Abbas
University of Nizwa, Oman

ABSTRACT

Camels are an important source of nutritious meat and meat products for people, and therefore play a major role in the national economies of many countries. In comparison with other red meats, camel meat generally contains less fat and ash, more moisture, and similar protein content. Camel meat products are receiving worldwide interest owing to its unique healthy features and the ability of camels to thrive in climatic regions of the world that may be a challenge to many other meat-producing species. Camel meat products contain many essential nutrients and some components with potential bioactive properties that could be beneficial for human health and wellbeing. Continued improvements in the understanding and optimization of the production processes of camel meat are required for successful industrial implementation and marketing. Advances in ingredient systems may be used to manufacture new meat products from camel meat where higher levels of nutrition are required to enhance consumer health and wellbeing. Camel meat as a functional food is one area that can be exploited.

DOI: 10.4018/978-1-7998-1604-1.ch013

INTRODUCTION

The perception of meat consumers has changed over recent decades from considering meat simply as a source of required nutrients and energy to seeing meat as including health-promoting components. Therefore, a significant effort in the meat industry has led towards improving and characterizing the quality and healthiness of meat and meat products (Decker & Park, 2010). Generally, hotter climates adversely affect livestock through heat-stress effects on health, productivity, and fertility, but camels have adapted to produce quality meat (Chapter 12), fibers and milk even in the hottest and least favorable environmental conditions (Al-Abri & Faye, 2019; Bouhaddaoui et al., 2019). Opportunities exist to improve the nutritional and health features of camel meat products through processing or natural production or addition of natural functional substances. The healthiness and functionality of camel meat may be increased by adding ingredients, but such processes need to be tested for changes in taste, flavor, appearance, and consistency to ensure consumer acceptance (Pogorzelska-Nowicka, Atanasov, Horba´nczuk, & Wierzbicka, 2018).

Camel meat products are well suited for consumers who are interested in nutritive values and health-boosting properties, while being averse to potentially toxic ingredients such as allergenic components, drug residues, intoxicants, and microbial contaminations, which may cause health problems. Conversely, consumers are interested in, and may pay more for, products enriched with health-promoting components such as bioactive compounds, which will improve their well-being.

This chapter aims to characterize the important nutrient components of camel meat and to consider future developments with camel meat and camel meat products. Approaches to enriching camel meat with natural health-boosting substances will be addressed.

NUTRIENT CONTENT OF CAMEL MEAT

An outline of the nutritional characteristics of camel meat is provided in Table 1 with an indication of why they are important for human nutrition and comments on special aspects with respect to the meat from camels. Details on individual nutrients are provided in subsequent sections.

Information on the proximate composition of camel meat and other meats in Table 2 illustrates that, except for fat content, camel meat composition is generally similar to meat from other meat-producing mammals such as cattle, sheep, and deer.

Moisture contents in camel meat widely varied (72.1 to 77.7%) with higher values generally being associated with lower fat percentages. Kadim et al. (2006) stated that with age, the moisture contents of the camel meat decreases. Ibrahim, Nour and Kadim (2015) reported small difference in moisture contents between 3-4- and 6-7-year-old camels across different muscles while Gheisari, Aminlari and Shekarforoush (2009) found no such difference in moisture contents between camel meat and meat from other species of similar gender and age. The protein content of camel meat ranges from 15.9 to 22.1% (Table 2), with meat from young camels containing similar protein percentages to those found in young cattle, goat and lamb meats (Kadim, Mahgoub & Purchas, 2008). Various studies have demonstrated that animal age affects fat content with higher fat contents found in camel meat from older animals (Kadim et al., 2006; Ibrahim, Nour & Kadim, 2015). Some other factors may also affect the fat content of camel meat within similar age groups (Kadim et al., 2006, 2008, 2009b, Kadim, Mahgoub, Al-Marzooqi, & Khalaf, 2009a). Camel meat has lower ash percentages than beef, goat and lamb meat (Kadim et al., 2008).

Table 1. Examples of meat characteristics of importance for human nutrition with comments on these for meat from camels. Variation in these characteristics due to factors such as genotype, animal diet and differences between muscles may often be important but are not considered in this broad overview.

Nutritional characteristic	Importance for human diets and presence in meat	Comments regarding camel meat
Protein concentration	Proteins are an essential requirement of the human diet, with meat being an important source for many people.	Protein concentrations are similar or slightly lower in camel meat than for other red meats (see Table 2).
The amino-acid balance within proteins and as free amino acids.	The balance of the 12 essential amino acids in meat is close to estimated requirements for humans.	A similar balance to that of meat from other mammals (see Table 4).
Digestibility and bioavailability[a] of proteins and amino acids.	Proteins must be digestible and absorbable to be useful. Generally, very high for most meat proteins when cooked with care. Some connective tissue proteins are an exception.	Highly digestible as with proteins in other meats.
Bioactivity[b] of proteins or their breakdown products.	There is increasing evidence that certain short-chain polypeptides from meat proteins have bioactive properties.	Limited research specifically with proteins of camel meat (see section on bioactive compounds).
Lipid (fat) concentration	Some lipid components are essential for humans, but fat is mainly a source of energy. Some lipids are undesirable nutritionally.	Concentrations are generally low in camel meats (see Table 2).
Fatty-acid proportions in lipid	Some fatty acids in meat are beneficial (eg: long-chain n3 FAs), while some are undesirable for humans (eg: certain saturated FAs and some trans fats).	The balance of fatty acids in camel meat is generally good but is dependent on camel diets and levels of fatness (see Table 3).
Other lipid components	Several lipid components such as certain vitamins in meat are beneficial to human health and nutrition.	Low concentrations expected because of the low-fat nature of camel meat.
Minerals	Many minerals are essential for humans with meat being an important source of several key minerals including iron and zinc. Potentially harmful minerals are usually absent.	Similar to other red meats (see Table 5).
Bioavailability of individual minerals.	Important minerals such as iron in meat are more bioavailable than for the same minerals in many other foods.	Expected to mirror the case for other red meats.
Water-soluble vitamins	Required components of human diets, with meat being an important source, especially for vitamin B_{12}. A poor source of vitamin C.	Similar to other red meats based on limited data (see Table 6).
Fat-soluble vitamins	Also required in the human diet, with levels depending to some extent on fat levels in the meat.	Will tend to be at lower levels due to low concentrations of lipid (see Table 6).
Other compounds with possible bioactive properties	A developing area with examples of compounds being evaluated in meat including coenzyme Q_{10}, taurine, lipoic acid, carnitine, carnosine, creatine, growth factors, etc.	Limited information is available, but expected to be similar to other red meats (see section on bioactive compounds).

[a]Bioavailability: The effectiveness with which components of the diet are taken up and effectively utilised by cells within the body.

[b]Bioactivity: A compound is said to be bioactive if it contributes to human health and wellbeing in some way over and above its effect as a nutrient.

Table 2. Chemical composition (g/100g) of muscles from different species of animals used for meat production

No./Animal Species	Muscle	Moisture	Protein	Fat	Ash	References
10 Red deer	LD	76.9	21.70	0.6	1.11	Zomborszky, Szentmihalyi, Sarudi, Horn, & Szabo (1996)
10 Fallow deer	LD	74.9	22.0	2.5	1.08	
10 Roe deer	LD	74.8	23.0	1.7	1.15	
11 Reindeer	LD	71.8	23.60	2.8	1.10	Wiklund, Finstad, Johansson, Aguiar, & Bechtel (2008)
Dromedary	LT	73.8	19.0	6.2	0.85	
Dromedary	IS	73.2	18.2	5.3	096	
Dromedary	TB	77.7	17.1	1.9	1.00	
Dromedary	ST	75.4	18.5	3.1	0.91	Kadim et al. (2013)
Dromedary	SM	73.0	22.1	2.5	0.93	
Dromedary	BF	74.3	20.8	2.5	1.00	
9 Bactrian	LT	72.1	17.0	10	0.9	
9 Bactrian	IS	78.5	18.0	2.5	1.0	
9 Bactrian	TB	78.4	17.6	3.0	1.0	
9 Bactrian	ST	78.0	18.8	2.2	1.0	Raiymbek et al. (2018)
9 Bactrian	SM	78.8	18.2	2.0	1.0	
9 Bactrian	BF	78.5	18.3	2.1	1.1	
15 Dromedary	LT	77.0	15.9	4.1	1.0	Kimassoum et al. (2016)
20 Lama	LT	73.9	23.1	0.5	2.40	Cristofanelli, Antonini, & Torres (2004)
40 Alpaca	LT	73.6	23.3	0.5	2.50	
70 Guanaco	LT	73.9	20.9	1.0	1.10	Gonzalez, Smulders, Paulsen, Skewes, & Konig (2004)
10 llama male		71.9	19.2	8.0	1.0	Perez et al. (2000)
10 Ilama female		72.2	21.4	5.5	1.0	
Kangaroo		75.5	20.3	0.8	1.20	Nuttab (2010)
6 Beef	LD	70.9	20.0	5.7	0.98	Moreira, de Souza, Matsushita, do Prado & Nascimento (2003)
17 Beef	BF	72.2	21.1	6.1	0.96	Purchas, Wilkinson, Carruthers, & Jackson (2014)

(LD = longissimus dorsi; LT = longissimus thoracis; IS = infraspinatus; TB = triceps brachii; ST = semitendinosus; SM = semimembranosus; BF = biceps femoris).

Fatty Acids

The fatty acid content of meat has important effects on human health, and consumer concern and knowledge about this characteristic has increased over recent decades (Blasbalg, Hibbeln, Ramsden, Majchrzak & Rawlings, 2011). Decreases in saturated fatty acid intake plays a role in reducing obesity, hypercholesterolaemia and in minimizing the risk of cancer (Chan, 2004). Camel meat contains relatively high levels of polyunsaturated fat acids (PUFAs) and low cholesterol levels (Kadim et al., 2008).

Generally, diet-related diseases such as coronary diseases are associated with higher contributions of animal fat in human diets (Mozaffarian, Micha & Wallace, 2010). Camel meat with its low intramuscular fat and low cholesterol content is a low meat-fat product (Kadim et al., 2008). The major saturated, monounsaturated and polyunsaturated fatty acids in camel meat are summarized in Table 3. Saturated fatty acids comprise on average 45.0% of total fatty acids in camel muscle, with approximately half as palmitic acid (C16:0), and a third as stearic acid (C18:0). Polyunsaturated fatty acids (PUFA) range from 7.2% to 12.8% of total fatty acids. Rawdah, El-Faer & Koreish (1994) reported levels of 18.9% oleic acid (C18:1) and 12.1% linoleic acid (C18:2) in camel meat. On the other hand, about twice the amount of oleic acid (C18:1) and less than half the amount of linoleic acid (C18:2) were reported by Al-Bachir & Zeinou (2009) and Kadim et al. (2011). Linoleic acid is derived entirely from the diet (Wood et al., 2008) and such differences are not unexpected from studies from different regions. Sinclair, Slattery & O'Dea (1982) reported that PUFAs were higher in camel meat (11.2%) than in beef (8.8%), but lower than in meat from deer (31.4%) and buffalo (28.6%). In camel meat, the linoleic to linolenic acids ratio is 13.9 which is much higher than cattle, sheep or goat meat (2.0, 2.4 and 2.8, respectively) (Sinclair et al., 1982). Maqsood, Manheem, Abushelaibil & Kadim (2014) found that the camel meat contains significant amount of health-promoting PUFA. However, the presence of PUFA along with high haem proteins (Hb and Mb) could make camel meat more prone to lipid oxidation as reflected by high PV and TBARS formation.

Cholesterol content of camel meat has been reported to be low compared to beef and lamb (Kadim et al., 2008; Raiymbek et al., 2019). This is particularly important to the Middle Eastern and African countries where eating habits and cooking styles are very different from Western ones and the use of animal fat in cooking is very common.

Amino Acids

The concentrations of essential amino acid in camel meat are equivalent to beef, goat and lamb meat (Table 4), but camel meat has a slightly higher percentage of methionine and lysine than ostrich meat (Al-Shabib & Abu-Tarboush, 2004). According to Casey (1993), the quality of muscle protein lies in the extent of the availability of essential amino acids such as lysine and leucine in proportions required by human. For a 70 kg adult the amount of camel meat to supply necessary essential amino acids is similar to that for lamb, beef and goat (Fig. 1).

The most abundant essential amino acid in camel meat was lysine, followed by leucine, methionine, isoleucine, threonine and phenylalanine (Raiymbek et al., 2018; Kadim et al, 2011; Abdelhadi et al, 2017). Table 4 shows that, relative to total protein, leucine (6.8-9.9%) and lysine (8.1- 9.9%) were the most abundant essential amino acids (Table 4). In the study of Dawood and Alkanhal (1995), essential amino acids (mg/100 g DM) varied slightly between muscles and between studies (Table 4). The concentration of tryptophan was lower in camel meat than other meats in the study of Dawood and Alkanhal (1995). However, a recent study on camel by Raiymbek et al. (2018) found tryptophan concentration was 0.83% of the total amino acids which was lower than values reported for camel (1.76%) (Kadim et al., 2008) and beef (1.28%) (Al-Shabib & Abu-Tarboush, 2004). However, these values were obtained from different studies; a study comparing amino acid profiles in camel and other red meats is required.

Non-essential amino acids contents also varied slightly between camel muscles (Table 4). Raiymbek et al. (2018) reported lower alanine concentrations in camel meat compared to other red meats, in contrast to later studies that did not report lower concentrations (Dawood & Alkanhal, 1995; Al-Shabib

Table 3. Fat, and fatty acid composition determined in meat from various species (see Table 2 for muscle abbreviations)

	Fatty acid (% of total fatty acids)										
Species/Muscle	**C14:0**	**C16:0**	**C18:0**	**C18:1**	**C18:2**	**C18:3**	**C20:4**	**TSFA[1]**	**TUFA[2]**	**TPUFA[3]**	
20 Lama LT	4.09	24.8	21.5	35.8	3.13	0.82	1.78	50.3	42.5	7.2	Polidori, Renieri, Antonini, Passamonti, & Pucclarelli (2007)
Dromedary IS	7.62	27.6	8.79	25.0	7.14	0.64	2.81	51.8	-	11.4	
Dromedary TB	7.78	27.3	8.90	26.3	7.83	0.43	2.72	50.8	48.2	11.6	
Dromedary LT	7.16	26.9	9.82	26.2	7.11	0.59	2.84	51.3	49.2	11.5	
Dromedary ST	7.24	25.1	8.71	26.4	7.79	0.62	2.83	48.6	48.7	12.3	Kadim et al. (2013)
Dromedary SM	7.48	26.5	8.37	26.8	7.98	0.54	2.55	49.9	50.4	11.9	
Dromedary BF	7.83	26.2	8.02	26.9	7.94	0.54	3.51	48.9	50.2	12.8	
Dromedary LT	8.88	26.1	12.0	25.9	12.7	1.22	-	48.9	51.1	15..4	
Dromedary BF	8.78	25.4	12.2	25.2	14.2	1.11	-	48.6	51.4	16.6	Ibrahim, Nour, Al-Maqbali & Kadim (2017)
Dromedary ST	8.91	26.4	12.6	23.4	14.0	1.64	-	50.0	50.0	15.9	
Dromedary SM	8.25	27.2	11.9	25.8	13.6	1.21	-	49.2	50.8	16.2	
Dromedary TB Dromedary ST	7.60 5.88	27.5 29.6	8.69 16.6	21.5 24.5	7.14 5.69	0.65 1.90	1.87	58.5	41.5	12.2	Magsoos et al. (2014)
Dromedary IS	7.35	25.3	8.76	26.3	7.83	0.64	-	-	-	-	
Dromedary BF Dromedary ST Dromedary LT Dromedary SM	7.13 7.46 7.81 7.84	27.4 26.8 27.7 27.3	9.80 8.40 8.18 8.95	26.6 27.1 26.8 21.3	7.10 7.66 7.68 7.88	0.66 0.56 0.54 0.44	- - - -	- - - -	- - - -	- - - -	
Bactrian TB Bactrian IS Bactrian BF Bactrian ST Bactrian LT Bactrian SM	6.34 6.19 6.01 6.03 5.73 5.15	19.5 17.4 20.5 18.6 17.9 16.9	6.90 6.31 7.74 5.17 9.15 6.08	21.4 21.8 21.2 20.4 17.8 20.3	10.1 9.96 10.1 10.3 9.61 10.0	0.92 0.91 0.84 0.85 0.84 0.81	- - - - - -	- - - - - -	- - - - - -	- - - - - -	Raimbek et al. (2019
Bactrian SM	7.40	25.1	8.99	29.4	14.7	1.22	4.60	43.4	56.6	21.8	
Bactrian IS	8.59	24.0	8.74	30.2	13.9	1.26	3.50	44.0	56.0	19.7	
Bactrian ST	8.42	25.8	7.19	28.9	14.4	1.19	3.32	43.3	56.7	21.5	
Bactrian TB	8.19	26.1	9.30	28.4	13.6	1.25	3.41	46.0	54.0	19.7	Raiymbek et al. (2018)
Bactrian LT	8.30	25.8	13.1	26.0	14.1	1.19	3.69	49.3	50.7	20.3	
Bactrian BF	7.85	26.9	10.1	28.2	13.2	1.10	3.06	47.8	52.2	18.6	

[1]TSFA: Total Saturated Fatty Acid,[2]TUFA: Total Unsaturated Fatty Acid, [3]TPUFA: Total Polyunsaturated Fatty Acid.

Figure 1. The amount of meat from different species required to supply the daily requirements of indispensable amino acids for adults (70 kg body weight) based on mean nitrogen requirement of 105 mg nitrogen/kg per day (0.66 g protein/kg per day) recommended by WHO (2002)

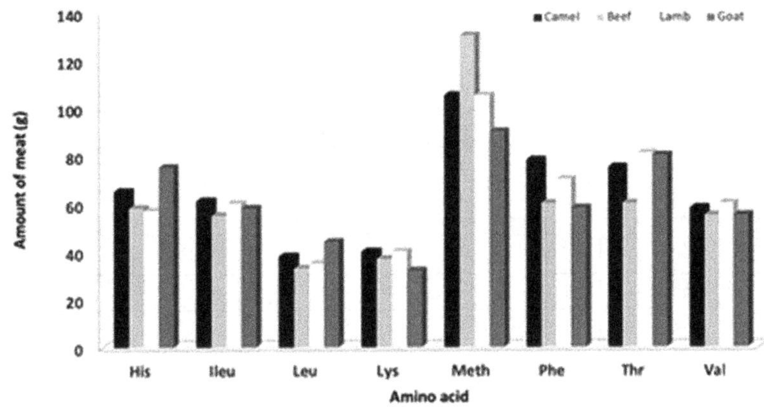

& Abu-Tarboush, 2004; Kadim et al., 2011). In general, it appears that camel meat may be a better, or at least as good, source of non-essential amino acids as beef, lamb and goat meats (Kadim et al, 2011; Dawood & Alkanhal, 1995; Al-Shabib & Abu-Tarboush, 2004; Raiymbek et al., 2018).

Minerals

Camel meat products are considered good sources of minerals for humans due to the natural characteristics of the feed consumed by camels. Minerals include those required essential elements for growth and health, and those that are toxic, but the latter will not be considered here.

Potassium is the major element in camel meat and other meats (Table 5), followed by phosphorus, sodium, sulphur and magnesium. Differences between muscles or cuts have been reported as shown in Table 5.

Iron is a vital component in human nutrition due to its multiple physiological functions including oxygen transport, the synthesis of enzymes, the regulation of immune functions and the energy production (Radlowski & Johnson, 2013). Iron also plays a crucial role in proper brain development of the fetus. Iron concentrations in camel meat tend to be higher than in pork, lamb or beef (Table 5) and the iron in muscle foods is more bioavailable than in many other foods. Iron concentrations in meat can be enhanced in processed products such as patties by adding iron compounds (Navas-Carretero, Pérez-Granados, Sarriá, & Vaquero, 2009), and iron concentrations increase with drying (Czerwonka & Szterk, 2015) and during cooking. Calcium is the most abundant mineral element in the body, and it is of importance for bone structure, muscle functions, nerve transmission, intracellular transmission, vascular contraction and vasodilation (Beto, 2015). Beef from cattle fed a Ca-enriched diet had higher calcium levels (Dikeman et al., 2003), but similar trials have not been conducted with camels.

Selenium being the part of selenoproteins regulates several physiological functions in humans and other animals, therefore it is equally important trace element for their health (Pogorzelska-Nowicka et al., 2018). Selenium supplements in animal feed, especially with organic selenium, increases its concentration in the meat of various animals (Polawska et al., 2016). The addition of selenium to animal

Table 4. Reported composition of the amino acids in camel meat muscles (LT = longissimus thoracic; IS = infraspinatus; TB = triceps brachii; ST = semitendinosus; SM = semimembranosus; BF = biceps femoris)

Factor	Essential Amino acids																	Reference
	His	Ileu	Leu	Lys	Met	Phe	Thr	Trp	Val	Ala	Arg	Asp	Glu	Gly	Pro	Ser	Tyr	
Bactrian camel																		
IS	4.2	6.8	7.4	9.7	6.6	6.3	5.9	0.8	5.2	4.2	6.8	9.8	15.2	-	5.2	3.1	3.5	
SM	5.1	6.8	7.3	9.7	7.3	6.4	5.5	0.8	5.3	4.0	7.1	10.0	15.9	-	5.9	3.8	3.5	
TB	4.5	6.8	6.9	8.1	6.6	5.5	5.8	0.8	5.2	3.9	7.1	10.0	15.7	-	5.8	3.8	3.7	
ST	4.2	7.0	6.9	8.7	7.6	4.4	6.0	0.8	5.6	4.0	7.8	10.3	16.3	-	5.0	4.1	4.0	Raiymbek et al. (2018)
BF	3.5	6.1	6.8	8.8	6.7	4.7	6.0	0.9	5.8	3.9	6.9	10.1	17.0	-	4.9	3.9	4.2	
LT	4.2	6.0	7.1	9.9	7.0	4.8	5.7	0.9	5.7	3.9	6.7	9.9	15.9	-	4.0	3.9	3.5	
Dromedary camel																		
LT	4.0	5.8	8.1	8.3	3.6	6.9	4.9	0.8	5.3	4.8	6.8	9.9	16.1	2.24	-	3.5	3.8	
BF	3.8	5.1	6.9	8.9	3.7	4.9	4.8	0.8	4.6	4.8	6.9	9.9	16.9	1.82	-	3.9	3.8	Ibrahim et al. (2017)
ST	4.1	5.7	7.0	7.9	3.6	5.0	4.9	0.7	5.1	4.9	7.0	9.9	16.7	2.39	-	3.8	3.8	
SM	3.8	5.1	6.9	8.7	3.7	5.0	5.0	0.7	4.9	4.9	7.0	10	16.9	2.11	-	3.9	3.9	
LT	4.4	4.7	8.3	9.4	2.9	4.3	4.5	-	5.6	6.5	6.6	9.3	15.9	4.3	3.9	3.6	3.5	Kadim et al. (2011)*
Loin	3.4	4.2	7.1	9.1	1.6	5.6	4.8	1.6	4.7	-	-	-	-	-	-	-	-	Al-Shabib andAbu-Tarboush (2004)
Leg	3.4	4.3	8.4	9.1	1.3	5.5	4.8	1.9	4.6	-	-	-	-	-	-	-	-	
Chuck	4.7	5.3	8.6	8.4	2.6	4.1	4.2	0.5	4.9	6.3	7.5	9.3	17.1	6.0	5.4	3.5	3.0	
Ribeye	4.3	5.4	8.3	8.6	2.2	4.4	4.7	0.7	5.3	6.2	7.1	9.3	17.3	5.9	4.9	3.8	3.4	Dawood and Alkanhal (1995)
Leg	4.5	4.9	8.3	8.3	2.5	4.2	4.2	0.6	5.4	6.3	7.5	8.6	16.4	5.9	5.9	3.6	3.3	
Camel	5.6	5.9	9.5	8.9	3.5	4.7	4.8	-	6.3	3.9	7.1	10.8	18.6	6.1	3.9	3.2	3.8	
Beef	6.2	6.5	10.7	9.1	2.7	5.7	5.5	-	6.6	7.7	7.1	10.8	16.5	6.2	4.5	4.2	4.1	Elgasim and Alkanhal (1992)
Lamb	5.9	5.8	9.6	8.5	3.3	4.9	4.2	-	5.9	6.7	6.9	10.3	17.9	5.5	3.8	2.9	3.5	
Goat	4.7	6.0	7.9	11	3.9	6.5	4.4	-	6.8	4.7	7.1	10.8	15.6	5.2	3.8	3.6	5.9	
Camel	3.4	4.3	7.7	9.1	1.4	5.5	4.8	1.8	4.7	6.5	6.9	9.7	17.0	6.2	-	4.3	3.3	Al-Shabib and Abu-Tarboush (2004)
Ostrich	2.8	3.8	7.4	4.3	0.5	4.9	4.2	1.8	3.8	5.6	5.9	8.3	15.4	4.5	-	3.7	2.8	

*= calculated from mg/100 DM values using the average DM and protein contents.

feeds increases lipid oxidation stability, delays microbial growth (Kim et al., 2010), and increases the firmness and chewiness of meat (Miezeliene, Alencikiene, Gruzauskas, & Barstys, 2011). Selenium can also be added directly to meat products.

Zinc is an essential trace element for human health, with over 100 enzymes being zinc-dependent. It is important in protein and cell membrane maintenance and regulatory gene expression functions in cells. Long-term insufficient intake leads to anemia, diarrhea, pneumonia, disturbed brain development, and abnormalities in fetal growth (Roohani, Hurrell, Kelishadi, & Schulin, 2013). Camel meat along with other red meats is an important source of Zn, and adequate meat levels can decrease fat oxidation, reduce cooking loss, increase crude protein content and increase total antioxidant capacity (Yang et al., 2016).

Table 5. Mineral concentrations in camel meat (mg/100g fresh weight) (see Table 2 for muscle abbreviations)

	Mineral[1]											
Factor	**Ca**	**Cu**	**Fe**	**K**	**Mg**	**Mn**	**Sl**	**Na**	**P**	**S**	**Zn**	
Rump	-	0.12	2.5	-	-	-	-	-	-	-	-	Badiei, Mostaghni, Pourjafar, & Parchami (2006)
Loin	10.2	0.16	2.86	446	28.0	0.16	-	189	-	-	3.7	
Leg	9.8	0.26	3.39	548	42.5	0.19	-	313	-	-	3.9	
Chuck	11.5	-	3.2	249	17.4	-	-	73.5	-	-	3.7	Dawood & Alkanhal (1995)
Loin	8.1	-	2.9	231	16.3	-	-	67.1	-	-	3.7	
Limb	10.3	-	3.4	251	17.1	-	-	69.7	-	-	3.9	
Shoulder	5.1	0.07	1.2	357	20.6	0.01	-	69.1	196	56.1	3.5	El-Faer, Rawdah, Attar, & Dawson (1991)
Thigh	5.4	0.09	1.4	361	21.0	0.01	-	70.4	199	55.0	3.1	
Ribs	4.7	0.07	1.2	324	18.5	0.01	-	84.1	181	58.0	3.9	
Neck	5.6	0.09	1.4	338	18.5	0.01	-	87.3	181	64.4	4.8	
Camel	5.9	-	-	193	12.9	-	-	45.3	105	-	-	Kadim et al. (2009a)
Beef	6.2	-	-	416	20.5	-	-	51.0	162	-	-	
Camel	4.9	0.04	1.9	228	17.7	0.01	-	47.9	-	-	3.2	Elgasim & Alkanhal (1992)
LT[2]	13.3	4.11	3.25	797	37.1	0.15	-	149	352	-	5.11	
ST[3]	14.1	4.41	3.55	751	34.9	0.14	-	139	355	-	4.98	Ibrahim et al. (2017)
SM[4]	14.4	4.55	3.89	778	35.6	0.13	-	141	389	-	5.49	
BF[5]	13.6	4.99	3.22	759	35.9	0.14	-	141	393	-	5.58	
Llama	11.6	-	3.3	447	28.4	106	-	-	379	-	4.4	Polidori et al. (2007)
Alpaca	8.8	-	3.0	412	23.1	92.8	-	-	338	-	3.9	
Beef BF	4.7	-	1.91	325	20.7	0.02	-	50.4	181	-	3.7	Purchas et al. (2014)
Lamb LT	9.7	-	-	328	22.2		4.5	71.8	187	-	3.02	

1 Mineral: Ca: Calcium; Cu: Copper; Fe: Iron; K: Potassium; Mg: magnesium; Mn. Manganese; Sl Selnium, Na: Sodium; P; Phosphorus; S; Sulfate Zn: Zinc.[2]LT: longissimus thoracis, [3]ST: semitendinosus, [4]semimembranosus, [5]biceps femoris

Vitamins

Camel meat has low intramuscular fat (Kadim *et al,* 2008), so vitamin A will be low (Table 6) compared to other red meats with higher fat contents. In the study of Raiymbek et al., (2018), it was found that camel meat contained 9.97 to 10.5 µg vit A/100g.

Vitamin E (Table 6) is a group of chemically similar compounds including tocopherols and tocotrienols with antioxidant characteristics (Pearce & Jacob, 2004). The most pronounced protective effect of vitamin E is against oxidation of the plasma lipoproteins and polyunsaturated fatty acid (PUFA) components of cell membranes (Horba ´nczuk & Wierzbicka, 2016). Metmyoglobin formation was inhibited by vitamin E addition to Hanwoo cattle forage thereby improving meat color (Lee, Kim, Liang, & Song, 2003). Additionally, vitamin E decreases toughness (lowering shear force) (Carnagey et al., 2008), increases

Table 6. Vitamin concentrations in camel meat (see Table 2 for muscle abbreviations)

		Vitamin[1]									
Species	Muscle	B_1	B_2	B_3	B_5	B_6	B_{12}	A	D	E	
	IS	0.09	-	-	0.88	0.64	4.64	10.5	-	0.85	
	TB	0.08	-	-	0.89	0.62	4.74	10.3	-	0.89	
Bactrian	LT	0.08	-	-	0.86	0.66	4.83	11.2	-	0.92	Raiymbek et al., (2018)
	ST	0.09	-	-	0.87	0.65	4.86	9.99	-	0.82	
	SM	0.09	-	-	0.82	0.61	4.98	10.1	-	0.86	
	BF	0.08	-	-	0.84	0.67	4.53	9.97	-	0.87	
Dromedary	LT	0.11	0.23		0.78	0.59	4.64	10.5		0.85	Ibrahim, ., Nour, Al-Maqbali, & Kadim (2018)
	ST	0.08	0.22		0.76	0.61	4.77	11.2		0.92	
	SM	0.09	0.26		0.72	0.61	4.68	10.1		0.86	
	BF	0.09	0.26		0.77	0.62	4.69	9.99		0.83	
Beef	Several	0.05	0.10	3.49	0.39	0.27	1.69	9.38	0.15	0.45	Purchas et al., (2014)
Lamb	Several	0.10	0.16	5.13	0.50	0.15	1.85	4.69	0.04	0.29	

[1]B_1: Thiamine (mg/100g), B_2: Riboflavin (mg/100r), B_3: Niacin (mg/100g), B_5: Pantothenic acid (mg/100g), B_6: Pyridoxine (mg/100g), B_{12}: Cyanocobalamin (µg/100g), A: Retinol (µg/100g), D: D_3 Cholecalciferol (µg/100g), E: Alpha-Tocopherol (E) (mg/100g)

tenderness (improved collagen solubility) (Maiorano et al., 2007), increases water-holding capacity and has an impact on the profile of volatile compounds in meat (Brodowska et al., 2016).

Vitamin D levels in meat are low (Table 6) compared with recommended target intakes of 10–20 µg/day. Feeding animals with vitamin D-enriched forage may increase levels in meat (Montgomery et al., 2004) and improve meat colour (Wiegand et al., 2002).

Meat is an important source of the B vitamins with vitamin B_{12} being particularly important because it is not present in most foods. Camel meat contained 4.75µg/100 g vit B_{12} (Table 6), which is higher than for sheep (0.25 mg/100g) and veal meats (0.18 mg/100g) (Ono et al, 1984; Ono, Berry. & Douglass, 1986).

ANTIOXIDANTS

Antioxidants are present in meat (see the next section on bioactive compounds) but are not as strong as those found in plants. Polyphenols from plants have strong antioxidant properties and are responsible for the flavor, taste and color of plants. Antioxidants prevent of various diseases such as ischemic heart diseases, Alzheimer's disease, diabetes, ischemic heart diseases, allergies, liver disorders, and bowel diseases in human (Tewari et al., 2018). Polyphenols inclusion in animal feed has achieved some success, but positive effects of polyphenol addition to meat or meat products on color (Kim, Cho, & Han, 2013) and sensory properties (Fan, Chen, Sun & Zheng, 2014) has been reported with no adverse effect on textural properties (Hayes, Stepanyan, Allen, O'Grady & Kerry, 2011). Further research should be conducted with camel meat products.

BIOACTIVE COMPOUNDS

Several bioactive compounds have been measured in meat (Arihara, 2006) and may be useful in marketing. For example, carnosine and anserine are important dipeptides which are found in high concentrations in the muscle and brain of mammalian and avian species (Tomonaga et al., 2006). They function as antioxidants and putative neurotransmitters in the brain (Tomonaga et al., 2006). High concentrations of about 365 and 400 mg/100 g have been reported in beef and lamb, respectively (Purchas, Rutherfurd, Pearce, Vather & Wilkinson, 2004) and in red deer, 290 and 329 mg/ 100g (Purchas, Triumf, & Egelandsdal, 2010). The average levels of carnosine and anserine (mmol/kg dry matter) in camel middle gluteal muscles are shown in Fig. 2. On a fresh weight basis, camel middle gluteal muscle had 181.7 mg carnosine /100 g fresh weight and 268.6 mg anserine /100 g fresh weight (Dunnett, Harris, Soliman & Suwar, 1997; Dunnett & Harris, 1997). Carnosine concentrations varies between muscles in beef and lamb (Purchas, et al., 2004; Purchas & Busboom, 2005) and similar variations in carnosine and anserine have been found between camel muscles. This have been attributed to differences in metabolic activity and diet (Dunnett et al., 1997), thus, the concentrations of these bioactives in different camel muscles and how that compares to other animal species under similar environment requires more research.

L-carnitine plays an important physiological role in producing energy during exercise through transporting long-chain fatty acids across the inner mitochondrial membranes. The L-carnitine concentrations in chicken, pork, beef, horse and venison have been reported as 0.69 to 4.95 µmol/g fresh weights (Shimada et al., 2004). Alhomida, Duhaiman, A1-Jafari & Junaid (1995) reported 5.17, 2.60 and 7.77 µmol/g fresh weight of free carnitine, acylcarnitine and total carnitine respectively in camel meat (Figure 3). While the significance of these results from different laboratories need to be repeated in a controlled experiment, it is possible that camel meat may be a good source of L-carnitine. In the study of Abdelhadi et al., (2017), no significant effect of gender on nutritive value of meat was observed except that female camel's muscles had significantly higher arginine contents than males. Moreover, higher percentage of cis 9, trans 11 (18:2) was found in female muscles (Abdelhadi et al., 2017).

Figure 2. The average concentrations of carnosine, anserine, taurine and balenine in camel middle gluteal muscle
From Dunnett et al. (1997) and Dunnett and Harris (1997)

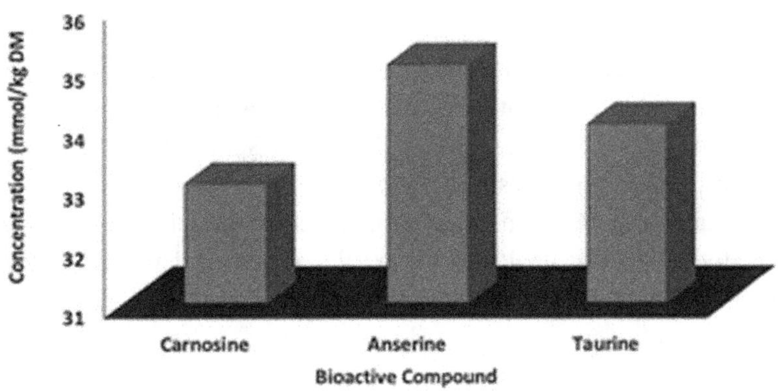

Figure 3. Average concentrations of free carnitine, acylcarnitine and total carnitine in camel muscle tissue (Alhomida et al., 1995)

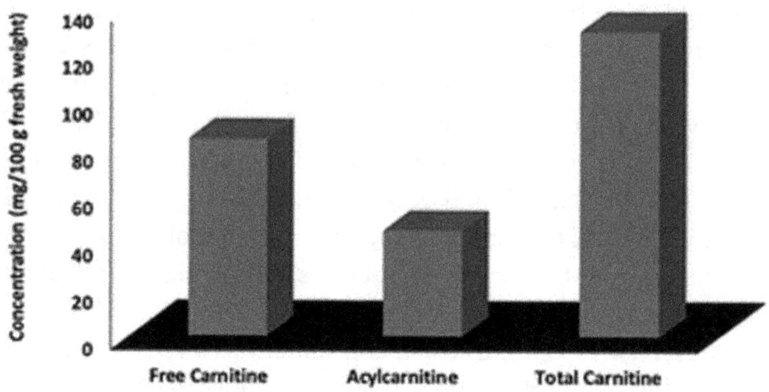

CONTAMINANTS

Various studies investigated the concentrations of organochlorine pesticides in meat, liver and kidney samples from camel, cattle and sheep (Sallam & Morshedy, 2008; Ibrahim et al., 2018; Jurjanz, Nurseitova, Toregozhina, Konuspayeva, & Faye, 2018). Despite the longer life span of camels compared to cattle and sheep, lower levels of contaminates were found in camel meat. The low bioaccumulation of pesticides in camel meat (Sallam & Morshedy 2008) is of interest because many African countries still have major problems with the use of organochlorine products. The advantage of camel in polluting areas is that, because pesticides are lipophilic, the contaminants are concentrated in the hump and not in the meat (Jurjanz et al., 2018). The same authors concluded that chronic exposure of camels to PCBs would lead to contamination of the hump. Camel meat being essentially free from most pesticides and antibiotics indicates that it is safe for human consumption. This favorable picture may indicate an ability of camel to detoxify organochlorines more efficiently compared with cattle and sheep, but this needs to be confirmed in properly designed experiments. Camels are generally reared in arid regions where the use of pesticides is limited, so it might be the lack of exposure rather than natural low bioaccumulation that is the cause of the low organochlorines observed by Sallam & Morshedy (2008).

HEALTH BENEFITS OF CAMEL MEAT

Camel meat is rich in many essential amino acids, minerals, vitamins, bioactive compounds such as carnosine, anserine, glutathione and essential fatty acids such as omega 3 fatty acids (Williams, 2007; Schonfeldt & Gibson, 2008; Abrhaley & Leta, 2018; Kadim & Sahi, 2018). Apart from its nutrient content, camel meat provides new experiences of eating unlike other protein sources. Camel meat protein contents are considered equal or better than other meats on commercial basis in Africa, Middle East and some Asian countries. Studies relating health problems like obesity and high saturated fat and cholesterol owing to increased use of animal products (Biesalski, 2005; Chao et al., 2005) has recommended smaller portions and less frequently (Schonfeldt & Gibson, 2008) or replacing red meat with white meat. The camel meat with low cholesterol and fat contents along with comparatively higher levels of unsaturated fatty acids prove that it is a good alternative to mutton and beef with more fat and cholesterol (Kadim et al., 2008).

Generally, meat is considered as a cure for many diseases and to improve performance in many cultures around the world based mainly on anecdotal evidence (Migdal & Živković, 2007). Camel meat and offal such as liver are considered to have medicinal properties (Bin Saeed, Al-Hamdan, & Fontaine, 2005). It has been noted that Somalis and Indians believe in the health benefits of consuming camel meat (Kadim et al., 2008). Among many African and Asian countries, camel meat has traditionally been used to cure diseases such as seasonal fever, sciatica and shoulder pain, as well as for removing freckles, and camel meat soup has been used to cure corneal opacity and to strengthen eyesight. Large number of camel meat consumers consider it a healthier option during the dry season in which cattle are often infected with various zoonotic diseases (Kurtu, 2004). This belief probably originated from the historical use of organs and meat from animals in folklore and traditional medicine. Lev (2006) cited the use of camel meat in remedial formulations by Al-Tabari, Al-Kindi & Al-Qazwini which indicate the roots of some of the current beliefs.

PROCESSED MEATS

Processed meat products are defined here as meat that has been physically treated in some way (grinding, drying, emulsifying, etc.) with or without the addition of items intended to enhance its eating quality, keeping quality, appearance, and/or health-promoting properties. Meat that has been cooked without any other treatment is not normally considered as processed meat. Examples of processed meat products that may include camel meat are listed in Table 7.

Table 7. Examples of processed-meat products that may include camel meat with or without additives[a]

Type of processed meat product	Process(s) involved	Features
Patties & meat balls	Grinding/mincing with or without additives[a].	Used alone or in burgers or casseroles with many options in terms of additives[a] (Farouk & Bekhit, 2013; Heba, Abdel-Haeem Hussein & Mohamed, 2016).
Dried products such as jerky	Controlled drying with or without additives	The level of drying varies, but usually an enhanced shelf life without refrigeration (Lonnecker et al., 2010).
Cured meat products as sausages	Curing often combined with mincing or emulsifying. Curing additives[a] as well as others.	Curing enhances the shelf life and colour of meat, but there is some consumer resistance to the processes.
Product in cans or sealed containers.	Heating for sterilization with or without additives[a].	Enhanced keeping quality without need for refrigeration. A wide choice of additives[a] (Legarreta, 2010).
Smoked products	Smoking step often combined with heating and additives[a]	Characteristic smoke flavour often with improved keeping quality.

[a]Additives may include items intended to enhance product properties such as eating quality, keeping quality, appearance, and/or health-promoting properties.

Camel sausages fermented by using *Lb. plantarum*, exhibited higher antioxidant, antihypertensive and cytotoxicity properties than beef sausages. This probiotic can be utilized in the fermented meat industry on commercial basis (Ayyash et al., 2019). In another study, Khezrian and co-worker prepared novel films composed of nanomontmorillonite-chitosan (MMT-Ch) and nanomontmorillonite-carboxymethyl cellulose (MMT-CMC). These films prevent microbial spoilage and thus have industrial application to improve quality of minced meat and also delay the oxidation of lipid and protein during storage (Khezrian & Shahbazi, 2018). Furthermore, Maqsood, Al Haddad and Mudgil (2016) found that vacuum packaging was very effective in retarding lipid oxidation, microbial growth and protein degradation, as well as maintaining the higher redness (a*) values of camel meat. Vacuum packaging can maintain the quality of the camel meat for longer period by limiting the microbial load, lipid oxidation and preserving the colour of the meat, therefore, it can be applied as an effective preservation strategy for displaying the fresh camel meat on the refrigerated shelves as well as transportation of the meat from one country to another without freezing the meat.

CONCLUSION

Camel meat has comparable nutritional values to other red meats. It has higher amino acid and mineral contents than other animal meats while intramuscular fat level is lower. Camel meat has been processed into burgers, sausages, patties, and shawarma in order to add value. The quality characteristics of camel meat are similar to those of beef from animals of similar ages. According to the composition and quality parameters of camel meat, it can be successfully marketed alongside that of cattle, deer, sheep and goat. Future research is needed for exploiting the potential of the camel meat through multidisciplinary research into efficient production systems, and improved meat technology and marketing. The emerging properties of camel meat as a healthy meat provide the foundation for the expansion and marketing of camel processed products. With the increasing demand for high-protein and low-fat shelf stable products for recreational activities, the potential of some traditional products (such jerky, Qwanta, and pastirma) to be marketed internationally is very high.

REFERENCES

Abdelhadi, O. M. A., Babiker, S. A., Bauchart, D., Listrat, A., Re'mond, D., Hocquette, J. F., & Faye, B. (2017). Effect of gender on quality and nutritive value of dromedary camel (*Camelus dromedarius*) longissimus lumborum muscle. *Journal of the Saudi Society of Agricultural Sciences*, *16*(3), 242–249. doi:10.1016/j.jssas.2015.08.003

Al-Abri, M. A., & Faye, B. (2019). Genetic improvement in dromedary camels: Challenges and opportunities. *Frontiers in Genetics*, *10*, 167. doi:10.3389/fgene.2019.00167 PMID:30915101

Al-Bachir, M., & Zeinou, R. (2009). Effect of gamma irradiation on microbial load and quality characteristics of minced camel meat. *Meat Science*, *82*(1), 119–124. doi:10.1016/j.meatsci.2008.12.012 PMID:20416783

Al-Shabib, N. A., & Abu-Tarboush, H. M. (2004). Nutritional value and some functional properties of protein in Ostrich and Camel meat. *Arab Journal of Food Nutrition*, *5*, 6–20.

Alhomida, A. S., Duhaiman, A. S., Al-Jafari, A. A., & Junaid, M. A. (1995). Determination of L-carnitine, acylcarnitine and total carnitine levels in plasma and tissues of camel (*Camelus dromedarius*). *Comparative Biochemistry and Physiology*, *111B*(3), 441–445. doi:10.1016/0305-0491(95)00014-Y PMID:7613767

Arihara, K. (2006). Strategies for designing novel functional meat products. *Meat Science*, *74*(1), 219–229. doi:10.1016/j.meatsci.2006.04.028 PMID:22062731

Ayyash, M., Liu, S. Q., Al Mheiri, A., Aldhaheri, M., Raeisi, B., Al-Nabulsi, A., & Olaimat, A. (2019). In vitro investigation of health-promoting benefits of fermented camel sausage by novel probiotic Lactobacillusplantarum: A comparative study with beef sausages. *Lebensmittel-Wissenschaft + Technologie*, *99*, 346–354. doi:10.1016/j.lwt.2018.09.084

Badiei, M., Mostaghni, K., Pourjafar, M., & Parchami, A. (2006). Serum and tissue trace elements in Iranian camels (Camelus dromedaries). *Comparative Clinical Pathology*, *15*(1), 58–61. doi:10.100700580-006-0610-x

Beto, J. A. (2015). The Role of Calcium in Human Aging. *Clinical Nutrition Research*, *4*(1), 1–8. doi:10.7762/cnr.2015.4.1.1 PMID:25713787

Biesalski, H. (2005). Meat as a component of a healthy diet – Are there any risks or benefits if meat is avoided in the diet? *Meat Science*, *70*(3), 509–524. doi:10.1016/j.meatsci.2004.07.017 PMID:22063749

Bin Saeed, A. A., Al-Hamdan, N. A., & Fontaine, R. E. (2005). *Plague from Eating Raw Camel Liver. Emerg.Inbfec. bDis.bb11*. Available from http://www.cdc.gov/ncidod/EID/vol11no09/05-0081.htm

Blasbalg, T. L., Hibbeln, J. R., Ramsden, C. E., Majchrzak, S. F., & Rawlings, R. R. (2011). Changes in consumption of omega-3 and omega-6 fatty acids in the United States during the 20th century. *The American Journal of Clinical Nutrition*, *93*(5), 950–962. doi:10.3945/ajcn.110.006643 PMID:21367944

Bouhaddaoui, S., Chabir, R., Errachidi, F., El Ghadraoui, L., El Khalfi, B., Benjelloun, M., & Soukri, A. (2019). Study of the Biochemical Biodiversity of Camel Milk. *The Scientific World Journal*, *2019*, 1–7. doi:10.1155/2019/2517293 PMID:31093015

Brodowska, M., Guzek, D., Kołota, A., Głabska, D., Górska-Horczyczak, E., Wojtasik-Kalinowska, I., & Wierzbicka, A. (2016). Effect of diet on oxidation and profile of volatile compounds of pork after freezing storage. *Journal of Food and Nutrition Research*, *55*, 40–47.

Carnagey, K. M., Huff-Lonergan, E. J., Trenkle, A., Wertz-Lutz, A. E., Horst, R. L., & Beitz, D. C. (2008). Use of 25-hydroxyvitamin D3 and vitamin E to improve tenderness of beef from the longissimus dorsi of heifers. *Journal of Animal Science*, *86*(7), 1649–1657. doi:10.2527/jas.2007-0502 PMID:18344288

Casey, N. H. (1993). Carcass and meat quality. In C. Maree & N. H. Casey (Eds.), *Livestock production systems; principles and practice* (pp. 306–333). Brooklyn, South Africa: Agri-Development Foundation.

Chan, W. (2004). Macronutrients in meat. In W. K. Jensen, C. Devine, & M. Dikeman (Eds.), *Encyclopedia of meat science* (pp. 614–618). Oxford, UK: Elsevier Academic Press. doi:10.1016/B0-12-464970-X/00235-X

Chao, A., Thun, M., Connell, C., McCullough, M., Jacobs, E., & Flanders, W. (2005). Meat consumption and risk of colorectal cancer. *Journal of the American Medical Association*, *293*(2), 172–182. doi:10.1001/jama.293.2.172 PMID:15644544

Cristofanelli, S., Antonini, M., Torres, D., Polidori, P., & Renieri, C. (2004). Meat and carcass quality form Peruvian llama (lama glama) and alpaca (*lama pacos*). *Meat Science*, *66*(3), 589–593. doi:10.1016/S0309-1740(03)00174-8 PMID:22060868

Czerwonka, M., & Szterk, A. (2015). The effect of meat cuts and thermal processing on selected mineral concentration in beef from Holstein–Friesian bulls. *Meat Science*, *105*, 75–80. doi:10.1016/j.meatsci.2015.03.011 PMID:25828160

Dawood, A., & Alkanhal, M. A. (1995). Nutrient composition of Najdi- Camel Meat. *Meat Science*, *39*(1), 71–78. doi:10.1016/0309-1740(95)80008-5 PMID:22059764

Decker, E. A., & Park, Y. (2010). Healthier meat products as functional foods. *Meat Science*, *86*(1), 49–55. doi:10.1016/j.meatsci.2010.04.021 PMID:20580991

Dikeman, M. E., Hunt, M. C., Addist, P. B., Schoenbeck, H. J., Pullen, M., Katsanidis, E., & Yancey, E. J. (2003). Effects of postexsanguination vascular infusion of cattle with a solution of saccharides, sodium chloride, and phosphates or with calcium chloride on quality and sensory traits of steaks and ground beef. *Journal of Animal Science*, *81*(1), 156–166. doi:10.2527/2003.811156x PMID:12597386

Dunnett, M., & Harris, R. C. (1997). High-performance liquid chromatographic determination of imidazole dipeptides, histidine, 1 -methylhistidine and 3- methylhistidine in equine and camel muscle and individual muscle fibres. *Journal of Chromatography. B, Biomedical Sciences and Applications*, *688*(1), 47–55. doi:10.1016/S0378-4347(97)88054-1 PMID:9029312

Dunnett, M., Harris, R. C., Soliman, M. Z., & Suwar, A. A. S. (1997). Carnosine, anserine and taurine contents in individual fibres from the middle gluteal muscle of the camel. *Research in Veterinary Science*, *62*(3), 213–216. doi:10.1016/S0034-5288(97)90192-2 PMID:9300536

El-Faer, M. Z., Rawdah, T. N., Attar, K. M., & Dawson, M. V. (1991). Mineral and proximate composition of the meat of the one-humped camel (*Camelus dromedaries*). *Food Chemistry*, *42*(2), 139–143. doi:10.1016/0308-8146(91)90029-N

Elgasim, E. A., & Alkanhal, M. A. (1992). Proximate composition, amino acids and inorganic mineral content of Arabian Camel meat: Comparative study. *Food Chemistry*, *45*(1), 1–4. doi:10.1016/0308-8146(92)90002-J

Fan, W., Chen, Y., Sun, J., & Zheng, Y. (2014). Effects of tea polyphenol on quality and shelf life of pork sausages. *Mboxemph Journal of Food Science and Technology*, *51*(1), 191–195. doi:10.100713197-013-1076-x PMID:24426069

Farouk, M. M., & Bekhit, A. E. (2013). Processing Camel meats. In I. T. Kadim, O. Mahgoub, B. Faye, & M. M. Farouk (Eds.), *Camel Meat and Meat production* (pp. 186–203). CABI. doi:10.1079/9781780641010.0186

Gheisari, H. R., Aminlari, M., & Shekarforoush, S. S. (2009). A comparative study of the biochemical and functional properties of camel and cattle meat during frozen storage. *Veterinarski Arhiv*, *79*, 51–68.

Gonzalez, F., Smulders, F. J. M., Paulsen, P., Skewes, O., & Konig, H. E. (2004). Anatomical investigations on meat cuts of guanacos (Lama guanicoe, Muller, 1776) and chemical composition of selected muscles. *Wiener Tierärztliche Monatsschrift, 91*, 77–84.

Hayes, J. E., Stepanyan, V., Allen, P., O'Grady, M. N., & Kerry, J. P. (2011). Evaluation of the effects of selected plant-derived nutraceuticals on the quality and shelf-life stability of raw and cooked pork sausages. *Lebensmittel-Wissenschaft + Technologie, 44*, 164–172.

Heba, H. S., Hussein, A.-H., & Mohamed, M. H. (2016). Improving the physico-chemical and sensory characteristics of camel meat burger patties using ginger extract and papain. *Meat Science, 118*, 52–60.

Horbanczuk, O. K., & Wierzbicka, A. (2016). Technological and nutritional properties of ostrich, emu and rhea meat quality. *Journal of Veterinary Research (Pulawy), 60*, 279–286.

Ibrahim, G. A., Nour, I. A., & Al-Maqbali, R. (2018). Determination of pesticide and antibiotic residues in musclkes of Sudanese camel (Camelus dromedaries). *Journal of Camel Practice and Research, 25*(2), 163–169. doi:10.5958/2277-8934.2018.00023.1

Ibrahim, G. A., Nour, I. A., Al-Maqbali, R., & Kadim, I. T. (2017). Effect of age on concentrations of nutrients in four muscles of Sudanese dromedary (Camelus dromedaries) camel. *Journal of Applied Animal Research, 45*(1), 577–584. doi:10.1080/09712119.2016.1232266

Ibrahim, G. A., Nour, I. A., & Kadim, I. T. (2015). Effect of age on quality characteristics and composition of muscles of Sudanese camel (Camelus dromedaries). *Journal of Camel Practice and Research, 22*(2), 209–216. doi:10.5958/2277-8934.2015.00033.8

Jurjanz, S., Nurseitova, M., Toregozhina, Z., Konuspayeva, G., & Faye, B. (2018). Kinetics of polychlorinated biphenyls in Bactrian camels. *Emirates Journal of Food and Agriculture, 30*(4), 312–319. doi:10.9755/ejfa.2018.v30.i4.1667

Kadim, I. T., Al-Ani, M. R., Al-Maqbaly, R. S., Mansour, M. H., Mahgoub, O., & Johnson, E. H. (2011). Proximate, amino acid, fatty acid and mineral composition of raw and cooked camel (Camelus dromedarius) meat. *British Food Journal, 113*(4), 482–493. doi:10.1108/00070701111123961

Kadim, I. T., Al-Karousi, A., Mahgoub, O., Al-Marzooqi, W., Al-Maqbaly, R., Khalaf, S. K., & Raiymbek, G. (2013). Physical, chemical, quality and histochemical characteristics of infraspinatus, triceps brachii, longissimus thoraces, biceps femoris, semitendinosus, and semimembranosus of dromedary camel (Camelus dromedaries) muscles. *Meat Science, 93*, 564–571. doi:10.1016/j.meatsci.2012.11.028 PMID:23273465

Kadim, I. T., & Mahgoub, O. (2008). Effect of age on quality and composition of one-humped camel Longissimus thoracis muscle. Intern. *Journal of Post-Harvest Technology Innovation, 1*(3), 327–336. doi:10.1504/IJPTI.2008.021467

Kadim, I. T., Mahgoub, O., Al-Marzooqi, W., Al-Zadgali, S., Annamali, K., & Mansour, M. H. (2006). Effects of age on composition and quality of muscle Longissimusthoracisofthe Omani Arabian Camel (Camelus dromedarius). *Meat Science, 73*(4), 619–625. doi:10.1016/j.meatsci.2006.03.002 PMID:22062561

Kadim, I. T., Mahgoub, O., Al-Marzooqi, W., & Khalaf, S. K. (2009a). Effect of low voltage electrical stimulation and splitting carcass on histochemical and meat quality characteristics of the one-humped camel (Camelus dromedaries) Longissimus thoracis muscle. *Journal of Camelid Science*, *2*, 30–40.

Kadim, I. T., Mahgoub, O., Al-Marzooqi, W., Khalaf, S. K., Mansour, M. H., Al-Sinani, S. S. H., & Al-Amri, I. S. (2009b). Effects of electrical stimulation on histochemical muscle fiber staining, quality, and composition of camel and cattle Longissimus thoracis muscles. *Journal of Food Science*, *74*(1), S44–S52. doi:10.1111/j.1750-3841.2008.00992.x PMID:19200120

Kadim, I. T., Mahgoub, O., & Purchas, R. W. (2008). A review of the Growth, and of the Carcass and Meat Quality Characteristics of the One-humped Camel (Camelus dromedaries). *Meat Science*, *73*, 619–625. doi:10.1016/j.meatsci.2006.03.002 PMID:22063567

Kadim, I. T., & Sahi, A. B. A. (2018). Health aspects of camel meat: A review of literature. *Advances in Animal and Veterinary Sciences*, *6*(7), 271–272. doi:10.17582/journal.aavs/2018/6.7.271.272

Khezrian, A., & Shahbazi, Y. (2018). Application of nanocompostie chitosan and carboxymethyl cellulose films containing natural preservative compounds in minced camel's meat. *International Journal of Biological Macromolecules*, *106*, 1146–1158. doi:10.1016/j.ijbiomac.2017.08.117 PMID:28847602

Kim, S. J., Cho, A. R., & Han, J. (2013). Antioxidant and antimicrobial activities of leafy green vegetable extracts and their applications to meat product preservation. *Food Control*, *29*(1), 112–120. doi:10.1016/j.foodcont.2012.05.060

Kimassoum, D., Bawe, N. M., Nadjilem, D., Nji, A. M., Tidjani, A., Bughe, R. N., & Mbacham, W. F. (2016). Evaluation of some nutritional and physicochemical properties of camel meat originating from Chad. *African Journal of Food Science*, *10*(12), 368–373.

Kurtu, M. Y. (2004). An assessment of the productivity for meat and carcass yield of camel (Camelus dromedaries) and the consumption of camel meat in the Eastern region of Ethiopia. *Tropical Animal Health and Production*, *36*(1), 65–76. doi:10.1023/B:TROP.0000009520.34657.35 PMID:14979560

Lee, S. K., Kim, Y. S., Liang, C. Y., & Song, Y. H. (2003). Effects of dietary vitamin E supplementation on color stability, lipid oxidation and reducing ability of Hanwoo (Korean cattle) beef during retail display. *Asian-Australasian Journal of Animal Sciences*, *10*(10), 1529–1534. doi:10.5713/ajas.2003.1529

Legarreta, I. G. (2010). Canned products and Pâté. In F. Toldra (Ed.), *Handbook of Meat Processing* (pp. 337–349). Ames, IA: Wiley-Blackwell. doi:10.1002/9780813820897.ch19

Lev, E. (2006). Healing with animals in the Levant from the 10th to the 18th century. *Journal of Ethnopharmacology and Ethnomedicine*, *2*. doi:10.1186/1746-4269-2-11 PMID:16504024

Lonnecker, S., Boyle, E. A., Getty, K. J. K., Buege, D. R., Ingham, S. C., Searls, G., & Harper, N. M. (2010). Production methods and product characteristics of jerky produced by small and very small meat processing businesses. *Journal of Muscle Foods*, *21*(4), 826–833. doi:10.1111/j.1745-4573.2010.00222.x

Maiorano, G., Cavone, C., Mccormick, R. J., Ciarlariello, A., Gambacorta, M., & Manchisi, A. (2007). The effect of dietary energy and vitamin E administration on performance and intramuscular collagen properties of lambs. *Meat Science*, *76*(1), 182–188. doi:10.1016/j.meatsci.2006.11.001 PMID:22064205

Maqsood, S., Al Haddad, N. A., & Mudgil, P. (2016). Vacuum packaging as an effective strategy to retard off-odour development, microbial spoilage, protein degradation and retain sensory quality of camel meat'. *Lebensmittel-Wissenschaft + Technologie*, *72*, 55–62.

Maqsood, S., Manheem, K., Abushelaibil, A., & Kadim, I. T. (2014). Characterization of the lipid and protein fraction of fresh camel meat and the associated changes during refrigerated storage. *Journal of Food Composition and Analysis*, *41*, 212–220. doi:10.1016/j.jfca.2014.12.027

Miezeliene, A., Alencikiene, G., Gruzauskas, R., & Barstys, T. (2011). The effect of dietary selenium supplementationon meat quality of broiler chickens. *Biotechnologie, Agronomie, Société et Environnement*, *15*, 61–69.

Migdal, W., & Žirković, B. (2007). Meat–from functional food to disease of modern civilization. *Biotechnology in Animal Husbandry*, *23*, 19–31.

Montgomery, J. L., King, M. B., Gentry, J. G., Barham, A. R., Barham, B. L., Hilton, G. G., ... Miller, M. F. (2004). Supplemental vitamin D3 concentration and biological type of steers. II. Tenderness, quality, and residues of beef. *Journal of Animal Science*, *82*(7), 2092–2104. doi:10.2527/2004.8272092x PMID:15309957

Moreira, F. B., de Souza, N. E., Matsushita, M., do Prado, I. N., & Nascimento, W. G. (2003). Evaluation of carcass characteristics and meat chemical composition of Bos indicus and Bos indicus x Bos taurus crossbred steers fi nished in pasture systems. *Brazilian Archives of Biology and Technology*, *46*(4), 609–616. doi:10.1590/S1516-89132003000400016

Mozaffarian, D., Micha, R., & Wallace, S. (2010). Effects on Coronary Heart Disease of Increasing Polyunsaturated Fat in Place of Saturated Fat: A Systematic view and Meta-Analysis of Randomized Controlled Trials. *PLoS Medicine*, *7*(3), e1000252. doi:10.1371/journal.pmed.1000252 PMID:20351774

Navas-Carretero, S., Pérez-Granados, A. M., Sarriá, B., & Vaquero, P. M. (2009). Iron absorption from meat pate fortified with ferric pyrophosphate in iron-deficient women. *Nutrition (Burbank, Los Angeles County, Calif.)*, *25*(1), 20–24. doi:10.1016/j.nut.2008.07.002 PMID:18752926

NUTTAB. (2010). *Nutrient data tables*. Food Standard Australia New Zealand (FSANZ). Accessed Aug. 2, 2012. http://www.foodstandards.gov.au/consumerinformation/nuttab2010/

Ono, K., Berry, B., Johnson, H. K., Russek, E., Parker, C. F., Cahill, V., & Althouse, P. (1984). Nutrient composition of lamb of two age groups. *Journal of Food Science*, *49*(5), 1233–1239. doi:10.1111/j.1365-2621.1984.tb14961.x

Ono, K., Berry, B. W., & Douglass, L. W. (1986). Nutrient content of some fresh and retail cuts of veal. *Journal of Food Science*, *51*(5), 1352–1357. doi:10.1111/j.1365-2621.1986.tb13120.x

Pearce, K., & Jacob, R. (2004). Saltbush lifts sheep meat vitamin content. *Farming Ahead*, *153*, 63.

Perez, P., Maino, M., Guzman, R., Vaquero, A., Kobrich, C., & Pokniak, J. (2000). Carcass characteristics of liama (*Lama glama*) reared in central Chile. *Small Ruminant Research*, *37*(1-2), 93–97. doi:10.1016/S0921-4488(99)00127-3 PMID:10818308

Pogorzelska-Nowicka, E., Atanasov, A. G., Horba ´nczuk, J., & Wierzbicka, A. (2018). Review: Bioactive compounds in functional meat products. *Molecules (Basel, Switzerland)*, *23*(2), 307. doi:10.3390/molecules23020307

Poławska, E., Zdanowska-Sa̦siadek, Z., Horbanczuk, J. O., Pomianowski, J., Józ˙wik, A., Tolik, D., ... De Smet, S. (2016). Effect of dietary organic and inorganic selenium supplementation on chemical, mineral and fatty acid composition of ostrich meat. *CYTA: Journal of Food*, *14*(1), 84–87. doi:10.1080/19476337.2015.1046940

Polidori, P., Renieri, C., Antonini, M., Passamonti, P., & Pucclarelli, F. (2007). Meat fatty acid composition of llama (lama glama) reared in the Andean highlands. *Meat Science*, *75*(2), 356–358. doi:10.1016/j.meatsci.2006.07.010 PMID:22063670

Purchas, R. W., & Busboom, J. R. (2005). The effect of production system and age on levels of iron, taurine, carnosine, coenzyme Q10, and creatine in beef muscles and liver. *Meat Science*, *70*(4), 589–596. doi:10.1016/j.meatsci.2005.02.008 PMID:22063884

Purchas, R. W., Rutherfurd, S. M., Pearce, P. D., Vather, R., & Wilkinson, B. H. P. (2004). Concentrations in beef and lamb of taurine, carnosine, coenzyme Q10, and creatine. *Meat Science*, *66*(3), 629–637. doi:10.1016/S0309-1740(03)00181-5 PMID:22060873

Purchas, R. W., Triumf, E. C., & Egelandsdal, B. (2010). Quality characteristics and composition of the Longissimus muscle in the short-loin from male and female farmed red deer in New Zealand. *Meat Science*, *86*(2), 505–510. doi:10.1016/j.meatsci.2010.05.043 PMID:20584574

Purchas, R. W., Wilkinson, B. H. P., Carruthers, F., & Jackson, F. (2014). A comparison of the nutrient content of uncooked and cooked lean from New Zealand beef and lamb. *Journal of Food Composition and Analysis*, *35*(2), 75–82. doi:10.1016/j.jfca.2014.04.008

Radlowski, E. C., & Johnson, R. W. (2013). Perinatal iron deficiency and neurocognitive development. *Frontiers in Human Neuroscience*, *7*, 34–43. doi:10.3389/fnhum.2013.00585 PMID:24065908

Raiymbek, G., Faye, B., Kadim, I. T., Serikbaeva, A., & Konuspayeva, G. (2019). Comparative fatty acids composition and cholesterol content in Bactrian (*Camelus bactrianus*) and dromedary camel (*Camelus dromedaries*) meat. *Tropical Animal Health and Production*, *51*(7), 2025–2035. doi:10.100711250-019-01894-2 PMID:31011922

Raiymbek, G., Kadim, I. T., Al-Amri, I. S., Abdulaziz, Y. A., & Faye, B. (2018). Concentration of nutrients in six muscles of Bactrian (Camelus bacterianus) camel. *Journal of Camel Practice and Research*, *25*(1), 109–121. doi:10.5958/2277-8934.2018.00016.4

Raiymbek, G., Kadim, I. T., Al-Amri, I. S., AlKindi, A. Y., Faye, B., Khalaf, S. K., ... Purchas, R. W. (2018). Concentrations of nutrients in six muscles of Bactrian (*Camelus bactrianus*) Camels. *Journal of Camel Practice and Research*, *25*(1), 109–121. doi:10.5958/2277-8934.2018.00016.4

Rawdah, T. N., El-Faer, M. Z., & Koreish, S. A. (1994). Fatty acid composition of the meat and fat of the one-humped camel (*Camelus dromedarius*). *Meat Science*, *37*(1), 149–155. doi:10.1016/0309-1740(94)90151-1 PMID:22059419

Roohani, N., Hurrell, R., Kelishadi, R., & Schulin, R. (2013). Zinc and its importance for human health: An integrative review. *Journal of Research in Medical Sciences*, *18*, 144–157. PMID:23914218

Sallam, K. I., & Morshedy, A. E. M. A. (2008). Organochlorine pesticides residues in camel, cattle and sheep carcasses slaughtered in Sharkia province, Egypt. *Food Chemistry*, *18*(1), 154–164. doi:10.1016/j.foodchem.2007.10.066

Schönfeldt, H., & Gibson, N. (2008). Changes in the nutrient quality of meat in an obesity context. *Meat Science*, *80*(1), 20–27. doi:10.1016/j.meatsci.2008.05.025 PMID:22063166

Shimada, K., Sakuma, Y., Wakamatsu, J., Fukushima, M., Sekikawa, M., Kuchida, K., & Mikami, M. (2004). Species and muscle differences in L-carnitine levels in skeletal muscles based on a new simple assay. *Meat Science*, *68*(3), 357–362. doi:10.1016/j.meatsci.2004.04.003 PMID:22062403

Sinclair, A. J., Slattery, W. J., & O'Dea, K. (1982). The analysis of polyunsaturated fatty acids in meat by capillary gas-liquid chromatography. *Journal of the Science of Food and Agriculture*, *33*(8), 771–776. doi:10.1002/jsfa.2740330814

Tewari, D., Stankiewicz, A., Mocan, A., Sah, A., Huminiecki, L., Horba ́nczuk, J. O., & Atanasov, A. G. (2018). Ethnopharmacological approaches for management of dementia and the therapeutic significance of natural products and herbal drugs. *Frontiers in Aging Neuroscience*, *10*, 3. doi:10.3389/fnagi.2018.00003

Tomonaga, S., Kaneko, K., Kaji, Y., Kido, Y., Denbow, D. M., & Furuse, M. (2006). Dietary β-alanine enhances brain, but not muscle, carnosine and anserine concentrations in broilers. *Animal Science Journal*, *77*(1), 79–86. doi:10.1111/j.1740-0929.2006.00323.x

Wiegand, B. R., Sparks, J. C., Beitz, D. C., Parrish, F. C. Jr, Horst, R. L., Trenkle, A. H., & Ewan, R. C. (2002). Short-term feeding of vitamin D3 improves color but does not change tenderness of pork-loin chops. *Journal of Animal Science*, *80*, 2116–2121. PMID:12211380

Wiklund, E., Finstad, G., Johansson, L., Aguiar, G., & Bechtel, P. J. (2008). Carcass composition and yield of Alaskan reindeer (Rangifer tarandus tarandus) steers and effects of electrical stimulation applied during field slaughter on meat quality. *Meat Science*, *78*(3), 185–193. doi:10.1016/j.meatsci.2007.06.004 PMID:22062269

Williams, P. (2007). Nutritional composition of red meat. *Nutrition & Dietetics: the Journal of the Dietitians Association of Australia*, *64*(s4), S113–S119. doi:10.1111/j.1747-0080.2007.00197.x

Wood, J. D., Enser, M., Fisher, A. V., Nute, G. R., Sheard, P. R., Richardson, R. I., ... Whittington, F. M. (2008). Fat deposition, fatty acid composition and meat quality: A review. *Meat Science*, *78*(4), 343–358. doi:10.1016/j.meatsci.2007.07.019 PMID:22062452

Yang, W. L., Chen, Y. P., Cheng, Y. F., Li, X. H., Zhang, R. Q., Wen, C., & Zhou, Y. M. (2016). An evaluation of zinc bearing palygorskite inclusion on the growth performance, mineral content, meat quality, and antioxidant status of broilers. *Poultry Science*, *95*(4), 878–885. doi:10.3382/ps/pev445 PMID:26787924

Zomborszky, Z., Szentmihalyi, G., Sarudi, I., Horn, P., & Szabo, C. S. (1996). Nutrient composition of muscles in deer and boar. *Journal of Food Science*, *61*(3), 625–627. doi:10.1111/j.1365-2621.1996.tb13172.x

Chapter 14
Camel Gelatin Composition, Properties, Production, and Applications

Irwandi Jaswir
International Islamic University Malaysia, Malaysia

Hassan Abdullah Al-Kahtani
King Saud University, Saudi Arabia

Fitri Octavianti
Avicenna Dental Clinic, Malaysia

Widya Lestari
International Islamic University Malaysia, Malaysia

Nurlina Yusof
International Islamic University Malaysia, Malaysia

ABSTRACT

Gelatin is an important protein produced through partial hydrolysis of collagen from animal parts and byproducts such as cartilage, bones, tendons, and hides. The ability of gelatin to form a thermo-reversible gel at normal body temperature and high water content make it an exceptional food ingredient. A good quality gelatin is translucent, brittle, colorless (sometimes slightly yellow), bland in taste, and odorless. Gelatin has been found useful as stabilizer and filler in dairy products and other food industries. Recently, the global gelatin production net over 300,000 metric tons: 46% were from pigskin, 29.4% from bovine hides, 23.1% from bones, and 1.5% from other parts. Although camels have been recognized as source of meat and milk, utilization of camel bones and skins for gelatin production has not been fully explored. This chapter will discuss the processing of camel gelatin extraction.

DOI: 10.4018/978-1-7998-1604-1.ch014

INTRODUCTION

Gelatin is an important protein produced through partial hydrolysis of collagen from animal parts and byproducts such as cartilages, bones, tendons and hides. The ability of gelatin to form a thermo-reversible gel at normal body temperature and its ability to retain large amounts of water makes it a unique food ingredient. A good quality gelatin is translucent, brittle, colorless (sometimes slightly yellow), bland in taste and odorless. Gelatin has been found useful as a stabilizer and filler in dairy products (see Chapter 5) and other food industries (Mariod & Adam, 2013). Recently, the net global gelatin production was over 300,000 metric tons; 46% were from pigskin, 29.4% from bovine hides, 23.1% from bones and 1.5% from other parts or animals (Zilhadia, Harahap, Jaswir, & Effionora, 2018). Although camels have been recognized as a source of meat (see Chapter 12 and 13) and milk (see Chapter 2), utilization of camel's bones and skins for gelatin production has not been fully explored.

Bone gelatin is primarily used for pharmaceutical purposes because of its high level of purity. Prior to extraction of gelatin from bone samples, the bones must be demineralized using dilute acid solution to remove inherent calcium that is part of the bone matrix (Harahap, Jaswir, & Anwar, 2016). Structurally, the function of calcium salt deposited in the organic matrix of bone is to maintain the bone integrity by holding the scaffolds and crosslinks that improves bone strength and rigidity. Removal of calcium salt from bone through acidulation with dilute acid is an essential step towards successful gelatin production since the results of the acid treatment produces bone protein (collagen) which contained water-soluble gelatin. Extraction temperature, pH and extraction period are common operating parameters influencing gelatin production (Gehan, El-Bassyouni, & Abdel-Fattah, 2013). The effect of processing conditions on the properties of gelatin from fish bone with pretreatment with hydrochloric acid has been reported (Taheri, Abedian Kenari, Gildberg, & Behnam, 2009). Adoption of specific processing parameters and raw material sources often improve the consistency in functionality of gelatin or collagen.

Recently, there has been increase interest in the effective use of underutilized resources and industrial wastes to reduce production cost and environmental hazards. Utilization of animal bone for gelatin production offers opportunities including waste to wealth and waste minimization.

Gelatins from bovine and porcine sources are becoming less acceptable because of increasing allergen cases and tradition or religious believes. This has called for production of gelatin from other sources. Therefore, camel bone gelatin can be a good alternative source of gelatin. However, there has been less effort to identify processing conditions for demineralization of camel bone. The developed demineralization processing conditions for cattle bone are kept as company secret, and conflicting values have been reported. This Chapter will discuss various aspects of the processing of gelatin, particularly camel gelatin extraction, regulations and standards, physico-chemical characteristics, as well as the application of gelatins.

MANUFACTURING OF GELATIN

The typical commercial sources of gelatin are of mammalian origin, mainly pigs and cows. Their bones, skins, and hides are used. Gelatin from these sources form strong gels with good properties. However, there has been a rise in concerns that gelatin might transmit diseases such as mad cow disease and for religious reasons, i.e., various prohibitions against the use of pigs and cows along with the need for using only animals slaughtered appropriately and such materials being kept separate. This leads to alternative sources such as from insects which exploits sorghum and melon bugs, and different fish species such as tilapia and pollock (Karim & Bhat, 2009).

Industrial, gelatin is used in various trades due to its versatile applications. In food industry, gelatin is used as an aroma carrier to control the flavor release and also as a food additive to stabilize, thicken, and emulsify (see Chapter 5). Due to its mechanical properties and the health and environmental benefits, gelatin can replace petroleum-based polymers for packaging purposes (Zilhadia et al. 2018). The application of gelatin in soft gels for tableting has already been established in the pharmaceutical industry and in laboratories, gelatin is also used in assays of microbiological studies as well as forensic sciences (Schrieber & Gareis, 2007).

In general, manufacturing of gelatin involves three steps; chemical treatment of the raw materials, gelatin extraction (thermal hydrolysis), and drying and purification of final product (Sockalingam, Idris, & Abdullah, 2016). At the first stage, treatment of the materials using chemical solutions aims to remove non-collagenous materials and to solubilize native collagen by disrupting the non-covalent bonds that hold structures of protein by means of swelling (Karim & Bhat, 2009). Preceded by treatment of raw materials, the elimination of non-collagenous proteins by using alkaline solution increases the purity of gelatin produced besides inactivating proteases that are involved in degrading collagen. Subsequent removal of fat from the source of collagen with high level of fat helps in minimizing negative effects on gelatin (Ardekani, Mahmoodani, See, Yusop, & Babji, 2013).

There are two types of pre-treatment processes which are acid process and alkaline process, and it mainly depends on the raw materials. The acid process is suitable for Type A raw materials with low quantities of stable intermolecular cross-links such as pig skin and fish skin, while alkaline method is used to hydrolyse protein in the liming process generating type B gelatin. Acid treatment disintegrates the covalent crosslinks in collagen in which during extraction, releasing free α-chains. The disruption of intra-chain amide bonds in collagen by enzymatic reaction is reduced as the acid treatment inactivates protease to some extent. This leads to longer chain length of collagen which is proportional to the quality of gelatin as fewer amino acid residues are lost (Benjakul, Kittiphattanabawon, & Regenstein, 2012). Since fish skin is highly soluble and low in concentration of intra and inter-chain non-reducible cross-links, a mild acid pre-treatment is usually used in present production of fish gelatin. There were several types of acid that have been incorporated in the acid pre-treatment. However citric acid is mainly used because it does not cause unwanted odour and colour to the final product (Gomez-Guillen, Gimenez, Lopez-Caballero, & Montero, 2011)

CHEMICAL COMPOSITION AND PHYSICAL PROPERTIES OF COLLAGEN AND GELATIN

Gelatin is a water-soluble macromolecule composing of a mixture of heterologous polypeptides as a result of thermal destruction of structure of collagen in a partial hydrolysis process. It contains all the essential amino acids except tryptophan with the important residues being amino acids (proline and hydroxyproline) and glycine. The basis of gelatin is collagen, the insoluble structural protein in extra-cellular matrix and connective tissues, which makes up 25%-35% of the total body protein content in vertebrates (Gomez-Guillên et al., 2002).

Gelatin can be classified according to two types based of the treatment performed. Acquirement via acid treatment with isoelectric point (pI) of 8-9 and alkaline treatment with pI of 4-5 is categorized as Type A and Type B gelatin, respectively. Pretreatment is an important step in hydrolysis process of collagen in order to disintegrate the non-covalent bonds and in turn the polypeptide structure which leads to increase in solubility of collagen. Thermal denaturation on the other hand disrupts the hydrogen and hydrophobic bonds causing collagen units to detach. The hydrolysis process then disintegrates the intramolecular linking that hold the three helical chains (Gómez-Guillén et al., 2009).

Structurally, collagen consists of three α-chains that could be either homo-trimer or hetero-trimer, determined by the types and sources of collagen. Out of the 27 types of collagens discovered, Type I is the most abundant in connective tissues. Also known as major fibrillar collagen, Type I collagen is a heterotrimer with two α1 and one α2 chains. On its own, α-chain is structurally a left-hand helix and eventually forms right hand triple super-helical structure when the three α-chains intertwines by means of hydrogen bonding. The structure composes of triplet repeating units of Gly-X-Y where X and Y is proline and hydroxyproline, respectively. In order to form such conformation, glycine is a key factor where the non-polar residue acts as the center part of the super-helical structure and conforms to no steric hindrance due to its R group being a hydrogen atom enabling the three chains to pack tightly with a hydrophobic core. The telo-peptide units which situate at the carboxyl and amino terminal of the helix with 25 and 16 amino acid residues respectively depicts the absenteeism of the repeating units of Gly-X-Y (Ferraro, Anton, & Santĕ-lhoutellier, 2016). The collagen molecules ultimately align head to tail which permits repeating cross linking to occur at telopeptide forming the foundation of collagen fibrils present in connective tissues, tendons, bones, and skins which are the major sources of gelatin (Liu, Nikoo, Boran, Zhou, & Regenstein, 2015).

Although gelatin is derived from collagen, their molecule arrangements are different due to denaturation that causes alterations of the molecular compositions of amino acid residues (Duconseille, Astruc, Quintana, Meersman, & Sante-Lhoutellier, 2015). During extraction process, the conformation of helixes of fibrils was changed due to heating and form either three α-chains, one α-chain and one β-chain, and γ-chain. These are known as secondary structure of gelatin while primary structure shows configuration similar to that of native collagen (Mariod & Adam, 2013). Some of the factors influencing the change of gelatin structure includes humidity rate, temperature, concentration, raw material, and molecular weight distribution where the latter is proportional with the cross- link degree of collagen (Ahmad et al., 2017).

REGULATIONS AND STANDARD QUALITY TEST METHODS

Gelatin is originated from animals by product and one of the foodstuffs that undergo the comprehensive investigation and stringently controlled on the market. Manufacture of gelatin must follow strict regulations in order to ensure that supplies of gelatin comply with all required physical, chemical, microbiological, and technical production and quality standards. Every process, from fresh raw materials until delivery of the product will be monitored and documented. For that, all gelatin manufacturers need to have established certified Quality Management Systems according to the worldwide standard ISO 9000. Most of the countries have their own regulatory requirements that need to be fulfilled strictly. For example, production on gelatin for pharmaceutical uses have adhere strict regulations from FDA, the European CPMP's and European Pharmacopoeia (Schrieber & Gareis, 2007).

Possibility of mammalian by-product to carry the animal disease is a bit alarming. Therefore, monitoring the potential risk of animal-derived products and other similar risk areas was done by the Food and Drug Administration (FDA), with the support of the TSE Advisory Committee since 1997. Research done by European and American research institute shows that there is no trace of bovine spongiform encephalopathy (BSE) in the gelatin produced by several manufacturing methods and it safe to be consumed. After that, in 2003, the Scientific Steering Committee (SSC) of the European Union had confirmed the previous finding and stated that the BSE in gelatin is almost zero. Later in 2006, the European Food Safety Authority (EFSA) was agreed with the SSC opinion, that the BSE risk was very small and there is no support for the request to exclude the skull and vertebrae of bovine origin older than 12 months from the material used in the production of gelatin (Shahaj, Monguidi, & Stoicescu, 2019).

Standard Quality Test

Besides quality test, standard tests also were done by the gelatin manufacturer, such as gel strength, viscosity test, physicochemical test and purity test. Gel strength is the most important characteristic in determine the quality of the gelatin. It used to measure the rigidity of the gelatin gel formed. Determination of gel strength was done using Bloom test that was patented in 1925 by O. T. Bloom (US Patent No. 1 540 979). The procedure has been standardized by AOAC, GMIA and GME and it is important to strictly follow the steps to ensure the reliability of results.

The 6.67% gel was prepared by dissolving the 6.67 g of dry gelatin in 100 ml of water and stand at room temperature for maximum 3 hours for complete swelling. To ensure that gelatin powder dissolve completely, the mixture was exposed at high temperature (up to 65°C) for not more than 15 min. To improve the hardness of the gel, the sample was let to stand at room temperature for 15 – 20 min before letting it for maturing in 10°C water bath for 16-18 hours. The analysis was done using texture analyzer with the 12.7 mm diameter flat-bottomed cylindrical plunger to depress the surface of a gelatin gel to a depth of 4 mm. The force was measured in bloom grams and it represent the rigidity of the gelatin. The range of standard gelatin is between 50 to 300 g, where high bloom range between 200 to 300 g, medium-Bloom and that of 50 to 100 g as low-Bloom. The analysis is always carried out in triplicate to ensure the accurate and reproducible results. (Haug & Draget, 2011).

CHEMICAL COMPOSITION AND PHYSICAL PROPERTIES OF GELATIN

Properties of gelatin highly depends on the species of the raw materials, pretreatment method and extraction method.

Rheological Properties

Generally rheological properties involve studies on the flow and deformation of materials under applied forces, applicable to all materials, which is measured using a rheometer. From dynamic rheological tests of gelatin samples, two main parameters can be identified which are (1) the elastic modulus, which test the solid-like response to materials, and (2) viscous modulus, which exam the liquid like response of the material. The interactions or bonds between the chains in gelatin is physical in nature (van der Waal's bonds), thus gelatin is a physical gel. The bonding energy in gelatin is weak, thus it can form thermos-reversible gels. Other characteristics of gelatin includes it solubility in water and the ability to form thermally reversible gels. Gelatin gels start to melt when the temperature increase above gel melting point (usually lower than human body temperature). Gelation of gelatin occurs when collagen molecules aggregates and forms fibrils induced by factors such as pH, ionic strength and temperature. The term thermoreversible refers to the ability of collagen to form gelatin and vice versa. Similarly, collagen gels melt by lowering the temperature, while gelatin gel melts when the temperature is raised. Besides that, the main difference between mammalian and fish gelatin are also the viscosities, where fish gelatin has higher viscosity than that of mammals.

Physical Properties

Gel strength, which also known as bloom strength is one of the principal properties of gelatin. By defining value of bloom strength around 50-300, it gives the information about the grade of gelatin as well as the suitable application of the gelatin. Higher bloom value indicates higher gelling and melting temperature and therefore, stronger gel. Gel strength is influenced by molecular characteristics of gelatin such as amino acid constitution (proline and hydroxyproline composition), ratio of α/β- chains in gelatin, and molecular weight distribution. Increase in the concentration of gelatin is proportional to the gel strength. Gel strength primarily depicts the stiffness of gelatin gel formed. Ultimately, gelatin that contains more a-chains exhibits higher gel strength.

Viscosity determines the average molecular weight of gelatin sample more than bloom strength does. It is partly regulated by molecular weight and polydispersity. It increases proportionally to the gelling temperature, melting temperature, melting point, and gel strength. Gelatin is water soluble and forms thermoreversible gel which can melt when the temperature increases above the gel melting point, which is usually lower than human body temperature. Depending on habitual temperature of raw materials of gelatin, melting point can be impacted by the lower content of amino acid causing the reduction of the tendency of formation of intermolecular helix. Gelling point is affected by the origin of raw material and conditions of extraction. Use of high concentration of acid and alkali influences the gel-forming ability of gelatin due to the impact to the degree of crosslinking in collagen. It can form film due to gelatin shrinkage with great force on drying. The range of gelling temperature might be caused by the leftover chemicals post processing and from raw material.

Colour properties of gelatin is affected by the raw materials used and it is indicated by three tests that are Hunter L (brightness), a (redness), and b (yellowness) colour values. It is recorded that fish gelatin have higher L values compared to mammalian gelatin but lower a and b values. Higher turbidity value depicts poor quality of gelatin which is the result of inadequate filtration.

Chemical Properties

Proximate composition of gelatin involves moisture, ash, protein, and fat contents. High protein content and low moisture, ash, and fat contents depend on the raw material besides chemical leftovers post processing as well as the likelihood of mixing with other substances. Gelatin with high quality contains 0.5% ash or less (Abouheif, Basmaeil, & Bakkar, 1990). The variety in ash content is determined by the amount of minerals present in raw materials as well as difference in extraction methods. Percentage of ash present can be lowered by means of demineralization before extraction process. Meanwhile, the moisture content in gelation should not exceed 15%. The amount of moisture differs from gelatin to gelatin due to the degree of drying, humidity during storage, and absorbency of moisture by packaging material. The yield of gelatin can be predicted by the content of crude protein of collagenous materials and amount of lipid can be lowered by process of degreasing prior to extraction (Jakhar et al., 2012; Ratnasari, Sudarmindo, Nusyam, & Widjanarko, 2014; See, Hong, Ng, Wan Aida, Babji, 2010; Sow & Yang, 2015).

The net proline and hydroxyproline content differs from species to species whereby generally, warm blooded animals and those in warm habitats have higher content of such amino acids compared to animals living in a cold environment (Haug & Draget, 2009). High percentage of hydroxyproline contributes to better gel properties due to the residue's importance in renaturing of subunits of gelatin during gel formation. Hydroxyproline helps in stabilizing the triple helical collagen structure by hydrogen bonding through hydroxyl group (Silva, Bandeira, & Pinto, 2014). Low content of iminoacid could lead to meagre gelling ability (Ardekani et al., 2013). This causes low melting point of gelatin compared to high iminoacid content due to less sterically hindered helix (Ratnasari, Yuwono, Nusyam, & Widjanarko, 2013). Acid pre-treatment causes gelatin with higher isoionic points caused by the less occurrence of deamination of asparagine and glutamine. Meanwhile, lower isoionic points caused by extended alkaline treatment causes deamidation of the aforementioned residues due to the exposure of collagenous materials to acid or alkali. Therefore, the type and strength of acid or alkali used give different pH value of gelatin. (See et al., 2010). Molecular weight distribution plays an important role in determining the gel strength of gelatin which contains a blend of peptide fragments with molecular weight ranging from 80 to over 250 kDa (Liu, Han, & Guo, 2009). Higher percentage of α-chains contributes to desirable properties of gelatin while high amount of β-chain affects gelatin negatively by lowering the viscosity and melting point of gelatin. High β- and γ-chains on the other hand contribute to systematized assembly with high gel strength. γ-chain helps in maintaining the stability of gelatin molecule (Margarida Figueiredoa et al., 2011).

Antimicrobial Properties

Gelatin is a growing option for environmentally friendly food packaging. Integration of gelatin with various active compounds increases its antimicrobial properties which is crucial to prevent against undesirable changes to the food as well as food safety. Naturally occurring antimicrobials such as chitosan, various essential oils derived from plants, nanometals and mixtures of the aforementioned compounds (Zilhadia et al., 2018). Antimicrobial activity of gelatin is assayed by using the agar diffusion method and the positive result is depicted by the presence of inhibition zones of gram negative and positive bacteria colonies (Harahap, Jaswir, & Anwar, 2016). For example, in an experiment conducted by the incorporation of cinnamon essential oil nanopolisome in fish gelatin has constant antimicrobial stability after some time compared to only adding cinnamon essential oil. This is due to the long process of the release of bioactive compounds in nanopolisomes. The increase in stability might be contributed by the lipophilic substance interaction and the phospholipid membrane components of microorganisms causing changes in the film structure.

In another research where the development of bioactive nanocomposite film incorporating chitosan nanoparticles was enhanced with addition of oregano essential oil. Without the latter compound, gelatin-chitosan nanoparticles exhibits nil antimicrobial activity due to the strong hydrogen bonds formation between functional groups of gelatin (hydroxyl group, carboxyl end groups and amino group, and the side groups) and CSNPs (groups of hydroxyl and amino of chitosan) cause slow diffusion of nanoparticles from the gelatin matrix into agar medium. The side chain amino groups contribute to the antimicrobial activity in gelatin due to the presence of oligopeptide chains as a result of hydrolysis (Muyonga, Cole, & Duodu, 2004).

THE EXTRACTION OF GELATIN FROM CAMEL BONE

In line with the current development of world halal industry, in the last few years we have extensively developed method to extract gelatin from camel. The procedure and processes discussed in this book chapter are of our own experiments (Al-Kahtani et al., 2017).

Camel Bone Extraction

Bones of camel were obtained from sacrificed healthy animals; muscles, periosteum and adherent soft tissues were removed from the specimen and bone marrow was discarded.

Demineralization of bone was conducted according to flow chart in Figure 1. Dried bones were cleaned by washing with tap water and drained afterwards. Bone samples were then crushed into small particle size, and demineralization process was carried out by soaking in acid solution (Al-Kahtani et al., 2017). Quality assessment included determination of ash content, gel strength, FTIR spectrum, and morphology and elemental analyses.

QUALITY OF THE CAMEL BONE GELATIN

Demineralization of Camel Bone

Bone gelatin production depends on efficient removal of calcium from the apatite through acid demineralization. Demineralization process is a critical process that removes as many inorganic chemical components in form of hydroxyapatite from the bone matrix and releases the organic collagen (ossein). Since ash content measures the amount of inorganic minerals in bones, it was therefore adopted as a measure of demineralization process. Bone demineralization depends on concentration of acid and soaking period. There was reduction in ash content of all demineralized sample (Figure 2). Initial rate of ash reduction was rapid for the first day in all demineralized samples possibly due to acute surface washing of mineral ions.

The present result was corroborated by observation of other workers that opined increased HCl concentration and elevated treatment period could result in release of ossein. A sharp continuous reduction in ash content was observed for 6.0% HCl up to day 4 and then stabilized afterwards. This observation

Figure 1. Flow chart for ossein and gelatin preparation form camel bone

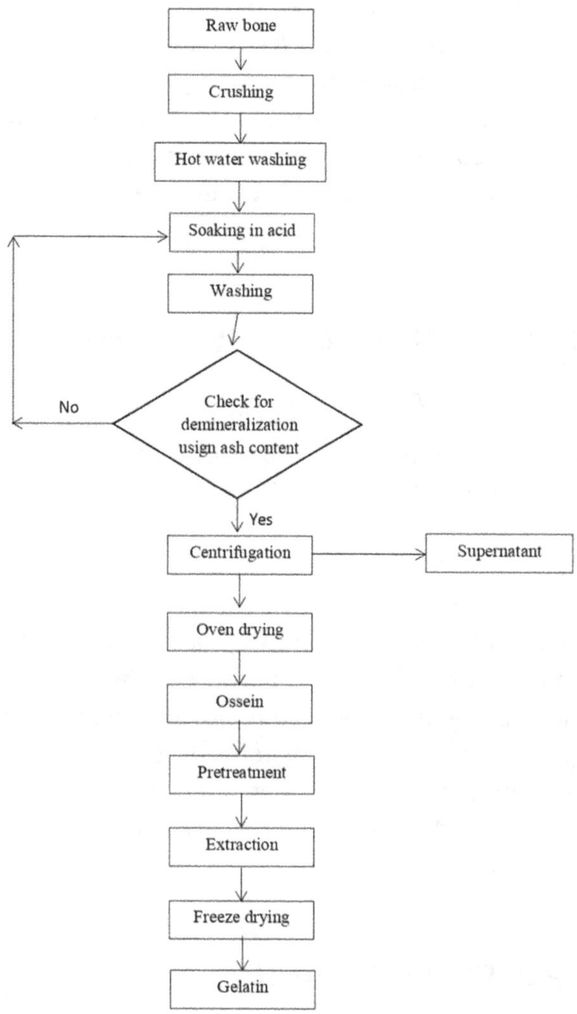

was consistent with other investigation where it was postulated that calcium removal depends on HCl concentration and duration of treatment. Therefore, in order to produce ossein with adequate demineralization from camel bone, 6.0% HCl for 5 or 6 days at room temperature was the appropriate condition (Gehan, El-Bassyouni, & Abdel-Fattah, 2013).

Effect of Demineralization on Chemical Structures of Camel Bone

FTIR was used to determine structural changes resulting from demineralization of camel bone (Figueiredo, Martins, & Gamelas, 2012). Figure 3 shows FTIR spectra of the control and the demineralized sample. There were variations in the peaks and their intensities between the two spectra. Higher peak intensity was observed in demineralized sample compared to the control. This is possibly due to increase in vibration of the functional groups after demineralization. Spectra peak that are more than 1500 cm^{-1} are assigned to vibrations from the amide groups from ossein. The intense peak at 3544 cm^{-1} corresponds

Figure 2. Demineralization kinetic of camel bone using different HCI concentrations

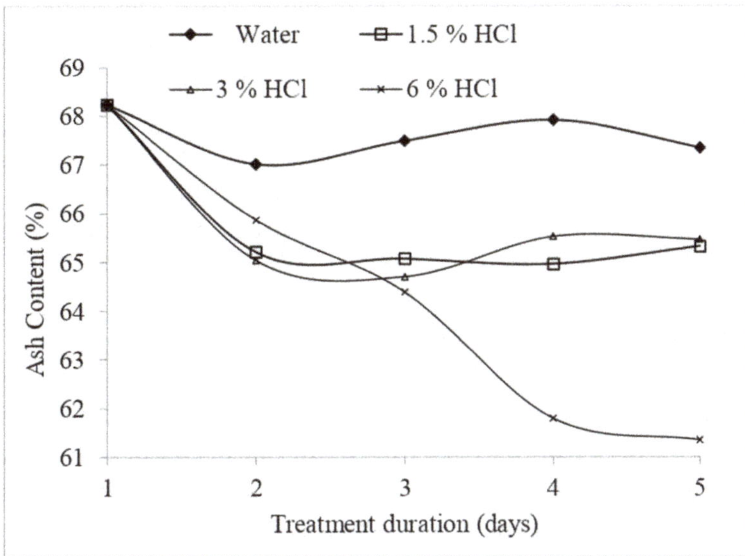

Figure 3. FTIR spectra of camel bone and ossein

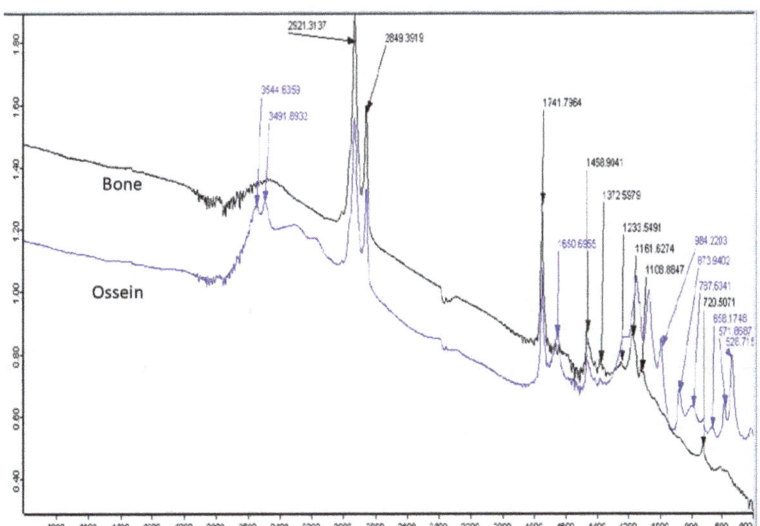

to OH^- vibrations while carbonate replacement in the resulting apatite originate a peak at 873 cm^{-1} and a double band in the 1372–1459 cm^{-1} signified CH_2 wag and bend respectively. Higher spectra intensity at 787 cm^{-1}, 873 cm^{-1} and 984 cm^{-1} were assigned for skeletal stretch, CO_3^{2-} bending and symmetrical PO_4^{3-} stretching of ossein respectively. (Wang et al., 2008). Comparatively, the appearance of new peaks corresponding to collagen showed that demineralization impacted the camel bone and released huge calcium thus, ease vibration of molecules most especially proteins fingerprint from the original bone.

Energy-Dispersive X-Ray Spectra of Minerals Analyses of Camel Bone

Energy-dispersive X-ray (EDX) spectroscopy is used for rapid detection and measurement (qualitative and quantitative) of the energy permits elemental analysis of a mineral dense sample (Horneman, Ottens, Hoorneman, van der Wielen, & Tesson, 2004). EDX spectroscopy was used to analyze the elemental composition of camel bone and ossein (bone treated with 6% HCl for 6 days). The result show presence C, N, O, Au and Ca (Table 1). Bone demineralization led to removal of oxygen-containing-anions (CO_3^{2-} to CO_2 and PO_4^{3-}) because they are converted to soluble compounds thus suggesting the observed reduction of oxygen.

Morphology of Camel Bone and Ossein

Scanning electron microscope was used to obtain morphological characteristic of camel bone and ossein (Khalil, Beheri, & Fattah, 2002). Figure 4 shows morphology changes of camel-bone due to demineralization. The initial smooth and intact surface of camel bone was lost during to demineralization. After 2 days, the resulting matter surface become rough which increase after 5 days of demineralization. Ca salts –hydroxyapatite inherent in bone structures is responsible for strengthening of the matrix and crosslinks. Hence, removal of Ca salts during HCl-demineralization led to disorganized bone scaffolds. Surface roughness dominated with observed crevices and apertures might be due to loss in Ca-salt (Khalil, Beheri, & Fattah, 2002).

Table 1. Elemental composition of camel bone and ossein

Sample	Minerals (%)				
	Carbon	Nitrogen	Oxygen	Calcium	Gold
Camel bone	29.7	27.6	31.3	7.2	4.1
Ossein	41.9	31.8	22.5	0.4	3.4

Figure 4. Morphological analysis of camel bone and ossein

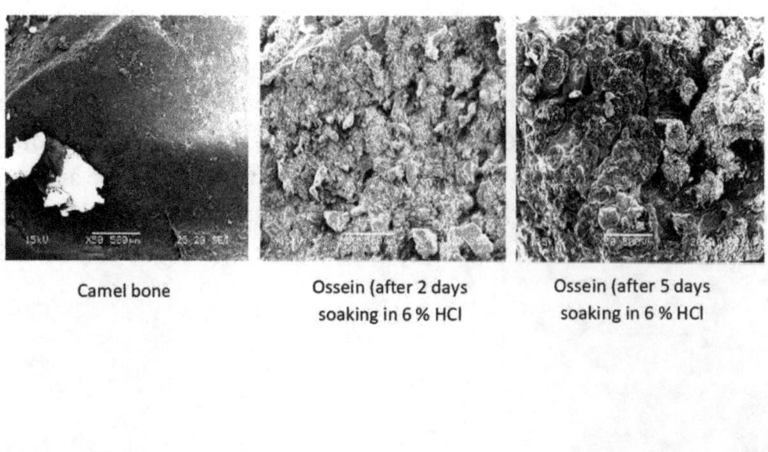

Camel bone

Ossein (after 2 days soaking in 6 % HCl

Ossein (after 5 days soaking in 6 % HCl

Gelatin Extraction from Ossein (Demineralized Camel Bone)

In order to obtained high gelatin yield, three processing conditions (temperature, pH and time) were investigated using center composite design (CCD) in random surface methodology (RSM). The yield of gelatin range from 8.54 – 25.33% for bone (Table 2). Significant ($P < 0.05$) effects were observed at quadratic level of time and pH for gelatin extraction from ossein. The effect of extraction time might be due to the additional time required to uncoil the crosslink in collagen prior to gelatin formation.

The estimated model coefficients were calculated by regression analysis on the yield of gelatin from camel bone. Statistical analysis revealed that the model was significant ($P<0.05$), suggesting that the model is suitable for prediction of gelatin yields from bone (Equation 1) samples.

$$\text{Camel bone gelatin yield} = +0.13 +0.27A - 0.18B+0.20C + 0.12A^2 + 0.30B^2 + 0.046\,C^2 + 0.021AB + 0.27AC + 0.029BC \quad (1)$$

where A is temperature, B is pH and C is extraction time.

Graphical format (Figures 5a – 5b) of the response of the optimization study is easy to visualize the optimum regions. The figures show that optimum regions were achieved at certain points within the

Table 2. Optimization result: Yield of gelatin from camel bone

A: Temperature (°C)	B: pH	C: Time (min)	Yield Bone gelatin (%)
80	7	0.5	8.5
60	4	0.5	16.4
60	4	2.0	25.3
80	4	2.0	20.5
80	1	0.5	9.5
60	4	2.0	25.3
40	4	2.0	18.9
40	1	3.5	16.2
60	4	2.0	25.3
60	4	3.5	11.4
80	7	3.5	15.0
60	7	2.0	14.3
60	4	2.0	25.3
60	4	2.0	25.3
40	1	0.5	11.4
40	7	3.5	14.0
80	1	3.5	10.8
60	4	2.0	25.3
60	1	2.0	18.5
40	7	0.5	9.5

Figure 5. Three dimension plot of optimization of yield (%) for extraction of gelatin from camel ossein as affected by processing factors (a: temperature and time – b: pH and time)

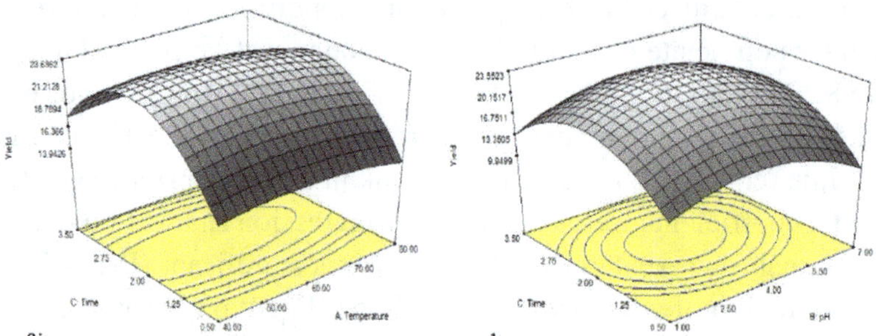

a: b

range of extraction conditions. The model describing the effects of investigated parameters was highly significant (p˂0.05). Extraction temperature, pH and extraction time linearly significantly contributed to the optimum gelatin yield. All extraction factors exhibited optimum region towards the center points with obvious oval shape at their respective contour lines. Further statistical analysis gave optimum conditions (Table 3) for high gelatin yield (23.66%) from camel-ossein. Validation of the optimized process gave gelatin yield of 21.33% which is very close to theoretical yield (Harahap et al., 2016).

Gel Strength of Camel Bone Gelatin

Gel strength –a measure of firmness, is an important mechanical property of gelatin that is often used for quality assessment. It measures of the amount of force required to push a plunger through a depression of 4 mm into the matured gelatin. The value of the force (in gram) is referred to as Bloom number (Zilhadia et al., 2018). Based on the optimum extraction conditions reported in Table 4, the gel strength of optimized camel bone gelatin reached 205.74±2.6 g. The result obtained for camel bone gelatin falls within that range of commercial gelatin obtained from mammals. The gelling strength of commercial

Table 3. Analysis of variance for the optimization of gelatin yield of camel bone

Source	Sum of squares	DF	Mean square	F-value	Prob > F
Model	2.91	9	0.32	15.62	< 0.0001
A	0.74	1	0.74	35.71	0.0001
B	0.32	1	0.32	15.47	0.0028
C	0.39	1	0.39	18.81	0.0015
A^2	0.042	1	0.042	2.04	0.184
B^2	0.25	1	0.25	11.99	0.0061
C^2	0.01	1	0.01	0.28	0.608
AB	0.00	1	0.00	0.17	0.693
AC	0.57	1	0.57	27.67	0.0004
BC	0.01	1	0.01	0.33	0.581

A = temperature, B = pH, C = extraction time

Table 4. Gelatin yield and optimum conditions for camel bone gelatin extraction

Parameters		Theoretical optimum value	Experimental optimum values (Validation)
Extraction condition	pH	5.26	5.3
	Temperature (°C)	71.9	72
	Time (h)	2.58	2.5
Yield (%)	Camel bone	23.7	21.3

gelatins ranges from 100 to 300g, but gelatins with Bloom values of 250-260 are most desired (Charlier et al., 2010). Gelatin used in food usually runs from 125 to 250 Bloom; the unflavored gelatin sold in supermarkets is at the higher end of this range. The highest grade in commerce is around 300 Bloom, which is used in food applications and to make special effects makeup artists to create prostheses, such as fake wounds. Gelatins with low Bloom numbers are used to clear cloudiness in beverages (Abdullah Amqizal, Al-Kahtani, Ismail, Hayat, & Jaswir, 2017).

Gelatin Extraction from Camel Skin

The extraction of gelatin from camel skin has been conducted separately from the gelatin extraction of camel bones explained above. Both samples are different in nature and need different pretreatments to be done.

Camel hides were procured from sacrificed healthy animals and muscles, periosteum and adhering soft tissues were removed. Clean camel skin was air dried and salted prior to preservation in airtight container for subsequent use. The salted skin was is stripped of its hair by soaking the skin in sodium sulphide solution for 3 days at 10 °C before size reduction (Abouheil et al., 1991). The depilated camel skins were treated with HCl for three days and the acid was thoroughly removed by rinsing with clean water. Camel hair structure, properties and commercial products is discussed in this book in Chapter 15.

The pre-treated camel skin was mixed with distilled water (at a ratio of 1/3, w/v) and gelatin was extraction was conducted under different conditions following the design layout obtained from response surface methodology, implemented in Design expert software 6.0.8 by Minneapolis (Table 5).

Quality analyses performed included amino acid composition, foaming properties, gel strength, and film formation.

QUALITY OF THE CAMEL SKIN GELATIN

Optimization of Gelatin Extraction from Camel Skin

Yield of gelatin ranges from 9.57 – 28.59% (Table 5). The pronounced effect of extraction time might be due to the additional time required to uncoil the crosslink in collagen prior to gelatin formation. Equation 2 is the estimated model coefficients were calculated by regression analysis on the yield of gelatin from camel skin.

Table 5. Optimization result: Yield of gelatin from camel skin

A: Temperature (°C)	B: pH	C: Time (min)	Yield of Skin gelatin (%)
80	7	0.5	9.6
60	4	0.5	11.1
60	4	2.0	28.6
80	4	2.0	24.9
80	1	0.5	9.2
60	4	2.0	28.6
40	4	2.0	13.5
40	1	3.5	25.9
60	4	2.0	28.6
60	4	3.5	25.7
80	7	3.5	28.0
60	7	2.0	14.9
60	4	2.0	28.6
60	4	2.0	28.6
40	1	0.5	10.7
40	7	3.5	27.2
80	1	3.5	16.4
60	4	2.0	28.6
60	1	2.0	27.3
40	7	0.5	9.7

$$\text{Camel skin gelatin yield} = +26.34 + 0.11A - 8.738E - 003B + 7.29C - 3.72A^2 - 1.83B^2 - 4.54C^2 + 1.44AB - 0.88AC + 1.69BC \quad (2)$$

where A is temperature, B is pH and C is extraction time.

For easy understanding, Figures 6a and 6b, a graphical format, was adopted to depict superimpose multiple responses and useful for optimization study to visualize the optimum regions. The figures show that optimum regions were achieved at certain points within the range of extraction conditions.

Physical Characteristics of Camel Gelatin: Bloom

Among the important parameters of gelatin is bloom value (gel strength) which indicate the firmness of gels. It measures the force required to cause 4mm depression of specific type of plunger into the matured gelatin. The gel strength of camel skin gelatin was 340±0.5 g. A high value of gel strength suggests that camel skin gelatin is higher than the range of commercial mammalian gelatin. The gelling strength of commercial gelatins ranges from 100 to 300g, but gelatins with Bloom values of 250-260 are most desired. Gelatin used in food usually runs from 125 Bloom to 250 Bloom; the unflavored gelatin sold in supermarkets is at the higher end of this range. The highest grade in commerce is around 300 Bloom,

Figure 6. Three dimensional plot of optimization of yield (%) for extraction of gelatin form camel skin

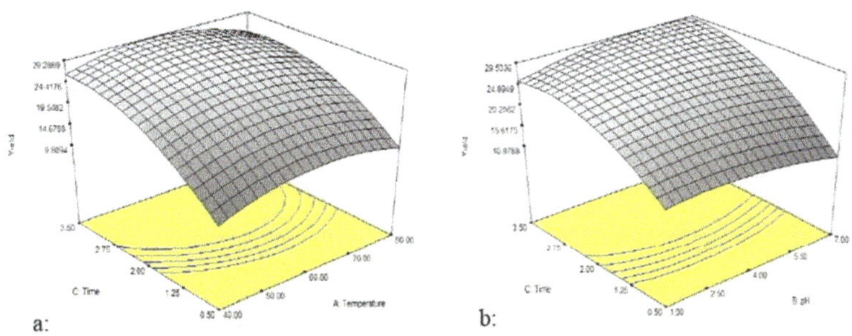

which is used, for example, by special effects makeup artists to create prostheses, such as fake wounds. Gelatins with low Bloom numbers are used to clear cloudiness in beverages.

Film Formation

Gelatin based film is gaining increase acceptability for coating for foods (e.g fruits, meats and deli items) to protect them from drying and exposure to light and oxygen. In agreement with previous reports, thickness of gelatin films produced from camel skin and bone in this study fall within the range reported for that of bovine-hide and tuna-skin, i.e. 0.5 cm.

Amino Acid Profile of Gelatin From Camel Skin and Bone

Similar to other protein, the functional properties of gelatin are the result of its Amino acid profile (Abdullah Amqizal et al., 2017). The amino acid profiles of camel skin contain high amount of glycine, threonine, alanine and leucine (Table 6). The sample presented highest content of Glycine – a typical observation for gelatin – which usually occupy every third position of amino-acid chain and nearly one-third of its residues. According to the previous review on biofilm properties of gelatin, amino acid profile (mostly glycine, proline and hydroxyproline) play a significant role on the quality gelatin-based-films. Presence of high amount of proline and hydroxyproline in gelatin give film with low deformation values possibly due to their role in the structure of collagen. Proline and hydroxyproline are responsible for the unique secondary structure of collagen as they limit rotation of the polypeptide backbone thus contribute to stability of triple helix (Harahap et al., 2016).

APPLICATIONS OF GELATIN

Food Industry

Gelatin has unique properties, which broaden it used in the various industries including foods, pharmaceutical and cosmetics. In food industry, gelatin act as gelling agent, gelatin is used as food additive to stabilize, thicken, and emulsify the food. It also acts as aroma carrier to control the flavour release. Gelatin is the main ingredient for jelly and gummy bears. Interaction between gelatin and sugar present

Table 6. Amino acid profiling of camel skin gelatin

	Amino acid mg/100 g
Aspartic acid/Asparagine	25
Glutamic acid/Glutamine	52
Serine	14
Glycine	101
Histidine	3
Arginine	17
Threonine	15
Alanine	15
Proline	57
Hydroxy Proline	49
Tyrosine	4
Valine	13
Methionine	4
Isoleucine	5
Leucine	20
Phenylalanine	11
Lysine	17
Tryptophan	ND [not determined]
Total	422.27

in the jelly formulation would determine the hardness of the jelly, due to their competitiveness to access to the water in the food system. In ice cream preparation, adding gel-foaming stabilizer gelatin inhibits the formation of ice crystal in the product's structure and produce the smooth creamy texture of ice cream (see Chapter 5). Combination of several properties such as physical, chemical and surface-active properties results produced melt-in-the-mouth property with the melting point behavior in the range of 10-30°C. Besides, gelatin ability to decrease the surface tension of the syrup and increase the foam stability upon cooling by increasing viscosity make it very useful property in marshmallow production. Different amount of gelatin will be used (approximately 2%-7%), depending on desired texture (GMIA, 2012).

In addition, gelatin is used in winemaking as clarifying agent due to its ability to induce the flocculation of floating particle through charged ion interactions. Gelatin is also used in the canned meat products such as canned pork, hams, cured, loaves, frankfurters and Vienna sausages. Its unique water absorbing property, where gelatin could absorb water up to 10 times of its volume, helps in absorb the exudates from the meat during cooking and was present as a gel when the canned was opened. Besides, by adding gelatin in the meat canned would increase the heat transfer medium and it hold the juice lost throughout the cooking process. These various functional properties have increased the demand for gelatin protein worldwide (Mariod & Adam, 2013)

Pharmaceutical Industry

Nearly 5% of gelatin was used in pharmaceutical industry in early 20th century and the number is increasing yearly. Its characteristics such as biodegradable, nontoxic and easy to crosslink and to modify chemically are the reasons on the high interest in gelatin in the industry. However, gelatin from fish skin has low gelling nature, caused it to shrink with great force on drying. Study done by Huang et al. (2017) shows that the addition of chemical crosslinker such as glutaraldehyde and transglutaminase has modified the structure of the gelatin polymer and gives better performance compared to unmodified particles. In addition, the structural alteration has improved its properties and characteristics, such as stability, insolubility at elevated temperatures, reduced swelling in water and lower permeability to cell membranes, making it an ideal component for carrying drugs (Mariod & Adam, 2013).

Main application of gelatin in pharmaceutical industry is it is used in production of two-piece hard capsules, soft elastic gelatin capsules, tableting, tablet coating, granulation, encapsulation and microencapsulation (GMIA, 2012) due to its film-forming property. The first capsule from gelatin was patented in 1834 by Mothes and DuBlanc. The advantages of capsule from are its odour and tasteless and has melt-in-the-mouth property. The soft capsule casing is usually made from gelatin with low gel strength (cold water fish) and it dissolves quickly and may be sensitive to the heat. In contrast, mammalian gelatin and modified gelatin are used in production of hard capsule and it represents majority of capsule products manufactured in the industry nowadays. Usually, the soft capsule contains the unpleasant-tasting liquid medication while the hard gelatin is filled with powder, granules and pellets. For microencapsulation of vitamins A, D and E, it used gelatin with bloom in the range of 0 to 140 (GMIA, 2013)

Besides being used in production of capsules, gelatin is also used as matrix for implants, in injectable drug-delivery microspheres and in intravenous infusions. Example of gelatin carrying drugs is H.P Acthar gel. The Acthar gel, containing adrenocorticotropic hormone, 0.5% phenol, not more than 0.1% cysteine (added), sodium hydroxide, and/or acetic acid to adjust pH and water for injection, is supplied as a sterile preparation in 16% gelatin. The drugs used to treat relapsing multiple sclerosis, infantile spasm and nephrotic syndrome and was released into human body through intramuscular or subcutaneous injection. The use of gelatin is to provide a prolonged release after the dose.

Apart from food and pharmaceutical industries, gelatin is also used widely in the cosmetic and photography industries. Gelatin is used the production of almost all items of cosmetics. The camel milk disguised cosmeceutical is discussed in Chapter 16. Its function here is less similar to the function of gelatin in food industry. While in the photography, gelatin is used in a process called 'gelatin silver process'. Gelatin silver process is the photographic process used with currently available black-and-white films and printing papers. A suspension of silver salts in gelatin is coated onto a support such as glass, flexible plastic or film, baryta paper, or resin-coated paper.

CONCLUSION

Gelatin is an ingredient used widely in various industries, such as food, cosmetics, pharmaceuticals, and photography industries. It may be produced from the skins or bones of animals. In order to extract gelatin from camel bone, camel bone needs to be demineralized through HCl-acidulation process at various concentrations. Energy Dispersive X-ray Spectroscopy (EDX) elemental-analysis revealed reduction in Ca and increase in N and H while O remain unaffected. Particulate characteristics by scanning electron microscope showed an increased surface roughness of bone after demineralization. Camel bone is suitable for production of gelatin with good potentials in food and non-food applications. We have also obtained gelatin from camel skin and bone using CCD-RSM to optimize extraction conditions (temperature, pH and extraction time) and the extracted gelatins were characterized successfully.

ACKNOWLEDGMENT

The authors would like to thank the National Plan for Science, Technology, and Innovation (NPST), Kingdom of Saudi Arabia, (Project No. 12-AGR2487-02) for funding this camel project and to Konsortium Institute Halal Malaysia (KIHIM) for funding this Chapter write-up.

REFERENCES

Abdullah Amqizal, H. I., Al-Kahtani, H. A., Ismail, E. A., Hayat, K., & Jaswir, I. (2017). Identification and verification of porcine DNA in commercial gelatin and gelatin containing processed foods. *Food Control*, *78*, 297–303. doi:10.1016/j.foodcont.2017.02.024

Abouheif, M., Basmaeil, S., & Bakkar, M. (1990). A standard method for jointing camel carcasses with reference to the effect of slaughter age on carcass characteristics in najdi camels. I1. Variation in lean growth and distribution. *Asian-Australasian Journal of Animal Sciences*, *3*(2), 97–102. doi:10.5713/ajas.1990.97

Abouheil, M., Basmaeil, S., & Bakkar, M. (1991). A standard method for jointing camel carcasses with reference to the effect of slaughter age on carcass characteristics in najdi camels. 3. partition and distribution of carcass fat. *Animal Science (Penicuik, Scotland)*, *4*(3), 219–225.

Ahmad, T., Ismail, A., Aqlima, S., Khalil, K. A., Kumar, Y., Adeyemi, K. D., & Sazili, A. Q. (2017). Recent advances on the role of process variables affecting gelatin yield and characteristics with special reference to enzymatic extraction : A review. *Food Hydrocolloids*, *63*, 85–96. doi:10.1016/j.foodhyd.2016.08.007

Al-Kahtani, H. A., Jaswir, I., Ismail, E. A., Ahmed, M. A., Hammed, A. M., Olorunnisola, S., & Octavianti, F. (2017). Structural characteristics of camel-bone gelatin by demineraization and extraction. *International Journal of Food Properties*, *20*(11), 2559–2568. doi:10.1080/10942912.2016.1244543

AOAC. (2019). *Official Methods of Analysis of AOAC International* (21st ed.). Arlington, VA: AOAC International.

Ardekani, V. S., Mahmoodani, F., See, S. F., Yusop, S. M., & Babji, A. S. (2013). Processing optimization and characterization of gelatin from catfish (*Clarias gariepinus*) skin. *Sains Malaysiana*, *42*(12), 1697–1705.

Benjakul, S., Kittiphattanabawon, P., & Regenstein, J. M. (2012). Fish gelatin. In B. K. Simpson (Ed.), *Food biochemistry and food processing* (2nd ed.; pp. 388–405). John Wiley & Sons. doi:10.1002/9781118308035.ch21

Chang, M. C., & Tanaka, J. (2002). FT-IR study for hydroxyapatitecollagen nanocomposite cross-linked by glutaraldehyde. *Biomaterials*, *23*(24), 4811–4818. doi:10.1016/S0142-9612(02)00232-6 PMID:12361620

Charlier, P., Huynh-Charlier, I., Munoz, O., Billard, M., Brun, L., & de la Grandmaison, G. L. (2010). The microscopic (optical and SEM) examination of dental calculus deposits (DCD). Potential interest in forensic anthropology of a bio-archaeological method. *Legal Medicine*, *12*(4), 163–171. doi:10.1016/j.legalmed.2010.03.003 PMID:20444636

Duconseille, A., Astruc, T., Quintana, N., Meersman, F., & Sante-Lhoutellier, V. (2015). Gelatin structure and composition linked to hard capsule dissolution: A review. *Food Hydrocolloids*, *43*, 360–376. doi:10.1016/j.foodhyd.2014.06.006

Ferraro, V., Anton, M., & Santé-lhoutellier, V. (2016). The "sisters" α-helices of collagen, elastin and keratin recovered from animal by-products: Functionality, bioactivity and trends of application. *Trends in Food Science & Technology*, *51*, 65–75. doi:10.1016/j.tifs.2016.03.006

Figueiredo, M. M., Gamelas, J. A. F., & Martins, A. G. (2012). Characterization of bone and bone-based graft materials using FTIR spectroscopy. *Infrared Spectroscopy: Life and Biomedical Sciences*. Retrieved from www.intechopen.com

Figueiredoa, M. S. C., Martinsa, G., Freitasb, J., Judasb, F., & Figueiredo, H. (2011). Influence of hydrochloric acid concentration on the demineralization of cortical bone. *Chemical Engineering Research*, *89*(1), 116–124. doi:10.1016/j.cherd.2010.04.013

Gehan, T., & El-Bassyouni, O. W. G. (2013). Morphological and macrostructural studies of dog cranial bone demineralized with different acids. *Current Applied Physics*, *13*(5), 864–874. doi:10.1016/j.cap.2012.12.026

GMIA. (2012). Gelatin handbook. New York: Gelatin Manufacturers Institute of America, GMIA.

Gómez-Guillén, M., Pérez-Mateos, M., Gómez-Estaca, J., López-Caballero, E., Giménez, B., & Montero, P. (2009). Fish gelatin: A renewable material for developing active biodegradable films. *Trends in Food Science & Technology*, *20*(1), 3–16. doi:10.1016/j.tifs.2008.10.002

Gómez-Guillén, M., Turnay, J., Fernández-Dıaz, M., Ulmo, N., Lizarbe, M., & Montero, P. (2002). Structural and physical properties of gelatin extracted from different marine species: A comparative study. *Food Hydrocolloids*, *16*(1), 25–34. doi:10.1016/S0268-005X(01)00035-2

Gomez-Guillen, M. C., Gimenez, B., Lopez-Caballero, M. E., & Montero, M. P. (2011). Functional and bioactive properties of collagen and gelatin from alternative sources: A review. *Food Hydrocolloids*, *25*(8), 1813–1827. doi:10.1016/j.foodhyd.2011.02.007

Harahap, Y., Jaswir, I., & Anwar, E. (2016). Physicochemical and functional properties of gelatin extracted from goat (*Capra hircus*) skin using the partial acid hydrolysis method. *Proceedings of the 3rd International Halal Conference (INHAC 2016)*, 565-576.

Haug, I. J., & Draget, K. I. (2009). Gelatin. In G. O. Phillips & P. A. Williams (Eds.), *Handbook of hydrocolloids* (2nd ed.; pp. 142–163). Cambridge, UK: Woodhead Publishing Limited. doi:10.1533/9781845695873.142

Haug, I. J., & Draget, K. I. (2011). Gelatin. In G. O. Phillips & P. A. Williams (Eds.), *Handbook of food proteins* (pp. 92–115). Cambridge, UK: Woodhead Publishing Limited. doi:10.1533/9780857093639.92

Horneman, D. A., Ottens, M., Hoorneman, M., van der Wielen, L. A., & Tesson, M. (2004). Reaction and diffusion during demineralization of animal bone. *AIChE Journal. American Institute of Chemical Engineers*, *50*(11), 2682–2690. doi:10.1002/aic.10264

Huang, T., Tu, Z., Wang, H., & Zhang, L. (2017). Rheological and structural properties of fish scales gelatin: Effects of conventional and ultrasound- assisted extraction. *International Journal of Food Properties*, *2912*.

Jakhar, J. K., Reddy, A. D., Maharia, S., Devi, M., Reddy, G. V. S., & Venkateshwarlu, G. (2012). Characterization of fish gelatin from blackspotted croaker (Protonibea diacanthus). *Archives of Applied Science Research*, *4*(3), 1353–1358.

Karim, A. A., & Bhat, R. (2009). Fish gelatin: Properties, challenges, and prospects as an alternative to mammalian gelatins. *Food Hydrocolloids*, *23*(3), 563–576. doi:10.1016/j.foodhyd.2008.07.002

Khalil, M. S., Beheri, H. H., & Fattah, W. I. A. (2002). Structural and electrical properties of zirconia/hydroxyapatite porous composites. *Ceramics International*, *28*(4), 451–458. doi:10.1016/S0272-8842(01)00118-3

Liu, D., Nikoo, M., Boran, G., Zhou, P., & Regenstein, J. M. (2015). Collagen and gelatin. *Annual Review of Food Science and Technology*, *6*(1), 527–557. doi:10.1146/annurev-food-031414-111800 PMID:25884286

Liu, H., Han, J., & Guo, S. (2009). Characteristics of the gelatin extracted from Channel Catfish (Ictalurus Punctatus) head bones. *Lebensmittel-Wissenschaft + Technologie*, *42*(2), 540–544. doi:10.1016/j.lwt.2008.07.013

Margarida Figueiredoa, Martinsa, Freitasb, Judasb, & Figueiredo. (2011). Influence of hydrochloric acid concentration on the demineralization of cortical bone. *Chemical Engineering Research and Design*, *89*, 116–124.

Mariod, A. A., & Adam, H. F. (2013). Review: Gelatin, source, extraction and industrial applications. *Acta Scientiarum Polonorum. Technologia Alimentaria*, *12*(2), 135–147.

Muyonga, J., Cole, C., & Duodu, K. (2004). Fourier transform infrared (FTIR) spectroscopic study of acid soluble collagen and gelatin from skins and bones of young and adult Nile perch (*Lates niloticus*). *Food Chemistry*, *86*(3), 325–332. doi:10.1016/j.foodchem.2003.09.038

Power, R. C., Salazar-García, D. C., Wittig, R. M., & Henry, A. G. (2014). Assessing use and suitability of scanning electron microscopy in the analysis of micro remains in dental calculus. *Journal of Archaeological Science*, *49*, 160–169. doi:10.1016/j.jas.2014.04.016

Ratnasari, I., Sudarminto, S. Y., Nusyam, H., & Widjanarko, S. B. (2014). Extraction process modification to enhance properties of skin gelatin of pangas catfish (Pangasius pangasius). *Food and Public Heath*, *4*(3), 140–150.

Ratnasari, I., Yuwono, S. S., Nusyam, H., & Widjanarko, S. B. (2013). Extraction and characterization of gelatin from different fresh water fishes as alternative sources of gelatin. *International Food Research Journal, 20*(6), 3085–3091.

Ridzoulis, C. (2013). *Introduction to the physical chemistry of foods* (J. Rhoades, Ed.). CRC Press, Taylor & Francis Group. doi:10.1201/b14705

Schrieber, R., & Gareis, H. (2007). *Gelatine handbook: Theory and industrial practice.* Weinheim: Wiley-VCH Verlag GmbH & Co. doi:10.1002/9783527610969

See, S. F., Hong, P. K., Ng, K. L., Wan Aida, W. M., & Babji, A. S. (2010). Physicochemical properties of gelatins extracted from skins of different freshwater fish species. *International Food Research Journal, 17*(3), 809–816.

Shahaj, A., Monguidi, M., & Stoicescu, A-V. (2019). Guidelines for reporting surveillance data on Transmissible Spongiform Encephalopathies (TSE) in the EU within the framework of Regulation (EC) No 999/2001. EFSA Supporting Publications.

Silva, R. S. G., Bandeira, S. F., & Pinto, L. A. A. (2014). Characteristics and chemical composition of skins gelatin from cobia (*Rachycentron canadum*). *Lebensmittel-Wissenschaft + Technologie, 57*(2), 580–585. doi:10.1016/j.lwt.2014.02.026

Sockalingam, K., Nelson, H., Idris, M. I., & Abdullah, H. Z. (2016). Effects of pre-treatment durations on properties of black tilapia (*Oreochromis Mossambicus*) skin gelatin. *Materials Science Forum, 840*, 146–150. doi:10.4028/www.scientific.net/MSF.840.146

Sow, L. C., & Yang, H. (2015). Effects of salt and sugar addition on the physicochemical properties and nanostructure of fish gelatin. *Food Hydrocolloids, 45*, 72–82. doi:10.1016/j.foodhyd.2014.10.021

Taheri, A., Abedian Kenari, A. M., Gildberg, A., & Behnam, S. (2009). Extraction and physicochemical characterization of greater lizardfish (*Saurida tumbil*) skin and bone gelatin. *Journal of Food Science, 74*(3), E160–E165. doi:10.1111/j.1750-3841.2009.01106.x PMID:19397722

Wang, L., An, X., Yang, F., Xin, Z., Zhao, L., & Hu, Q. (2008). Isolation and characterisation of collagens from the skin, scale and bone of deep-sea redfish (*Sebastes mentella*). *Food Chemistry, 108*(2), 616–623. doi:10.1016/j.foodchem.2007.11.017 PMID:26059140

Zilhadia, Y., Harahap, Y., Jaswir, I., & Effionora, A. (2018). Characterization and functional properties of gelatin extracted from goatskin. *International Food Research Journal, 25*(1), 275–281.

Chapter 15
Camel Hair Structure, Properties, and Commercial Products

Surong Hasi
Inner Mongolia Agricultural University, China

Guleng Amu
Inner Mongolia Agricultural University, China

Wenbin Zhang
Bactrian Camel Institute of Alxa, China

ABSTRACT

The camel coat can be divided into upper and lower layers based on the external shape. The upper layer is sparse and upright coarse wool; the lower layer is thick wool, which is mainly composed of camel cashmere mixed with small amount of coarse hair. This chapter introduces the basic characteristics of camel hair, such as morphological structure, microstructure, fiber type, and density. Then it introduces the process characteristics of camel wool, the net wool rate, camel hair grades, the photometric and thermodynamic properties of camel cashmere. Finally it gives some camel cashmere and hair products. All contents try to give detailed experimental data and images and insist on giving a more comprehensive and scientific explanation for camel hair.

INTRODUCTION

Camel hair is an animal fiber collected from the camel. The Bactrian camel gives more hair (wool) than the dromedary and is of higher quality, used for making padded cloth, quilts and mattresses, rope, clothes, tents, carpets, robes, saddle girths and blankets (Barat & Morteza, 2015). Therefore, the properties and applications of the Bactrian camel hair are mainly discussed in present chapter. Bactrian camel is a species with a history of several thousand years and closely related to human clothing, food, shelter, travel,

DOI: 10.4018/978-1-7998-1604-1.ch015

and special commercial use. According to incomplete statistics the total number of Bactrian camels in the world would be around 2.8 million (Bright, Jing, Heller, Sirigu & Mutu, 2017) although official number in FAO database is less than one million (Faye & Bonnet, 2012). However, distribution of Bactrian camel is very limited, and mainly distributed in Mongolia, China, Kazakhstan and Kyrgyzstan, adapted to specific weather conditions of desert and semi-desert regions (Galindar & Chagan, 2012; Feng, 2007). Bactrian camels are tall and strong, covered with hair coat with different lengths and thicknesses (Figure 1). The history, population and distribution of camels worldwide were discussed in Chapter 1.

Figure 1. The hair coat of a bactrian camel
Photo courtesy of Mr. Zhang Wenbin, Bactrian Camel Institute of Alasha, Inner Mongolia (2019)

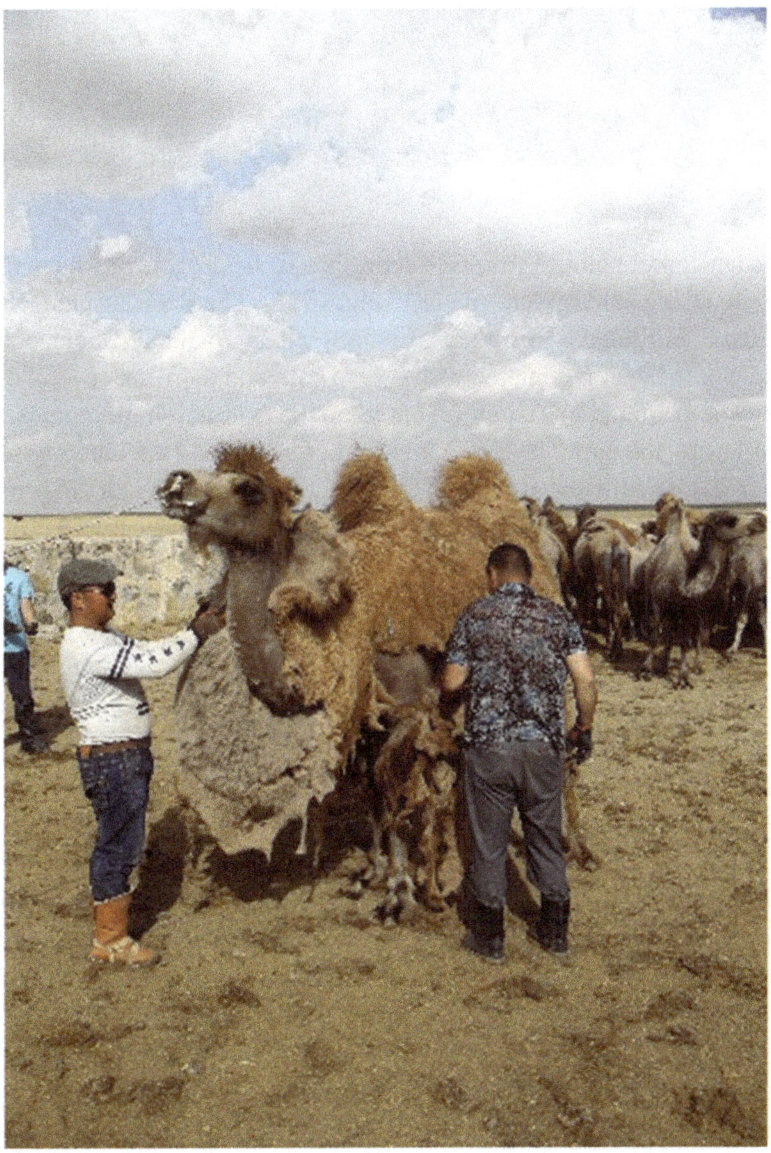

Figure 2. The two layers of hair coats of Bactrian camel
Photo courtesy of Mr. Zhang Wenbin, Bactrian Camel Institute of Alasha, Inner Mongolia (2019)

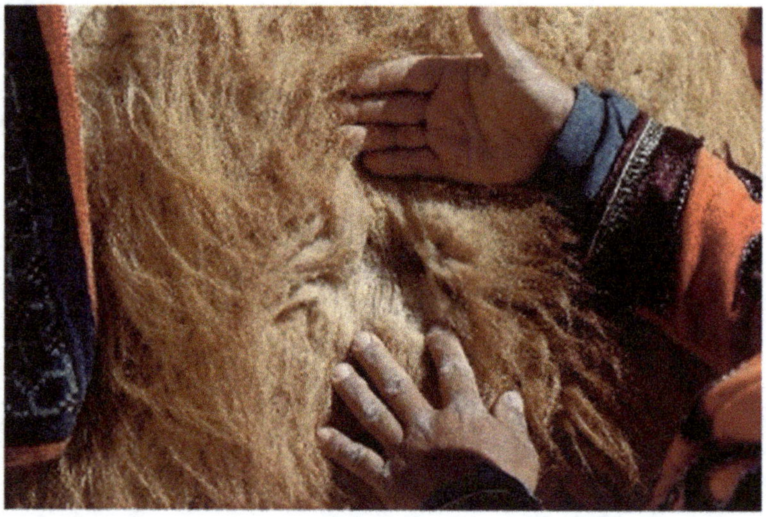

The coat of Bactrian camel belongs to mixed hair, that is, heterogeneous hair, including long hair, coarse hair and soft hair (Feng, 2007; Wei, Yin, & Wang, 1985). The Bactrian camel hair is irregular and has no obvious braided or clustered structure due to the slender camel hair fibers, curved and less of oil sweat. The hair bundle of the coat is centered on a coarse hair, and there are several or even a dozen soft hair with varying thickness around it. Therefore, based on the external shape, camel coat can be divided into upper and lower layers, the upper layer is composed of sparse and upright coarse hair (also contain long hair in certain areas), and the lower layer is composed of thick soft hair (Figure 2).

The total hair yield of Bactrian camel refers to the total amount of camel body hair. Long hair is usually collected by shearing or plucking from the end of February to mid-March. Coarse hair and soft hair were mixed into a mass peeled off together, collected and separated for spinning or knitting. The shedding of camel coats starts from early March of each year and finish at the end of June, and usually start from the region underarms, groin, abdomen and limbs, then the neck, forequarters, hindquarters, the back and body sides. The statistics of hair yield of Bactrian camels were obtained by weighing the completely collected hairs (Altansuhe, 1997). The hair yield statistics of adult Bactrian camels in different regions are as below: Alasha Bull camel's is 5.6~9.4 kg and female camel's is 3.3~5.8 kg, Sunid Bull camel's is 4.5~97.5 kg and female camel's is 3.8~6.0 kg. While, Xinjiang Bull camel's is 4.0~7.5 kg, female camel's is 3.5~5.0 kg, Mongolian Bull camel's is 6.6~12.6 kg. Moreover, female camel's is 3.5~7.8 kg, Kalmyk Bull camel's is 7.5~16.0 kg, female camel's is 4.5~10.0 kg, respectively (Tumenbayar, Erdemt, & Serendalai, 2015). The thickness of the hair layer refers to the natural distance from the surface of the skin to the top of the hair layer. Some average measured thickness of the hair layer in different parts of the Sunid Bactrian camel as below: neck 5.5±0.9 cm, shoulder 5.6±0.8cm, body side 4.7±0.7cm, thigh 3.6±0.7cm (Wei & Wu, 1983). As for dromedary camel, there is a similar hair distribution, not only the hair of different camels is very different, but also the hair of different parts of the same camel is very different (Egbal, Marwa-Babiker, Mohamed, & Ismail, 2017).

This chapter aims to introduce extensive information and knowledge of Bactrian camel hairs, including the morphological structure,microstructure,fiber types, process characteristics, net hair rate,grades,photometric and thermodynamic properties and products of the Bactrian Camel hair.

MORPHOLOGICAL STRUCTURE OF CAMEL HAIR FIBER

Bactrian camel hair can be divided into three parts: hair shaft, hair root and hair bulb in the morphological structure (Su, 1988) (Figure 3). The hair shaft is the part of hair fiber that expose the surface of the skin, often called hair. The hair root is the part within the skin of the hair fiber position, the upper end

Figure 3. Longitudinal section of hair fiber: 1-hair shaft; 2-hair root; 3-hair bulb; 4-hair dermal papilla; 5-hair sheath; 6-hair follicle; 7-sebaceous gland; 8- sweat gland; 9- arrector muscle; 10-scaly layer; 11-cortex layer; 12-medullary layer

Image cited from "Camel Raising Science" by Su Xuebin (1989), Agricultural College of Ningxia, and modified by Dr. Guleng Amu, Inner Mongolia agricultural University

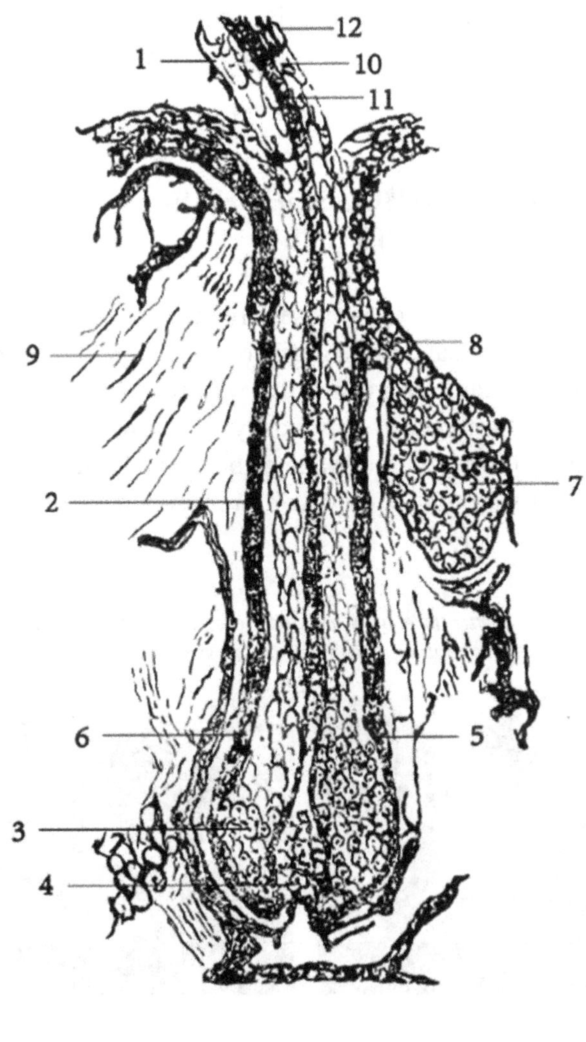

relates to the hair shaft, and the lower end relates to the hair bulb, which is the continuation part of the hair shaft in the hair follicle. The hair bulb, located in the deep layer of the skin, is the swelling part of the end of the hair fiber and the starting point of the hair fiber. As the cells in the hair bulb continue to proliferate, the hair fiber can continue to grow. In addition, there are certain organs that play a nutritional and protective role in the growth of hair fiber. The dermal papilla is an important organ that supplies hair fiber nutrition and plays a neuromodulating role in hair growth. The dermal papilla is connected to the hair bulb and consists of connective tissue, which contains dense capillaries and nerve endings, which ensure the nutrition and neuromodulation of the hair bulb cells, enabling them to proliferate continuously. The hair sheath is a round tube formed by several layers of epidermal cells, surrounding the hair root. The hair follicle is the connective tissue around the sheath, forming the outer membrane of the sheath. The sebaceous glands are located in the skin along both sides of the sheath, and the secretory tube opens in the sheath. This gland secretes oil, which acts to moisturize and protect hair fibers. The oil is mixed with sweat on the surface of the skin, so called oil sweat. The sweat gland is located deep in the skin and consists of epithelial cells. The secretory tube is directly open at the neck of the hair follicle above the level of the sebaceous gland. The physiological role of the sweat gland is a metabolite that regulates body temperature and excretes uselessness. The arrector muscle is a small smooth muscle bundle in the inner layer of the skin. One end is attached to the sheath at the lower part of the adipose gland, and the other end is connected to the epidermis. The contraction and relaxation of the vertebral muscles regulate the secretion of sebaceous glands and sweat glands and regulates blood and lymph circulation as well (Su, 1988).

CROSS-SECTION SHAPE OF CAMEL SOFT HAIR AND THE PROCESS CHARACTERISTICS

The cross-section shape of camel hair fiber is closely related to its process value. The shape of the cross-section of camel soft hair and goat cashmere fibers are different (Figure 4). The Camel soft hair and goat cashmere had a smaller diameter and smaller variation. Microscopic observation also found that the cross-section of the camel soft hair fiber is mostly elliptical and nearly circular, while the cross-section shape of the coarse hair fiber is in the shape of beans and polygons or other irregular shapes. In addition, the shape of the cross-section differs in different sections of the same camel hair fiber. For

Figure 4. Images of cross-section structure by scanning electron microscope (1000×)
Photo courtesy of Dr. Guleng Amu, Inner Mongolia agricultural University (2015)

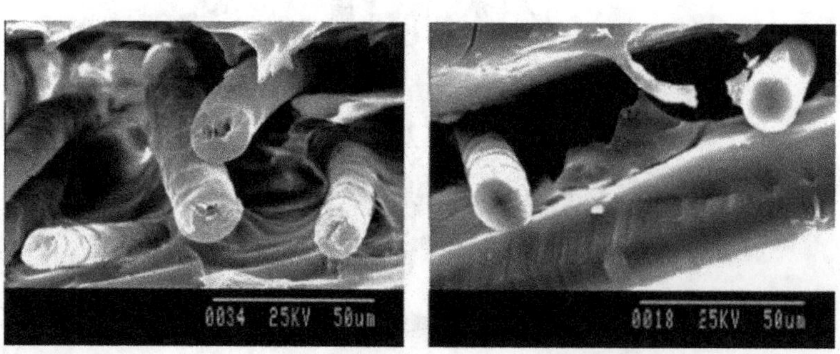

example, the cross section of the upper section (hair sheath) of a soft hair fiber is generally bean-shaped or elliptical, while the lower section (hair root) is nearly circular and elliptical. This difference is mainly caused by the unevenness of the diameter of the soft hair fibers and the large change in the cross-section diameter ratio. According to Tumenbayar (2015), the average diameters in the different sections of the body soft hair fibers of the Sunid Bactrian camel are as below: tip's is 20.72 μm, middle's 19.37 μm, root's 17.31μm and root tip's 3.42μmm. The diameter of the root and sheath of a camel soft hair fiber differs by 3.17 to 4.08 μm.

In wool textile industry, diameter ratio is used to represent the cross-section shape of wool fibers, that is, the ratio of large diameter to minimum diameter of wool fibers. It is used to describe the cross-section shape of wool fibers (Su, 1987; Jiang, 2005). The smaller the diameter ratio of wool fibers is, the more uniform and regular the wool fibers are, and the better the spinning performance is. The cross-section diameter ratio of the goat cashmere is generally 1:1.2 ~1.3, and that of the camel soft hair is generally about 1.2. According to the data of the wool textile industry, if the cross-section diameter ratio of the wool fibers is 1.2 or less, the wool fiber is the superior textile materials; if the diameter ratio is 1.2 to 1.22, the wool fiber is for the medium textile materials; and if the diameter ratio is 1.22 or higher, the wool fiber is the general textile material.

MICROSTRUCTURE OF THE CAMEL HAIR

The histological structure of Bactrian camel hair is observed under the microscope. It is similar to the histological structure of sheep wool. From the surface to the inside, it was divided into three layers: scale layer, cortex layer and medulla layer (Figure 3). The microstructure of the dromedary camel hair is very similar to Bactrian camel's coarse hair (Egbal, 2017).

Scale Layer

The scale layer is located at the outermost layer of the camel hair and consists of flat irregular keratinocytes. The cells of the scale layer are arranged in shape similar to fish scale, so it is called scale layer.

The scale layer of camel hair fiber, according to its arrangement characteristics and the size of the scale, can be generally divided into two types: annular scales and non-annular scales. Annular scales are more common in finer cashmere fibers, and non-circular scales are more common in thicker hair fibers, resembling pine bark. There is a significant difference between camel soft hair and goat cashmere on the scale layer (Figure 5), which largely determines the special properties of camel soft hair fiber. The scales of goat cashmere fiber are mainly composed of relatively regular circular arc and slanted, while the scale layers of the camel soft hair are more radians that close to triangular and partially slanted, with more morphological changes than goat cashmere (Liu, 2017). The scaly contour of the goat cashmere fiber is clear, while that of the camel soft hair is close to each other, and the edges of some tend to merge. Camel soft hair fiber has fewer scales and tightly surrounds the cortical layer. The number of scales in every 1 mm length of fibers is as follow: camel soft hair 40~90 slices, alpaca cashmere 70~150 slices, goat cashmere 60~70 slices, sheep fine wool 65~80 slices, and sheep coarse wool 45~60 slices (Su, 1987 and 1988). The role of the scale layer is to protect the camel soft hair fiber from various physical and chemical attacks. If the scale layer is destroyed, the strength, elongation, elasticity and other process characteristics of the camel soft hair fiber would be lost, and the textile would not be wearable or durable.

Figure 5. Images of the fiber scale structure of by Scanning electron microscope (2000×)
Photo courtesy of Dr. Guleng Amu, Inner Mongolia agricultural University (2015)

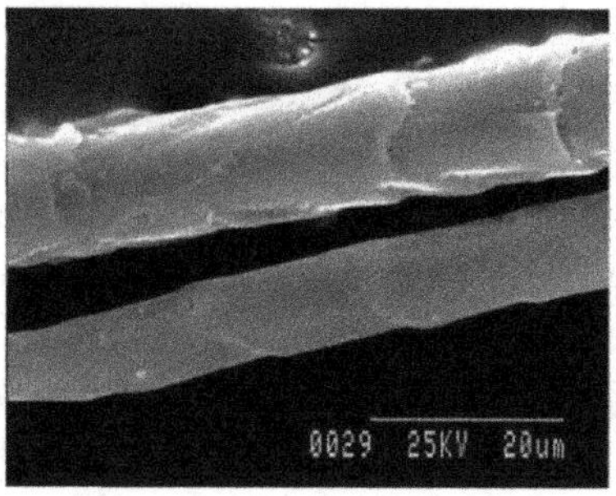

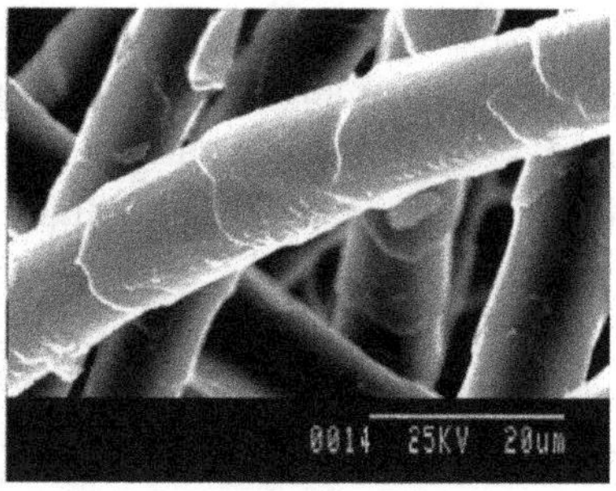

Cortical Layer

The cortical layer is the main body of the hair fibers, which is located below the scale layer and consists of flat and long spindle-shaped cells (Su, 1988).

The cortical cells of camel hair are thinner and longer than sheep's and are arranged along the longitudinal axis of the hair fibers, and the cells are closely connected to each other. The pigment particles are contained in the middle of the cells, thereby determining the color of the hair fibers. The cortical cells are bound by a gel, and the tightness of the gel to the cells determines the strength and elasticity of the fluff fibers. If the hair fibers were degreased with ether for more than 48 hours, the cortical layer showed a small cavity on the cross section.

When camel soft hair is magnified by 2000 times and the camel coarse hair is magnified by 1500 times, the cavity is much smaller and much less than the case when the goat cashmere is magnified by 1000 times. This indicates that the cortical cells of camel hairs are connected closely to each other, and the quality, strength and elasticity of the camel fibers are good, and belong to a superior textile raw material.

Medullary Layer

The medulla layer is below the cortical layer and is the central part of the camel hair fibers. Microstructural measurements showed that the Bactrian camel soft hair was non-medullary, and the coarse hair can be divided into medullary and non-medullary hair (Bai, 2014; Egbal, 2017). Most of the myelinated medulla are continuous medulla, and a few are intermittent medulla. The average fineness of continuous medullary hair is larger than that of intermittent medullary hair. Fineness of the body unmyelinated coarse hair of Alasha camel is 51.80±11.63 μm and that of Subei camel is 20.04±5.19 μm. While fineness of the body continuous myelinated coarse hair of Alasha camel is 75.43±23.13 μm and that of Subei camel is 58.69±13.19 μm. On the other hand, fineness of the side body discontinuous myelinated coarse hair of Alasha camel is 56.90±21.56 μm and that of Subei camel is 38.69±7.21 μm (Bai, 2014). The medullary shape can be roughly divided into four types: dotted line, slender, thick short and thick long. The first two medullas are more common in hair fibers below 50 microns, while the latter two medullas are found in hair fibers above 50.1 microns. The camel hair medulla is the same as sheep wool and is composed of spongy keratinocytes, which consists of a variety of cells and forms a honeycomb structure containing large amount of air. Well known, air is a poor heat conductor, which can reduce the thermal conductivity of the hair fibers. Therefore, the camel body temperature is well preserved in the cold winter and the camel body can be prevented from the hot summer. However, the coarse medullary hair fiber has poor strength, elongation, elasticity, bending and softness, easy to break, and so has low textile process value.

FIBER TYPE AND DENSITY OF CAMEL HAIR

Fiber Type of Camel Hair

The fiber type of camel hair refers to a single fiber. The classification of camel hair fiber type should be based on the shape and fineness of camel hair, while the histological structure and other conditions are auxiliary indicators of classification.

Classification According to the Morphology of the Hair Fibers

According to their shape, camel hair fibers generally are divided into three types: long hair, coarse hair and soft hair (Su, 1988; Zhang, 1982; Egbal, 2017). Long hair is long and thick and mainly distributed in the head crown, chest, neck, elbows, peaks, and tails. The chest hair is the longest one, about 40 ~ 50 cm; followed by elbow hair, about 20 ~ 30 cm; and then upper neck mane about 10 ~ 15 cm; the head crown hair, peak top hair and tail hairs are shorter hair, about 8 ~ 10 cm. The long hair of the bull camel is much longer than those of the female camel. This is also a manifestation of secondary sexual characteristics (Figure 6). The coarse hair (also called guard hair) is constituting the outer layer of the coat. This hair is median length, rare and inflexible, straight and smooth, coarse and brittle, and its medulla is relatively developed, which has a protective effect on the inner layer. The camel soft hair (also called fine hair, or undercoat, or camel cashmere) is an insulating undercoat. The fiber is short and dense, the texture is soft and fine, and the bending is more obvious. Especially the lower part of the soft hair fiber is curved and deep. The medulla at the upper section is generally quite thin and intermittent, which plays a warming role in the body of the Bactrian camel. Camel soft hair is a valuable raw material for wool

Figure 6. Bull camel and female camel
Photo courtesy of Dr. Surong Hasi, Inner Mongolia agricultural University (2015)

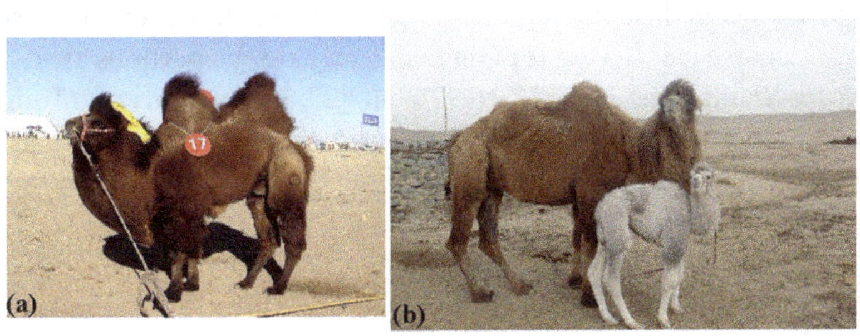

spinning industry and has a highly processability. The quality of this kind of hair fiber determines the breed quality of Bactrian camel in a large extent. In selective breeding process, it is mainly to increase the production of high-quality soft hair and supply raw materials for the wool textile industry.

Camel Hair Classification Based on the Diameter of the Hair Fibers

According to the diameter of the camel hair fiber, the camel hair can be divided into three types: fine hair (soft hair), coarse hair and half coarse hair (Su, 1988; Zhang, 1982). Fine hair refers to a thin, soft, fluffy fiber with a diameter of 14 to 30 μm, an average of 18 μm, and a natural length of 4.0 to 6.0 cm, and there are obviously irregular, inconsistent bends. The fibrous histological structure observed under the microscope, except for the scale layer and the cortical layer, most of the pile fibers have a dotted linear intermedullary layer. Most of the lower and upper section of the hair fibers are about 40 to 60 μm without medullary. However, there is a long and thin medulla in the upper or middle part of a few hair fibers. The soft hair account for about 70-80% of whole hair coat, but the proportion is varies greatly depending on the breed, age, sex and body parts of the region. Especially hair obtained from younger camel is finer and softer than that of from adult camel, and more suitable for excellent apparel purpose (Anjali, 2013).

Coarse hair refers to the coarse hair that is long and straight like a needle, and its diameter is generally 50.1 μm or more. The histological structure consists of three layers of scales, cortex and medulla, and the medulla is very developed, while the scales are not obvious and are arranged irregularly. The coarse hair and soft hair are mixed in the coats, and the coarse hair is exposed on the soft hair to form the outer layer of the coat. Its content is inversely proportional to the soft hair, meaning that if there are many fine hairs, the coarse hairs are relatively small; On the contrary, if the amount of fine hairs is small, the coarse hairs are relatively large. The content of coarse hair in Bactrian camel hair is generally 10-20%, however, this ratio varies with different conditions at the least 5-6% to the highest 30%.

Semi-coarse hair is a kind of hair fiber generally between coarse hair and fine hair, and its diameter is 30.1-50 μm, so it is also called two-type hair. The characteristics of semi-coarse hair fiber is that the upper section is thick and straight, without bending, and the medulla is long and developed, showing the characteristics of coarse hair. While the lower part is finer, with a small amount of irregular curvature, the medulla is thin and intermittent, and has the characteristics of soft hair. Because the coarse hair part of semi-coarse hair is short and the fine hair part is long, so it is easy to break. In the coat of Bactrian camels, the content of such hair fibers is very inconsistent, up to 30-40%, or only 7-8%. The contents of three kinds of camel hair in a whole camel coat are generally expressed by the ratio of the various hair numbers or the proportion of weights. The average ratio of the various hair number in the shoulder area of adult Bactrian camels in different regions of China is as follow: for camel soft hair is 82.97%, half coarse hair 12.52%, coarse hair 4.51%; for Qinghai camel, the proportions are 64.63%, 25.00%, and 10.37% respectively; for Sunid camel, 90.07%, 6.97% and 2.98% respectively (Tumenbayar, 2015). In fact, the average weight ratio of Bactrian camel hair is also changed greatly with age in the same area (Tumenbayar, 2015).

Density of Camel Hair and the Influencing Factors

The density of camel hair coat refers to the number of hair fibers per unit of surface area of the skin, for example, the number of hair fibers grown on one square centimeter of skin. The more the number of hairs, the greater the density and the higher of the hair yield. On the contrary, the number of hairs is small, the density is small, and the amount of hair production is low (Su, 1988).

In the inspection of the density of the hair coat, the hand feel method is used to inspect the density of hair coat. The hair is grasped by hand, and the density of the coat is determined according to the degree of compaction of the hair coat in the palm (Su, 1988). After grasping the hair, the tip of the finger cannot touch the palm, indicating dense hair. Instead, the tip of the finger can touch the palm, indicating thin hair. Secondly, it is also possible to peel the hair coat by hand and observe the size of the skin gap between the hair bundles. If the gap is small, it is dense, and if the gap is large, it is thin. Both above methods belong to the on-site estimation method and require some experience. The estimation error of experienced people is small, and the error of beginners is generally large (Tumenbayar et al., 2015).

The laboratory method uses a density clamp to take the hair from the neck, shoulders, side of the body and thighs of the same horizontal line of the camel body, take a 1 cm^2 hair sample, and calculate the amount or weight of the hair fiber per unit surface area. The density of Bactrian camel hair is varying with body sites due to differences in skin thickness, humidity, sebaceous glands, sweat glands, blood circulation and nerve distribution in various parts of the camel body. Where the skin is thick, the humidity is high, the sebaceous glands and sweat glands are more, and the blood vessels and nerve endings are densely distributed, the density of the coat is large, and vice versa. According to the preliminary measurements, the density of the hair coat of the adult Bactrian camel has 1800 to 3600 hair fibers on per cm^2 of area. The denser parts are neck, shoulder and thigh, then the body side, and then the lower part of the abdomen and lower extremities (Su, 1988; Wei & Wu, 1983).

PROCESS CHARACTERISTICS OF CAMEL HAIR

The difference in physical properties such as the fineness and elasticity of camel hair determines the value and use of camel hair fibers in the wool spinning industry, so often called this process characteristics (Jiang, 2005; Anjali & Suman, 2013). The process characteristics of camel hair is one of the criteria for assessing the quality of camel hair and identifying Bactrian camels in the camel production department, the commercial acquisition department and the wool textile industry. It is also one of the main characteristics of camel hair fibers differing from other fibers. It plays an important role in improving and guiding the production of camel industry.

There are many contents of the camel hair craftsmanship. Here we focus on the most commonly used indicators - fineness, length, uniformity, curvature, strength, elasticity, gloss and felting.

Fineness

The fineness of the camel hair refers to the diameter of the cross-section of the single hair fiber, measured in μm. Camel hair is a kind of heterogeneous hair. The diameter of various types of hair fibers is varying greatly. The average diameter of the soft hair is 18 μm, the range of variation is 14-30 μm; the diameter of coarse hair is above 50.1 μm; the diameter of the semi-coarse is 30.1 to 50 μm. For adult

Alasha Bactrian camel, the average diameter of the soft hair is 15.97 μm; the average diameter of the coarse hair is 66.75 μm, and the average diameter of the semi-coarse is 38.36 μm. For 2 to 4 years old young Bactrian camel, the average diameter of camel soft hair of is 14.78 μm (Su, 1988). Therefore, the diameter of the soft hair of the Bactrian camel is very close to that of the goat cashmere (Jiang, 2005; Liu, Xie, & Liu 2017).

However, the fineness of camel soft hair varies depending on the different breed, age, sex, body parts and the natural conditions of the pasture. In the adult Bactrian camel, the hair of the female camel and the castrated camel are thinner (Su, 1988). From the regional perspective, Alasha Bactrian camel's soft hair is finer (Su, 1988; Wei & Wu, 1983). From the body parts of the Bactrian camel, the femoral soft hair is the finest one, the shoulder soft hair is second, and the body side soft hair is relatively thick (Wei & Wu, 1983).

Length

Length of the camel hair is generally divided into two types: natural length and straight length. Natural length refers to the length of the hair bundle and the thickness of the hair layer in a natural state. Straight steel ruler is used to directly measure the distance from the skin surface to the tip of the soft hair or the coarse hair. However, as the coarse hair in the Bactrian camel hair coat is sparse, the thickness of the layer is usually used to represent the hair length. Straight length is the length of the single fiber when it was pulled until the curve disappears. Length of the straight length is directly related to the textile performance of the camel hair. Average straight length of adult Alasha Bactrian camel soft hair is 8.53±2.19 cm (Su, 1988). Straight length of castrated camel soft hair is longer than the female camel's, the neck's and shoulder's soft hairs are longest, and the body side's and the femoral's soft hairs are second, the lower part of the abdomen's and the lower limb's soft hairs are shortest (Su, 1988; Wei, Yin, & Wang, 1985). Length of camel coarse hair is closely related to the total hair yield. In the case of the same density, the length is proportional to hair yield, i.e. the longer the camel coarse hair, the higher the hair yield; otherwise, the hair yield is greatly affected.

The variation of the length of camel coarse hair is related to the types, nutritional status, age, gender and other factors. For example, Alasha Bactrian camel coarse hair is longer than Qinghai Bactrian camel's; in Bactrian camel with good nutrition, hair is longer than other camel's; for bull camel, coarse hair is thicker than other camels, but hairs in other parts are generally shorter than female camel and castrated camel. During the rainy years, the forage grows vigorously, and the hair of the Bactrian camel is longer and denser, whereas the hair is shorter and thinner during the drought year. (Su, 1988).

Evenness

Evenness refers to the degree of uniformity of the camel hair fibers in terms of fineness. On the same Bactrian camel hair coat, there are difference evenness for coarse hair and soft hair. However, if the difference between the evenness is too large, especially if the evenness of a same hair fiber is inconsistently, it will bring difficulties to the processing of the raw materials for the textile industry, thereby affecting the textile value and use of the camel hair. Therefore, in the breeding work of Bactrian camel, more attention should be pay on the evenness of camel hair, and strict selective breeding is necessary for improving the quality of camel soft hair (Su, 1988).

There are three main requirements for the evenness of camel hair: (i) the first one is the evenness of soft hair in various parts of the Bactrian camel, (ii) the second one is the evenness of the single hair fiber, for example, the difference in fineness from the root to tip of the one hair fiber, and (iii) the third one is the evenness of the hair layer, that is the difference in fineness of various hair fibers in the same hair tuft. In soft hair in various parts of the adult Bactrian camel, the fineness of the thigh hair is finer, the hair in shoulder is second, and hair in body side is thicker (Su, 1988). However, the difference in evenness did not exceed 3 μm, and the quality of hair still belong to the same grade.

For the fineness of each section of the soft hair fiber, in the upper section is thicker, in the middle section is second, and in the lower section is finer. From the difference between the fineness of the upper and lower sections, the finest reaches 5~7 μm, and the thickest reaches 10~12 μm. If measured by the quality count standard, the difference is 2~4 grades (Su, 1988). Due to the unevenness of the fineness of each section of the soft hair fiber, it will undoubtedly affect the spinning performance of the camel soft hair and reduce its utilization value. The main reason for this phenomenon is due to the extremely uneven nutrition in the four seasons in the desert (Su, 1989; Tumenbayar et al., 2015).

Tortuosity

Tortuosity refers to the number of bending of hair fibers in per unit length and the degree of bending. From the external form, the bending of the camel coarse hair fiber is generally not as regular as the bending of sheep wool. The occurrence of such irregular bending is mainly caused by the unevenness of the fineness of the camel coarse hair fibers. When the diameter of the hair fiber is about 10μm, the bending is more and deep, about 6 to 7 bends in the length of 1 cm, and the bending shape is mostly a deep bend, a narrow bend or a loop bend. When the diameter of the hair fiber is 20~30 μm, the number of bends is less and shallower than the former, mostly normal bend or shallow bend, and there are about 3~5 bends in the length of 1 cm. Most of the hair fibers with a diameter of more than 40 μm have no bends in the upper section, and only a small amount of shallow or flat bends in the lower section, only 1 to 3 bends in the length of 1 cm (Su, 1989; Tumenbayar et al., 2015).

For a single hair fiber, the tortuosity is also very different. In each camel hair fiber, many deep, narrow or loop bends are mainly concentrated in lower section (root section) of camel hair; and small number of large, shallow bends are distributed in middle section of hair, as well as, the small number of bends are distributed in the upper section (tip section) hair fiber. If it is a soft hair fiber, the curve is mostly flat and curved, while if it is a course hair, the tip is straight with no bending (Tumenbayar et al., 2015).

Strength and Extension

The strength of hair fibers refers to the weight that hair fibers can bear, that is, the force needed to break the fibers. There are two ways to express strength: one is absolute strength, which refers to the weight required to break one or a bundle of hair fibers, called the breaking strength, in grams or kilograms. The second is the relative strength, which refers to the force acting on the unit cross-sectional area when the camel coarse hair fiber is broken, expressed in kilograms per square centimeter (Su, 1989; Tumenbayar et al., 2015).

Whether wool textiles are strong and durable enough is closely related to the strength of wool fibers. Therefore, the wool textile industry ranks strength as an important indicator when selecting woolen raw materials. The strength of the wool fiber is closely related to its fineness. It is also affected by the feeding management and the method of preserving the wool fiber. Due to the large difference in fineness of camel hair, the range of intensity variation is also large. The strength of camel soft hair is 7 to 25 grams, and the strength of coarse hair is 45 to 60 grams (Su, 1989; Tumenbayar, et al.,2015).

If the stretched hair fiber is stretched again to break, it will increase in length. The percentage of this increased length to the original length of the hair fibers is referred to the extension. The extension of camel hair is generally 45-50%. Extension is one of the necessary conditions to determine the firmness of the hair. The fabric obtained from the hair fibers with less extension is easily broken in the corners and wrinkles after being made into clothes (Su, 1989; Tumenbayar et al., 2015).

Specific Gravity

The specific gravity of camel hair is also known as relative density. The greater the specific gravity, the greater the density. The specific gravity of camel coarse hair is close to sheep wool, but smaller than cotton, so camel coarse hair has a superior characteristic to cotton. The fabric obtained from the hair fibers with less extension is easily broken in the corners and wrinkles after being made into clothes. There is a certain correlation between strength and elongation, so the factors affecting the strength also affect the elongation (Su, 1988). The specific gravity of camel soft hair is 1.312, and the specific gravity of camel coarse hair is 1.284. Because of the developed coarse medulla and air in the medullary cavity, the specific gravity of camel coarse hair is relatively light (Wei, Yin, & Wang, 1985).

RAW HAIR COMPOSITION AND NET HAIR RATE

Raw Hair Composition

Hair removed from the body of the Bactrian camel without any processing or mechanical treatment is called the raw hair. In addition to hair fibers, the raw hair also contains various impurities (Figure 7). The impurities in camel hair can be divided into two categories: (i) **physiological impurities**, such impurities are oily sweat and dander, and the oily sweat content is generally about 4 to 5%, (ii) **living impurities**, mainly dust, mud sand, excrement, grass clippings, and dregs. Among them, sand accounts for the largest proportion, generally accounting for 15~25%, and the highest is more than 30% (Altansuhe,1997; Galindar & Chagan, 2012)

Net Hair Rate

After the raw hair is washed, the oily sweat, dust, mud sand, grass clippings, excrement, grass clippings and other impurities are removed, and the remaining hair fibers are net hair. The percentage of the weight of the net hair to the weight of the raw hair sample is called the net hair rate.

The method of measuring the net hair rate of camel hair is the same as that of sheep wool. First, take 50 grams of hair from all parts of the camel body, shake it well, and pick up sand, grass scraps and dregs. Secondly, it was soaked in water at about 30 °C, then washed twice at 30 °C in 0.3% alkali-soap mixed solution or 0.3% soap powder solution. Thirdly, wash it twice with clean water at about 30 °C. Finally, after the water is removed and dried under sunlight at 30-35 °C for 4 to 5 hours, the weight is measured, and the net hair ratio calculated (Su, 1988; Wei, 1983).

Figure 7. Various impurities in the camel raw hair
Photo courtesy of Mr. Zhang Wenbin, Bactrian Camel Institute of Alasha, Inner Mongolia (2019)

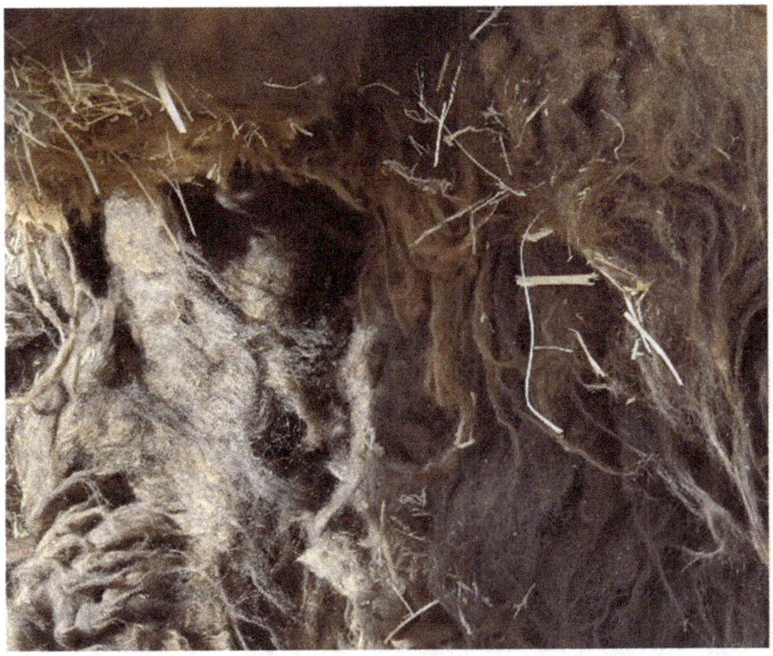

The average net hair rate of Sunid Bactrian camel after shake sand is more than 90% (Wei & Wu, 1983). If the raw hair is washed directly without shaking sand and removing soil, the net hair rate is about 75%, which indicates that the oily sweat content in raw hair is relatively low, while the sand and other impurities are more (Wei & Wu, 1983).

GRADE OF CAMEL HAIR

Classification and Grading Law of Camel Hair

According to "Chinese current draft of specifications for purchasing livestock products", camel hair can be classified into first grade, second grade and third grade based on the quality of hair fibers, but the color of camel hair is not graded (Su, 1988; Zhang, 1984; Su, 1989).

First grade hair (I) is soft, mainly composed of camel soft hair, and the hair fibers are slender, bright, apricot yellow, brown red, silver grey or white. Second grade hair (II) is coarse hair, shorter than first grade hair, with a small amount of soft hair content and dry dead hair. Third grade hair (III) is composed of long hair strands of different thickness, and the content of soft hair is very small (Figure 8).

Figure 8. Main distribution area on camel hair coat of difference grades
Photo courtesy of Dr. Surong Hasi, Inner Mongolia agricultural University (2010)

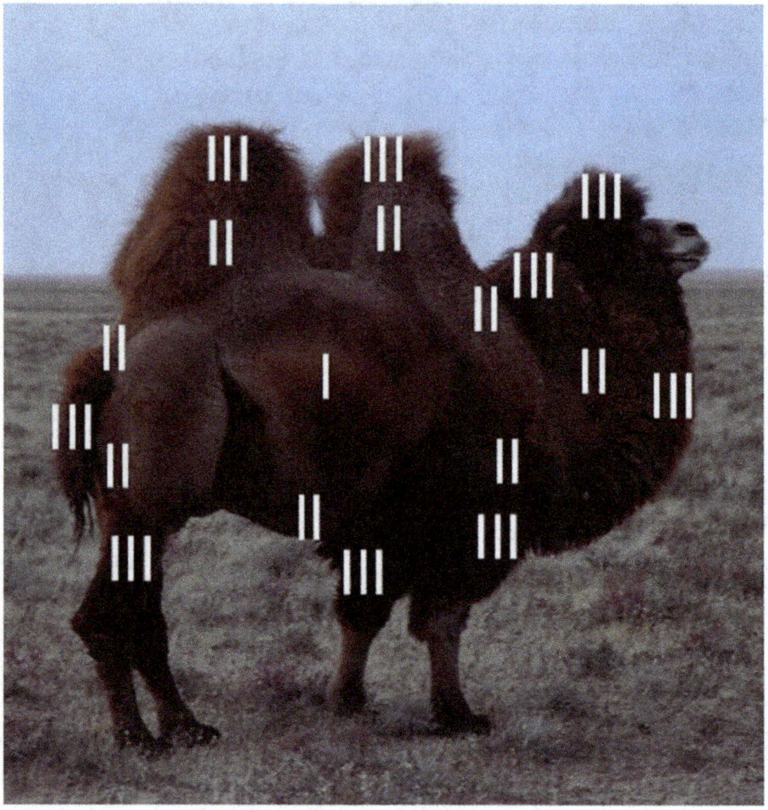

Difference of Regional Quality Ratio of Camel Hair

In China, Bactrian camels are mainly distributed in Inner Mongolia, Xinjiang, Qinghai, Gansu and Ningxia. The quality of camel hair varies due to different breeds and management conditions.

The quality of camel hair produced in Ordos, Bayannuur and Alasha of Inner Mongolia, Ningxia, Gansu and Northern Shaanxi is good, and the quality ratio difference is 100%. Among them, the quality of camel hair produced in Alasha area of Inner Mongolia is the best, characterized by the color of apricot yellow, slender and lustrous fibers. Quality ratio difference of camel hair in Shilingol, Chifeng and Northeast Province of Qinghai and Inner Mongolia is 95%. The quality of camel hair is characterized by yellowish color, short and thick fibers and poor luster. Camel coarse hair produced in Hebei, Shanxi and Beijing suburbs has poor quality ratio difference of 85%. It is characterized by dark color, thick fibers, gray-black and less luster (Bai & Feng, 2014).

THE PHOTOMETRIC AND THERMODYNAMIC PROPERTIES OF CAMEL SOFT HAIR

Anti-Ultraviolet (UV) Property of Camel Soft Hair

The anti-ultraviolet property of camel soft hair was studied by Bai and Amu (2019) and compared to that of goat cashmere and cotton. The standard of evaluation on anti UV properties of fabrics issued by the State Quality Inspection Bureau stipulates that as long as the Ultraviolet Protection Factor (UPF) value of the sample is greater than 30 and the transmittance (TR) of UVA is less than 5%, it can be called "anti-ultraviolet product", and these two conditions are indispensable. Preliminary qualitative experiments using YG(B)912E UV tester, the samples were tested every 5 nm in the wavelength range of about 280~400 nm. Figure 9 shows that the UV transmittance of camel soft hair is less than 2% in a large range of wavelength, so camel soft hair has the strongest UV protection property. The UPF of camel soft hair is high enough and transmittance of UVA and UVB is very low, so camel soft hair has stronger anti-ultraviolet property than other two samples (Bai & Amu, 2019).

Heat Transfer Property

Thermal conductivity K is an intrinsic property of material that indicates its ability to conduct the heat. It is the flux of heat (energy per unit area per unit time) divided by temperature gradient (temperature difference per unit length). In general, the lower the thermal conductivity K of the object, the weaker the thermal transfer performance of the object, and its thermal insulation is better. Thermal conductivity K of camel soft hair is very low, so the camel soft hair has better thermal insulation property (Bai & Amu, 2019).

Figure 9. Comparison of transmittance of different samples
Photo courtesy of Dr. Guleng Amu, Inner Mongolia agricultural University (2015)

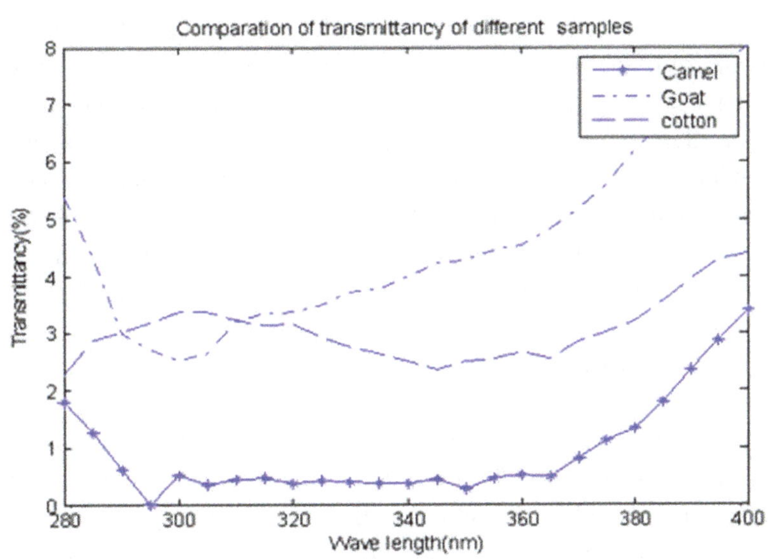

Thermal Contact Property

Thermal contact properties determine the feeling when the human skin touches an object for brief time. The more a material absorbs thermal energy, the more it acts as a thermal conductor, and the cooler it seems at the very first moment of contact with a warmer body. The characteristic value Q was proposed by Kawabata & Niwa (1989) and has been shown to estimate the temperature perception of the fabric. This value is the maximum rate of heat flux from a heated plate to the fabric and is convenient to measure. Q is usually measured with the KES-F7 (Kawabata Evaluation Systems for Fabrics). Large Q values correspond to cold sensations, and small Q values correspond to thermal sensations. That is, the larger the Q, the colder it is.

The heat Q obtained by each square centimeter for camel soft hair is very low, so camel soft hair has nice warm fleeing property (Bai & Amu, 2019).

Air Permeability of Camel Soft Hair

Air permeability (AP) is described as the rate of air flow through a known area under a prescribed air pressure differential between the two surfaces of material. Fabrics with small air permeability can prevent thermal divergence, which can also play a good thermal protective effect.

This experiment uses YG461E digital permeability meter to measure the air permeability of the sample, and each sample is measured 5 times. Camel soft hair has the lowest air permeability, so it emits water very well (Bai & Amu, 2019).

Experimental results show that Camel soft hair has strong anti-ultraviolet property, good thermal insulation, nice warm feeling, and high air permeability.

CAMEL HAIR PRODUCTS

Camel Soft Hair Products

Camel soft hair is a layer of short fluff close to the body of a Bactrian camel. After washing the raw hair, removing the coarse and semi-coarse hair, combing the remaining parts, the pure camel soft hair can be obtained (Figure 10). Due to the fineness, softness and curliness of the fibers, the flakes made from camel soft hair have the advantages of being light, thin, fluffy, windproof, mildewproof, breathable and warm. The garments made of camel soft hair is comfortable to wear and not as bloated as a down jacket. A variety of camel hair products can be made with camel soft hair, such as camel quilt, camel trousers, camel sweater, camel coat, camel socks, camel vest, camel knee pads, camel scarf, camel gloves, camel hat, camel blanket, camel insole, camel back waist strap, camel carpet, etc. (Figure 11).

Camel Coarse Hair Products

Camel coarse hair containing a large amount of coarse fiber has the advantages of keeping warm, windproof, mildewproof and breathable. However, compared with camel soft hair, the heating speed of camel coarse hair is slower. People like to use it as a filler for winter pants or camel coarse hair-padded mattress and use it also to make camel coarse hair carpets and camel hair ropes (Figure 12).

Figure 10. Combed pure camel soft hair
Photo courtesy of Mr. Zhang Wenbin, Bactrian Camel Institute of Alasha, Inner Mongolia (2019)

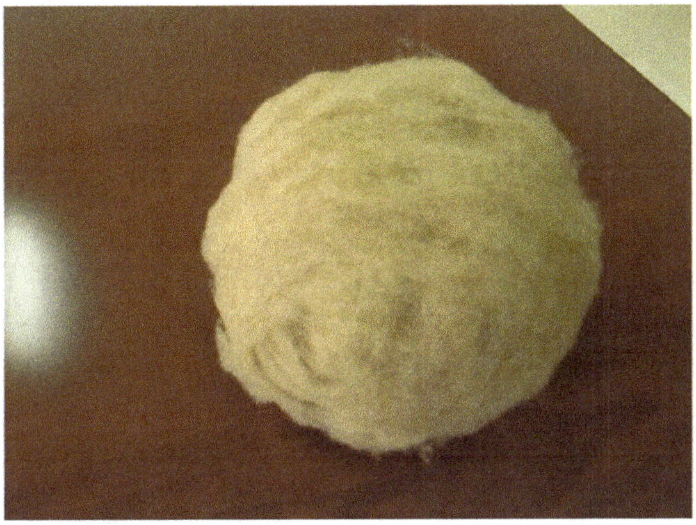

Figure 11. Camel soft hair products
Photo courtesy of Mr. Zhang Wenbin, Bactrian Camel Institute of Alasha, Inner Mongolia (2019)

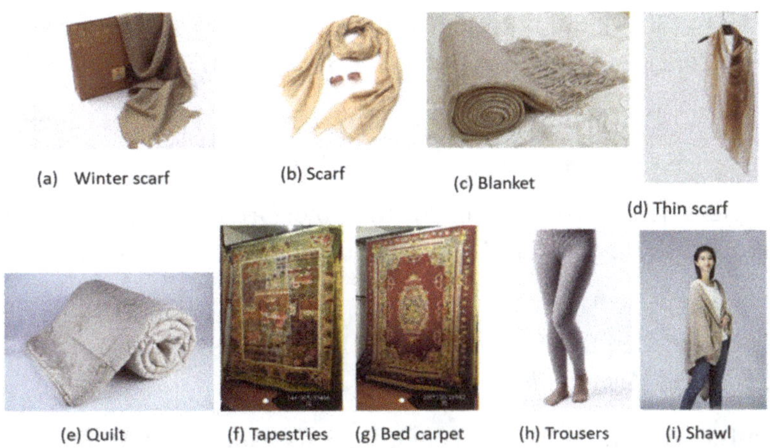

Figure 12. Camel coarse hair products
Photo courtesy of Mr. Zhang Wenbin, Bactrian Camel Institute of Alasha, Inner Mongolia (2019)

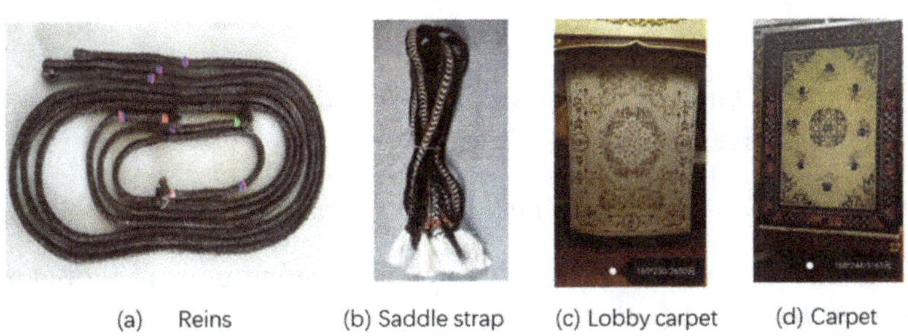

CONCLUSION AND PERSPECTIVES

Nowadays, with the development of science and technology, although there are many kinds of artificial fibers used for people, natural fibers are more and more preferred for daily clothing and bedding necessities. Bactrian camel hair has a high gross output, and its morphological structure, microstructure, fiber types determine good quality, strength and elasticity. Its photometric and thermodynamic properties show that camel soft hair has strong anti-ultraviolet property, good thermal insulation, nice warm feeling, and high air permeability. Bactrian camel hair belongs to a superior natural textile raw material.

In the process of writing this chapter, many research materials on camel hair were consulted. It was found that they were often limited to research reports, and not up to date for the last 5-10 years. Therefore, it is planned to achieve further studies on the physical and chemical properties of camel hair with high-precision modern instruments.

REFERENCES

Altansuhe. (1997). *Sunid Bactrian camel.* Inner Mongolia Peoples Publishing House.

Anjali, S., & Suman, P. (2013). Studies on camel hair -merino wool blended knitted fabrics. *Indian Journal of Fibre and Textile Research*, *38*, 317–319.

Bai, M. Z., & Amu, G. L. (2019). Study on Physical Properties of camel Cashmere. *Journal of Camel Practice and Research*, *26*(2), 113–116. doi:10.5958/2277-8934.2019.00030.4

Bai, L., & Feng, D. Z. (2014). Analysis of wool Quality and Fiber Types of Chinese Bactrian Camels. *Heilongjiang Animal Science and Veterinary Medicine*, *3*, 155-158.

Barat, A. Z. Y., & Morteza, K. (2015). Introduction to Camel Origin, History, Raising, Characterisctics, And Wool, Hair and Skin, A Review. *EPH - International Journal of Agriculture and Environmental Research*, *1*, 1–19.

Bright, L. Y., & Jing,, H., Heller, S., & Ri Mutu, J. (2017). Progress in Molecular Genetics of Bactrian Camel Origin and Evolution. *Acta Ecologiae Animalis Domastici*, *38*(3), 5–9.

Egbal, A. S., Marwa-Babiker, A. E., Mohamed, O. E., & Ismail, E. F. (2017). Morphology and Morphometry of Raw Camel Hair of Some Sudanese Camel types in Kordofan States. *Nova Journal of Medical and Biological Sciences*, *6*, 1–8.

Faye, B., & Bonnet, P. (2012). Camel sciences and economy in the world: current situation and perspectives. *Proc. 3rd ISOCARD conference*, 2-15.

Feng, D. Z. (2007). Study on Growth and Development and Production Model of Alashan Bactrian Camel. China Agricultural University.

Galindar & Chagan. (2012). *Gobi Bactrian camel.* Inner Mongolia Peoples Publishing House.

Jiang, P. E. (2005). An analysis on the factors influencing the spinning ability of camel hair. *Journal of Wenzhou Vocational and Technical College*, *5*, 39–40.

Kawabata, S., & Niwa, M. (1989). Fabric Performance in Clothing Manufacture. *Journal of the Textile Institute*, *80*(1), 19–50. doi:10.1080/00405008908659184

Liu, C., Xie, C. P., & Liu, X. J. (2017). Properties of Yak Wool in Comparison to Cashmere and Camel Hairs. *Journal of Natural Fibers*, *6*, 1–12.

Norbu, Z. (1988). Alasha Bactrian camel. Inner Mongolia Science and Technology Press.

Su, X. B. (1987). The histological structure of camel coarse hair and its character analysis. *Acta Veterinaria et Zootechnica Sinica*, *S1*, 52–58.

Su, X. B. (1988). Camel Raising Science. Agricultural Publishing House.

Su, X.B. (1989). Hair Characters and Ecological Environment of Bactrian Camels in China. *Livestock Ecology, 4*, 11-13.

Tumenbayar, E. S. (2015). Mongolian Bactrian camel. Menghe Text Publishing Company.

Wei, H. F., Yin, Z. C., & Wang, M. Q. (1985). Hair Characteristics and Fiber Types of Bactrian Camels. *Gansu Animal and Veterinary Sciences*, *1*, 10–12.

Wei, S. R., & Wu, J. G. (1983). Analysis of wool Quality of Sunid Bactrian Camel. *Zhongguo Xumu Zazhi*, *3*, 15–17.

Zhang, B. T. (1984). The property of camel hair. *Journal of China Textile Engineering Association*, *5*, 649–653.

Zhang, P. Y., Liu, G. L., & Bai, G. H. (1982). Physical Properties of Bactrian Camel coarse hair. *Zhongguo Xumu Zazhi*, *5*, 23–26.

Chapter 16
Camel Milk Disguised Cosmeceutical

Rajesh Datt Mehta
Department of Dermatology, Venereology, and Leprosy, S. P. Medical College, India

Ritika Agrawal
S.P.Medical College, Bikaner, India

ABSTRACT

This chapter conveys the untapped property of camel milk as cosmeceutical. The camel milk ingredients (i.e., water, ascorbic acid, alpha hydroxy acid, polyunsaturated fatty acid, peptides, and micronutrients) make it a cost-effective cosmeceutical with no adverse cutaneous or systemic reactions. It may be used as a photoprotective, moisturizing, anti-wrinkle, anti-aging skin softener. The bioactive ingredients may begin the new class of natural cosmeceutical when consumed orally or applied topically.

INTRODUCTION

The life on earth take place in a wonderful "ecological system" where the members of the animal kingdom exemplify great deal of interdependence. The symbiosis between the human (*Homo sapiens sapiens*) and the camel (*Camelus dromedaries and Camelus bactrianus*) is not an exception to this statement. Both serve each other for better co-existence. Camel and human are, therefore, good environmental friends. Camel repays, out of proportion to humans, through the medicinal values of milk and other properties (Al Haj & Al Kanhal, 2010). The potential therapeutic properties and disease preventing of camel milk was discussed in Chapter 7 and 8.

Camel, a precious species, is not only emblematic to certain geographical terrains but is also considered as a symbol of status and wealth. It was being used as mode of transport, communication and trade in historical sagas in arid zone. But in modern era too, camel is offering source of incomes to the camel producers. Camel milk, wool, dung, meat, leather, bones etc. are the viable source of livelihoods for the owners (Köhler-Rollefson & Rathore, 2004).

DOI: 10.4018/978-1-7998-1604-1.ch016

The chemical composition of camel milk (Kula & Tegegne, 2016; Galali & Hanee, 2019) makes it, a suitable candidate not only for health effect, but also for cosmeceuticals. Despite of synthetic compounds, certain natural ingredients of camel milk make it, a good cosmetic product (Rasheed, 2018). The dual advantage of camel milk lies in the fact that it cannot only be used topically but its ingestion also helps in enhancing beauty.

The use of pharmaceutical knowledge in the field of beautifying the skin and its appendages has created a new 'world' and 'word' of cosmeceuticals. Kligman coined this term to describe a good number of pharmacological products which had an evidence of proven biological activity to metamorphosize the aesthetic appearance of an individual. (Baumann, 2003; Draelos, 1995; Shah, 2005).

THE HUMAN SKIN CARE BY COSMETICALS

The normal skin care has got four pillars to maintain the health of inherited skin and to augment its beauty (Sachdeva & Khunger, 2010). These can be grouped as (i) cleansers, (ii) toners, (iii) moisturizers, and (iv) nutrients.

Cleansers are the products which are used to remove superficial dirt, grease, bacteria and desquamated keratinocytes. These include soaps, synthetic detergents, syndet bars and lipid free cleansing agents (Draelos, 2018). The chemical composition of soaps is fatty acids, glycerine, triglycerides, lanolin, paraffin, mineral acids, stearic acids, sodium lauryl sulphate, acrylate, propylene glycol etc.. The quality components in camel milk i.e. fatty acids, sterol, lanolin, make it, a versatile source for soap production (Mills, Berger & Baker,1993).

The **toners** are lotion or wash used to cleanse the skin and shrink the appearance of pores, usually used on the face by applying facial mask. Three types of skin toners are described: (i) fresheners (or skin bracers) containing water and humectant as glycerine and a little alcohol; the most popular toner being rosewater, (ii) skin tonics which contain up to 20% alcohol, water and humectant ingredient, used for normal and oily skin; orange flower is the more popular example, (iii) astringents which contain a high proportion of alcohol (up to 60%), antiseptic ingredients, water and a humectant ingredient; they are used to remove excess protective lipids. For this kind of products are not based on camel milk components.

Moisturizers are the cosmeceuticals which improve the hydration of skin, to make it, normal in appearance and give the person a normal or even euphoric feel, psychologically (Spencer, 1988). The components of a moisturizer are water, animal fats, silicon, phospholipids, hyaluronic acid, glycerine, propylene glycol, etc. Different combinations and permutations act synergistically to keep the skin hydrated and moist. This property of moisturizers creates an interface between skin and ultraviolet radiations thus providing a means of photoprotection. This mode acts as a preventive tool against photoaging (Wilhelm, Cua & Maibach, 1991). The high-water content (86-88%) of camel milk creates a vast scope to be used as basic constituent of moisturizer group of cosmeceuticals. Alpha lipoic acids, essential fatty acids (linoleic acid, linolenic acid and arachidonic acid), retinoids, vitamin c, vitamin e, peptides, animal oils (squalene, mink oil, lanolin, emu oil) act as moisturizers. Silicone and hyaluronic acid work as humectants. These may be derived from animal sources.

Nutrients are acting in the nutrition of skin. This is a very important factor to keep the skin glowing, smooth and give the 'ever young appearance (Mason, 2012). The essential nutrients required for maintaining the normal health of skin and improvising it, are vitamin A (Retinoids), β-carotene, vitamin C, vitamin D, vitamin E, protein, fats, oils and above all, water. The micronutrients, calcium, phosphorous, copper, iron, magnesium, manganese, sulphur, zinc, potassium and selenium are mandatory to make a cosmetic product, complete and perfect. These nutraceuticals have an added advantage of being effective in both ways, i.e, when consumed systemically or applied topically.

THE BENEFICIAL MILK COMPONENTS FOR COSMETICALS

The cosmeceuticals are aimed to provide the following benefits (Sachdeva, 2010):

1. Prevent ultraviolet rays' induced damage to the skin.
2. Reduction of free radicals.
3. Improvement of skin lipid barrier.
4. Providing glow to skin through brightening.
5. Uniformity of skin tone.
6. Decreasing the pore size.
7. Rhytids and fine wrinkles reduction.

The identification of the bioactive components of milk from different animal species is an imperative step to decide the domain of its public utility i.e. nutritional, immunological, or medicinal for such cosmeceutical matter. The gross composition of the camel milk is not highly different than the cow milk (Al Haj and Al Kanhal, 2010) and is widely described in Chapter 2 of the present book. The medicinal values of camel milk, widely described in the literature (Kula, 2016; Aref, 2018; Hammam, 2019) are also widely reported in the Chapters 7, 8 and 9 of the present book. But some fine components of the camel milk can also be used in topical formulations which may be tapped as cost effective and affordable cosmeceuticals. The components having potential cosmetic importance are water, proteins (peptides and amino acids), antioxidants (ascorbic acid and retinol), polyunsaturated Fatty Acids (PUFA), Alpha Hydroxy Acids (AHA), Hyaluronic Acid, and micronutrients.

Water

Water keeps the skin hydrated, protects it against the hazardous UV radiations, minimizes and delays the photoaging. Camel milk contains 86-90% of water. Surprisingly, water content of camel milk seems to increase in case of water restriction, overpassing 90% (Yagil & Etzion, 1980a and b). This fact is beneficial both for the dehydrated offspring as well as consumers of camel milk during dry and hot summers. The mechanism behind the rise in water content is linked to the increased ADH levels in dehydrated animal (Kula, 2016; Sisay & Awoke, 2015). Thus, the water availability in camel milk is at its probable maximum for cosmeticals during hot season. However, the effect of dehydration on water content of camel milk was not confirmed by Bekele & Dahlborn (2004) who found non-significant change in water content (87%) after 16 days dehydration and a decrease of milk production by 42%.

Proteins

Camel Milk Protein (CMP), either Camel Casein Protein (CCP) or Camel Whey Protein (CWP), may be fractionalised and hydrolysed into bioactive antioxidant peptides (Ibrahim, Isono & Miyata, 2018). These stimulate collagen production and prevent skin thinning. These peptides, derived from alpha casein, lactophorin and lactoferrin, may be used for treatment of peri-orbital hypermelanosis (POH), perioral rhytids (wrinkles), mottled pigmentation and photo damaged integument.

Amino Acid profiles in casein and whey proteins of camel milk (either essential or non-essential) were described in several publications (Salmen, Abu-Tarboush, Al-Saleh & Metwalli, 2012; Sabahelkheir, Faten & Hassan, 2012) showing that essential (Phe, Lys and His) and non-essential amino acids content was significantly higher in cow milk casein compared to camel casein of different camel breeds. However, there was high variability between camel breed. Moreover, an appropriate balance of branched chain amino acids (leu, ile and val) are present in camel milk casein and whey proteins (Sabahelkheir et al., 2012; Rafiq et al., 2016) (Figure 1). Leucine plays an important role in muscle protein synthesis via reversible phosphorylation. The leucine in camel milk is higher than in cow milk, and the immune protection with camel milk makes it superior (Figure 1).

The higher concentration of branched chain amino acids (BCAAs) in camel milk is useful to combat the catabolic actions and promoting repair of tissue. The amino acids containing sulphur, cysteine and methionine, boost the immune response through intracellular conversion to glutathione which have super-antioxidant property, making it a useful anti-aging compound.

Camel milk proteins in their hydrolysed form, are important components of personal care products. Protein *in totto*, whey proteins and sodium caseinate are used in 'Stay On or Leave On Preparations' of cosmeceutical groups. These formulations require more prolonged contact time for percutaneous absorption as compared to routinely used lotions, ointments, creams or gels. Sodium caseinate is also used in various kinds of sprays for hair, hand, face, neck and body. Hair conditioners and the deodorant sprays do have Sodium caseinate as a base. The hydrolysed formulations of camel milk proteins, rarely,

Figure 1. Branched chain amino acids (BCAA) concentration in human, camel, cow, goat and Sheep milk
From after Sabahelkheir et al. (2012)

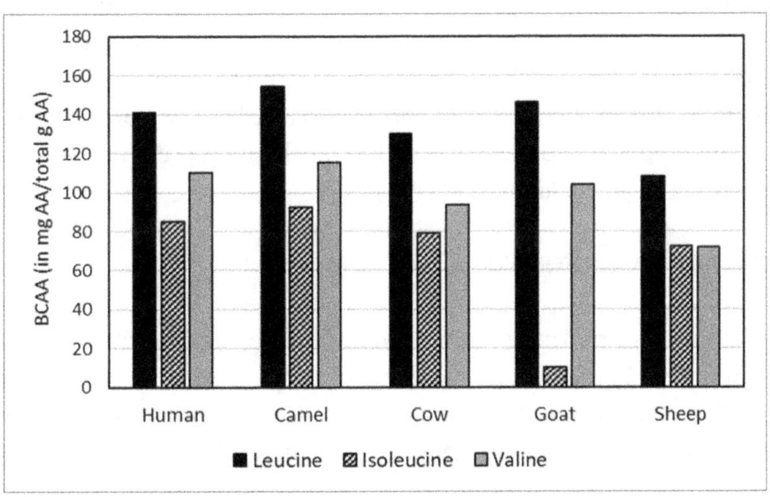

cause irritant contact dermatitis, allergic contact dermatitis or sensitization reactions (Korlepara, Kalla, Manthani & Keerthi,2017). The hypo-allergen properties of camel proteins (notably due to the lack of α-lactoglobulin) enhance the interest of the use of camel milk in cosmeceuticals (Maryniak, Hansen, Ballegaard, Sancho & Bøgh, 2018). This low-allergenicity of camel milk could be linked to the slower hydrolyse of α s-CN than β-CN (El-Agamy, Nawar, Shamsia, Awad & Haenlein, 2009). α-lactalbumin and phosphorus from camel milk are utilized for face and neck cosmeticals because of their low allergenic potency. These products rarely cause any adverse mucosal reactions even if they come in accidental contact with ophthalmic, oral or nasal mucosae.

Antioxidants

There are three types of local antioxidants which may be used on skin to prevent aging (i) the water soluble compounds like Vitamin C, cysteine, methionine, selenium and Glutathione; (ii) the lipid soluble antioxidants like Vitamin A, Vitamin E, carotenoids and Co-enzyme Q10; (iii) components having both water and lipid soluble properties like lipoic acid, polyphenols and flavonoids (Verschoore & Jerajani, 2015) which are in higher concentration in camel milk: 35.45 mg GAE /l of polyphenols compared to 28mg GAE /l only in cow milk, and 29.05mg EQ/l of flavonoids compared to 25.3mg EQ /l in cow milk (Bouhaddaoui et al., 2019).

These antioxidants fight the free radicals which play key role in aging. The cells produce free radicals through mitochondrial energetic catabolism, endogenously. Simultaneously certain exogenous factors like ultraviolet radiations from sunlight, pollution, stress, smoking and alcohol may aggravate the free radical production. Among all these antioxidant components, two of them (vitamins C and A) are widely used in cosmeticals.

Ascorbic Acid (Vitamin C)

Vitamin C is in topical ester form when it is applied or consumed systemically. It is a naturally available antioxidant in camel milk where it is present in high quantity. Indeed, its concentration in camel milk is three to ten times more than in cow milk. (Mal, Suchitra & Sahini, 2007; Haddadin, Gammoh & Robinson, 2008; Konuspayeva, Faye & Loiseau, 2011). It acts through scavenging the free radicals and inhibiting lipid peroxidation, thus protecting the skin from oxidative stress. It also minimizes the erythema induced by ultraviolet radiations. Vitamin C inhibits the production of Reactive Oxygen Species (ROS). Vitamin C also inhibits the induced Minimal Erythematous Dose (MED) of ultraviolet rays, hence preventing or delaying the photoaging (Catini, Savini & Rossi, 2005; Murray, Darr & Reich, 1999). Vitamin C is also being promoted as locally applicable demelanizing and brightening preparation with promising results in melasma and peri-orbital hypermelanosis.

Retinols (Vitamin A) and Carotenoids (Pro-Vitamin A)

Retinols and carotenoids are converted into retinoic acids, retinaldehyde and retinyl esters through metabolic pathways. This class of retinoids bind to specific nuclear receptors of keratinocytes to provide antiaging effects. The efficacy of retinoids can only be appreciated after a lag period of 8-24 weeks (Kligman & Grave, 1986). Retinols also check hyper pigmentation, by increasing the epidermal cell turnover time, thus decreasing the contact time between the melanocytes and keratinocytes. It promotes a decrease in melanosome transfer and a rapid loss of melanin via epidermopoiesis (Ortonne, 2006).

Rhytids (whether fine lines or wrinkles) may be also managed by retinoids, quite efficiently and effectively (Mukherjee et al., 2006; Serri & Lorrizo, 2008; Zussman, Ahdout & Kim, 2010). Retinoids decrease the collagen breakdown by decreasing the MMP enzymes (Matrix Metalloproteinases). On the other hand, collagen synthesis is promoted by glycosaminoglycan (GAG) with the help of retinoids. Here again, the advantage of camel milk retinoids is its availability, as a complete food. Despite of a relative lower concentration than in cow milk (Farah, Rettenmaier & Atkins, 1992), camel milk vitamin A is enough to reach the recommended daily allowance. Hence, camel milk acts as a systemic cosmeceutical. Obviously, the desired amounts of retinols can be extracted for topical preparations. Roughness reduction and smoothening of skin by retinoids is achieved by modulation of gene expressions for differentiation and proliferation. Indeed, retinoids are known to influence cellular processes, such as cellular growth and differentiation, cell surface alterations, and immune modulation. Many of their tissue effects are mediated by their interaction with specific cellular and nucleic acid receptors (Astrom et al., 1991).

Alpha-Tocopherol (Vitamin E)

Vitamin E is a lipid-soluble antioxidant that is present in the skin. A topical application of α-tocopherol exerts photoprotective effects by reducing the number of sunburn cells, reducing ultraviolet B (UVB)-induced damage, and inhibiting photocarcinogenesis (Gensler & Magdaleno, 1991). In humans, tocopherol 5%-8% cream applied to the face improved signs of photoaging and inhibit human macrophage metalloelastase, a member of the matrix metalloproteinase family involved in the degradation of elastin (Chung et al., 2002). The combination of vitamin E and A application can provide superior photoprotection (Boelsma, Hendriks & Roza, 2001). Vitamin E concentration in camel milk is comparable to that of cow milk: 56 vs 60 µg/100ml (Farah, Rettenmaier et Atkins 1992). In their comparative study, (Sboui, Djegham, Belhadj & Khorchani, 2016) found comparable values in camel (27.6 ±2.07) and cow milk (33.5 ±2.17 µg/100ml).

Polyunsaturated Fatty Acids (PUFA)

PUFA are in relative abundance in the camel milk (Konuspayeva, Lemarie, Faye, Loiseau & Montet, 2008). They help in combating the inflammatory cell damage. Omega-3 fatty acids (α-linolenic acid in particular) prevent the photo damage induced aging. As it is not a naturally occurring compound, its ingestion as a component of camel milk may postpone the cutaneous aging process (Pilkington, Watson, Nicolaou & Rhodes, 2011).

Liposomes

The liposomes are closed, spherical lipid bilayer, which forms an internal cavity capable of carrying aqueous solutions. The lipid bilayer is composed of two sheets of tightly arranged phospholipids. In camel milk, liposomes accentuate the rejuvenation of aged skin (Choi, Park, Kim, Lee & Kim, 2013). It acts by collagen and hyaluronan synthase-3 (HAS-3) gene expression. Simultaneously, elastase activity and matrix metalloproteinase (MMP-1) gene expression, implied in psoriasis lesion (Starodubtseva, Sobolev, Soboleva, Nikolaev & Bruskin, 2011) are modulated. It also helps to regenerate the Ultraviolet B damaged fibroblast. These phenomena make it an excellent anti-aging ingredient of camel milk.

Alpha Hydroxy Acid (AHA)

Alpha hydroxy acids are carboxylic acids derived from fruit sugars or milk. The most commonly used hydroxylated acids are glycolic and lactic acid because they have a special ability to penetrate the skin and allow facial rejuvenation by means of peelings. AHA acts through skin exfoliation, making the skin smoother and reducing the dyschromia (Babilas, Knie & Abels, 2012). Ample amounts of AHA in camel milk (Rasheed, 2017) might help to increase the collagen, elastin and glycosaminoglycan synthesis in the dermis; hence, increasing the dermal hydration (Tang & Yang, 2018). The extracted AHA from camel milk, when applied topically, may help to manage acne vulgaris, seborrheic keratosis and photoaging (Khunger & Gupta, 2017). Alpha-hydroxy acids act also through desquamation of Stratum corneum, the outer layer of integument. It works by cleavage of the cell to cell adhesions. Thus, new generation of cells migrate to the skin surface which are relatively more elastic, supple and younger in appearance. Anti-aging action of Alpha-Hydroxy Acid is further propagated by outer layers being thinned and lower dermis getting thickened. Hence, wrinkles, blemishes and dryness of aging skin gets addressed.

Hyaluronic Acid (HA)

Hyaluronic acid (HA), also known as, hyaluronan is the commonest glycosaminoglycan in skin tissue. It has important functions of controlling the hydration and maintaining the extracellular space through binding high amount of water (Laurent & Fraser, 1992). Hyaluronic acid, a big size molecule (2000 KDa) is fragmented into low molecular weight components up to 250-100 KDa. The process of fragmentation increases the penetration of water into the skin (Wegmann, Santonnat & Lersch, 2008). The low molecular weight hyaluronic acid reverses skin atrophy, a frequent and clinically relevant manifestation of aging, through the major cell-surface hyaluronate receptor, CD44 (Kaya et al., 2006). These combined mechanisms reverse the photodamaged aging skin to a great extent. This is further helped by hyaluronic acid's capacity to scavenge the free radicals produced by ultraviolet radiations inducing oxidative stress. Camel milk happens to be a very rich source of natural hyaluronic acid (Mohamed, Schaalan & El-Abhar, 2015). Ethnic population with type IV-VI, of Fitzpatrick's skin phototype classification (people who tends to present post-inflammatory hyperpigmentation, melasma, lentigines and freckles, nevus of Ota, and Hori nevus – Chan, Cohen, Da Cunha, & Maluf, 2018) may seek therapy for water volume repletion in skin. Indeed, those populations usually suffer from aging dependent volume and muscle loss in the photo exposed areas. Hyaluronic acid is one of the new generations of collagen filler by promoting collagen stimulation (Wang et al., 2007). It provides volumetric structural rejuvenation to the injected area. The filler injection may be given by lineal threading method rather than multiple injection technique to minimize the adversity and maximize the HA benefits (Christian, Khunger, Saraf & Clarie, 2015).

Micronutrients

Among the minerals which constitute 0.6 to 1% of camel milk (Al-Awadi & Srikumar, 2001; Konuspayeva, Faye & Loiseau, 2009; Abbas, Itifsa, Alia & Lubna, 2013), micronutrients as Zinc (Zn), Copper (Cu), Manganese (Mn), Iron (Fe), selenium (Se), cobalt (Co) and others are designated as Systemic Nutraceuticals. These elements when they are consumed as components of camel milk help to maintain the cutaneous health and prevent the environmental damage (Yadav, Kumar, Priyadarshini & Singh, 2015). The concentrations of camel milk in trace elements are highly variable, but globally camel milk appears richer in copper, iron and selenium while zinc and manganese are in similar quantity than cow milk (Faye & Bengoumi, 2018).

Most of the micronutrients are linked to specific proteins acting as metalloenzymes. For example, copper is associated to ceruloplasmin (Essamadi, Bengoumi, Tressol, Charcornac & Faye, 1998), zinc to superoxide dismutase (Bengoumi, Essamadi, Chacornac, Tressol, & Faye, 1998a) or selenium to glutathione-peroxidase (Bengoumi, Essamadi, Tressol, Chacornac, & Faye, 1998b). All these proteins act as antioxidant and are potentialized by the micronutrients. Micronutrients are also beneficial for recovering skin lesions after major burns (Berger & Shenkin, 1998). Among trace elements, zinc is particularly involved in skin protection. Topical zinc, in the form of divalent zinc ions, has been reported to provide antioxidant photoprotection for skin. Two antioxidant mechanisms have been proposed: (i) the replacement of redox active molecules by zinc ions at critical sites in cell membranes and proteins; (ii) alternatively, the induction of synthesis of metallothionein, sulfhydryl-rich proteins that protect against free radicals (Rostan, DeBuys, Madey & Pinnell, 2002).

CAMEL MILK CREAM PREPARATION FOR SKIN CARE

The methodology to prepare camel milk cream for skin care implies 3 steps: (i) evaporation and lyophilisation to get concentrate powder milk, (ii) precipitation and filtration, (iii) extraction, heat treatment and centrifugation (Kalejman & Sheva, 2011). Several adjuvants can be added in the final products to potentialize the antioxidant effects (Allemann & Baumann, 2008). The adjuvants could be animal or vegetal origin (Figure 2).

Mehta and Pathak (2012) in their pilot study, conducted at S. P. Medical College, Bikaner, in collaboration with National Research Centre on Camel, Bikaner (India), validated the cosmeceutical value of camel milk cream. It was found to be effective as smoothing, rejuvenating and photoprotective agent in most of the cases. In few cases (about 30%), it even had beneficial effect in combating photo-melanosis. Different formulations were proposed for the market (Figure 3).

Diseases like asteatosis, acne, psoriasis and eczema, may respond well, when camel milk cream is used as an adjuvant therapy (Loden, 2003). The use of such "natural" product is always preferred over artificial ones. Because its low allergenicity, camel milk stands as skin friendly raw material for class of cosmeceuticals whatever the gender, the age, the ethnic groups or socio-economic strata of the users. This is because people have become more concerned about their looks than before (Sadick, 2018).

Figure 2. Adjuvants to camel milk cosmetic cream

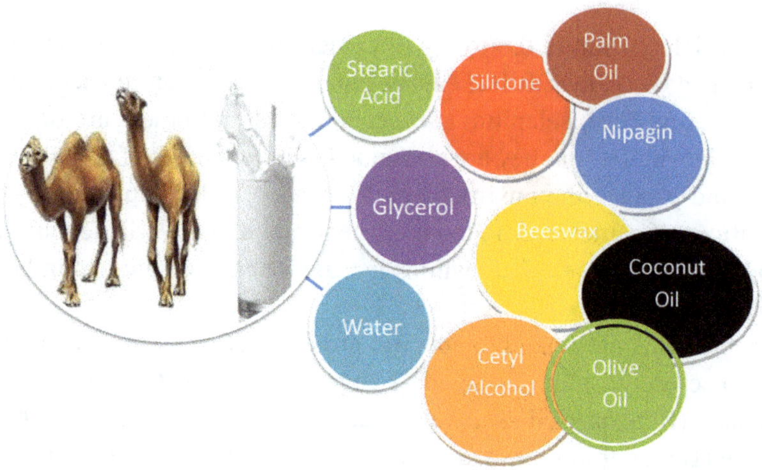

Figure 3. The cosmetic formulations derived from camel milk

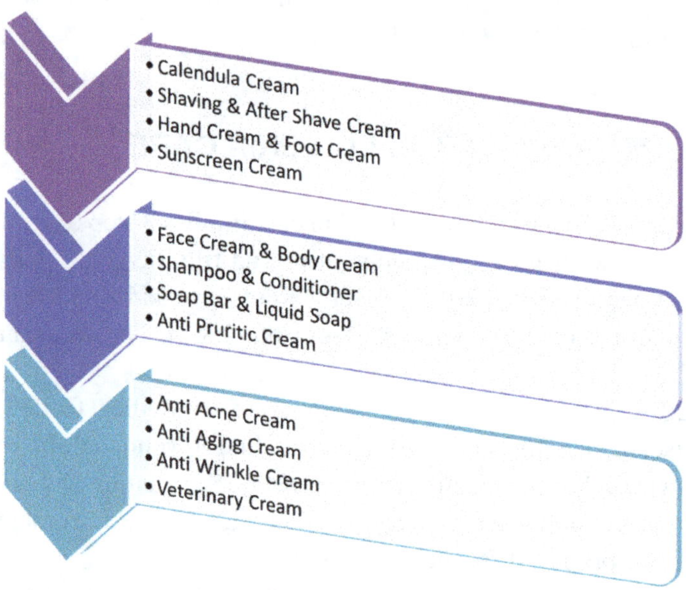

CONCLUSION

Camel milk, with its bioactive ingredients, may help to begin a new era of natural cosmeceutical when consumed orally or applied topically. This untapped resource prompts the researchers to discover a new ray of hope, with its properties of making the human skin, soft, supple, glowing and wrinkle free. Camel milk could be used for its anti-wrinkle, anti-aging, photo-protection, skin softener, anti-acne and moisturizer properties.

REFERENCES

Abbas, S., Ashraf, H., Nazir, A., & Sarfraz, L. (2013). Physio chemical analysis and composition of camel milk. *Intestinal Research*, *2*(2), 85–98.

Abrhaley, A., & Leta, S. (2018). Medicinal value of camel milk and meat. *Journal of Applied Animal Research*, *46*(1), 552–558. doi:10.1080/09712119.2017.1357562

Al-Awadi, F. M., & Srikumar, T. S. (2001). Trace elements and their distribution in protein fraction of camel milk in comparison to other commonly consumed milks. *The Journal of Dairy Research*, *68*(3), 463–469. doi:10.1017/S0022029901005003 PMID:11694048

Al Haj, O., & Al Kanhal, H. A. (2010). Compositional, technological and nutritional aspects of dromedary camel milk. *International Dairy Journal*, *20*(12), 811–821. doi:10.1016/j.idairyj.2010.04.003

Allemann, I. B., & Baumann, L. (2008). Antioxidants Used in Skin Care Formulations Skin. *Therapy Letter*, *13*(7), 5–8. PMID:18839043

Aref, A. R. (2018). Camel milk as complementary and alternative medicine. *International Journal of Scientific Research*, *7*(1), 435–439.

Astrom, A., Tavakkol, A., Pettersson, U., Cromie, M., Elder, J. T., & Voorhees, J. J. (1991). Molecular cloning of two human cellular retinoic acid-binding proteins (CRABP). Retinoic acid-induced expression of CRABP-II but not CRABP-I in adult human skin in vivo and in skin fibroblasts in vitro. *The Journal of Biological Chemistry*, *266*, 17662–17666. PMID:1654334

Babilas, P., Knie, U., & Abels, C. (2012). Cosmetic and dermatologic use of alpha hydroxy acid. *Journal der Deutschen Dermatologischen Gesellschaft*, *10*(7), 488–491. PMID:22916351

Baumann, L. (2003). Cosmeceuticals: Drugs versus cosmetics. In L. Baumann (Ed.), *Cosmetic dermatology principles and practice* (pp. 197–198). New York, NY: Tata Magraw.

Bekele, T., & Dahlborn, K. (2004). The effect of water deprivation on milk production of camels (*Camelus dromedarius*). *Journal of Animal and Feed Sciences*, *13*(Suppl. 1), 459–462. doi:10.22358/jafs/73965/2004

Bengoumi, M., Essamadi, A. K., Chacornac, J. P., Tressol, J. C., & Faye, B. (1998a). Comparative relationship between copper-zinc plasma concentration and superoxide dismutase activity in camels and cow. *Veterinary Research*, *29*, 557–565. PMID:9851012

Bengoumi, M., Essamadi, A. K., Tressol, J. C., Chacornac, J. P., & Faye, B. (1998). Comparative effect of selenium concentration and erythrocyte gluthatione peroxidase activity in cattle and camels. *Animal Science (Penicuik, Scotland)*, *67*, 461–466. doi:10.1017/S1357729800032872

Berger, M. M., & Shenkin, A. (1998). Trace elements in trauma and burns. *Current Opinion in Clinical Nutrition and Metabolic Care*, *1*(6), 513–517. doi:10.1097/00075197-199811000-00006 PMID:10565403

Boelsma, E., Hendriks, H. F., & Roza, L. (2001). Nutritional skin care: Health effects of micronutrients and fatty acids. *The American Journal of Clinical Nutrition*, *73*(5), 853–864. doi:10.1093/ajcn/73.5.853 PMID:11333837

Bouhaddaoui, S., Chabir, R., Errachidi, F., El Ghadraoui, L., El Khalfi, B., Benjelloun, M., & Soukri, A. (2019). Study of the Biochemical Biodiversity of Camel Milk. Hindawi, the Scientific World Journal.

Catini, M. V., Savini, I., Rossi, A., Melino, G., & Avigliano, L. (2005). Biological role of vitamin C in keratinocytes. *Nutrition Reviews*, *63*(3), 81–90. doi:10.1111/j.1753-4887.2005.tb00125.x PMID:15825810

Chakaravarthi, I. S., & Verschoore, M. (Eds.). (n.d.). *Basic sciences for modern cosmetic dermatology*. New Delhi, India: Jaypee Brothers Medical Publishers.

Chan, I. L., Cohen, S., da Cunha, M. G., & Maluf, L. C. (2018). Characteristics and management of Asian skin. *International Journal of Dermatology*, *2018*, 1–13. doi:10.1111/ijd.14153 PMID:30039861

Choi, S. K., Park, K. D., Kim, D. A., Lee, D. W., & Kim, Y. J. (2013). Preparation of camel milk liposome and its anti-aging effects. *Journal of Society of Cosmetic Scientists of Korea*, *40*(2), 155–161. doi:10.15230/SCSK.2014.40.2.155

Christian, O., Khunger, N., Saraf, V., & Clarie, B. (2015). *Peeling and fillers*. Academic Press.

Chung, J. H., Seo, J. Y., Lee, M. K., Eun, H. C., Lee, J. H., Kang, S., ... Voorhees, J. J. (2002). Ultraviolet modulation of human macrophage metalloelastase in human skin in vivo. *The Journal of Investigative Dermatology*, *119*(2), 507–512. doi:10.1046/j.1523-1747.2002.01844.x PMID:12190877

Draelos, Z. D. (1995). Photoaging, sunscreens and cosmeceuticals. In Z. D. Draelos (Ed.), *Cosmetics in dermatology* (pp. 233–244). New York, NY: Churchill Living Stone.

Draelos, Z. D. (2018). Cosmetics and cosmeceuticals. In J. L. Bolognia, J. V. Schaffer, & L. Cerroni (Eds.), *Dermatology* (pp. 2578–2580). New York, NY: Elsevier.

El-Agamy, E. I., Nawar, M., Shamsia, S. M., Awad, S., & Haenlein, G. F. W. (2019). Are camel milk proteins convenient to the nutrition of cow milk allergic children. *Small Ruminant Research*, *82*(1), 1–6. doi:10.1016/j.smallrumres.2008.12.016

Essamadi, K., Bengoumi, M., Tressol, J. C., Chacornac, J. P., & Faye, B. (1998). Comparative relationship of plasma copper concentration and ceruloplasmin activity of camel and cow. *Trends in Comparative Biochemistry & Physiology*, *5*, 211–220.

Farah, Z., Rettenmaier, R., & Atkins, D. (1992). Vitamin Content of Camel Milk. *International Journal for Vitamin and Nutrition Research*, 30–33. PMID:1587705

Faye, B. & Bengoumi, M. (2018). Camel clinical biochemistry and haematology. In *Trace-elements*. Springer Publ.

Galali, Y., & Al-Dmoor, H. M. (2019). Miraculous properties of camel milk and perspective of modern science. *Journal of Family Medicine and Disease Prevention*, *5*(1), 1–7.

Gensler, H. L., & Magdaleno, M. (1991). Topical vitamin E inhibition of immunosuppression and tumorigenesis induced by ultraviolet irradiation. *Nutrition and Cancer*, *15*(2), 97–106. doi:10.1080/01635589109514117 PMID:2038569

Haddadin, M. S. Y., Gammoh, S. I., & Robinson, R. K. (2008). Seasonal variations in the chemical composition of camel milk in Jordan. *The Journal of Dairy Research*, *75*(1), 8–12. doi:10.1017/S0022029907002750 PMID:17971263

Hammam, A. R. (2019). Compositional and therapeutic properties of camel milk: A review. *Emirates Journal of Food and Agriculture*, *31*(3), 148–152. doi:10.9755/ejfa.2019.v31.i3.1919

Ibrahim, H. R., Isono, H., & Miyata, T. (2018). Potential antioxidant bioactive peptides from camel milk protiens. *Animal Nutrition*, *4*(3), 273–280. doi:10.1016/j.aninu.2018.05.004 PMID:30175255

Kalejman, H., & Sheva, B. (2011). *United State Patent*. US Patent No. US7, 883, 691, B2.

Kaya, G., Tran, C., Sorg, O., Hotz, R., Grand, D., Carraux, P., & Saurat, J. H. (2006). Hyaluronate fragments reverse skin atrophy by a CD44- dependent mechanism. *PLoS Medicine*, *3*(12), 493. doi:10.1371/journal.pmed.0030493 PMID:17177600

Khunger, N., & Gupta, J. (2017). Approach to management of aging skin. In M. Venktaram (Ed.), *ACS(I) Textbook of cutaneous & aesthetic surgery* (pp. 711–715). New Delhi, India: Jaypee Brothers Medical Publisher.

Kligman, A. M., & Grave, G. L. (1986). Topical tretinoin for photoaged skin. *Journal of the American Academy of Dermatology*, *15*(4), 836–838. doi:10.1016/S0190-9622(86)70242-9 PMID:3771853

Köhler-Rollefson, I., & Rathore, H. S. (2004). The camel in Rajasthan: Agrobiodiversity under threat. *Annals of Arid Zone*, *43*(3&4), 401–412.

Konuspayeva, G., Faye, B., & Loiseau, G. (2009). The composition of camel milk: A meta-analysis of the literature data. *Journal of Food Composition and Analysis*, *22*(2), 95–101. doi:10.1016/j.jfca.2008.09.008

Konuspayeva, G., Faye, B., & Loiseau, G. (2011). Variability of vitamin C content in camel milk from Kazakhstan. *Journal of Camelid Science*, *4*, 63–69.

Konuspayeva, G., Lemarie, E., Faye, B., Loiseau, G., & Montet, D. (2008). Fatty acid and cholesterol composition of camel's (Camelus bactrianus, Camelus dromedarius and hybrids) milk in Kazakhstan. *Dairy Science & Technology*, *88*(3), 327–340. doi:10.1051/dst:2008005

Korlepara, R. G., Kalla, A. M., Manthani, V., & Keerthi, S. (2017). Camel milk a white gold of desert: A review. *International Archive of Applied Sciences and Technology*, *8*(3), 74–83.

Kula, J. (2016). Camel milk and its therapeutic effects: A review. *Global Veterinaria*, *16*(4), 378–388.

Kula, J., & Tegegne, D. (2016). Chemical composition and medicinal value of camel milk. *International Journal of Research Studies in Bioscience*, *4*(4), 13–25.

Laurent, T. C., & Fraser, J. R. (1992). Hyaluronan. *The FASEB Journal*, *6*(7), 2397–2404. doi:10.1096/fasebj.6.7.1563592 PMID:1563592

Loden, M. (2003). Role of topical emollients and moisturizers in the treatment of dry skin barrier disorders. *American Journal of Clinical Dermatology*, *4*, 771–788. doi:10.2165/00128071-200304110-00005 PMID:14572299

Mal, G., Suchitra, D. S., & Sahani, M. S. (2007). Changes in chemical and macro-minerals content of dromedary milk during lactation. *Journal of Camel Practice and Research*, *14*(2), 195–197.

Maryniak, N., Hansen, E., Ballegaard, A.S., Sancho, A., & Bøgh, K. (2018). Comparison of the Allergenicity and Immunogenicity of Camel and Cow's Milk—A Study in Brown Norway Rats. *Nutrients*, *10*(12), 1-18.

Mason, J. (2012). Vitamins, trace minerals and other micronutrients. In L. Goldman & A. I. Schafer (Eds.), *Cecil textbook of medicine* (pp. 1–10). Philadelphia: Saunders.

Mehta, R. D., & Pathak, K. M. L. (2012). *Camel milk cream: The candidate cosmeceutical* (A Pilot Study, Unpublished).

Mills, O. H., Berger, R. S., & Baker, M. D. (1993). A controlled comparison of skin cleansers in photoaged skin. *Journal of Geriatric Dermatology*, *1*, 173–179.

Mohamed, W. A., Schaalan, M. F., & El-Abhar, H. S. (2015). Camel Milk: Potential Utility as an Adjunctive Therapy to Peg-IFN/RBV in HCV-4 Infected Patients in Egypt. *Nutrition and Cancer*, *67*(8), 1307–1315. doi:10.1080/01635581.2015.1087041 PMID:26492130

Mukherjee, S., Date, A., Patarvale, V., Korting, H. C., Roeder, A., & Weindl, G. (2006). Retinoids in the treatment of skin aging: An overview of clinical efficacy & clinical interventions in aging. *Clinical Interventions in Aging*, *1*, 327–348. doi:10.2147/ciia.2006.1.4.327 PMID:18046911

Murray, J., Darr, D., & Reich, J. (1991). Topical vitamin C treatment reduces UV radiation-induced erythema in human skin. *The Journal of Investigative Dermatology*, *96*, 587.

Ortonne, J. P. (2006). Retinoid therapy for pigmentary disorders. *Dermatologic Therapy*, *19*(5), 280–288. doi:10.1111/j.1529-8019.2006.00085.x PMID:17014483

Pilkington, S. M., Watson, R. E., Nicolaou, A., & Rhodes, L. E. (2011). Omega-3 polyunsaturated fatty acids: Photoprotective macronutrients. *Experimental Dermatology*, *20*(7), 537–543. doi:10.1111/j.1600-0625.2011.01294.x PMID:21569104

Rafiq, S., Huma, N., Pasha, I., Sameen, A., Mukhtar, O., & Khan, M. I. (2016). Chemical composition; nitrogen fraction and amino acid profile of milk from different animal species. *Asian-Australasian Journal of Animal Sciences*, *29*(7), 1022–1028. doi:10.5713/ajas.15.0452 PMID:26954163

Rasheed, Z. (2017). Medicinal values of bioactive constituents of camel milk: A concise report. *International Journal of Health Sciences*, *11*(5), 1–2. PMID:29114185

Rostan, E. F., DeBuys, H. V., Madey, D. L., & Pinnell, S. R. (2002). Evidence supporting zinc as an important antioxidant for skin. *International Journal of Dermatology*, *41*(9), 606–611. doi:10.1046/j.1365-4362.2002.01567.x PMID:12358835

Sabahelkheir, M. K., Faten, M. M., & Hassan, A. A. (2012). Amino acid composition of human and animal's milk (camel, cow, sheep and goat). *Journal of Science and Technology*, *2*(2), 32–34.

Sachdeva, M. (2010). Cosmeceuticals. In N. Khunger & M. Sachdeva (Eds.), *Practical manual of cosmetic dermatology and surgery* (pp. 213–223). New Delhi, India: Mehta Publishers.

Sachdeva, M., & Khunger, N. (2010). Principles of normal skin care. In N. Khunger & M. Sachdeva (Eds.), *Practical manual of cosmetic dermatology and surgery* (pp. 1–15). New Delhi, India: Mehta Publishers.

Sadick, N. S. (2018). The pathophysiology of the male aging face and body. In N. S. Sadick & B. H. Thiers (Eds.), *Dermatologic clinics cosmetic dermatology for men* (pp. 1–4). New York, NY: Elsevier. doi:10.1016/j.det.2017.08.002

Salmen, S. H., Abu-Tarboush, H. M., Al-Saleh, A. A., & Metwalli, A. A. (2012). Amino acids content and electrophoretic profile of camel milk casein from different camel breeds in Saudi Arabia. *Saudi Journal of Biological Sciences*, *19*(2), 177–183. doi:10.1016/j.sjbs.2011.12.002 PMID:23961177

Sboui, A., Djegham, M., Belhadj, O. & Khorchani, T. (2016). Le lait de chamelle: qualités nutritives et effet sur les variations de la glycémie. *Options Méditerranéennes*, *A*, 487-492.

Serri, R., & Lorrizo, M. (2008). Cosmeceuticals: Focus on topical in photoaging. *Clinics in Dermatology*, *26*(6), 633–638. doi:10.1016/j.clindermatol.2007.09.016 PMID:18940544

Shah, R. A. (2005). Cosmeceuticals. In S. Savant, D. Gore, R. A. Shah, & K. Sarangi (Eds.), *Textbook of dermato-surgery & cosmetology* (pp. 519–524). Mumbai, India: ASCAD.

Sisay, F., & Awoke, K. (2015). Review on production quality and use of camel milk in Ethiopia. *Journal of Fisheries & Livestock Production*, *3*(3), 155–162.

Spencer, T. S. (1988). Dry skin and skin moisturizers. *Clinics in Dermatology*, *6*(3), 24–28. doi:10.1016/0738-081X(88)90028-4 PMID:3071400

Starodubtseva, N. L., Sobolev, V. V., Soboleva, A. G., Nikolaev, A. A., & Bruskin, S. A. (2011). Genes expression of metalloproteinases (MMP-1, MMP-2, MMP-9, and MMP-12) associated with psoriasis. *Russian Journal of Genetics*, *47*(9), 1117–1123. doi:10.1134/S102279541109016X PMID:22117411

Tang, S. C., & Yang, J. H. (2018). Dual effects of alpha hydroxy acids on the skin. Molecules, 23(4), 863. doi:10.3390/molecules23040863

Verschoore, M., & Jerajani, H. (2015). Skin aging and antiaging cosmetics. In S. Chakaravarthi & M. Verschoore (Eds.), Basic sciences for modern cosmetic dermatology (pp. 148-161). New Delhi, India: Jaypee Brothers Medical Publishers.

Wang, F., Garza, L. A., Kang, S., Varani, J., Orringer, J. S., Fisher, G. J., & Voorhees, J. J. (2007). In Vivo Stimulation of De Novo Collagen Production Caused by Cross-linked Hyaluronic Acid Dermal Filler Injections in Photodamaged Human Skin. *Archives of Dermatology*, *143*(2), 155–163. doi:10.1001/archderm.143.2.155 PMID:17309996

Wegmann, M., Santonnat, B., & Lersch, P. (2008). Low molecular weight hyaluronic acid: Its effect on epidermal gene expression and skin aging. *SOFW-Journal*, *134*, 17–22.

Wilhelm, K. P., Cua, A. B., & Maibach, H. I. (1991). Skin aging: Effect on trans-epidermal water loss, stratum corneum hydration, skin surface pH, and casual sebum content. *Archives of Dermatology*, *127*(12), 1806–1809. doi:10.1001/archderm.1991.04520010052006 PMID:1845280

Yadav, A. K., Kumar, R., Priyadarshini, L., & Singh, J. (2015). Composition and medicinal properties of camel milk: A Review. *Asian Journal of Dairy and Food Research*, *34*(2), 83–91. doi:10.5958/0976-0563.2015.00018.4

Yagil, R., & Etzion, Z. (1980). Effect of drought condition on the quality of camel milk. *The Journal of Dairy Research*, *47*(02), 159–166. doi:10.1017/S0022029900021026

Yagil, R., & Etzion, Z. (1980a). Milk yield of camels (Camelus dromedarius) in drought areas. *Comparative Biochemistry and Physiology. Part A, Physiology*, *67*(1), 207–209. doi:10.1016/0300-9629(80)90433-8

Zussman, J., Ahdout, J., & Kim, J. (2010). Vitamin and photoaging: Do scientific data support their use. *Journal of the American Academy of Dermatology*, *63*(3), 507–525. doi:10.1016/j.jaad.2009.07.037 PMID:20189681

Chapter 17
Interaction Between Camel Farming and Environment

Bernard Faye
https://orcid.org/0000-0002-5762-5453
Independent Researcher, France

ABSTRACT

The close adaptation of camel to its desert environment could explain its weak expansion out of the arid lands of the world. This adaptation can contribute to the desertification combat, attesting to its small ecological footprint with traditional extensive farming. The camel population in the world, despite its active growth, remains marginal, and its contribution to the greenhouse gas emission is negligible. However, the current trends to the intensification of camel productions could change the impact of the species on the environment and on animal metabolism. The necessity to expect a better productivity face to the growing demand could lead to a "specialization" of the camel farms and a specific selection of the camel. Such trends require care with a possible erosion of the camel biodiversity and the consequences on the interactions between the emerging camel production system and the environment.

INTRODUCTION

According to FAO report published in 2006 (FAO, 2006), livestock was regarded as the cause of many environmental problems and responsible of some emblematic "hots-spots" in the planet, notably global climate warming, land degradation, pollution of the atmosphere and water, and loss of biodiversity. Nevertheless, the same report showed that 80 percent of the livestock sector growth is the result of industrial systems, the part of extensive livestock farming (which is still the case of camel farming) in these environmental impacts remains relatively low. However, data on camel species are lacking to accurately assess the specific effects of its farming. Among different interactions between livestock and environment (overgrazing, deforestation, gaseous emissions of livestock, animal waste management, domestic animal diversity), the camel, animal particularly adapted to desert ecosystem (Wilson, 1989) is mainly confronted to the desertification process (Faye, 2011). Obviously, its world distribution is closely linked to the arid zones of the old world (map 1). Face to the "hot-spot" of the desertification

DOI: 10.4018/978-1-7998-1604-1.ch017

Figure 1. World distribution of the dromedary (λ) and Bactrian (+) camel population (left map) and of the arid lands (right map) where rainfall is less than 250 mm/year

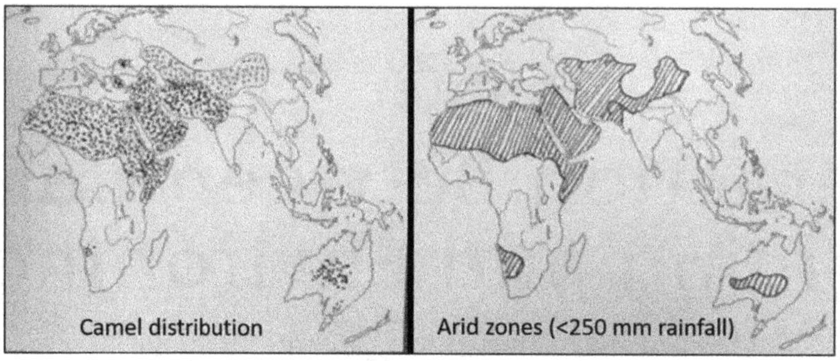

in arid lands (Steinfeld, De Haan & Blackburn, 2003), the camel farming systems can be regarded as a problem, but also as a solution. Indeed, the interaction between livestock and environment is complex and cannot be limited to negative externalities. Because its well-known adaptation to desert environment, the camel farming, especially camel pastoralism can contribute also to the desertification combat. However, in the same time, camel farming is under the influence of new trends including intensification and "peri-urbanization" process (Faye, 2016 and 2018). Such evolutions could greatly contribute to alter the interactions between camel breeding and the environment.

These different topics are discussed in the present chapter. It will be addressed successively (I) the adaptive peculiarities of the camel in arid contexts, (ii) its contribution to desertification combat, (iii) its contribution to greenhouse gas emissions, (iv) the consequences of the intensification on camel production systems and (v) the challenges of camel biodiversity.

THE CAMEL: AN ANIMAL ADAPTED TO ARID LANDS

It is amazing to observe that most of the scientific papers regarding camel, whatever the topic, start by a phrase such as "the camel is well adapted to harsh conditions" or "camel is the ship of desert". Obviously, large camelids are inextricably linked to the desert ecosystems. The description regarding anatomical and physiological mechanisms of adaptation of camels to the arid conditions was largely achieved for long time in scientific literature (Gauthier-Pilters, 1961). The desert being characterized by high nictemeral variation of the ambient temperature, permanent drought, rarity of water resources, and poor nutritive values of pastoral resources. The camel has developed along its evolution, a large capacity to resist to such conditions (Gebreyohanes & Assen, 2017). Among them, we could cite:

- **The resistance to the thirst** through two main mechanisms (i) decrease of the water loss by decreasing urine excretion, stopping sweating, slowing down basal metabolism, varying body temperature in relation to external temperature, and (ii) maintenance of the homeostasis by limiting variation of the vital blood parameters and by excreting efficiently the metabolic wastes (Bengoumi & Faye, 2002; Faye & Bengoumi, 2018);

- **The resistance to the heat stress** possible thanks to different (i) anatomical characteristics as concentration of fat storage in the hump facilitating the cutaneous dissipation of the body heat, long legs in standing animal and sternal pad in sitting animal allowing air circulation around the body, coat with thick fleece in winter becoming thin in summer, (ii) physiological mechanisms as thick skin with sweat glands activated when the external temperature is above 42°C, variability of internal temperature between 34 to 42°C according to ambient temperature, maintenance of blood fluidity in case of dehydration for maintaining the heat transfer from the periphery to the hearth (Yagil, 1985), general decreasing of the metabolism by hypothyroidism (Etzion, Alfassi, Lavi & Yagil, 1987), and (iii) specific behavior as sitting face to sun to decrease the surface of skin exposed to the sun, grazing trees at the hottest time of the day (Faye & Tisserand, 1989).
- **The adaptation to low-nutritive feeding** as a consequence of a remarkable digestive physiology including for example (i) the tolerance to salt allowing the use of halophytes often unpalatable for other herbivores (Yagil, 1985), (ii) the better cellulolytic activity of ruminal flora and longer retention times of solid particles in the forestomach leading to a better digestion of organic matter and of the cellulosic fractions of the diet (Al-Jassim & Hogan, 2012), (iii) the more efficient nitrogen recycling compared to other ruminants allowing to maintain a minimal production of microbial proteins when dietary nitrogen is insufficient (Mousa, Ali & Hume, 1983), and finally (iii) a higher digestibility of low-nutritive forages by 4-5% than in other ruminants receiving the same diet (Jouany, 2000).
- **The adaptation to widespread resources** thanks to the feeding behavior of the camel notably (i) grazing of a wide variety of plants at different levels of the pasture, from grasses to trees up to 3.5 m height thanks to its long neck leading to a lower pressure on the floristic biodiversity in desert (Rutagwenda, Lechner-Doll, Schwartz, Schultka & Von Engelhardt, 1990), (ii) convenient management of the anatomical parts of the desert plants thanks to its very flexible tongue (Tayeb, 1950), able to reach leaves without damaging the branches, (iii) presence of a corneal mucous membrane inside the cheeks allowing to graze all sorts of very spinous plants, and overall (iv) the practice of "ambulatory grazing" characterized by a continuous moving during feeding time even in case of abundant biomass after rain, contributing to an evenly distribution of the carrying capacity of the camel herd in grazing area especially since the lack of gregarious instinct of the camel herd (Richard, 1985).

All these characteristics are proper to large camelids and are the marks of their adaptation to the environmental and climatic conditions of the desert areas, but the adaptability is also a matter of the camel farming, and a consequence of the camel management by the humans in such hostile environment. Indeed, the cameleers used camels for surviving in low-productive milieu and can produce zootechnical values, notably through milk, meat, wool and power production (Faye, 2016). In present book, camel based products are discussed in details in Chapter 5, 12, 14, 15, and 16. The most important aspect of the adaptation of camel farming to desert environment is obviously the mobility. This mobility can be random (solely linked to the water and pasture availability) or pendular (between two home territories) leading to nomad or transhumant system respectively. By the mobility, the cameleers rely on the camel behavior (ambulatory pasture, selection of a high variety of plants) as mentioned above. Traditionally, the camel farming systems based on the mobility of the herd allow a simple categorization into nomad or transhumant system in opposition to sedentary systems mainly linked to oasis implementation (Faye, Senoussi & Jaouad, 2017). However, such classification appears no longer convenient to cover the current changes in camel farming systems (Faye, 2018), the mobility can be transient, based on commercial opportunity, linked to climatic crisis (drought) or other events (political insecurity), can include all the family or a part only (Azoulay, Ancey, Dormoy, Crenn, Mangu & Thomashausen, 2014). These changes lead to a high complexity of the camel farming systems confronted to different evolutions including various degree of intensification of the productions, permanent or transient "peri-urbanization" of the camel herd, tendency to multi-activity of the camel owner, complex interactions between peri-urban and pastoral areas and various levels of market integration. Such changes make obsolete the classic typology in nomadic, transhumant and sedentary system (Faye, 2018). Overall, those trends change also the interactions between camel farming and environment.

THE ADDED-VALUE OF CAMEL FARMING IN DESERTIFICATION COMBAT

Nowadays, especially in relation to the international concern on desertification process, desert is regarded as a complex ecosystem and is the object of a scientific discipline named "eremology" (Monod, 1992). In this ecosystem, the camel by its adaptative peculiarities listed above and the cameleers, thanks to the proper management of their production system, can contribute significantly to combat desertification (Stiles, 1988) or to the sustainable development of the arid lands (Faye, Chaibou & Vias, 2012).

Thus, the ability of camel to manage long intervals between watering allows the camel herds using rangelands far away from the water points, and thus decrease the pressure around them, while cattle and small ruminants, unable to stay more than 2 days without drinking water, provoke often an overgrazing around the water points. Such concentrations of cattle herds around wells can lead to mineral imbalance in animals, provoking osteophagy and diseases like botulism, described as "disease of drilling" (Brown, 2006).

The browser behavior of camels is valorizing the floristic biodiversity in a large area. Consuming approximately 2-3 kg of fresh forage per hour in favorable season, and 1-1.5 kg in dry season by moving 1-2 km/h, they will consume finally few grasses in one place, contributing to a more rational use of pastoral areas by limiting local overgrazing. Furthermore, thanks to the slower transit of nutrients in the digestive tract of camel, the seeds rejected in the feces have higher germinability than with other herbivores reared in arid areas. Such peculiarity can promote the spread and regeneration of the desert plants (Trabelsi, Chehma, Senoussi & Faye, 2012). Moreover, contrary to cattle, small ruminants and equines, the camel has soft feet without hoof. So, walking camel herd is less aggressive for the soil.

However, the added value of camel farming in not limited to the consequences of the adaptative peculiarities of the animals. It includes also the ability to contribute to the desert productivity despite the low level of its resources (Chaibou, 2005). Indeed, camel farming can provide livelihood in desert ecosystem (Faye, 2011) contributing not only to the "desertification" combat, but also to the "desertion" combat by maintaining rural economic activity in remote areas of the earth. Typically, multi-purpose animal (Ornas & Hussein, 1993), the camel is not limited to packing or riding use, but also reared for its zootechnical productions (milk, meat, wool). In addition, the diversification of camel activities as auxiliary of agricultural activities in crop-livestock systems is increasing, not only in countries where such use is common as in south Asia (Rathore, 1986), but also in Africa for different practices as ploughing, harrowing or seeding (Vias, Ibrahim, Vall & Faye, 2004). Such agricultural activities are linked to the geographical expansion of camel rearing in relationships to the recurrent drought affecting notably Sahelian countries

(Faye et al., 2012), and illustrates the camel's ability to maintain rural activities in poor ecosystems and to contribute to the growth of agricultural productivity not only in the desert margins but more and more in sub-humid areas in Africa (Mankor & Koussou, 2015) as well as in Asia (Wilson, 2019).

According to the recent FAO data (FAOstat, 2019), camels provide, in 2017, 2.85 million tons of milk and 312,000 tons of meat, i.e. 0.36% of the total milk and 0.62% of the total red meat produced in the world. However, such proportion is increasing regularly (it has doubled for the last 50 years) for both milk and meat (Faye & Bonnet, 2012) and the part of camel production could represent more than 10% of the total livestock production in some countries like those of the Horn of Africa. For the last 50 years, the annual growth of camel milk and meat production was 6.3 and 5.3% respectively, i.e. in higher proportion than for other dairy species (except buffalo) or meat species (except goat). Moreover, those products are included nowadays in regional or even international market, contributing significantly to the incomes of the camel stakeholders and integrating the desert zones in national economies. Finally, the role of camel in desert is not limited to their primary production. Combating desertification doesn't regard only the ability of desert to deal with "zootechnical productivity" (Chaibou & Faye, 2005), but also with the ability of camel producers to market their products. However, the integration to market as well as the increase of the camel population (see Chapter 1) in the world in higher proportion than for other domestic animals (Faye & Bonnet, 2012) raise the problem of the potential negative impact of the camel stock on the environment. Indeed, even if the camel population (35 million heads in 2017 according to FAOstat, 2019) is marginal compared to other domestic animals, this population was multiplied by 2.7 since 1961 *vs* 1.6 for cattle, 1.2 for sheep, 2.3 for Buffalo, 1.0 for horse, and 1.7 for lama. Only goat population has a higher growth (x3 since 1961, date of the first word wide statistics). So, the question of impact on the greenhouse gas production must be emphasized.

THE IMPACT OF CAMEL FARMING ON THE GREENHOUSE GAS EMISSION

The Australian government proposed some years ago "to kill the Australian feral camels for saving the planet" by contributing therefore to the decrease of methane emission. Indeed, based on the extrapolation of data collected on cattle, the estimation of the contribution of camel to this emission is far from negligible especially as the feral camel population was estimated to be more than one million heads (Metcalfe & Bui, 2016). However, living in low-density areas and representing less than 3.5% of the Domestic Herbivorous Biomass (BHD) in the country, the contribution of camel to methane emission appears marginal. Moreover, a recent publication confirmed that the dromedary camel, Bactrian camel, and small camelids (lama and vicuna) emit less methane than the other ruminants. The camels produce 0.32l/kg LW/day methane vs 0.58l/kg on average for cattle and sheep (Dittman, Runge, Lang, Moser, Galeffi, Kreuzer, & Clauss, 2014). So, in Australia, the contribution of the camels to the methane emission by livestock is less than 2%. At the world level, the contribution of camelids (small and large) in the emission of methane is approximately 1% vs 72% for cattle (Faye, 2012). The camelids (large and small) represent only 2% of world BHD while cattle account for 65%. Moreover, considering that the whole livestock is responsible for 37% of the anthropic emission of methane (Steinfeld et al., 2003), the contribution of all camelids is representing less than 0.5% of the total emission.

In the same way, even if its contribution to the climatic warming is less important, the emission of ammonia in a stable of adult camels is estimated at 5-6 kg of ammonia/head/year, corresponding to about 50% of what makes a dairy cow. Moreover, if manure management is included in the calculation ammonia emissions are not more than 1.5-2.0 kg/animal/year i.e., 10 to 20% only of what produces a cow (Smits & Montety, 2009).

More widely, the impact of camel on environment can be estimated by its "ecological footprint", including not only the greenhouse gas emission but also its environmental carrying capacity i.e. the ratio between the whole population and the available resources (water, feeding, land) for maintaining the livestock production (Alemayehu, Amede, Böhme & Peters, 2012). With an estimated population in 2017 (FAO, 2019) of 35 million (camel) and 9 million heads (small camelids), the camelids represent approximately 1% of the total herbivorous population in the world. Even considering the relative importance of the camel population growth for the last 50 years, the pressure of this population on the environment appears marginal. Moreover, the camel density is low. The highest densities observed in the Horn of Africa and the United Arab Emirates are around 2 camels/km^2 and in Sahelian countries they don't overpass 1 camel/km^2. However, the ecological footprint of the camelid stock could appear more acute in certain regions of the world. For example, the weak management of feral camels in Australia leads to regard them as a pest (Dennis, Russell & Edwards, 2010). Obviously, it is the balance between the growth in camelid population and the ability to maintain a sustainable use of the resources that must be reached. For example, compared to intensive dairy system, camel Bedouin system will expense less water for producing on liter of milk in a proportion of 1:9 (Faye, 2016).

The "traditional life" in the desert is regarded as a "harmonious, symbiotic relationship with the environment" (Breulmann et al., 2007), the pastoralists managing their fragile rangelands without over-exploiting them (Olsvig-Whittaker, Frankenberg, Perevolotsky & Ungar, 2006). However, does such proximity to the nature including the emotional links with the camels be maintained despite the changes in the farming systems to intensification?

THE INTERACTIONS BETWEEN CAMEL INTENSIFICATION AND ENVIRONMENT

As mentioned above, the camel farming is traditionally associated to extensive mode in remote areas of the desert thanks to the adaptative capacities of the animal. However, a clear trend to intensification process is occurring in almost all camel countries face to the increasing demand for camel products as it is underlined above. The intensification in livestock is a process aiming to increase the productivity of the animal and/or of the farm by optimizing the production factors (land, labor, management). The consequences for camel farming are usually the stopping of the mobility, a rational feeding system based on the use of high nutritive value forage and concentrates, the improvement of the numerical productivity by the use of biotechnology (assisted reproduction, veterinary control), of the zootechnical productivity (milk production, growth), and the increase of labor productivity (use of fence to avoid guarding, milking machine, rational feed distribution). The consequences of intensification process of camel farm management and overall on the camel physiology, metabolism and health are obviously a big matter of issue, however insufficiently investigated by camel scientists. From a multipurpose animal, the camel is submitted to a specialization of its production: for example, camel dairy farms for milk production, feed-lots for meat production, racing stables. But except for race, the animals were rarely selected for such limited purpose.

Some effects of intensive management in camel farming are discussed below. Those effects involve either the animal itself (its metabolism, its health, its physiology) or the environment of the farm. Regarding the feeding for example, in pastoral ranges, the camel grazes a wide variety of plants, including halophytes plants, grasses, bushes and trees, and spend more than 8 hours/day grazing to satisfy its needs. At reverse, in intensive farm, camel becomes settled and is fed with monotonous diet (for example alfalfa hay with barley or commercial concentrates) distributed twice a day. Consequently, camel spends few times for eating and increases its feed intake, from approximately 1.8-2.2 kg DM/100 kg LW up to 2.5-3.0 kg/DM/100 kg LW (Faye, 2016). The effects on its digestive physiology (nitrogen recycling, intestinal transit, rumen flora) could be important but the consequences of a more limited feeding variability and more spaced meals on the rumen flora, on the feeding conversion, on the fattening, or on metabolic disorders are not sufficiently assessed by camel sciences. The distribution of a high proteo-energetic diet to camel, generally accustomed to valorizing poor nutritive grasses, could lead to an excess of fat storage remarkable by a body condition score reaching the maximum (BCS n°5= obesity) with higher risk of emergence of metabolic diseases and infertility (Benaissa, Faye & Kaidi, 2015).

Another aspect could regard the impact of such impoverished diet (in terms of floristic diversity) on the true or supposed medicinal virtues of the camel milk (Konuspayeva, Loiseau & Faye, 2004; Kaskous, 2015). Indeed, the nomads attribute those health effect to the milk composition linked to the desert plants (see Chapter 7, 8 and 9). All studies show that the type of farming (traditional or intensive) and the nature of feeding could have significant effect on composition of camel milk (see Chapter 2), notably on vitamin C and fatty acids composition (Benmohamed, Siboukeur & Edoub, 2018). Similar observations could be done for camel meat functional properties (see Chapter 13), the feeding management having effect on fine composition of the meat (Kadim, 2013).

The impact on water management must be taken also into account. Indeed, the use of irrigated forages to feed camel in in-door system for example, at the place of desert plant in out-door system has considerable consequence on the water expense. In a study achieved in Saudi Arabia comparing Bedouin (camel mobility, low inputs, pastoral feeding) to intensive farming system (irrigated feedstuffs, settlement, high market integration), it was reported that the water consumption increased from 3000 to 35,000 m^3/ha with a biomass productivity passing from 5 to 18 tons/ha (Faye, 2013). Over 50 years, the water consumption increased by 55% in Bedouin system while it was multiplied by 122 in intensive systems (Faye, 2013). Thus, the intensification process in camel sector has a strong effect on water demand which could be an important constraint for sustainable development. To limit the water expense in intensive systems, some alternatives were suggested by using agro-food by-products as the introduction of olive cake (Faye, Konuspayeva, Narmuratova, Serikbaeva, Musaad & Mehri, 2013) or date blocks (Faye, Konuspayeva, Almasaud, Alafaliq & Ben Abdallah, 2018) widely available in arid agriculture industry. Alternative ingredients for feeding high-yield camel like fodder produced under salty water irrigation was also proposed for contributing to a better balance between natural resources and camel production (Abu-Alrub, Marcum, Kabir, Aran & Al Hammadi, 2018).

The intensification is linked to the increase of metabolic diseases as said above but could explain also the onset of emerging diseases like MERS-coronavirus or prion disease with a risk of transboundary contamination through the regional market of live camel export (Younan, Bornstein & Gluecks, 2016), especially well-developed between the Horn of Africa and the Arabian Peninsula (Alary & Faye, 2016). Thus, camel is suspected to be involved in the transmission of MERS-Cov to human (Gossner et al., 2015), and the virus would have mutated due to changes in camel management (Hemida et al., 2015). According to a large panel of experts, the changes in camel husbandry in Arabian Peninsula where regular new coming camels from Africa occur, could be a potential risk factor for the camel-human transmission of the virus (Funk et al., 2016). Recently, a prion-disease was detected in camel from Algeria (Babelhadj et al., 2018). Despite the lack of intensification in camel husbandry in this environment, the significant change occurring in the camel "feeding" due to the rarefaction of the pastoral resources could be a hypothesis for prion disease emergence. Indeed, in this country the disease was detected in the region of Ouargla, close to oil basin of Hassi-Messaoud where the camels spend longer time in garbage dumps close to oil extractive areas.

Other emerging outbreaks provoking over-mortalities were described, especially in the Horn of Africa, but without clear relationships with a change in camel husbandry (Khalafalla et al., 2010; Roger et al., 2000) although the important movements linked to live camels' export could play a role. In Saudi Arabia, again, the origin of Rift Valley Fever outbreak occurring in the years 2000 and killing several hundred people was attributed to the importation of live animals (small ruminants and camels) from the Horn of Africa (Balkhy & Memish, 2003).

THE PRESERVATION OF CAMEL BIODIVERSITY

Face to the current changes in camel environment, the question of the genetic adaptation of this animal to such new conditions is raised. Indeed, up to recently, the selection pressure by human on the camel was less important than for other ruminants, except maybe, as mentioned above, for the racing camels in the Emirates by the wide use of embryo-transfer techniques (Anouassi & Tibary, 2013). The multipurpose functions of the camel have limited the selection pressure to obtain a "specialized" animal. At most, along the domestication process, the cameleers have "selected" a few types of animals for riding, packing or milking (most of the time regarded as a by-product). Thus, Blanc & Ennesser (1989) have differentiated eight types of camel based on their size (high, medium and short), their global conformation (longilineal or brevilineal) and their environment (flat or mountainous areas, sandy or rocky desert, etc). However, in the same publication, 52 "breeds" were defined although a huge confusion appears in the denomination, rather based on tribe belonging or on the coat color than on correct phenotype description (Legesse et al., 2018). Attempts of clarification to determine camel phenotypes were recently achieved in Saudi Arabia (Abdallah & Faye, 2012), Sudan (Ishag, Eisa & Ahmed, 2011), Tunisia (Chniter, Hammadi, Khorchani, Krit, Benwahada & Hamoud, 2013), Algeria (Oulad Belkhir, Chehma & Faye, 2013), India (Makhdoomi, Gazi, Nabi & Ahmed, 2013) or Pakistan (Shah, Qureshi & Reissmann, 2014), but there were no international rules regarding convenient body measurements. Coat color which is used often to distinguish camel names doesn't appear a discriminant trait for describing breeds. And despite the proposal for a linear scoring of udder morphology in relationships with milk yield potential, there is no application at any local or national level (Ayadi, Aljumaah, Samara, Faye & Caja, 2015).

Recent advances in camel genomics (Almathen et al., 2011; Fitak, Mohandesan, Corander & Burger, 2016; Ramadan & Inoue-Murayama, 2017) let expect possible genetic improvement of the species if relationships between production traits and performances could be assessed through performances control at a large scale. Unfortunately, only limited number of studies have addressed camel production performances according to genetic traits. In fact, most of the available literature has mainly focused on non-genetic (Al-Mutairi, Boujenane, Musaad & Awad-Acharari, 2010a) rather than on genetic factors of variability (breed effect) except few references for example regarding dairy performances (Gaili, Al-Eknah & Sadek, 2000), milk composition (Aljumaah, Almutairi, Ismail, Alshaikh, Sami & Ayadi, 2012), meat performances and composition (Al-Atiyat et al., 2016) or reproductive performances (Deen, 2013). Moreover, no study has investigated relations between camel breed and disease resistance/resilience, or environmental adaptation. Only few observations on the difference in trypanosomosis prevalence between camels types was published (El-Wathig, Faye, Thevenon, Ravel & Bossard, 2016).

Yet, the studies performed in camel underlined the relatively high variability of the performances. For example, regarding dairy performances, three main groups were identified (Alhadrami & Faye, 2016): the high-producing dairy camels with an annual milk production of more than 3000 liters; the medium with production between 1500 liters and 3000 liters and the poor producers with less than 1500 liters per year. Usually the high producing camels (for example Marecha breed in Pakistan, Al-Majaheem in Saudi Arabia, Sirtawi in Libya, Arvana in Turkmenistan) are characterized by large body size (up to 2.40 m at withers height), prominent mammary vein and well-developed udder. The medium-producing dairy camel are usually dual-purpose animals (milk and meat or packing/riding) as for example Hoor in Somalia, Al-Homor in Saudi Arabia, Anafi in Sudan, Dankali in Ethiopia), but also in Sahelian countries (for example Azbin in Niger or Birabish, in Mauritania). The milk production improvement is less sensitive to feeding supplementation, the animals having the tendency to accumulate fat in their hump rather to produce more milk. The low-producing camels are used for other purposes than milk. A part of this variability can be attributed to genetic as attested by the heritability of some traits like growth rate (Al-Sobayil, Khalil, Al-Jobeile, Mohamed & Salal, 2006) or milk yield (Al-Mutairi Boujenane, Musaad & Awad-Acharari, 2010b). These heritabilities show that the respective traits can be improved through specific selection (Al-Abri & Faye, 2019). Nevertheless, the low anthropic pressure on camel selection along the domestication process has led to avoid the invasion of one high-performance breed: there is no "camel-Holstein" or "camel-Angus" and a certain camel biodiversity is, for the moment, maintained. To preserve this biodiversity, genetic characterization is essential, notably for protecting some ecotypes having low herd size or living in specific environment like the wild Bactrian camel (Silbermayr et al., 2010), Adhana camel breed in Saudi Arabia limited to mountains area (Faye, Abdallah, Almathen, Harzallah & Al-Mutairi, 2011; Abdallah & Faye, 2012) or Raigi camel breed in Pakistan (Raziq, Tareen & de Verdier, 2011). Some breeds could have specific physiological peculiarities interesting to be investigated for a better understanding of adaptation process as for example the comparison of Manga and Azarghaf camel breed in Niger which are characterized by two different reproduction cycles probably due to different ovarian activities (Vias et al., 2006).

The preservation of camel biodiversity includes also the protection of wild Bactrian camel and the management of hybridization between dromedary and Bactrian camel. Wild Bactrian camel (*Camelus bactrianus ferus*), a species listed as Critically Endangered by IUCN, is recognized as a separate species after several investigations of its genome (Jirimutu et al., 2012; Mohandesan et al., 2017). The hybridization between dromedary (one-humped) and Bactrian (double-humped) is a common practice in Central Asia, formerly to get robust animals for commercial caravan, and nowadays, to improve the milk production by heterosis effect (Faye & Konuspayeva, 2012). However, the crossbreeding between two F1 giving one animal difficult to manage, the hybrid F1 cannot be fixed and requires the maintenance of pure Bactrians and dromedaries herd.

CONCLUSION

The interactions of the camel with its environment is something complex as for other animal species domesticated by human. We can summarize these interactions at three main levels. First, by the proper characteristics of the camel who have an anatomy, physiology and metabolism entirely turned to its surviving in the harsh conditions of the desert. By these dispositions evoked in the present chapter, the camel has finally a low ecological footprint, especially because its demography is quite less important than for other domestic ruminants. Second, the camel can valorize the remote areas of the world thanks to its production and its services to human. The arid lands occupy more than 35% of terrestrial surface, and in such areas, camel farming is an opportunity to maintain rural activities, the other speculations as agriculture being more difficult or having a deleterious effect on the environment, especially on water resources as shown by the development of irrigated cereals in Saudi Arabia for example. Third, by its progressive integration to regional or international market, those camel productions could contribute to the world economy and support the participation of the stakeholders living in desert or desert margins. However, the current changes in camel farming, limiting the traditional mobility of the herds, and more and more oriented to a certain intensification of the production system could modify this fragile balance between the meagre resources of the desert and the pressure of camel rearing. Camel scientists and developers must take in account this new equation in the development plan of the camel farming.

REFERENCES

Abdallah, H. R., & Faye, B. (2012). Phenotypic classification of Saudi Arabian camel (*Camelus dromedarius*) by their body measurements. *Emirates Journal of Food and Agriculture*, *24*(3), 272–280.

Abu-Alrub, I., Marcum, K. B., Kabir, N., Aran, A., & Al Hammadi, M. (2018). Productivity and nutritional value of four forage grass cultivars compared to Rhodes grass irrigated with saline water. *Australian Journal of Crop Science*, *12*(02), 203–209. doi:10.21475/ajcs.18.12.02.pne571

Al-Abri, M. A., & Faye, B. (2019). Genetic improvement in dromedary camels: challenges and opportunities. Frontiers in Genetic, 10.

Al-Atiyat, R. M., Suliman, G., AlSuhaibani, E., El-Waziry, A., Al-Owaimer, A., & Basmaeil, S. (2016). The differentiation of camel breeds based on meat measurements using discriminant analysis. *Tropical Animal Health and Production*, *48*(5), 871–878. doi:10.100711250-015-0990-5 PMID:26922738

Al-Hadrami, G., & Faye, B. (2016). Animal that produced dairy food: camel. In Reference Module in Food Science (2nd ed.; pp. 1-12). Elsevier.

Al Jassim, R., & Hogan, J. (2012). The digestive system of the camel, its anatomical, histological and functional characteristics: A comparative approach. In *Proceedings of 3rd ISOCARD Conference* (pp. 75-86). Muscat, Oman: Sultan Qaboos University.

Al-Mutairi, S. E., Boujenane, I., Musaad, A., & Awad-Acharari, F. (2010a). Non-genetic factors influencing reproductive traits and calving weight in Saudi camels. *Tropical Animal Health and Production*, *42*(6), 1087–1092. doi:10.100711250-010-9529-y PMID:20195755

Al-Mutairi, S. E., Boujenane, I., Musaad, A., & Awad-Acharari, F. (2010b). Genetic and nongenetic effects for milk yield and growth traits in Saudi camels. *Tropical Animal Health and Production*, *42*(8), 1845–1853. doi:10.100711250-010-9647-6 PMID:20617460

Al-Sobayil, K. A., Khalil, M. H., Al-Jobeile, H. S., Mohamed, K. M., & Salal, S. A. (2006). Quantitative genetic analysis and evaluation for early growth performance in Saudi camels. In *Proceedings of the International Scientific Conference on Camels* (pp. 201). Qassim, Saudi Arabia: Academic Press.

Alary, V., & Faye, B. (2016). The camel chains in East Africa- Importance of gaps between the data and the apparent reality. *Journal of Camelid Science*, *9*, 1–22.

Alemayehu, M., Amede, T., Böhme, M., & Peters, K. J. (2012). Increasing livestock water productivity under rain fed mixed crop/livestock farming scenarios of sub-Saharan Africa: A review. *Journal of Sustainable Development*, *5*(7), 1–10. doi:10.5539/jsd.v5n7p1

Aljumaah, R. S., Almutairi, F. F., Ismail, E., Alshaikh, M. A., Sami, A., & Ayadi, M. (2012). Effects of production system, breed, parity and stage of lactation on milk composition of dromedary camels in Saudi Arabia. *Journal of Animal and Veterinary Advances*, *11*, 141–147. doi:10.3923/javaa.2012.141.147

Almathen, F., Charruau, P., Mohandesan, E., Mwaharo, J. M., Orozco-Terwengel, P., Pitt, D., ... Burger, P. (2016). Ancient and modern DNA reveal dynamics of domestication and cross-continental dispersal of the dromedary. *Proceedings of the National Academy of Sciences of the United States of America*, *113*(24), 6707–6712. doi:10.1073/pnas.1519508113 PMID:27162355

Anouassi, A., & Tibary, A. (2013). Development of a large commercial camel embryo transfer program: 20 years of scientific research. *Animal Reproduction Science*, *136*(3), 211–221. doi:10.1016/j.anireprosci.2012.10.012 PMID:23153626

Ayadi, M., Aljumaah, R., Samara, S., Faye, B., & Caja, G. (2015). Udder typology of Arabian dairy camels and proposal of a linear scoring system for assessing their udder traits for machine milking. *Scientific and Practical Journal Veterinariya, 2*(42).

Azoulay, G., Ancey, V., Dormoy, D., Crenn, C., Mangu, A., & Thomashausen, A. (2014). *Mobilités et migrations: figures et enjeux contemporains: Pluralité des regards et des disciplines*. Paris, France: L'Harmattan.

Babelhadj, B., Di Bari, M. A., Pirisinu, L., Chiappini, B., Gaouar, S., Riccardi, G., ... Vaccari, G. (2018). Prion Disease in Dromedary Camels, Algeria. *Emerging Infectious Diseases*, *24*(6), 1029–1036. doi:10.3201/eid2406.172007 PMID:29652245

Balkhy, H. H., & Memish, Z. A. (2003). Rift Valley fever: An uninvited zoonosis in the Arabian Peninsula. *International Journal of Antimicrobial Agents*, *21*(2), 153–157. doi:10.1016/S0924-8579(02)00295-9 PMID:12615379

Benaissa, M. H., Faye, B., & Kaidi, R. (2015). Reproductive abnormalities in female camel (Camelus dromedarius) in Algeria: Relationship with age, season, breed and body condition score. *Journal of Camel Practice and Research*, *22*(1), 67–73. doi:10.5958/2277-8934.2015.00010.7

Bengoumi, M., & Faye, B. (2002). Adaptation du dromadaire à la déshydratation. *Sécheresse*, *13*, 121–129.

Benmohamed, C., Siboukeur, O., & Edoud, A. (2018). Influence of feeding on some physicochemical and biochemical characteristics of camel milk (*Camelus dromadarius*). *Emirates Journal of Food and Agriculture*, *30*(4), 251–255. doi:10.9755/ejfa.2018.v30.i4.1658

Blanc, C. P., & Hennesser, Y. (1989). Approche zoogéographique de la différenciation infraspécifique chez le dromadaire Camelus dromedarius Linné, 1766 (Mammalia: Camelidae). *Revue d'Élevage et de Médecine Vétérinaire des Pays Tropicaux*, *42*, 573–587.

Breulmann, M., Boer, B., Wernery, U., Wernery, R., El-Shaer, H., Alhadrami, G., ... Norton, J. (2007). *The camel, from tradition to modern times*. Doha, Qatar: UNESCO Doha Publ.

Brown, K. (2006). Tropical medicine and animal diseases: Onderstepoort and the development of veterinary science in South Africa 1908-1950. *South African Studies*, *31*(3), 513–529. doi:10.1080/03057070500202139 PMID:16628249

Chaibou, M. (2005). *Productivité zootechnique du désert: le cas du bassin laitier d'Agadez au Niger* (PhD thesis). Université de Montpellier.

Chaibou, M., & Faye, B. (2005). Fonctionnement des élevages camelins de la zone périurbaine d'Agadez au Niger: Enquête typologique. *Revue d'Élevage et de Médecine Vétérinaire des Pays Tropicaux*, *58*(4), 273–283. doi:10.19182/remvt.9922

Chniter, M., Hammadi, M., Khorchani, T., Krit, R., Benwahada, A., & Hamoud, M. B. (2013). Classification of Maghrebi camels (Camelus dromedarius) according to their tribal affiliation and body traits in southern Tunisia. *Emirates Journal of Food and Agriculture*, *25*(8), 625–634. doi:10.9755/ejfa.v25i8.16096

Deen, A. (2013). Reproductive performance in camel (*Camelus dromedarius*). *Camel: An International Journal of Veterinary Sciences*, *1*, 13–27.

Dennis, E., Russell, L., & Edwards, G. (2010). Feral camels in the Australian rangelands (2010). In *Proceedings of the 16th Biennial Conference of the Australian Rangeland Society*. Australian Rangeland Society.

Dittmann, M.T., Runge, U., Lang, R.A., Moser, D., Galeffi, C., Kreuzer, M., & Clauss, M. (2014). Methane emission by camelids. *Plos One*, *9*(4).

El Wathig, M., Faye, B., Thevenon, S., Ravel, S., & Bossard, G. (2016). Epidemiological surveys of camel trypanosomosis in Al-jouf, Saudi Arabia based on PCR and ELISA. *Emirates Journal of Food and Agriculture*, *28*(3), 212–216. doi:10.9755/ejfa.2015-09-759

Etzion, Z., Alfassi, Z., Lavi, N., & Yagil, R. (1987). Halide concentration in camel plasma in various state of dehydration. *Biological Trace Element Research*, *12*(1), 411–418. doi:10.1007/BF02796697 PMID:24254620

FAO. (2006). *Livestock's long shadow. Environmental issues and options*. FAO publ.

Faye, B. (2011). Combating desertification: The added value of the camel farming. *Annals of Arid Zone*, *50*(3&4), 1–11.

Faye, B. (2013). Camel Farming Sustainability: The Challenges of the Camel Farming System in the XXIth Century. *Journal of Sustainable Development*, *6*(12), 74–82. doi:10.5539/jsd.v6n12p74

Faye, B. (2016). The camel, new challenges for a sustainable development. *Tropical Animal Health and Production*, *48*(4), 689–692. doi:10.100711250-016-0995-8 PMID:26922737

Faye, B. (2018). What future for camel pastoralism in the world? In *Proceedings of the 5th Conference ISOCARD "Recent advances in camelids biology, health and Production"* (pp. 32-38). Laâyoune, Morocco: IAV Hassan II.

Faye, B., Abdallah, H., Almathen, F., Harzallah, B., & Al-Mutairi, S. (2011). Camel biodiversity. Camel phenotypes in the Kingdom of Saudi Arabia. In Camel Breeding, Protection and Improvement Center. project UTF/SAU/021/SAU. FAO publ.

Faye, B., & Bengoumi, M. (2018). *Camel clinical biochemistry and hematology*. New York: Springer. doi:10.1007/978-3-319-95562-9

Faye, B., & Bonnet, P. (2012). Camel sciences and economy in the world: Current situation and perspectives. In *Proceedings of the 3rd ISOCARD Conference. Keynote presentations* (pp. 2-15). Muscat, Oman: Sultan Qaboos University.

Faye, B., Chaibou, M., & Vias, G. (2012). Integrated impact of climate change and socioeconomic development on the evolution of camel farming systems. *British Journal of Environment and Climatic Change*, *2*(3), 227–244. doi:10.9734/BJECC/2012/1548

Faye, B., & Konuspayeva, G. (2012). The Encounter between Bactrian and Dromedary Camels in Central Asia. In E.-M. Knoll & P. A. Burger (Eds.), *Camels in Asia and North-Africa- Interdisciplinary perspectives on their past and present significance* (pp. 27–33). Wien: Austrian Academy of Sciences Press.

Faye, B., Konuspayeva, G., Narmuratova, M., Serikbaeva, A., Musaad, A. M., & Mehri, H. (2013). Effect of crude olive cake supplementation on camel milk production and fatty acid composition. *Dairy Science & Technology*, *93*(3), 225–239. doi:10.100713594-013-0117-6

Faye, B., Konuspayeva, G. S., Almasaud, A., Alafaliq, A., & Ben Abdallah, A. (2018). The effect of date-urea blocks as supplementary feeding on growth of young camels. *Emirates Journal of Food and Agriculture*, *30*(4), 320–325. doi:10.9755/ejfa.2018.v30.i4.1668

Faye, B., Senoussi, H., & Jaouad, M. (2017). Le dromadaire et l'oasis: Du caravansérail à l'élevage périurbain. *Cahiers Agricultures*, *26*(1), 14001. doi:10.1051/cagri/2017005

Faye, B., & Tisserand, J. L. (1989). Problèmes de la détermination de la valeur alimentaire des fourrages prélevés par le dromadaire. In Séminaire sur la nutrition et l'alimentation du dromadaire. Ouargla, Algérie: Options Méditerranéennes.

Fitak, R. R., Mohandesan, E., Corander, J., & Burger, P. A. (2016). The de novo genome assembly and annotation of a female domestic dromedary of north african origin. *Molecular Ecology Resources*, *16*(1), 314–324. doi:10.1111/1755-0998.12443 PMID:26178449

Funk, A., Goutard, F., Miguel, E., Bourgarel, M., Chevalier, V., Faye, B., ... Roger, F. (2016). Mers-coV at the animal–human interface: Inputs on exposure Pathways from an expert-Opinion elicitation. *Frontiers in Veterinary Science*, *3*, 88. doi:10.3389/fvets.2016.00088 PMID:27761437

Gaili, E. S. E., Al-Eknah, M. M., & Sadek, M. H. (2000). Comparative milking performance of three types of Saudi camels (Camelus dromedarius). *Journal of Camel Practice and Research*, *7*, 73–76.

Gauthier-Pilters, H. (1961). Observations sur l'écologie du dromadaire dans le Sahara nord-occidental. *Mammalia*, *25*(2), 195–280. doi:10.1515/mamm.1961.25.2.195

Gebreyohanes, M. G., & Assen, A. M. (2017). Adaptation mechanisms of camels (Camelus dromedarius) for desert environment: a review. Journal of Veterinary Science & Technology, 8(6).

Gossner, C., Danielson, N., Gervelmeyer, A., Berthe, F., Faye, B., Kaasik-Aaslav, K., ... Coulombier, D. (2015). Human–Dromedary Camel Interactions and the Risk of Acquiring Zoonotic Middle East Respiratory Syndrome Coronavirus Infection. *Zoonoses and Public Health*, *12171*. doi:10.1111/zph PMID:25545147

Hemida, M. G., Elmoslemany, A., Al-Hizab, F., Alnaeem, A., Almathen, F., Faye, B., ... Peiris, M. (2015). Dromedary Camels and the Transmission of Middle East Respiratory Syndrome Coronavirus (MERS-CoV). *Transboundary and Emerging Diseases*, 1–10. PMID:26256102

Hjört af Ornäs, A., & Ali Hussein, M. (1993). Camel herd dynamics in southern Somalia: Long term development and milk production implications. In A. Hjort af Ornäs (Ed.), The Multi-Purpose Camel: Interdisciplinary Studies on Pastoral Production in Somalia (pp. 31-42). Uppsala University.

Ishag, I. A., Eisa, M. O., & Ahmed, M.-K. A. (2011). Phenotypic characteristics of Sudanese camels (*Camelus dromedarius). Livestock Research for Rural Development*. Retrieved from http://www.lrrd.org/lrrd23/4/isha23099.htm

Jirimutu, W. Z. (2012). Genome sequences of wild and domestic Bactrian camels. *Nature Communications*, *3*(1), 1202. doi:10.1038/ncomms2192 PMID:23149746

Jouany, J. P. (2000). La digestion chez les camélidés; comparaison avec les ruminants. *Productions Animales*, *13*(3), 165–176.

Kadim, I. (2013). A Review of the Nutritive Value and Meat Quality Characteristics of the Dromedary (*Camelus dromedaries*) Camel Meats. *CAMEL: International Journal of Veterinary Science*, *1*(2), 129–156.

Kaskous, S. (2015). Importance of camel milk for human health. *Emirates Journal of Food and Agriculture*, *28*(3), 158–163. doi:10.9755/ejfa.2015-05-296

Khalafalla, A. I., Saeed, I. K., Ali, Y. H., Abdurrahman, M. B., Kwiatek, O., Libeau, G., ... Abbas, Z. (2010). An outbreak of peste des petits ruminants (PPR) in camels in the Sudan. *Acta Tropica*, *116*(2), 161–165. doi:10.1016/j.actatropica.2010.08.002 PMID:20707980

Konuspayeva, G., Loiseau, G., & Faye, B. (2004). La plus-value « santé » du lait de chamelle cru et fermenté: L'expérience du Kazakhstan. *Rencontre Recherches Ruminants*, *11*, 47–50.

Legesse, Y. W., Dunn, C. D., Mauldin, M. R., Ordonez-Garza, N., Rowden, G. R., Gebre, Y. M., ... Bradley, R. D. (2018). Morphometric and genetic variation in 8 breeds of Ethiopian camels (*Camelus dromedarius*). *Journal of Animal Science*, *96*(12), 4925–4934. PMID:30189034

Makhdoomi, D. M., Gazi, M. A., Nabi, S., & Ahmed, S. (2013). Morphometric studies on adult double humped camel of Ladakh, India. *Emirates Journal of Food and Agriculture*, *25*(7), 544–548. doi:10.9755/ejfa.v25i7.15999

Mankor, A., & Koussou, M. O. (2015). *Etude du sous-secteur camelin du Tchad*. N'Djamena, Chad: Rapport FAO.

Metcalfe, D., & Bui, E. (2016). Land: Resources and capacity for management. In *Australia state of the environment*. Canberra: Australian Government Department of the Environment and Energy. Retrieved from https://soe.environment.gov.au/theme/land/topic/2016/resources-and-capacity-management

Mohandesan, E., Fitak, R. R., Corander, J., Yadamsuren, A., Chuluunbat, B., Abdelhadi, O., ... Burger, P. A. (2017). Mitogenome sequencing in the genus Camelus reveals evidence for purifying selection and long term divergence between wild and domestic Bactrian camels. *Scientific Reports*, *7*(1), 9970. doi:10.103841598-017-08995-8 PMID:28855525

Monod, T. (1992). Du désert. *Sécheresse*, *1*(3), 7–24.

Mousa, H. M., Ali, K. E., & Hume, I. D. (1983). Effects of water deprivation on urea metabolism in camels, desert sheep and desert goats fed dry desert grass. *Comparative Biochemistry and Physiology*, *74A*(3), 715–720. doi:10.1016/0300-9629(83)90574-1 PMID:6132716

Olsvig-Whittaker, I., Frankenberg, E., Perevolotsky, A., & Ungar, E. D. (2006). Grazing, overgrazing and conservation. Changing concepts and practices in the Negev rangelands. *Sécheresse*, *17*, 195–199.

Oulad Belkhir, A., Chehma, A., & Faye, B. (2013). Phenotypic variability of two principal Algerian camel's populations (Targui and Sahraoui). *Emirates Journal of Food and Agriculture*, *25*(3), 231–237. doi:10.9755/ejfa.v25i3.15457

Ramadan, S., & Inoue-Murayama, M. (2017). Advances in camel genomics and their applications: A review. *The Journal of Animal Genetics*, *45*(2), 49–58. doi:10.5924/abgri.45.49

Rathore, G. S. (1986). *Camels and their Management. ICAR publ.*

Raziq, A., Tareen, A. M., & de Verdier, K. (2011). Characterization and significance of Raigi camel, a livestock breed of the Pashtoon pastoral people in Afghanistan and Pakistan. *Journal of Livestock Science*, *2*, 11–19.

Richard, D. (1985). *Le dromadaire et son élevage. In IEMVT, Coll. « études et synthèses*. Montpellier, France: CIRAD.

Roger, F., Diallo, A., Yigezu, L. M., Hurard, C., Libeau, G., Mebratu, G. Y., & Faye, B. (2000). Investigations of a new pathological condition of camels in Ethiopia. *Journal of Camel Practice and Research*, *7*(2), 163–166.

Rutagwenda, T., Lechner-Doll, M., Schwartz, H. J., Schultka, W., & Von Engelhardt, W. (1990). Dietary preference and degrability of forage on a semi-arid thornbush savannah indigenous ruminants, camels and donkeys. *Animal Feed Science and Technology*, *35*(3-4), 179–192. doi:10.1016/0377-8401(90)90123-P

Shah, M. G., Qureshi, A. S., & Reissmann, M. (2014). *Phenotypic and genetic differentiation of Pakistani camel breeds*. Lambert Academic Publishing.

Silbermayr, K., Orozco-terWengel, P., Charruau, P., Enkhbileg, D., Walzer, C., Vogl, C., ... Burger, P. A. (2010). High mitochondrial differentiation levels between wild and domestic Bactrian camels: A basis for rapid detection of maternal hybridization. *Animal Genetics*, *41*(3), 315–318. doi:10.1111/j.1365-2052.2009.01993.x PMID:19968638

Smits, M. G., & Montety, G. J. (2009). Ammonia emission from camel dairy in the Netherlands. *Journal of Camel Practice and Research*, *16*(2), 139–142.

Steinfeld, H., De Haan, C., & Blackburn, H. (2003). Livestock - Environment Interactions: issues and options. FAO publ.

Stiles, N. (1988). Le dromadaire contre l'avancée du désert. *La Recherche*, *201*, 948–952.

Tayeb, M. A. F. (1950). La cavité buccale du chameau. *Revue d'Élevage et de Médecine Vétérinaire des Pays Tropicaux*, *4*(3), 157–160. doi:10.19182/remvt.6884

Trabelsi, H., Chehma, A., Senoussi, A., & Faye, B. (2012). The Contribution of the dromedary in the spontaneous plant seeds transfer in the northern Algerian Sahara. *Journal of Life Science*, *6*(3), 300–303.

Vias, G., Faye, B., Kane, Y., Diarra, A., Laouali, G., & Daouda, H. (2006). Performances de reproduction de la femelle dromadaire (*Camelus dromedarius*) dans la zone pastorale de Zinder (Niger). *Revue Africaine de Santé et Productions Animales*, *4*, 111–116.

Vias, G., Ibrahim, Y., Vall, E., & Faye, B. (2004). La traction caméline, un apport important dans l'évolution des pratiques de traction animale au Niger. *Revue d'Élevage et de Médecine Vétérinaire des Pays Tropicaux*, *57*(3-4), 177–179. doi:10.19182/remvt.9888

Wilson, R. T. (1989). *Ecophysiology of the Camelidae and desert ruminants*. Berlin, Germany: Springer-Verlag. doi:10.1007/978-3-642-74483-9

Wilson, R. T. (2019). The one-humped camel in Bangladesh. *Journal of Camel Practice and Research*, *26*(1), 11–13. doi:10.5958/2277-8934.2019.00002.X

Yagil, R. (1985). *The desert camel: comparative physiological adaptation. In Comparative animal nutrition*. Basel, Germany: Karger.

Younan, M., Bornstein, S., & Gluecks, I. V. (2016). MERS and the dromedary camel trade between Africa and the Middle East. *Tropical Animal Health and Production*, *48*(6), 1277–1282. doi:10.100711250-016-1089-3 PMID:27324244

Compilation of References

Aadvik. (2019). *Welcome to Aadvik foods*. Retrieved in 22nd May, 2019 from https://www.indiamart.com/aadvikfoodsproducts/

Abbas, M., & Mahasneh, A. (2014). Isolation of Lactobacillus strains with probiotic potential from camel's milk. *African Journal of Microbiological Research*, *8*(15), 1645–1655. doi:10.5897/AJMR2013.6598

Abbas, S., Ashraf, H., Nazir, A., & Sarfraz, L. (2013). Physico-chemical analysis and composition of camel Milk. *Intestinal Research*, *2*, 85–98.

Abbas, S., Ashraf, H., Nazir, A., & Sarfraz, L. (2013). Physio chemical analysis and composition of camel milk. *Intestinal Research*, *2*(2), 85–98.

Abd El-Fattah, A. M., Ragab Abd Rabo, F. H., El-Dieb, S. M., & El-Kashef, H. A. S. (2014). Preservation methods of buffalo and bovine colostrum as a source of bioactive components. *International Dairy Journal*, *39*(1), 24–27. doi:10.1016/j.idairyj.2014.04.008

Abd El-Salam, M. H., & El-Shibiny, S. (2011). A comprehensive review on the composition and properties of buffalo milk. *Dairy Science & Technology*, *91*(6), 663–699. doi:10.100713594-011-0029-2

Abd El-Salam, M. H., & El-Shibiny, S. (2013). Bioactive Peptides of Buffalo, Camel, Goat, Sheep, Mare, and Yak Milks and Milk Products. *Food Reviews International*, *29*(1), 1–23. doi:10.1080/87559129.2012.692137

Abd El-Salam, M. H., & El-Shibiny, S. (2017). Preparation, properties, and uses of enzymatic milk protein hydrolysates. *Critical Reviews in Food Science and Nutrition*, *57*(6), 1119–1132. doi:10.1080/10408398.2014.899200 PMID:25880259

Abdalla, E. B., Ashmawya, A. E. A., Salama, O. A. E., Farouk, M. H., Khalila, F. A., Seioudy, A. E., & Caja, G. (2016). Effect of milking interval on milk partitioning between udder compartments, milk yield and milk composition in Maghrebi camels. *Small Ruminant Research*, *136*, 214–220. doi:10.1016/j.smallrumres.2016.02.001

Abdallah, H. R., & Faye, B. (2012). Phenotypic classification of Saudi Arabian camel (Camelus dromedarius) by their body measurements. *Emirates Journal of Food and Agriculture*, *24*(3), 272–280.

AbdAlmageed, E. (2005). *Properties of milk powder made from the milk of cow, goat and camel* (Unpublished MSc. thesis). Umdurman Islamic University, Sudan.

Abdel Galil, M. (2016). The unique medicinal properties of camel products: A review of the scientific evidence. *Journal of Taibah University Medical Sciences*, *11*(2), 98–103. doi:10.1016/j.jtumed.2015.12.007

Abdelgadir, W., Ahmed, T., & Dirar, H. (1998). The traditional fermented milk products of the Sudan. *International Journal of Food Microbiology*, *44*(1-2), 1–13. doi:10.1016/S0168-1605(98)00090-7 PMID:9849779

Abdelgadir, W., Nielsen, D. S., Hamad, S., & Jakobsen, M. (2008). A traditional Sudanese fermented camel's milk product, Gariss, as a habitat of Streptococcus infantarius subsp. Infantarius. *International Journal of Food Microbiology*, *127*(3), 215–219. doi:10.1016/j.ijfoodmicro.2008.07.008

Abdelhadi, O. M. A., Babiker, S. A., Bauchart, D., Listrat, A., Re'mond, D., Hocquette, J. F., & Faye, B. (2017). Effect of gender on quality and nutritive value of dromedary camel (*Camelus dromedarius*) longissimus lumborum muscle. *Journal of the Saudi Society of Agricultural Sciences*, *16*(3), 242–249. doi:10.1016/j.jssas.2015.08.003

Abdel-Rahman, I. (2007). *Biochemical changes in camel milk fermented by bacterial starter cultures* (Unpublished doctoral dissertation). University of Khartoum, Sudan.

Abdullah Amqizal, H. I., Al-Kahtani, H. A., Ismail, E. A., Hayat, K., & Jaswir, I. (2017). Identification and verification of porcine DNA in commercial gelatin and gelatin containing processed foods. *Food Control*, *78*, 297–303. doi:10.1016/j.foodcont.2017.02.024

Abdulrahman, A. O., Ismael, M. A., Al-Hosaini, K., Rame, C., Al-Senaidy, A. M., Dupont, J., & Ayoub, M. A. (2016). Differential effects of camel milk on insulin receptor signalling – towards understanding the insulin-like properties of camel milk. *Frontiers in Endocrinology*, *7*, 4. doi:10.3389/fendo.2016.00004

Abeiderrahmane, N. (1997). Camel milk and modern industry. *Journal of Camel Practice and Research*, *4*(2), 223–228.

Abera, T., Legesse, Y., Mummed, B., & Urga, B. (2016). Bacteriological quality of raw camel milk along the market value chain in Fafen zone, Ethiopian Somali regional state. *BMC Research Notes*, *9*(1), 285–285. doi:10.118613104-016-2088-1

Abirached, C., Medrano, C., Araujo, A., Moyna, P., Añón, M., & Panizzolo, L. (2012). Comparison of interfacial and foaming properties of soy and whey protein isolates. *Journal of Food Science and Engineering*, *2*, 376–381.

Abouheif, M., Basmaeil, S., & Bakkar, M. (1990). A standard method for jointing camel carcasses with reference to the effect of slaughter age on carcass characteristics in najdi camels. I1. Variation in lean growth and distribution. *Asian-Australasian Journal of Animal Sciences*, *3*(2), 97–102. doi:10.5713/ajas.1990.97

Abouheil, M., Basmaeil, S., & Bakkar, M. (1991). A standard method for jointing camel carcasses with reference to the effect of slaughter age on carcass characteristics in najdi camels. 3. partition and distribution of carcass fat. *Animal Science (Penicuik, Scotland)*, *4*(3), 219–225.

Abrahamson, D. R. (1986). Recent studies on the structure and pathology of basement membranes. *The Journal of Pathology*, *149*(4), 257–278. doi:10.1002/path.1711490402 PMID:2944999

Abrhaley, A., & Leta, S. (2018). Medicinal value of camel milk and meat. *Journal of Applied Animal Research*, *46*(72), 552–558. doi:10.1080/09712119.2017.1357562

Åbrink, M., Larsson, E., Gobl, A., & Hellman, L. (2000). Expression of lactoferrin in the kidney: Implications for innate immunity and iron metabolism. *Kidney International*, *57*(5), 2004–2010. doi:10.1046/j.1523-1755.2000.00050.x PMID:10792619

Abu Lehia, I., & Abu Tarboush, H. (1995). Milk fat products and ice cream. Academic Press.

Abu-Alrub, I., Marcum, K. B., Kabir, N., Aran, A., & Al Hammadi, M. (2018). Productivity and nutritional value of four forage grass cultivars compared to Rhodes grass irrigated with saline water. *Australian Journal of Crop Science*, *12*(02), 203–209. doi:10.21475/ajcs.18.12.02.pne571

Abuelgasim, K. A., Alsharhan, Y., Alenzi, T., Alhazzani, A., Ali, Y. Z., & Jazieh, A. R. (2018). The use of complementary and alternative medicine by patients with cancer: A cross-sectional survey in Saudi Arabia. *BMC Complementary and Alternative Medicine*, *18*(1), 88. doi:10.118612906-018-2150-8 PMID:29530034

Abu-Lehia, H. (1991). Nitrogen distribution and mineral contents of camel colostrum. *Australian Journal of Dairy Technology*, *46*, 82–84.

Abu-Lehia, I. H. (1989). Physical and chemical characteristics of camel milk fat and its fractions. *Food Chemistry*, *34*(4), 267–271. doi:10.1016/0308-8146(89)90103-9

Abu-Lehia, I. H., Al-Mohizea, I. S., & El-Beheri, M. (1989). Physical and chemical characteristics of camel colostrum. *Australian Journal of Dairy Technology (Australia)*, *44*(23), 34–36.

Abu-Lehia, I., Al-Mohiezea, I., & El-Behry, M. (1989). Studies on the production of ice cream from camel milk products. *Australian Journal of Dairy Technology*, *44*, 31–34.

Abu-Qatouseh, L., Mallah, E., Issa, H., Sabri, I., & Shihab, P. (2019). Antimicrobial And Anti-Inflammatory Activity Of Camel Milk Derived Immune Proteins And Peptides Against Propionibacterium Acnes. *International Journal of Biology. Pharmacy and Allied Sciences*, *8*, 163–173.

Abushelaibi, A., Al-Mahadin, S., El-Tarabily, K., Shah, N. P., & Ayyash, M. (2017). Characterization of potential probiotic lactic acid bacteria isolated from camel milk. *Lebensmittel-Wissenschaft + Technologie*, *79*, 316–325. doi:10.1016/j.lwt.2017.01.041

Abu-Taraboush, H. M., Al-Dagal, M. M., & Al-Royli, M. A. (1998). Growth, viability, and proteolytic activity of Bifidobacteria in whole camel milk. *Journal of Dairy Science*, *81*(2), 354–361. doi:10.3168/jds.S0022-0302(98)75584-5 PMID:9532489

Accolas, J., Deffontaines, J., Aubin, F., Grosclaude, F., Kuzdzal-Savoie, S., Langlois, D., & Jeunet, R. (1975). Rural activities in the Mongolian Peoples' Republic II Dairy Products (Fr.). *Etudes Mongoles*, *6*, 7–98.

Adams, C. M. (2013). Patient report: Autism spectrum disorder treated with camel milk. *Global Advances in Health and Medicine: Improving Healthcare Outcomes Worldwide*, *2*(6), 78–80. doi:10.7453/gahmj.2013.094 PMID:24349886

Adams, J. B., & Holloway, C. (2004). Pilot study of a moderate dose multivitamin/mineral supplement for children with autistic spectrum disorder. *Journal of Alternative and Complementary Medicine (New York, N.Y.)*, *10*(6), 1033–1039. doi:10.1089/acm.2004.10.1033 PMID:15673999

Adongo, A. O., Coppock, D. L., & Wayua, F. O. (2013). Simple evaporative cooling method reduces bacterial content of traditionally marketed camel milk in Isiolo County, Kenya. *African Journal of Food, Agriculture, Nutrition and Development*, *13*(01), 7213–7224. doi:10.18697/ajfand.56.12460

Adugnaa, M., Seifub, E., Kebededd, A., & Doluschitze, R. (2013). Quality and safety of camel milk along the value Chain in Eastern Ethiopia. *International Journal of Food Studies*, *2*(2), 150–157. doi:10.7455/ijfs/2.2.2013.a2

Afolabi, L., Onilude, H., & Afolabi, M. O. (2013). Assessment of microbiological quality of yogurt sold by street vendors in Onitsha metropolis, Anambra state, Nigeria. *British Microbiology Research Journal*, *3*(2), 198–20. doi:10.9734/BMRJ/2013/1801

Agrawal, R. P., Budania, S., Sharma, P., Gupta, R., & Kochar, D. K. (2007b). Zero prevalence of diabetes in camel milk consuming Raica community of northwest Rajasthan, India. *Diabetes Research and Clinical Practice*, *76*, 290-296.

Agrawal, R. P., Saran, S., Sharma, P., Gupta, R., Kochar, D. K., & Sahani, M. S. (2007a). Effect of camel milk on residual β-cell function in recent onset type 1 diabetes. *Diabetes Research and Clinical Practice*, *77*, 494-495.

Agrawal, P., Swami, S., Beniwal, R., Kochar, D., Sahani, M., Tuteja, F., & Ghouri, S. (2003). Effect of camel milk on glycemic control, risk factors and diabetes quality of life in type-1 diabetes: A randomised prospective controlled study. *Journal of Camel Practice and Research*, *10*(1), 45–50.

Agrawal, R. P., Beniwal, R., Sharma, S., Kochar, D. K., Tuteja, F. C., Ghorui, S. K., & Sahani, M. S. (2005). Effect of raw camel milk in type 1 diabetic patients: 1year randomised study. *Journal of Camel Practice and Research*, *12*(1), 27–31.

Agrawal, R. P., Kochar, D. K., Sahani, M. S., Tuteja, F. C., & Ghouri, S. K. (2004b). Hypoglycemic activity of camel milk in streptozotocin induced diabetic rats. *International Journal of Diabetes in Developing Countries*, *24*, 47–49.

Agrawal, R. P., Saran, S., Sharma, P., Gupta, R. P., Kochar, D. K., & Sahani, M. S. (2007). Effect of camel milk on residual β-cell function in recent onset type 1 diabetes. *Diabetes Research and Clinical Practice*, *77*(3), 494–495. doi:10.1016/j.diabres.2007.01.012 PMID:17320238

Agrawal, R. P., Sharma, P., & Gafoorunissa, S. J. (2011). Effect of camel milk on glucose metabolism in adults with normal glucose tolerance and type 2 diabetes in Raica community: A crossover study. *Acta Bio Medica Atenei Parmensis*, *82*(3), 181–186. PMID:22783713

Agrawal, R. P., Sharma, P., Jain, S., Gafoorunissa, S. A., Ibrahim, B., Shah, D., ... Kaur, T. (2011). Effect of camel milk on glucose metabolism in adults with normal glucose tolerance and type 2 diabetes in Raica community: A crossover study. *Acta Biomedica*, *82*(3), 181–186.

Agrawal, R. P., Singh, G., Nayak, K. C., Kochar, D. K., Sharma, R. C., Beniwal, R., ... Gupta, R. (2004a). Prevalence of diabetes in camel milk consuming 'RAICA' Rural Community of North West Rajasthan. *International Journal of Diabetes in Developing Countries*, *24*, 109–114.

Agrawal, R. P., Swami, S. C., Beniwal, R., Kochar, D. K., Sahani, M., Tuteja, F. C., & Ghouri, S. K. (2003). Effect of camel milk on glycemic control, risk factors and diabetes quality of life in type-1 diabetes: A randomized prospective controlled study. *Journal of Camel Practice and Research*, *10*(1), 45–50.

Agrawal, R., Budania, S., Sharma, P., Gupta, R., Kochar, D. K., Panwar, R. B., & Sahani, M. S. (2007). Zero prevalence of diabetes in camel milk consuming Raica community of northwest Rajasthan, India. *Diabetes Research and Clinical Practice*, *76*(2), 290–296. doi:10.1016/j.diabres.2006.09.036 PMID:17098321

Agrawal, R., Jain, S., Shah, S., Chopra, A., & Agarwal, V. (2011). Effect of camel milk on glycemic control and insulin requirement in patients with type 1 diabetes: 2-years randomized controlled trial. *European Journal of Clinical Nutrition*, *65*(9), 1048–1052. doi:10.1038/ejcn.2011.98 PMID:21629270

Agrawal, R., Sahani, M., Tuteja, F., Ghouri, S., Sena, D., Gupta, R., & Kochar, D. K. (2005). Hypoglycemic activity of camel milk in chemically pancreatectomized rats-an experimental study. *International Journal of Diabetes in Developing Countries*, *25*(3), 75–79. doi:10.4103/0973-3930.22776

Agrawal, R., Singh, G., Nayak, K., Kochar, D., Sharma, R., Beniwal, R., ... Gupta, R. (2004). Prevalence of diabetes in camel milk consuming 'RAICA'Rural Community of North West Rajasthan. *International Journal of Diabetes in Developing Countries*, *24*, 109–114.

Agrawal, R., Swami, S., Beniwal, R., Kochar, D., Sahani, M., Tuteja, F., & Ghorui, S. (2003). Effect of camel milk on glycemic control, lipid profile and diabetes quality of life in type 1 diabetes: A randomised prospective controlled cross over study. *The Indian Journal of Animal Sciences*, *73*(10), 1105–1110.

Agrawal, R., Swami, S., Beniwal, R., Kochar, D., Sahani, M., Tuteja, F., & Ghouri, S. (2003). Effect of raw camel milk on glycemic control, risk factors and diabetes quality of life in type-1 diabetes: A randomized prospective controlled study. *Journal of Camel Practice and Research*, *10*, 45–50.

Ahmad, S., Yaqoob, M., Bilal, M. Q., Khan, M. K., Muhammad, G., Yang, L.-G., & Tariq, M. (2012). Factors affecting yield and composition of camel milk kept under desert conditions of central Punjab, Pakistan. *Tropical Animal Health and Production*, *44*(7), 1403–1410. doi:10.100711250-012-0079-3 PMID:22270241

Ahmad, T., Ismail, A., Aqlima, S., Khalil, K. A., Kumar, Y., Adeyemi, K. D., & Sazili, A. Q. (2017). Recent advances on the role of process variables affecting gelatin yield and characteristics with special reference to enzymatic extraction : A review. *Food Hydrocolloids*, *63*, 85–96. doi:10.1016/j.foodhyd.2016.08.007

Ahmed, A. I., Mohamed, B. E., Eyousif, N. M., Faye, B., Loiseau, G., & Montet, D. (2015). Effect of production site, seasonality and age of fermented camel (Camelus dromedarius) milk gariss on fatty acids profile. *Journal of Advances in Food Science & Technology*, *2*(1), 1–8.

Ahmed, A. I., Mohamed, B. E., Yousif, N. M. E., Faye, B., & Loiseau, G. (2012). Antimicrobial activity and antibiotic resistance of LAB isolated from Sudanese traditional fermented camel (*Camelus dromedarius*) milk *gariss*. *International Journal of Biosciences*, *2*(11), 129–136.

Ahmed, A., & El Zubeir, I. (2015). Microbiological and sensory properties of low fat ice cream from camel milk using natural additives. *Annals. Food Science and Technology (Valahia University of Târgoviste)*, *16*(1), 236–244.

Ahmed, M., Alhassan, A., & Elobeid, E. (2017). Comparison of chemical composition, major metals and vitamin C of camel. *International Journal of Advanced Research*, *5*(3), 712–717. doi:10.21474/IJAR01/3562

Ahmed, N. A. A., & El-Zubeir, E. M. (2011). Effect of salt level on some physical and chemical properties and acceptability of camel milk cheese. *Journal of Camelid Science*, *4*, 40–48.

Ahmed, N., & Zubeir, I. E. (2011). Effect of Salt Level on Some Physical and Chemical Properties and Acceptability of Camel Milk Cheese. *Journal of Camelid Science*, *4*, 40–48.

Ahmed, S., Haroun, R., & Eisa, M. (2010). Banana frozen yogurt from camel milk. *Pakistan Journal of Nutrition*, *9*(10), 955–956. doi:10.3923/pjn.2010.955.956

Ajarem, J., Allam, A., Ebaid, H., Maodaa, S., AL-Sobeai, S. M., Rady, A. M., ... Sabri, M. I. (2015). AL-Sobeai S, Rady A, Metwalli A, Altoom N, Ibrahim, & Sabri M (2015) Neurochemical, structural and neurobehavioral evidence of neuronal protection by whey proteins in diabetic albino mice. *Behavioral and Brain Functions*, *11*(1), 7. doi:10.118612993-015-0053-0 PMID:25888881

Ajlouni, S., Michelle, R., Senaka, R., & Timothy, D. (2017).. . *Archives of the International Society of Antioxidants in Nutrition and Health*, *5*(2), 1–4.

Akalın, A., Kesenkas, H., Dinkci, H., Unal, G., Ozer, E., & Kınık, O. (2018). Enrichment of probiotic ice cream with different dietary fibers: Structural characteristics and culture viability. *Journal of Dairy Science*, *101*(1), 37–46. doi:10.3168/jds.2017-13468 PMID:29103712

Akanova, A., Kikebayev, N., Shaikenova, K., Seiitkazhy, Z., & Okuskhanov, E. (2017). Nutritive and Biological Value of Mares Milk Ice Cream. *Pakistan Journal of Nutrition*, *16*(6), 457–462. doi:10.3923/pjn.2017.457.462

Akhmetsadykova, S., Konuspayeva, S., Loiseau, G., Baubekova, A., Kanayat, S., Akhmetsadykov, N., & Faye, B. (2012) Protection against lead contamination by strains of Lactic Acid Bacteria (LAB) from fermented camel milk. *Proceedings of the 3rd conference of the international society of camelid research and development*, 420–22. Retrieved from https://www.academia.edu/4489898/Farmers_Attitude_Towards_Interventions_Regarding_Camel_Calf_Health_Care

Akhmetsadykova, Sh., Baubekova, A., Konuspayeva, G., Akhmetsadykov, N., Faye, B., & Loiseau, G. (2015). Lactic acid bacteria biodiversity in raw and fermented camel milk. *African Journal of Food Science and Technology*, *6*(3), 84–88.

Akhmetsadykova, Sh., Baubekova, A., Konuspayeva, G., Akhmetsadykov, N., & Loiseau, G. (2014). Microflora identification of fresh and fermented camel milk from Kazakhstan. *Emirates Journal of Food and Agriculture*, *26*(4), 327–332. doi:10.9755/ejfa.v26i4.17641

Akhu-Zaheya, L. M., & Alkhasawneh, E. M. (2012). Complementary alternative medicine use among a sample of Muslim Jordanian oncology patients. *Complementary Therapies in Clinical Practice*, *18*(2), 121–126. doi:10.1016/j.ctcp.2011.10.003 PMID:22500850

Al haj, O. A. & Al Kanhal, H. A. (2010). Compositional, technological and nutritional aspects of dromedary camel milk. *International Dairy Journal, 20*, 811-821.

Al haj, O. A., & Al Kanhal, H. A. (2010). Compositional, technological and nutritional aspects of dromedary camel milk. *International Dairy Journal, 20*, 811-821.

Al Haj, O. A., & Al Kanhal, H. A. (2010). Compositional, technological and nutritional aspects of dromedary camel milk. A review. *International Dairy Journal*, *20*, 811–821.

Al Jassim, R., & Hogan, J. (2012). The digestive system of the camel, its anatomical, histological and functional characteristics: A comparative approach. In *Proceedings of 3rd ISOCARD Conference* (pp. 75-86). Muscat, Oman: Sultan Qaboos University.

Alabdulkarim, B. (2012). Effect of camel milk on blood glucose, cholesterol, triglyceride and liver enzymes activities in female albino rats. *World Applied Sciences Journal*, *17*(11), 1394–1397.

Al-Abri, M. A., & Faye, B. (2019). Genetic improvement in dromedary camels: challenges and opportunities. Frontiers in Genetic, 10.

Al-Abri, M. A., & Faye, B. (2019). Genetic improvement in dromedary camels: Challenges and opportunities. *Frontiers in Genetics*, *10*, 167. doi:10.3389/fgene.2019.00167 PMID:30915101

Alais, C. (1984). Les lipides. In Sciences du Lait. Principes des Techniques Laitidres, (pp. 61-106). Sepaic.

Al-Amoudi, S., Cañas, J., Hohl, S. D., Distelhorst, S. R., & Thompson, B. (2015). Breaking the Silence: Breast Cancer Knowledge and Beliefs Among Somali Muslim Women in Seattle, Washington. *Health Care for Women International*, *36*(5), 608–616. doi:10.1080/07399332.2013.857323 PMID:24351062

Alaoui Ismaili, M., Saidi, B., Zahar, M., Hamama, A., & Ezzaier, R. (2019). Composition and microbial quality of raw camel milk produced in Morocco. *Journal of the Saudi Society of Agricultural Sciences*, *18*(1), 17–21. doi:10.1016/j.jssas.2016.12.001

Alary, V., & Faye, B. (2016). The camel chains in East Africa- Importance of gaps between the data and the apparent reality. *Journal of Camelid Science*, *9*, 1–2.

Al-Atiyat, R. M., Suliman, G., AlSuhaibani, E., El-Waziry, A., Al-Owaimer, A., & Basmaeil, S. (2016). The differentiation of camel breeds based on meat measurements using discriminant analysis. *Tropical Animal Health and Production*, *48*(5), 871–878. doi:10.100711250-015-0990-5 PMID:26922738

Al-Attabi, Z., D'arcy, B. R., & Deeth, H. C. (2009). Volatile sulphur compounds in UHT milk. *Critical Reviews in Food Science and Nutrition*, *49*(1), 28–47. doi:10.1080/10408390701764187 PMID:18949597

Al-Aubaidy, H. A., & Jelinek, H. F. (2014). Oxidative stress and triglycerides as predictors of subclinical atherosclerosis in prediabetes. *Redox Report*, *19*(2), 87–91. doi:10.1179/1351000213Y.0000000080 PMID:24520969

Alavi, F., Salami, M., & Emam-Djomeh, Z. (2018). Nutraceutical properties of camel milk. In *Nutrients in Dairy and Their Implications for Health and Disease* (pp. 451–468). Academic Press.

Alavi, F., Salami, M., Emam-Djomeh, Z., & Mohammadian, M. (2017). Neutraceutical properties of camel milk. In R. Watson, R. Collier, & V. Preedy (Eds.), *Nutrients in dairy and their implications for health and disease* (pp. 451–468). New York: Academic Press. doi:10.1016/B978-0-12-809762-5.00036-X

Al-Ayadhi & Elamin. (2015). *Camel milk as a potential therapy as an antioxidant in autism spectrum disorder (ASD)*. Apple Academic Press.

Al-Ayadhi, Halepoto, Al-Dress, Mitwali, & Zainah. (2015). Behavioral benefits of camel milk in subjects with autism spectrum disorder. *Journal of the College of Physicians and Surgeons--Pakistan*, *25*(11), 819–823. PMID:26577969

AL-Ayadhi, L., & Elamin, N. E. (2013). Camel milk as a potential therapy as an antioxidant in autism spectrum disorder (ASD). *Evidence-Based Complementary and Alternative Medicine*, 1–8. PMID:24069051

Al-Bachir, M., & Zeinou, R. (2009). Effect of gamma irradiation on microbial load and quality characteristics of minced camel meat. *Meat Science*, *82*(1), 119–124. doi:10.1016/j.meatsci.2008.12.012 PMID:20416783

AlBedah, A., Khalil, M., Elolemy, A. T., Al, A. M., Al, S. E., Al-Yahia, O. A., ... Henary, B. Y. (2013). The use of and out-of-pocket spending on complementary and alternative medicine in Qassim province, Saudi Arabia. *Annals of Saudi Medicine*, *33*(3), 282–289. doi:10.5144/0256-4947.2013.282 PMID:23793433

Albrecht, S., Lane, J. A., Marin, K., Al Busadah, K. A., Carrington, S. D., Hickey, R. M., & Rudd, P. M. (2014). A comparative study of free oligosaccharides in the milk of domestic animals. *British Journal of Nutrition*, *111*(7), 1313–1328. doi:10.1017/S0007114513003772 PMID:24635885

Alemayehu, M., Amede, T., Böhme, M., & Peters, K. J. (2012). Increasing livestock water productivity under rain fed mixed crop/livestock farming scenarios of sub-Saharan Africa: A review. *Journal of Sustainable Development*, *5*(7), 1–10. doi:10.5539/jsd.v5n7p1

Aleme, A., & Yusuf, M. (2014). Traditional consumption, therapeutic value and its derived dairy products of dromedary camel (*Camelus dromedaries*) milk in Somali regional state, eastern Ethiopia: A review. *Global Journal of Animal Scientific Research*, *3*(1), 240–246.

Al-Gedan, M. M., Al-Aguili, H., Alomayri, A., Konuspayeva, G., & Faye, B. (2015). Monitoring of camel milk production and composition in intensive dairy farm. *Scientific and Practical Journal Veterinariya*, *2*(42), 164-166.

Al-Ghsyar, M. A., Salem, S. A., & Ahmad, S. H. (2018). Studies on Physiochemical and functional properties of Protein Co-Precipitates from Camel's and Goat's Milk. *Health Science Journal*, *12*(5), 587–594.

Algruin, K., & Konuspayeva, G. (2015). Making leben with camel milk. *Scientific and Practical Journal Veterinariya*, *2*(42), 398

Al-Hadrami, G., & Faye, B. (2016). Animal that produced dairy food: camel. In Reference Module in Food Science (2nd ed.; pp. 1-12). Elsevier.

Alhaider, A. A., Abdel Gader, A. G. M., Almeshaal, N., & Saraswati, S. (2014). Camel milk inhibits inflammatory angiogenesis via downregulation of proangiogenic and proinflammatory cytokines in mice. *APMIS*, *122*(7), 599–607. doi:10.1111/apm.12199 PMID:24320686

Alhaj, O. A., Al-Khalifa, A. S., Metwalli, A. A., Ismail, E. & Ali, H. S. (2017). *Method of making a fermented dairy product from camel milk*. Patent Number: 9623057.

Alhaj, O., Al-Khalifa, A., Metwalli, A., Ismail, E., & Ali, H. (2017). *Method of making a fermented dairy product from camel milk*. United States Patent, Number US9,623,057B1.

Alhaj, O. A. (2017). Identification of potential ACE-inhibitory peptides from dromedary fermented camel milk. *CYTA: Journal of Food, 15*(2), 191–195. doi:10.1080/19476337.2016.1236353

Alhaj, O. A., Kanekanian, A., & Peters, A. (2007). Investigation on whey proteins profile of commercially aviabale milk-based probiotics health drinks using fast protein liquid chromatography (FPLC). *British Food Journal, 109*(6), 469–480. doi:10.1108/00070700710753526

Alhaj, O. A., Metwalli, A. A. M., & Ismail El, A. (2011). Heat Stability of Camel Milk Proteins after Sterilisation Process. *Journal of Camel Practice and Research, 18*(2), 277–282.

Alhaj, O. A., Metwalli, A. A., & Ismail, E. A. (2011). Heat stability of camel milk proteins after sterilization process. *Journal of Camel Practice and Research, 18*, 277–282.

Alhaj, O., & Al Kanhal, H. A. (2010). Compositional, technological and nutritional aspects of dromedary camel milk. *International Dairy Journal, 20*(12), 811–821. doi:10.1016/j.idairyj.2010.04.003

Alhaj, O., Kanekanian, A., Peters, A., & Tatham, A. (2010). Hypocholesterolemic effect of *Bifidobacterium animalis* subsp. *Lactis* (Bb12) and trypsin casein hydrolysate. *Food Chemistry, 123*(2), 430–435. doi:10.1016/j.foodchem.2010.04.061

Alhaj, O., Metwalli, A., & Ismail, E. (2011). Heat stability of camel milk proteins after sterilisation process. *Journal of Camel Practice and Research, 18*, 277–282.

Alhaj, O., Metwalli, A., Ismail, E., Ali, H., Al-khalifa, A., & Kanekanian, A. (2018). Angiotensin converting enzyme-inhibitory activity and antimicrobial effect of fermented camel milk (*Camelus dromedarius*). *International Journal of Dairy Technology, 17*(1), 27–35. doi:10.1111/1471-0307.12383

Alhaj, O., Taufik, E., Handa, Y., Fukuda, K., Saito, T., & Urashima, T. (2013). Chemical characterization of oligosaccharides in commercially pasteurized dromedary camel (*camelusdromedarius*) milk. *International Dairy Journal, 28*(2), 70–75. doi:10.1016/j.idairyj.2012.08.008

Al-Harbi, M. M., Qureshi, S., Ahmed, M. M., Raza, M., Baig, M. Z. A., & Shah, A. H. (1996). *Effect of camel urine on the cytological and biochemical changes induced by cyclophosphamide in mice*. doi:10.1016/0378-8741(96)01399-2

Alhomida, A. (1996). Total, free, short-chain and long-chain acyl carnitine levels in Arabian camel milk (Camelus dromedarius). *Annals of Nutrition & Metabolism, 40*(4), 221–226. doi:10.1159/000177925 PMID:8886250

Alhomida, A. S., Duhaiman, A. S., Al-Jafari, A. A., & Junaid, M. A. (1995). Determination of L-carnitine, acylcarnitine and total carnitine levels in plasma and tissues of camel (*Camelus dromedarius*). *Comparative Biochemistry and Physiology, 111B*(3), 441–445. doi:10.1016/0305-0491(95)00014-Y PMID:7613767

Al-Humaid, A., Mousa, H., El-Mergawi, R., & Abdel-Salam, A. (2010). Chemical composition and antioxidant activity of dates and dates-camel-milk mixtures as a protective meal against lipid peroxidation in rats. *American Journal of Food Technology, 5*(1), 22–30. doi:10.3923/ajft.2010.22.30

Alimi, D., Hajaji, S., Rekik, M., Abidi, A., Gharbi, M., & Akkari, H. (2016). First report of the in vitro nematicidal effects of camel milk. *Veterinary Parasitology, 228*, 153–159. doi:10.1016/j.vetpar.2016.09.003 PMID:27692318

Alinovi, M., Cordioli, M., Francolino, S., Locci, F., Ghiglietti, R., Monti, L., ... Giraffa, G. (2018). Effect of fermentation-produced camel chymosin on quality of Crescenza cheese. *International Dairy Journal, 84*, 72–78. doi:10.1016/j.idairyj.2018.04.001

Al-Juboori, A., Mohammed, M., Rashid, J., Kurian, J., & El Refaey S. (2013). Nutritional and medicinal value of camel (Camelus Dromedarius) milk. *Food & Environment II, 170*, 221-232.

Al-Juboori, A. T., Mohammed, M., Rashid, J., Kurian, J., & El Refaey, S. (2013). Nutritional and medicinal value of camel (*Camelus dromedarius*) milk. *WIT Transactions on Ecology and the Environment*, *170*, 221–232. doi:10.2495/FENV130201

Aljumaah, R. S., Almutairi, F. F., Ismail, E., Alshaik, M. A., Sami, A., & Ayadi, M. (2012). Effects of production system, breed, parity and stage of lactation on milk composition of dromedary camels in Saudi Arabia. *Journal of Animal and Veterinary Advances*, *11*(1), 141–147. doi:10.3923/javaa.2012.141.147

Al-Kahtani, H. A., Jaswir, I., Ismail, E. A., Ahmed, M. A., Hammed, A. M., Olorunnisola, S., & Octavianti, F. (2017). Structural characteristics of camel-bone gelatin by demineraization and extraction. *International Journal of Food Properties*, *20*(11), 2559–2568. doi:10.1080/10942912.2016.1244543

Al-Khdier, A. M., Al-Saleh, A. A., Abu-Tarboush, H. M., Ismail, E. A., & Metwalli, A. (2014). The ability of some starter cultures to increase the conjugated linoleic acid level in cow and camel milks. *Journal of Pure & Applied Microbiology*, *8*, 363–370.

Allemann, I. B., & Baumann, L. (2008). Antioxidants Used in Skin Care Formulations Skin. *Therapy Letter*, *13*(7), 5–8. PMID:18839043

Almahdy, O., EL-Fakharany, E. M., EL-Dabaa, E., Ng, T. B., & Redwan, E. M. (2011). Examination of the activity of camel milk casein against hepatitis C virus (genotype-4a) and its apoptotic potential in hepatoma and hela cell lines. *Hepatitis Monthly*, *11*(9), 724–730. doi:10.5812/kowsar.1735143X.1367 PMID:22235215

Al-Majali, A., Ismail, Z., & Al-Hami, Y. (2007). Lactoferrin concentration in milk from camels (*Camelus dromedarius*) with and without subclinical mastitis. *International Journal of Applied Research in Veterinary Medicine*, *5*, 120.

Almathen, F., Charruau, P., Mohandesan, E., Mwacharo, J. M., Orozco-ter Wengel, P., Pitt, D., & ... Burger, P.A. (2016) Ancient and modern DNA reveal dynamics of domestication and cross-continental dispersal of the dromedary. *Proceedings of the National Academy of Sciences* USA, *113*, 6707-12. 10.1073/pnas.1519508113

Almehdar, H. A., El-Baky, N. A., Alhaider, A. A., & Redwan, E. M. (2019). Immunogenicity comparison of lactoferrin purified from Saudi Arabia camel clans milk. *Human Antibodies*, 1–6. PMID:30372672

Al-Mutairi, S. E., Boujenane, I., Musaad, A., & Awad-Acharari, F. (2010a). Non-genetic factors influencing reproductive traits and calving weight in Saudi camels. *Tropical Animal Health and Production*, *42*(6), 1087–1092. doi:10.100711250-010-9529-y PMID:20195755

Al-Mutairi, S. E., Boujenane, I., Musaad, A., & Awad-Acharari, F. (2010b). Genetic and nongenetic effects for milk yield and growth traits in Saudi camels. *Tropical Animal Health and Production*, *42*(8), 1845–1853. doi:10.100711250-010-9647-6 PMID:20617460

Al-Nasseri, R. H., Al-Ruqashi, H., Al-Sabahi, J., Al-Harrasi, A., Kanekanian, A., Banerjee, Y., ... Hassan, N. (2019). Lipids derived from camel milk regulate NLRP3 inflammasome subunit-dependent inflammatory responses in human macrophages. *Functional Foods in Health and Disease*, *9*(4), 224–240. doi:10.31989/ffhd.v9i4.567

Al-Numair, S., Chandramohan, G., Kamalakkannan, N., Alsaif, M. A., & Sundaraselvan, G. (2010). Effect of camel milk on the activities of ATPases in normal and streptozotocin-diabetic rats. *Polish Journal of Food and Nutrition Sciences*, *60*(4), 375–380.

Al-Omari, M. M., Al-Ghariebeh, R. B., Alhaija, A. A. A., Al-Zoubi, H., & Al-Qaoud, K. M. (2019). Camel milk whey inhibits inflammatory colorectal cancer development via down regulation of pro-inflammatory cytokines in induced AOM/DSS mouse model. *Emirates Journal of Food and Agriculture*, *31*(4), 256–262. doi:10.9755/ejfa.2019.v31.i4.1935

Alrowais, N. A., & Alyousefi, N. A. (2017). The prevalence extent of Complementary and Alternative Medicine (CAM) use among Saudis. *Saudi Pharmaceutical Journal, 25*(3), 306–318. doi:10.1016/j.jsps.2016.09.009 PMID:28344484

Al-Saleh, A. (1996). Heat coagulation of camel milk. *Journal of King Saud University, 8*, 107–117.

Al-Saleh, A., Metwalli, A., Ismail, E., & Alhaj, O. (2014). Antioxidative activity of camel milk casein hydrolysates. *Journal of Camel Practice and Research, 21*(2), 229–237. doi:10.5958/2277-8934.2014.00041.1

Al-Shabib, N. A., & Abu-Tarboush, H. M. (2004). Nutritional value and some functional properties of protein in Ostrich and Camel meat. *Arab Journal of Food Nutrition, 5*, 6–20.

Alshaikh, M. A., & Salah, M. S. (1994). Effect of milking interval on secretion rate and composition of camel milk in late lactation. *The Journal of Dairy Research, 61*(4), 451–456. doi:10.1017/S0022029900028375 PMID:7829750

Al-Shamsi, K. A., Mudgil, P., Hassan, H. M., & Maqsood, S. (2017). Camel milk protein hydrolysates with improved technofunctional properties and enhanced antioxidant potential in in vitro and in food model systems. *Journal of Dairy Science, 101*(1), 47–60. doi:10.3168/jds.2017-13194 PMID:29128226

Al-Sobayil, K. A., Khalil, M. H., Al-Jobeile, H. S., Mohamed, K. M., & Salal, S. A. (2006). Quantitative genetic analysis and evaluation for early growth performance in Saudi camels. In *Proceedings of the International Scientific Conference on Camels* (pp. 201). Qassim, Saudi Arabia: Academic Press.

Altansuhe. (1997). *Sunid Bactrian camel.* Inner Mongolia Peoples Publishing House.

Altay, F., Karbancıoglu-Güler, F., Daskaya-Dikmen, C., & Heperkan, D. (2013). A review on traditional Turkish fermented non-alcoholic beverages: Microbiota, fermentation process and quality characteristics. *International Journal of Food Microbiology, 167*(1), 44–56. doi:10.1016/j.ijfoodmicro.2013.06.016 PMID:23859403

Al-Wabel, N. A. (2008). Mineral contents of milk of cattle, camels, goats and sheep in the central region of Saudi Arabia. *Asian Journal of Biochemistry, 3*(6), 373–375. doi:10.3923/ajb.2008.373.375

Al-Wabel, N., Hassan, A., Abbas, H., & Muosa, H. (2012). Antiulcerogenic effect of camel milk against ethanol induced gastric ulcers in rats. *WebmedCentral Veterinary Medicine, 3*(3), WMC002804.

Al-Yousef, N., Gaafar, A., Al-Otaibi, B., Al-Jammaz, I., Al-Hussein, K., & Aboussekhra, A. (2012). *Camel urine components display anti-cancer properties in vitro.* doi:10.1016/j.jep.2012.07.042

Al-Zoreky, N. S., & Al-Otaibi, M. M. (2015). Suitability of camel milk for making yogurt. *Food Science and Biotechnology, 24*(2), 601–606. doi:10.100710068-015-0078-z

Ameen, S. H., & Hameed, A. K. (2019). Therapy Role of Camel Milk for the Treatment of Hepatitis Mice Which Induces via Listeria Monocytogenes. *Indian Journal of Public Health Research & Development, 10*(2), 537. doi:10.5958/0976-5506.2019.00347.4

Amr, A., Takruri, H., Shomaf, M., Alhaj, O., & Faris, M. (2018). Fermented Camel (*Camelus dromedarius*) and Bovine Milk Attenuate Azoxymethane-induced Colonic Aberrant Crypt Foci in Fischer 344 Rats. *Pakistan Journal of Nutrition, 17*(4), 179–189. doi:10.3923/pjn.2018.179.189

Anema, S. G., & Li, Y. (2003). Association of denatured whey proteins with casein micelles in heated reconstituted skim milk and its effect on casein micelle size. *The Journal of Dairy Research, 70*(1), 73–83. doi:10.1017/S0022029902005903 PMID:12617395

Anema, S. G., Lowe, E. K., & Stockman, R. (2005a). Particle size changes and casein solubilization in high-pressure-treated skim milk. *Food Hydrocolloids, 19*(2), 257–267. doi:10.1016/j.foodhyd.2004.04.025

Anema, S. G., Stockman, R., & Lowe, E. K. (2005b). Denaturation Of Β-Lactoglobulin In Pressure Treated Skim Milk. *Journal of Agricultural and Food Chemistry*, *53*(20), 7783–7791. doi:10.1021/jf050326x PMID:16190631

Angulo, L., Lopez, E., & Lema, C. (1993). Microflora present in kefir grains of the Galician region (north-west of Spain). *The Journal of Dairy Research*, *60*(2), 263–267. doi:10.1017/S002202990002759X PMID:8320374

Anjali, S., & Suman, P. (2013). Studies on camel hair -merino wool blended knitted fabrics. *Indian Journal of Fibre and Textile Research*, *38*, 317–319.

Anonymous. (1986). *A/S Niro Atomizer: Technical doc.* Copenhagen: Wilentation.

Anouassi, A., & Tibary, A. (2013). Development of a large commercial camel embryo transfer program: 20 years of scientific research. *Animal Reproduction Science*, *136*(3), 211–221. doi:10.1016/j.anireprosci.2012.10.012 PMID:23153626

AOAC. (2019). *Official Methods of Analysis of AOAC International* (21st ed.). Arlington, VA: AOAC International.

Aqib, A. I., Kulyar, M. F.-A., Ashfaq, K., Bhutta, Z. A., Shoaib, M., & Ahmed, R. (2019). Camel milk Insuline: Pathophysiological and molecular Repository. *Trends in Food Science & Technology*, *88*, 497–504. doi:10.1016/j.tifs.2019.04.009

Arab, H. H., Salama, S. A., Eid, A. H., Omar, H. A., Arafa, E.-S. A., & Maghrabi, I. A. (2014). *Camel's milk ameliorates TNBS-induced colitis in rats via downregulation of inflammatory cytokines and oxidative stress.* doi:10.1016/j.fct.2014.04.032

Arbuckle, W. (1966). Ice cream. Avi Publ. Co. Inc.

Arbuckle, W. S. (1986). Calculating Cost and Percentage of Overrun. In *Ice Cream*. Boston, MA: Springer. doi:10.1007/978-1-4615-7222-0_10

Ardekani, V. S., Mahmoodani, F., See, S. F., Yusop, S. M., & Babji, A. S. (2013). Processing optimization and characterization of gelatin from catfish (*Clarias gariepinus*) skin. *Sains Malaysiana*, *42*(12), 1697–1705.

Aref, A. R. (2018). Camel milk as complementary and alternative medicine. *International Journal of Scientific Research*, *7*(1), 435–439.

Ariano, M. A., Armstrong, R. B., & Edgerton, V. R. (1973). Hind limb muscle fibre populations of five mammals. *The Journal of Histochemistry and Cytochemistry*, *21*(1), 51–55. doi:10.1177/21.1.51 PMID:4348494

Arias, M., Lopez-Fandino, R., & Olano, A. (2000). Influence of PH on the Effects of High Pressure on Milk. *Milchwissenschaft*, *55*(4), 191–194.

Arihara, K. (2006). Strategies for designing novel functional meat products. *Meat Science*, *74*(1), 219–229. doi:10.1016/j.meatsci.2006.04.028 PMID:22062731

Arthur, P. G., Smith, M., & Hartmann, P. (1989). Milk lactose, citrate and glucose as markers of lactogenesis in normal and diabetic women. *Journal of Pediatric Gastroenterology and Nutrition*, *90*(4), 488–496. doi:10.1097/00005176-198911000-00016 PMID:2621526

Asghar, A., & Pearson, A. M. (1980). Influence of ante- and postmortem treatments upon muscle composition and meat quality. *Advances in Food Research*, *26*, 53–213. doi:10.1016/S0065-2628(08)60318-3

Asha, A., Pareek, K., & Shah, S. (2016). In silico physico-chemical comparative study of human and camel insulin. *IOSR Journal of Pharmacy*, *6*(11), 50–53.

Ashmaig, A., Hasan, A., & El Gaali, E. (2009). Identification of lactic acid bacteria isolated from traditional Sudanese fermented camel's milk (Gariss). *African Journal of Microbiological Research*, *3*(8), 451–457.

Ashmore, C. R., Tompkins, G., & Doerr, L. (1972). Postnatal development of muscle fibre types in domestic animals. *Journal of Animal Science*, *4*(1), 37–41. doi:10.2527/jas1972.34137x PMID:4258174

Asresie, A., Eyassu Seifu, E., & Kurtu, M. (2013). Churning efficiency and microbial quality of butter made from camel milk alone and blending it with goat milk. *Net Journal of Agricultural Science*, *1*(3), 75–80.

Asresie, A., & Yusuf, M. (2014). Traditional Consumption, Therapeutic Value and Its Derived Dairy Products of Dromedary Camel (Camelus Dromedaries) Milk in Somali Regional State, Eastern Ethiopia: A Review. *Global Journal of Animal Scientific Research*, *3*, 240–246.

Astrom, A., Tavakkol, A., Pettersson, U., Cromie, M., Elder, J. T., & Voorhees, J. J. (1991). Molecular cloning of two human cellular retinoic acid-binding proteins (CRABP). Retinoic acid-induced expression of CRABP-II but not CRABP-I in adult human skin in vivo and in skin fibroblasts in vitro. *The Journal of Biological Chemistry*, *266*, 17662–17666. PMID:1654334

Aswad, D. W., Paranandi, M. V., & Schurter, B. T. (2000). Isoaspartate in peptides and proteins: Formation, significance, and analysis. *Journal of Pharmaceutical and Biomedical Analysis*, *21*(6), 1129–1136. doi:10.1016/S0731-7085(99)00230-7 PMID:10708396

Aswal, P., Shukla, A., & Priyadarshi, S. (2012). Yoghurt: Preparation, characteristics and recent advancements. *Cibtech Journal of Bio-Protocols*, *1*(2), 32–44.

Attia, H., Kherouatou, N., & Dhouib, A. (2001). Dromedary milk lactic acid fermentation: Microbiological and rheological characteristics. *Journal of Industrial Microbiology & Biotechnology*, *26*(5), 263–270. doi:10.1038j.jim.7000111 PMID:11494100

Attia, H., Kherouatou, N., Fakhfakh, N., Khorchani, T., & Trigui, N. (2000). Dromedary milk fat: Biochemical, microscopic and rheological characterics. *Journal of Food Lipids*, *7*(2), 95–112. doi:10.1111/j.1745-4522.2000.tb00164.x

Augustin, M. A. (2000). Mineral salts and their effect on milk functionality. *Australian Journal of Dairy Technology*, *55*, 61–64.

Awad, H., El Zubeir, I., & Babiker, S. (2006). Microbiology of camel fermented milk (Gariss) in Sudan. *Research Journal of Microbiology*, *1*(2), 160-165.

Ayadi, M., Aljumaah, R., Samara, S., Faye, B., & Caja, G. (2015). Udder typology of Arabian dairy camels and proposal of a linear scoring system for assessing their udder traits for machine milking. *Scientific and Practical Journal Veterinariya, 2*(42).

Ayadi, M., Hammadi, M., Casals, R., Atigui, M., Khorchani, T., Samara, E. M., ... Caja, G. (2019). Influence of management type and stage of lactation on the performance and milk fatty acid profile of dairy camels (*Camelus dromedarius*). *The Journal of Agricultural Science*, *156*(9), 1111–1122. doi:10.1017/S0021859618001065

Ayadi, M., Musaad, A., Aljumaah, R. S., Samara, E. M., Abelrahman, M. M., Alshaikh, M. A., ... Faye, B. (2013). Relationship between udder morphology traits, alveolar and cisternal milk compartments and machine milking performances of dairy camels (Camelus dromedarius). *Spanish Journal of Agricultural Research*, *11*(3), 790–797. doi:10.5424jar/2013113-4060

Ayoub, M. A., Palakkott, A. R., Ashraf, A., & Iratni, R. (2018). The molecular basis of the anti-diabetic properties of camel milk. *Diabetes Research and Clinical Practice*, *146*, 305–312. doi:10.1016/j.diabres.2018.11.006

Ayyash, M., Abu-Jdayil, B., Hamed, F., & Shaker, R. (2018). Rheological, textural, microstructural and sensory impact of exopolysaccharide-producing Lactobacillus plantarum isolated from camel milk on low-fat akawi cheese. *Lebensmittel-Wissenschaft + Technologie*, *87*, 423–431. doi:10.1016/j.lwt.2017.09.023

Ayyash, M., Abushelaibi, A., Al-Mahadin, S., Enan, M., El-Tarabily, K., & Shah, N. (2018a). *In-vitro* investigation into probiotic characterisation of *Streptococcus* and *Enterococcus* isolated from camel milk. *Lebensmittel-Wissenschaft + Technologie*, *87*, 478–487. doi:10.1016/j.lwt.2017.09.019

Ayyash, M., Al-Dhaheri, A. S., Al Mahadin, S., Kizhakkayil, J., & Abushelaibi, A. (2018b). In vitro investigation of anticancer, antihypertensive, antidiabetic, and antioxidant activities of camel milk fermented with camel milk probiotic: A comparative study with fermented bovine milk. *Journal of Dairy Science*, *101*(2), 900–911. doi:10.3168/jds.2017-13400 PMID:29224862

Ayyash, M., Al-Nuaimi, A. K., Al-Mahadin, S., & Liu, S. Q. (2018b). *In vitro* investigation of anticancer and ACE-inhibiting activity, α-amylase and α-glucosidase inhibition, and antioxidant activity of camel milk fermented with camel milk probiotic: A comparative study with fermented bovine milk. *Food Chemistry*, *239*, 588–597. doi:10.1016/j.foodchem.2017.06.149 PMID:28873609

Ayyash, M., Liu, S. Q., Al Mheiri, A., Aldhaheri, M., Raeisi, B., Al-Nabulsi, A., & Olaimat, A. (2019). In vitro investigation of health-promoting benefits of fermented camel sausage by novel probiotic Lactobacillusplantarum: A comparative study with beef sausages. *Lebensmittel-Wissenschaft + Technologie*, *99*, 346–354. doi:10.1016/j.lwt.2018.09.084

Azoulay, G., Ancey, V., Dormoy, D., Crenn, C., Mangu, A., & Thomashausen, A. (2014). *Mobilités et migrations: figures et enjeux contemporains: Pluralité des regards et des disciplines*. Paris, France: L'Harmattan.

Azwai, S. M., Carter, S. D., & Woldehiwet, Z. (1996). Immunoglobulins of camel (*Camelus dromedarius*) colostrum. *Journal of Comparative Pathology*, *114*(3), 273–282. doi:10.1016/S0021-9975(96)80049-1 PMID:8762585

Baba, A. (2019). *Emirates Industry for camel milk & products factory*. Retrieved in 22nd May, 2019 from: https://ae1043581272.fm.alibaba.com/company_profile.html?spm=a2700.9099375.35.3.5e2b762cUmDTL4#top-nav-bar

Babelhadj, B., Di Bari, M. A., Pirisinu, L., Chiappini, B., Gaouar, S., Riccardi, G., ... Vaccari, G. (2018). Prion Disease in Dromedary Camels, Algeria. *Emerging Infectious Diseases*, *24*(6), 1029–1036. doi:10.3201/eid2406.172007 PMID:29652245

Babiker, S. A., & Yousif, O. K. (1990). Chemical composition and quality of camel meat. *Meat Science*, *27*(4), 283–287. doi:10.1016/0309-1740(90)90066-F PMID:22055364

Babiker, W. I. A., & El-Zubeir, I. E. M. (2014). Impact of husbandry, stages of lactation and parity number on milk yield and chemical composition of dromedary camel milk. *Emirates Journal of Food and Agriculture*, *26*(4), 333–341. doi:10.9755/ejfa.v26i4.17664

Babilas, P., Knie, U., & Abels, C. (2012). Cosmetic and dermatologic use of alpha hydroxy acid. *Journal der Deutschen Dermatologischen Gesellschaft*, *10*(7), 488–491. PMID:22916351

Badawy, A. A., El-Magd, M. A., & Alsadrah, S. A. (2018). Therapeutic Effect of Camel Milk and Its Exosomes on MCF7 Cells In Vitro and In Vivo. *Integrative Cancer Therapies*. doi:10.1177/1534735418786000 PMID:29986606

Badiei, M., Mostaghni, K., Pourjafar, M., & Parchami, A. (2006). Serum and tissue trace elements in Iranian camels (Camelus dromedaries). *Comparative Clinical Pathology*, *15*(1), 58–61. doi:10.100700580-006-0610-x

Badr, G. (2013). Camel whey protein enhances diabetic wound healing in a streptozotocin-induced diabetic mouse model: The critical role of b-Defensin-1, -2 and -3. *Lipids in Health and Disease*, *12*(1), 46. doi:10.1186/1476-511X-12-46

Badr, G., Mohany, M., & Metwalli, A. (2011). Effects of undenatured whey protein supplementation on CXCL12- and CCL21-mediated B and T cell chemotaxis in diabetic mice. *Lipids in Health and Disease*, *9*(10), 203. doi:10.1186/1476-511X-10-203 PMID:22070978

Badr, G., Sayed, L. H., Omar, H. E.-D. M., Abd El-Rahim, A. M., Ahmed, E. A., & Mahmoud, M. H. (2017). Camel whey protein protects B and T cells from apoptosis, by suppressing activating transcription factor-3 (ATF-3)-mediated oxidative stress and enhancing phosphorylation of AKT and IjB-a in type I diabetic mice. *Cellular Physiology and Biochemistry*, *41*(1), 41–54. doi:10.1159/000455935

Bai, L., & Feng, D. Z. (2014). Analysis of wool Quality and Fiber Types of Chinese Bactrian Camels. *Heilongjiang Animal Science and Veterinary Medicine*, *3*, 155-158.

Bai, M. Z., & Amu, G. L. (2019). Study on Physical Properties of camel Cashmere. *Journal of Camel Practice and Research*, *26*(2), 113–116. doi:10.5958/2277-8934.2019.00030.4

Baio, J., Wiggins, L., Christensen, D. L., Maenner, M. J., Daniels, J., Warren, Z., ... White, T. (2018). Prevalence of autism spectrum disorder among children aged 8 years—autism and developmental disabilities monitoring network, 11 sites, United States, 2014. *MMWR. Surveillance Summaries*, *67*(6), 1–23. doi:10.15585/mmwr.ss6706a1 PMID:29701730

Bai, Y. H., Zhao, D. B., & Zhang, H. P. (2009). Physiochemical properties and amino acid composition of Alxa bactrian camel milk and shubat. *Journal of Camel Practice and Research*, *16*(2), 249–255.

Bajad, D., Kalyankar, S., Dehmukh, M., Bachanti, P., & Bajad, G. (2016). Impact of physico-chemical properties of mix on the final quality of ice-cream. *Asian Journal of Dairy & Food Reserch*, *35*(4), 293–297.

Baker, D. M., & Santer, R. M. (1990). Development of a quantitative histochemical method for determination of succinate dehydrogenase activity in autonomic neurons and its application to the study of aging in the autonomic nervous system. *The Journal of Histochemistry and Cytochemistry*, *38*(4), 525–531. doi:10.1177/38.4.2319123 PMID:2319123

Bakheit, S. A., Majid, A. A., & Nikhala, A. M. (2008). Camels (Camelus dromedarius) under pastoral systems in North Kordofan, Sudan: Seasonal and parity effects on milk composition. *Journal of Camelid Science*, *1*, 32–36.

Balkhy, H. H., & Memish, Z. A. (2003). Rift Valley fever: An uninvited zoonosis in the Arabian Peninsula. *International Journal of Antimicrobial Agents*, *21*(2), 153–157. doi:10.1016/S0924-8579(02)00295-9 PMID:12615379

Balny, C., & Masson, P. (1993). Effects of High Pressure on Proteins. *Food Reviews International*, *9*(4), 611–628. doi:10.1080/87559129309540980

Baragob, A. E. A. (2015). Composition and hypoglycemic effect of camel milk in streptozotocin–induced diabetic rats. *Biochemistry and Biotechnology Research*, *3*, 38–42.

Barat, A. Z. Y., & Morteza, K. (2015). Introduction to Camel Origin, History, Raising, Characterisctics, And Wool, Hair and Skin, A Review. *EPH - International Journal of Agriculture and Environmental Research*, *1*, 1–19.

Barbas, C., & Herrera, E. (1998). Lipid composition and vitamin E content in human colostrum and mature milk. *Journal of Physiology and Biochemistry*, *54*, 167–174. PMID:10217214

Barłowska, J., Szwajkowska, M., Litwińczuk, Z., & Król, J. (2011). Nutritional Value and Technological Suitability of Milk from Various Animal Species Used for Dairy Production. *Comprehensive Reviews in Food Science and Food Safety*, *10*(6), 291–302. doi:10.1111/j.1541-4337.2011.00163.x

Barrett, J. S., Irving, P., Shepherd, S. J., Muir, J. G., & Gibson, P. R. (2009). Comparison of the prevalence of fructose and lactose malabsorption across chronic intestinal disorders. *Alimentary Pharmacology & Therapeutics*, *30*(2), 165–174. doi:10.1111/j.1365-2036.2009.04018.x PMID:19392860

Barthe, L. (1905). La composition du lait de chamelle. *Journal de Pharmacie et de Chimie*, *21*, 386–388.

Bashir, S., & Al-Ayadhi, L. Y. (2014). Effect of camel milk on thymus and activation-regulated chemokine in autistic children: Double-blind study. *Pediatric Research, 75*(4), 559–563. doi:10.1038/pr.2013.248 PMID:24375082

Baubekova, A., Kalimbetovaa, S., Akhmetsadykova, O., Konuspayeva, & Faye, B. (2015). Comparison of D. Lactate and L. lactate content in cow and camel milk. *Scientific and Practical Journal Veterinarya, 2*, 397-398.

Baubekova, A., Akhmetsadykova, S., Konuspayeva, G., Akhmetsadykov, N., Faye, B., & Loiseau, G. (2015). Biodiversity study of the yeast in fresh and fermented camel and mare's milk by denaturing gradient gel electrophoresis. *Journal of Camel Practice and Research, 22*(1), 91–95. doi:10.5958/2277-8934.2015.00014.4

Bauman, D., Mather, I., Wall, R., & Lock, A. (2006). Major advances associated with the biosynthesis of milk. *Journal of Dairy Science, 89*(4), 1235–1243. doi:10.3168/jds.S0022-0302(06)72192-0 PMID:16537956

Baumann, L. (2003). Cosmeceuticals: Drugs versus cosmetics. In L. Baumann (Ed.), *Cosmetic dermatology principles and practice* (pp. 197–198). New York, NY: Tata Magraw.

Beg, O. U., von Bahr-Lindström, H., Zaidi, Z. H., & Jörnvall, H. (1986). A camel milk whey protein rich in half-cystine: Primary structure, assessment of variations, internal repeat patterns, and relationships with neurophysin and other active polypeptides. *European Journal of Biochemistry, 159*(1), 195–201. doi:10.1111/j.1432-1033.1986.tb09852.x

Bekele, B., Hansen, E. B., Eshetu, M., Ipsen, R., & Hailu, Y. (2019). Effect of starter cultures on properties of soft white cheese made from camel (*Camelus dromedarius*) milk. *Journal of Dairy Science, 102*(2), 1108–1115. doi:10.3168/jds.2018-15084 PMID:30591338

Bekele, T., & Dahlborn, K. (2004). The effect of water deprivation on milk production of camels (*Camelus dromedarius*). *Journal of Animal and Feed Sciences, 13*(Suppl. 1), 459–462. doi:10.22358/jafs/73965/2004

Bekhit, A. E., & Farouk, M. M. (2013). Nutritive and health value of camel meat. In I. T. Kadim, O. Mahgoub, B. Faye, & M. M. Farouk (Eds.), *Camel Meat and Meat Products* (pp. 205–223). CAB International. doi:10.1079/9781780641010.0205

Bellamy, W., Takase, M., Wakabayashi, H., Kawase, K., & Tomita, M. (1992). Antibacterial spectrum of lactoferricin B, a potent bactericidal peptide derived from the N-terminal region of bovine lactoferrin. *The Journal of Applied Bacteriology, 73*(6), 472–479. doi:10.1111/j.1365-2672.1992.tb05007.x PMID:1490908

Bell, J. G., Miller, D., MacDonald, D. J., MacKinlay, E. E., Dick, J. R., Cheseldine, S., ... O'Hare, A. E. (2010). The fatty acid compositions of erythrocyte and plasma polar lipids in children with autism, developmental delay or typically developing controls and the effect of fish oil intake. *British Journal of Nutrition, 103*(8), 1160–1167. doi:10.1017/S0007114509992881 PMID:19995470

Benabdelkamel, H., Masood, A., Alanazi, I., Alzahrani, D., Alrabiah, D., AlYahya, S., & Alfadda, A. (2017). Proteomic profiling comparing the effects of different heat treatments on camel (*Camelus dromedarius*) milk whey proteins. *International Journal of Molecular Sciences, 18*(4), 721. doi:10.3390/ijms18040721 PMID:28350354

Benaissa, M. H., Faye, B., & Kaidi, R. (2015). Reproductive abnormalities in female camel (Camelus dromedarius) in Algeria: Relationship with age, season, breed and body condition score. *Journal of Camel Practice and Research, 22*(1), 67–73. doi:10.5958/2277-8934.2015.00010.7

Bengoumi, M., Faye, B., & Tressol, J. C. (1998). Composition minérale du lait de chamelle du Sud marocain. In Actes de l'atelier « Chameaux et dromadaires, animaux laitiers », 24-26 Oct. 1994, Nouakchott. CIRAD (coll. Colloques).

Bengoumi, M., Essamadi, A. K., Chacornac, J. P., Tressol, J. C., & Faye, B. (1998a). Comparative relationship between copper-zinc plasma concentration and superoxide dismutase activity in camels and cow. *Veterinary Research, 29*, 557–565. PMID:9851012

Bengoumi, M., Essamadi, A. K., Tressol, J. C., Chacornac, J. P., & Faye, B. (1998). Comparative effect of selenium concentration and erythrocyte gluthatione peroxidase activity in cattle and camels. *Animal Science (Penicuik, Scotland)*, *67*, 461–466. doi:10.1017/S1357729800032872

Bengoumi, M., & Faye, B. (2002). Adaptation du dromadaire à la déshydratation. *Sécheresse*, *13*, 121–129.

Benjakul, S., Kittiphattanabawon, P., & Regenstein, J. M. (2012). Fish gelatin. In B. K. Simpson (Ed.), *Food biochemistry and food processing* (2nd ed.; pp. 388–405). John Wiley & Sons. doi:10.1002/9781118308035.ch21

Benkerroum, N., Mekkaoui, M., Bennani, N., & Kamal, H. (2004). Antimicrobial activity of camel's milk against pathogenic strains of Escherichia coli and Listeria monocytogene. *International Journal of Dairy Technology*, *57*(1), 39–43. doi:10.1111/j.1471-0307.2004.00127.x

Benmohamed, C., Siboukeur, O., & Edoud, A. (2018). Influence of feeding on some physicochemical and biochemical characteristics of camel milk (*Camelus dromadarius*). *Emirates Journal of Food and Agriculture*, *30*(4), 251–255. doi:10.9755/ejfa.2018.v30.i4.1658

Bennett, R. M., & Kokocinski, T. (1978). Lactoferrin content of peripheral blood cells. *British Journal of Haematology*, *39*(4), 509–521. doi:10.1111/j.1365-2141.1978.tb03620.x PMID:359033

Berg, E. H. (1992). *Reaction of lactose during heat treatment of milk: A quantitative study* (Ph.D Thesis). Wageningen Agricultural University, The Netherlands.

Berger, M. M., & Shenkin, A. (1998). Trace elements in trauma and burns. *Current Opinion in Clinical Nutrition and Metabolic Care*, *1*(6), 513–517. doi:10.1097/00075197-199811000-00006 PMID:10565403

Berhe, T., Ipsen, R., Seifu, E., Kurtu, M. Y., Eshetu, M., & Hansen, E. B. (2018). Comparison of the acidification activities of commercial starter cultures in camel and bovine milk. *LWT*, *89*, 123–127. doi:10.1016/j.lwt.2017.10.041

Berhe, T., Seifu, E., Ipsen, R., Kurtu, M. Y., & Hansen, E. B. (2017). Processing challenges and opportunities of camel dairy products. *International Journal of Food Sciences*, *2017*, 9061757. doi:10.1155/2017/9061757 PMID:29109953

Beriain, M.J., Bass, P., Purroy, A., & Treacher, T. (2000). Effect of animal and nutritional factors and nutrition on lamb meat quality. *Centre international de hautes études agronomiques méditerranéennes*, 75-86.

Bernard, F., & Pascal, B. (2012). Camel sciences and economy in the world: current situation and perspectives. *Proc. 3rd ISOCARD Conference. Keynote Presentations, 2*–15.

Beto, J. A. (2015). The Role of Calcium in Human Aging. *Clinical Nutrition Research*, *4*(1), 1–8. doi:10.7762/cnr.2015.4.1.1 PMID:25713787

Beukes, E. M., Bester, B. H., & Mostert, J. F. (2001). The microbiology of South African traditional fermented milks. *International Journal of Food Microbiology*, *63*(3), 189–197. doi:10.1016/S0168-1605(00)00417-7

Biesalski, H. (2005). Meat as a component of a healthy diet – Are there any risks or benefits if meat is avoided in the diet? *Meat Science*, *70*(3), 509–524. doi:10.1016/j.meatsci.2004.07.017 PMID:22063749

Bin Saeed, A. A., Al-Hamdan, N. A., & Fontaine, R. E. (2005). *Plague from Eating Raw Camel Liver. Emerg.Inbfec. bDis.bb11*. Available from http://www.cdc.gov/ncidod/EID/vol11no09/05-0081.htm

Bin Saeed, A. A., Al-Hamdan, N. A., & Fontaine, R. E. (2005). Plague from Eating Raw Camel Liver. *Advances in Food Research*, *26*, 53–213. PMID:16229781

Biratu, K., & Seifu, E. (2016). Chemical composition and microbiological quality of Dhanaan: Traditional fermented camel milk produced in eastern Ethiopia. *International Food Research Journal*, *23*(5), 2223–2228.

Birchal, V., Passos, M., Wildhagen, G., & Mujumdar, A. (2005). Effect of spray-dryer operating variables on the whole milk powder quality. *Drying Technology*, *23*(3), 611–636. doi:10.1081/DRT-200054153

Blanc, C. P., & Hennesser, Y. (1989). Approche zoogéographique de la différenciation infraspécifique chez le dromadaire Camelus dromedarius Linné, 1766 (Mammalia: Camelidae). *Revue d'Élevage et de Médecine Vétérinaire des Pays Tropicaux*, *42*, 573–587.

Blasbalg, T. L., Hibbeln, J. R., Ramsden, C. E., Majchrzak, S. F., & Rawlings, R. R. (2011). Changes in consumption of omega-3 and omega-6 fatty acids in the United States during the 20th century. *The American Journal of Clinical Nutrition*, *93*(5), 950–962. doi:10.3945/ajcn.110.006643 PMID:21367944

Bloomer, R. J., Butawan, M., Farney, T. M., & McAllister, M. J. (2019). An Overview of the Dietary Ingredient Carnitine. In *Nutrition and Enhanced Sports Performance* (pp. 605–617). Elsevier. doi:10.1016/B978-0-12-813922-6.00051-5

Blum, J. W., & Hammon, H. (2000). Colostrum effects on the gastrointestinal tract, and on nutritional, endocrine and metabolic parameters in neonatal calves. *Livestock Production Science*, *66*(2), 151–159. doi:10.1016/S0301-6226(00)00222-0

Boehm, G., & Stahl, B. (2003). Oligosaccharides. In Functional Dairy Products (pp. 203-243). Cambridge, UK: Woodhead Publishers.

Boehm, G., & Stahl, B. (2007). Oligosaccharides from Milk. *The Journal of Nutrition*, *137*(3), 847S–849S. doi:10.1093/jn/137.3.847S PMID:17311985

Boelsma, E., Hendriks, H. F., & Roza, L. (2001). Nutritional skin care: Health effects of micronutrients and fatty acids. *The American Journal of Clinical Nutrition*, *73*(5), 853–864. doi:10.1093/ajcn/73.5.853 PMID:11333837

Bolotin, A., Quinquis, B., Renault, P., Sorokin, A., Ehrlich, S. D., Kulakauskas, S., ... Hols, P. (2004). Complete sequence and comparative genome analysis of the dairy bacterium Streptococcus thermophilus. *Nature Biotechnology*, *22*(12), 1554–1558. doi:10.1038/nbt1034

Bornaz, S., Sahli, A., Attalah, A., & Attia, H. (2009). Physicochemical Characteristics and Renneting Properties of Camels' Milk: A Comparison with Goats', Ewes' and Cows' Milks. *International Journal of Dairy Technology*, *62*(4), 505–513. doi:10.1111/j.1471-0307.2009.00535.x

Borschell, M., Elkin, R., Kirksey, A., Story, J., Galal, O., Harrison, G., & Jerome, N. (1986). Fatty acid composition of mature human milk of Egyptian and American women. *The American Journal of Clinical Nutrition*, *44*(3), 330–335. doi:10.1093/ajcn/44.3.330 PMID:3751954

Boudjenah-Haroun, S., Laleye, L., Moulti-Mati, F., Si Ahmed, S., Mahboub, N., Siboukeur, O. E., & Mati, A. (2011). Comparative study of milk clotting activity of crude gastric enzymes extracted from camels' abomasum at different ages and commercial enzymes (rennet and pepsin) on bovine and camel milk. *Emirates Journal of Food and Agriculture*, *23*, 301–310.

Bouhaddaoui, S., Chabir, R., Errachidi, F., El Ghadraoui, L., El Khalfi, B., Benjelloun, M., & Soukri, A. (2019). Study of the Biochemical Biodiversity of Camel Milk. Hindawi, the Scientific World Journal.

Bouhaddaoui, S., Chabir, R., Errachidi, F., El Ghadraoui, L., El Khalfi, B., Benjelloun, M., & Soukri, A. (2019). Study of the Biochemical Biodiversity of Camel Milk. The Scientific World Journal.

Bouhaddaoui, S., Chabir, R., Errachidi, F., El Ghadraoui, L., El Khalfi, B., Benjelloun, M., & Soukri, A. (2019). Study of the Biochemical Biodiversity of Camel Milk. *The Scientific World Journal*. PMID:31093015

Boulanger, A., Grosclaude, F., & Mahé, M. F. (1984). Polymorphisme des caséines αs1 et αs2 de la chèvre (Capra hircus). *Génétique, Sélection. Evolution; International Journal of Organic Evolution*, *16*(2), 157–176.

Boumpa, T., Tsioulpas, A., Grandison, A. S., & Lewis, M. J. (2008). Effects of phosphates and citrates on sediment formation in UHT goats' milk. *The Journal of Dairy Research*, *75*(2), 160–166. doi:10.1017/S0022029908003166 PMID:18474132

Bracco, U., Hidalgo, J., & Bohren, H. (1972). Lipid composition of the fat globule membrane of human and bovine milk. *Journal of Dairy Science*, *55*(2), 165–172. doi:10.3168/jds.S0022-0302(72)85454-7 PMID:4672739

Breitling, L. (2002). Insulin and anti-diabetes activity of camel milk. *Journal of Camel Practice and Research*, *9*(1), 43–45.

Breitling, L. (2002). Insulin and anti-diabetic activity of camel milk. *Journal of Camel Practice and Research*, *9*, 43–45.

Breulmann, M., Boer, B., Wernery, U., Wernery, R., El-Shaer, H., Alhadrami, G., ... Norton, J. (2007). *The camel, from tradition to modern times*. Doha, Qatar: UNESCO Doha Publ.

Brezovečki, A., Cagalj, M., Dermit, Z. F., Mikulec, N., Ljoljić, D., &Antunac, N. (2015). *Camel milk and milk products. Mljekarstvo/Dairy*, *65*(2), 81-90.

Brezovečki, A., Čagalj, M., Dermit, Z. F., Mikulec, N., Ljoljić, D. B., & Antunac, N. (2015). Camel Milk and Milk Products. *Camel Milk. Mljekarstvo*, *65*, 81–90.

Bright, L. Y., & Jing,, H., Heller, S., & Ri Mutu, J. (2017). Progress in Molecular Genetics of Bactrian Camel Origin and Evolution. *Acta Ecologiae Animalis Domastici*, *38*(3), 5–9.

Brodowska, M., Guzek, D., Kołota, A., Głabska, D., Górska-Horczyczak, E., Wojtasik-Kalinowska, I., & Wierzbicka, A. (2016). Effect of diet on oxidation and profile of volatile compounds of pork after freezing storage. *Journal of Food and Nutrition Research*, *55*, 40–47.

Brondino, N., Fusar-Poli, L., Rocchetti, M., Provenzani, U., Barale, F., & Politi, P. (2015). Complementary and alternative therapies for autism spectrum disorder. *Evidence-Based Complementary and Alternative Medicine*. PMID:26064157

Brooke, M. H., & Kaiser, K. K. (1970). Three myosin ATPase systems, the nature of their pH lability and sulfhydral dependence. *The Journal of Histochemistry and Cytochemistry*, *18*, 670–672. doi:10.1177/18.9.670 PMID:4249441

Brown, K. (2006). Tropical medicine and animal diseases: Onderstepoort and the development of veterinary science in South Africa 1908-1950. *South African Studies*, *31*(3), 513–529. doi:10.1080/03057070500202139 PMID:16628249

Brückner, H., & Fujii, N. (2010). *D-Amino Acids in Chemistry, Life Sciences and Biotechnology*. Weinheim, Germany: Verlag Helvetica ChimicaActa, Zürich, Switzerland and Wiley-VCH.

Brueckner, H., & Hausch, M. (1990). D-amino acids in dairy products: Detection, origin and nutritional aspects. I. Milk, fermented milk, fresh cheese and acid crude cheese. *Milchwissenschaft. Milk Science International*, *45*, 357–360.

Buchheim, W., & Abou El Nour, A. M. (1992). Induction of Milkfat Crystallisation In the Emulsified State by High Hydrostatic Pressure. *Fett Wissenschaft Technologie*, *94*(10), 369–373. doi:10.1002/lipi.19920941003

Buchta, R. (1991). Ovine lactoferrin: Isolation from colostrum and characterization. *The Journal of Dairy Research*, *58*(2), 211–218. doi:10.1017/S0022029900029757 PMID:1856354

Buffa, M., Trujillo, A. J., & Guamis, B. (2001a). Rennet Coagulation Properties of Raw, Pasteurised And High Pressure-Treated Goat Milk. *Milchwissenschaft. Milk Science International*, *56*(5), 243–246.

Buffa, M., Trujillo, A. J., & Guamis, B. (2001b). Changes in Textural, Microstructure, And Colour Characteristics During Ripening of Cheeses Made from Raw, Pasteurised Or High-Pressure-Treated Goats' Milk. *International Dairy Journal*, *11*(11–12), 927–934. doi:10.1016/S0958-6946(01)00141-8

Bühler, C., Hammon, H., Rossi, G. L., & Blum, J. W. (1998). Small intestinal morphology in eight-day-old calves fed colostrum for different durations or only milk replacer and treated with long-R3-insulin-like growth factor I and growth hormone. *Journal of Animal Science*, *76*(3), 758–765. doi:10.2527/1998.763758x PMID:9535335

Bukovics, S., Hucker, A., & Szafner, G. (2015). Impact of microfiltration on camel milk's microbiological and organoleptic characteristics. *Scientific and Practical Journal Veterinariya, 2*(42), 168-170.

Bulca, S. (2017). Functional properties of camel milk and their influences on technological applications. *Scientific Bulletin. Series F. Biotechnologies*, *21*, 275–283.

Bulliet, R. W. (1975). *The camel and the wheel.* Cambridge, MA: Harvard University Press.

Buonopane, G. J., Kilara, A., Smith, J. S., & McCarthy, R. D. (1992). Effect of skim milk supplementation on blood cholesterol concentration, blood pressure, and triglycerides in a free-living human population. *Journal of the American College of Nutrition*, *11*(1), 56–67. doi:10.1080/07315724.1992.10718197 PMID:1541797

Burger, P. (2016). The history of old world camelids in the light of molecular genetics. *Tropical Animal Production*, *48*(5), 905–913. doi:10.100711250-016-1032-7 PMID:27048619

Burger, P., Ciani, E., & Faye, B. (2019). Old World camels in a modern world – a balancing act between conservation and genetic improvement. *Animal Genetics*, *50*(6), 598–612. doi:10.1111/age.12858 PMID:31532019

Businco, L., Bruno, G., Giampietro, P., & Cantoni, A. (1992). Allergenicity and nutritional adequacy of soy protein formulas. *The Journal of Pediatrics*, *121*(5), S21–S28. doi:10.1016/S0022-3476(05)81402-7 PMID:1447630

Bussa, N., Belayneh, A., & Deressa, M. (2017). The Potential of Camel Milk and Extracts of Major Plants Browsed by the Animal for Diabetes Treatment. *East African Journal of Sciences*, *11*(2), 129–138.

Butikofer, U., Meyer, J., Sieber, R., & Wechsler, D. (2007). Quantification of the angiotensinconverting enzyme-inhibiting tripeptides Val Pro-Pro and Ile-Pro-Pro in hard, semi-hard and soft cheeses. *International Dairy Journal*, *17*(8), 968–975. doi:10.1016/j.idairyj.2006.11.003

Butz, P., Zielinski, B., Ludwig, H., & Tauscher, B. (1999). The Influence of High Pressure on The Autoxidation of Major Unsaturated Fatty Acid Constituents of Milk. In H. Ludwig (Ed.), *Advances in High Pressure Bioscience and Biotechnology* (pp. 453–456). Heidelberg, Germany: Springer. doi:10.1007/978-3-642-60196-5_82

Buyong, N., Kok, J., & Luchansky, J. B. (1998). Use of a Genetically Enhanced, Pediocin-Producing Starter Culture, Lactococcus lactis subsp. Lactis MM217, To Control Listeria monocytogenes in Cheddar Cheese. *Applied and Environmental Microbiology*, *64*(12), 4842–4845.

Bylund, G. (1983). Dairy Processing Handbook. Tetra Pack Processing Systems.

Bylund, G. (2003). *Dairy processing handbook.* Tetra Pak Processing Systems AB.

Cadesky, L., Walkling-Ribeiro, M., Kriner, K. T., Karwe, M. V., & Moraru, C. I. (2017). Structural changes induced by high-pressure processing in micellar casein and milk protein concentrates. *Journal of Dairy Science*, *100*(9), 7055–7070. doi:10.3168/jds.2016-12072 PMID:28647329

Calkin, C. R., Dutson, T. R., Smith, G. C., Carpenter, Z. I., & Davis, G. W. (1981). Relationship of fibre type composition to marbling and tenderness of bovine muscle. *Journal of Food Science*, *46*(3), 708–710. doi:10.1111/j.1365-2621.1981.tb15331.x

Camel cookies®. (2019). *Camel cookies.* Retrieved in 19th May from https://web.facebook.com/pg/camelcookiespage/about/?ref=page_internal

Camel milk South Africa®. (2019). *Organic camel milk.* Retrieved from https://camelmilksouthafrica.co.za/

Camel, O. Dairy®. (2019). *Camel Milk Soap, Skincare and Chocolate.* Retrieved in 13th May, 2019 from: https://camel-dairy.com/shop?olsPage=products

Camelait®. (2019*). Al Ain – the leading producer of Camel Milk in the UAE.* Retrieved in 22nd May, from: http://camelait.asia/

Cameron, A. J., Shaw, J. E., & Zimmet, P. Z. (2004). The metabolic syndrome: Prevalence in worldwide populations. *Endocrinology and Metabolism Clinics, 33*(2), 351–375. doi:10.1016/j.ecl.2004.03.005 PMID:15158523

Camier, B., Beaucher, E., Gaucheron, F., Konuspayeva, G., & Faye, B. (2014). Fabrication et caractérisation physico-chimique d'un fromage « blanc » fabriqué à partir de lait de chamelle-une comparaison avec le lait de vache. Actes des 1ères rencontres internationales "le lait, vecteur de développement", 105.

Camilk®Dairy. (2019). *About camel milk & all natural camel milk products.* Retrieved in 22nd May, 2019 from: https://www.camilkdairy.com/pages/faq

Capellas, M., Mor-Mur, M., & Needs, E. C. (2001). *Physical Properties of Yoghurt from Pressurised Concentrated and Fortified Milks.* In Eurocaft Meeting, Berlin, Germany.

Cardak, A. D., Yetismeyen, A., & Brückner, H. (2003). Quantitative comparison of free fatty acids in camel, goat and cow milk. *Milchwissenschaft. Milk Science International, 58*, 127–130.

Cardoso, R. R. A., Santos, R., Cardoso, C., & Carvalho, M. (2010). Consumption of camel's milk by patients intolerant to lactose: A preliminary study. *Revista Alergia Mexico, 57*, 3–26. PMID:20857626

Cardoso, R., Santos, R., Cardoso, C., & Carvalho, M. (2010). 12 Consumption of camel's milk by patients intolerant to lactose. A preliminary study. 13. *Revista Alergia Mexico, 57*, 26–32. PMID:20857626

Carnagey, K. M., Huff-Lonergan, E. J., Trenkle, A., Wertz-Lutz, A. E., Horst, R. L., & Beitz, D. C. (2008). Use of 25-hydroxyvitamin D3 and vitamin E to improve tenderness of beef from the longissimus dorsi of heifers. *Journal of Animal Science, 86*(7), 1649–1657. doi:10.2527/jas.2007-0502 PMID:18344288

Carter, D. C., & Ho, J. X. (1994). Structure of serum albumin. In C. B. Anfinsen, J. T. Edsall, F. M. Richards, & D. S. Eisenberg (Eds.), *Advances in protein chemistry* (pp. 153–203). New York: Academic Press.

Casey, N. H. (1993). Carcass and meat quality. In C. Maree & N. H. Casey (Eds.), *Livestock production systems; principles and practice* (pp. 306–333). Brooklyn, South Africa: Agri-Development Foundation.

Cassens, R. G., & Cooper, C. (1971). Red and white muscle. *Advances in Food Research, 19*, 1–45. doi:10.1016/S0065-2628(08)60030-0 PMID:5000245

Castro-Gómez, M. P., Rodriguez-Alcalá, L. M., Calvo, M. V., Romero, J., Mendiola, J. A., Ibañez, E., & Fontecha, J. (2014). Total milk fat extraction and quantification of polar and neutral lipids of cow, goat, and ewe milk by using a pressurized liquid system and chromatographic techniques. *Journal of Dairy Science, 97*(11), 6719–6728. doi:10.3168/jds.2014-8128 PMID:25200790

Catini, M. V., Savini, I., Rossi, A., Melino, G., & Avigliano, L. (2005). Biological role of vitamin C in keratinocytes. *Nutrition Reviews, 63*(3), 81–90. doi:10.1111/j.1753-4887.2005.tb00125.x PMID:15825810

Cauvain, S. P. (2016). Cookies, Biscuits and Crackers: Formulation, Processing and Characteristics. In C. Wrigley, H. Corke, K. Seetharaman, & J. Faubion (Eds.), *Encyclopedia of Food Grains* (2nd ed.; pp. 37–43). Oxford, UK: Academic Press. doi:10.1016/B978-0-12-394437-5.00119-4

Cavallini, D. C., Bedani, R., Bomdespacho, L. Q., Vendramini, R. C., & Rossi, E. A. (2009). Effects of probiotic bacteria, isoflavones and simvastatin on lipid profile and atherosclerosis in cholesterol-fed rabbits: A randomized double-blind study. *Lipids in Health and Disease*, *8*(1), 1. doi:10.1186/1476-511X-8-1

CDC. (2019). *Data & Statistics on Autism Spectrum Disorder*. Retrieved from https://www.cdc.gov/ncbddd/autism/data.html

Cecchi, G. W., Shaw, W., Marletta, A., Mattioli, A., & Robinson, T. (2010). Geographic distribution and environmental characterization of livestock production systems in Eastern Africa. *Agriculture, Ecosystems & Environment*, *135*(1-2), 98–110. doi:10.1016/j.agee.2009.08.011

Cekici, H., & Sanlier, N. (2019). Current nutritional approaches in managing autism spectrum disorder: A review. *Nutritional Neuroscience*, *22*(3), 145–155. doi:10.1080/1028415X.2017.1358481 PMID:28762296

Cenci-Goga, B. T., Karama, M., Sechi, P., Iulietto, M. F., Novelli, S., Selvaggini, R., & Mattei, S. (2015). Growth Inhibition of Selected Microorganisms by an Association of Dairy Starter Cultures and Probiotics. *Italian Journal of Animal Science*, *14*(2), 3745. doi:10.4081/ijas.2015.3745

Chaibou, M. (2005). *Productivité zootechnique du désert: le cas du bassin laitier d'Agadez au Niger* (PhD thesis). Université de Montpellier.

Chaibou, M., & Faye, B. (2005). Fonctionnement des élevages camelins de la zone périurbaine d'Agadez au Niger: Enquête typologique. *Revue d'Élevage et de Médecine Vétérinaire des Pays Tropicaux*, *58*(4), 273–283. doi:10.19182/remvt.9922

Chakaravarthi, I. S., & Verschoore, M. (Eds.). (n.d.). *Basic sciences for modern cosmetic dermatology*. New Delhi, India: Jaypee Brothers Medical Publishers.

Chandan, R. C., Shahani, K. M., & Holly, R. G. (1964). Lysozyme Content of Human Milk. *Nature*, *204*(4953), 76–77. doi:10.1038/204076a0 PMID:14240122

Chang, M. C., & Tanaka, J. (2002). FT-IR study for hydroxyapatitecollagen nanocomposite cross-linked by glutaraldehyde. *Biomaterials*, *23*(24), 4811–4818. doi:10.1016/S0142-9612(02)00232-6 PMID:12361620

Chan, I. L., Cohen, S., da Cunha, M. G., & Maluf, L. C. (2018). Characteristics and management of Asian skin. *International Journal of Dermatology*, *2018*, 1–13. doi:10.1111/ijd.14153 PMID:30039861

Chan, W. (2004). Macronutrients in meat. In W. K. Jensen, C. Devine, & M. Dikeman (Eds.), *Encyclopedia of meat science* (pp. 614–618). Oxford, UK: Elsevier Academic Press. doi:10.1016/B0-12-464970-X/00235-X

Chao, A., Thun, M., Connell, C., McCullough, M., Jacobs, E., & Flanders, W. (2005). Meat consumption and risk of colorectal cancer. *Journal of the American Medical Association*, *293*(2), 172–182. doi:10.1001/jama.293.2.172 PMID:15644544

Chaplin, L. C., & Lyster, R. L. J. (1988). Effect of Temperature on The Ph Of Skim Milk. *The Journal of Dairy Research*, *55*(2), 280. doi:10.1017/S0022029900026108

Chapman, M. J. (1991). Camels. *Biologist, 38*, 41-44.

Charlier, P., Huynh-Charlier, I., Munoz, O., Billard, M., Brun, L., & de la Grandmaison, G. L. (2010). The microscopic (optical and SEM) examination of dental calculus deposits (DCD). Potential interest in forensic anthropology of a bioarchaeological method. *Legal Medicine*, *12*(4), 163–171. doi:10.1016/j.legalmed.2010.03.003 PMID:20444636

Chawla, R., Patil, G. R., & Singh, A. K. (2011). High hydrostatic pressure technology in dairy processing: A review. *Journal of Food Science and Technology*, *48*(3), 260–268. doi:10.100713197-010-0180-4 PMID:23572744

Cheftel, J. C. (1995). Review: High-Pressure, Microbial Inactivation and Food Preservation. *Food Science & Technology International*, *1*(2–3), 75–90. doi:10.1177/108201329500100203

Chen, B. Y., Grandison, A. S., & Lewis, M. J. (2012). Comparison of Heat Stability of Goat Milk Subjected to Ultra-High Temperature and In-Container Sterilization. *Journal of Dairy Science*, *95*(3), 1057–1063. doi:10.3168/jds.2011-4367 PMID:22365189

Chen, C., Wang, P., Zhang, N., Zhang, W., & Ren, F. (2019). Improving the textural properties of camel milk acid gel by treatment with trisodium citrate and transglutaminase. *Lebensmittel-Wissenschaft + Technologie*, *103*, 53–59. doi:10.1016/j.lwt.2018.12.063

Chiang, M.-L., Chen, H.-C., Wang, S.-Y., Hsieh, Y.-L., & Chen, M.-J. (2011). Use of Taiwanese Ropy Fermented Milk (TRFM) and Lactococcus lactis subsp. Cremoris Isolated from TRFM in Manufacturing of Functional Low-Fat Cheeses. *Journal of Food Science*, *76*(7), M504–M510. doi:10.1111/j.1750-3841.2011.02320.x

Chilliard, Y., Ferlay, A., & Doreau, M. (2001). Contrôle de la qualité nutritionnelle des matières grasses du lait par l'alimentation des vaches laitières: Acides gras trans, polyinsaturés, acide linoléique conjugué. *Productions Animales*, *14*, 323–335.

Chniter, M., Hammadi, M., Khorchani, T., Krit, R., Benwahada, A., & Hamoud, M. B. (2013). Classification of Maghrebi camels (Camelus dromedarius) according to their tribal affiliation and body traits in southern Tunisia. *Emirates Journal of Food and Agriculture*, *25*(8), 625–634. doi:10.9755/ejfa.v25i8.16096

Choi, S., Park, K., Kim, D., Lee, D., & Kim, Y. (2013). Preparation of Camel Milk Liposome and Its Anti-Aging Effects. *Journal of the Society of Cosmetic Scientists of Korea*, *40*(2), 155–161. doi:10.15230/SCSK.2014.40.2.155

Christian, O., Khunger, N., Saraf, V., & Clarie, B. (2015). *Peeling and fillers*. Academic Press.

Chung, J. H., Seo, J. Y., Lee, M. K., Eun, H. C., Lee, J. H., Kang, S., ... Voorhees, J. J. (2002). Ultraviolet modulation of human macrophage metalloelastase in human skin in vivo. *The Journal of Investigative Dermatology*, *119*(2), 507–512. doi:10.1046/j.1523-1747.2002.01844.x PMID:12190877

Chuvakova, Z., Beisembayeva, R., Puzyrevskaya, Saubenouva, O., Shamenova, M., Glebova, M., … Baimenov, E. K. (2000). Chemical Composition, Microbial Control and Antiviral Properties of Freshly Made and Conserved Shubat "Bota." *Proc. 2nd International Camelid Conference Agro economics of Camelid Farming*, 8-12.

Cissé, H., Muandze-Nzambe, J. U., Somda, N. S., Sawadogo, A., Drabo, S. M., Tapsoba, F., ... Savadogo, A. (2019). Assessment of safety and quality of fermented milk of camels, cows, and goats sold and consumed in five localities of Burkina Faso. *Veterinary World*, *12*(2), 295–304. doi:10.14202/vetworld.2019.295-304

Claeys, W. L., Cardoen, S., Daube, G., De Block, J., Dewettinck, K., Dierick, K., ... Herman, L. (2013). Raw or heated cow milk consumption: Review of risks and benefits. *Food Control*, *31*(1), 251–262. doi:10.1016/j.foodcont.2012.09.035

Claeys, W. L., Verraes, C., Cardoen, S., De Block, J., Huyghebaert, A., Raes, K., & Herman, L. (2014). Consumption of raw or heated milk from different species: An evaluation of the nutritional and potential health benefits. *Food Control*, *42*, 188–201. doi:10.1016/j.foodcont.2014.01.045

Clark, K. A., McElhinny, A. S., Beckerle, M. C., & Gregorio, C. C. (2002). Striated muscle cytoarchitecture: An intricate web of form and function. *Annual Review of Cell and Developmental Biology*, *18*(1), 637–706. doi:10.1146/annurev.cellbio.18.012502.105840 PMID:12142273

Colville, T., & Bassert, J. M. (2002). *Clinical Anatomy and Physiology for Veterinary Technicians*. St Louis, MO: Mosby, Inc.

Conesa, C., Sanchez, L., Rota, C., Pérez, M. D., Calvo, M., Farnaud, S., & Ewans, R. W. (2008). Isolation of lactoferrin from milk of different species: Calorimetric and antimicrobial studies. *Comparative Biochemistry & Physiology, Part B., 150*(1), 131–139. doi:10.1016/j.cbpb.2008.02.005 PMID:18387837

Considine, T., Patel, H. A., Anema, S. G., Singh, H., & Creamer, L. K. (2007). Interactions of milk proteins during heat and high hydrostatic pressure treatments— A Review. *Innovative Food Science & Emerging Technologies, 8*(1), 1–23. doi:10.1016/j.ifset.2006.08.003

Contarini, G., Povolo, M., Leardi, R., & Toppino, P. M. (1997). Influence of heat treatment on the volatile compounds of milk. *Journal of Agricultural and Food Chemistry, 45*(8), 3171–3177. doi:10.1021/jf960849s

Contarini, G., Povolo, M., Pelizzola, V., Monti, L., Bruni, A., Passolungo, L., ... Degano, L. (2014). Bovine colostrum: Changes in lipid constituents in the first 5 days after parturition. *Journal of Dairy Science, 97*(8), 5065–5072. doi:10.3168/jds.2013-7517 PMID:24931528

Coroian, A., Erler, S., Matea, C. T., Mireşan, V., Răducu, C., Bele, C., & Coroian, C. O. (2013). Seasonal changes of buffalo colostrum: Physicochemical parameters, fatty acids and cholesterol variation. *Chemistry Central Journal, 7*(1), 40. doi:10.1186/1752-153X-7-40 PMID:23442377

Corrieu, G., & Béal, C. (2016). Yogurt: The Product and its Manufacture. In Encyclopedia of Food and Health (Vol. 5, pp. 617–624). Elsevier. doi:10.1016/B978-0-12-384947-2.00766-2

Cosentino, C., Labell, C., & Elshafie, H. S. (2016). Effects of different heat treatments on lysozyme quantity and antimicrobial activity of jenny milk. *Journal of Dairy Science, 99*(7), 5173–5179. doi:10.3168/jds.2015-10702 PMID:27157571

Costabel, L. M., Bergamini, C., Vaudagna, S. R., Cuatrin, A. L., Audero, G., & Hynes, E. (2016). Effect of high-pressure treatment on hard cheese proteolysis. *Journal of Dairy Science, 99*(6), 4220–4232. doi:10.3168/jds.2015-9907 PMID:27016833

Cristofanelli, S., Antonini, M., Torres, D., Polidori, P., & Renieri, C. (2004). Meat and carcass quality form Peruvian llama (lama glama) and alpaca (*lama pacos*). *Meat Science, 66*(3), 589–593. doi:10.1016/S0309-1740(03)00174-8 PMID:22060868

Cronshaw, H. B. (1947). *Dairy Information*. London: Dairy Industries Ltd.

Czerwonka, M., & Szterk, A. (2015). The effect of meat cuts and thermal processing on selected mineral concentration in beef from Holstein–Friesian bulls. *Meat Science, 105*, 75–80. doi:10.1016/j.meatsci.2015.03.011 PMID:25828160

D'Aniello, G., Grieco, N., Filippo, M., Capiello, F., Topo, E., D'Aniello, E., & Ronsini, S. (2007). Reproductive implication of D-aspartic acid in human pre-ovulatory follicular fluid. *Human Reproduction (Oxford, England), 22*(12), 3178–3183. doi:10.1093/humrep/dem328 PMID:17951582

Darwish, H. A., Abd Raboh, N. R., & Mahdy, A. (2012). *Camel's milk alleviates alcohol-induced liver injury in rats*. doi:10.1016/j.fct.2012.01.016

Datta, N., & Deeth, H. C. (2007). *Advances in Thermal and Non-Thermal Food Preservation*. Ames, IA: Blackwell Publishing. doi:10.1002/9780470277898.ch4

Datta, N., Elliott, A. J., Perkins, M. L., & Deeth, H. C. (2002). Ultra-high-temperature (UHT) treatment of milk: Comparison of direct and indirect mods of heating. *Australian Journal of Dairy Technology, 57*(3), 211–227.

Davis, J. G. (1955). *A Dictionary of Dairying (2nd ed.)*. London: Leonard Hill.

Dawood, A. (1995). Physical and Sensory characteristics of Najdi camel meat. *Meat Science*, *39*(1), 59–69. doi:10.1016/0309-1740(95)80007-7 PMID:22059763

Dawood, A., & Alkanhal, M. A. (1995). Nutrient composition of Najdi- Camel Meat. *Meat Science*, *39*(1), 71–78. doi:10.1016/0309-1740(95)80008-5 PMID:22059764

De Vuyst, L., Zamfir, M., Mozzi, F., Adriany, T., Marshall, V., Degeest, B., & Vaningelgem, F. (2003). Exopolysaccharide-producing Streptococcus thermophilus strains as functional starter cultures in the production of fermented milks. *3rd NIZO Dairy Conference - Dynamics of Texture, Process and Perception (Part 1)*, *13*(8), 707–717. 10.1016/S0958-6946(03)00105-5

Decker, E. A., & Park, Y. (2010). Healthier meat products as functional foods. *Meat Science*, *86*(1), 49–55. doi:10.1016/j.meatsci.2010.04.021 PMID:20580991

Deen, A. (2013). Reproductive performance in camel (*Camelus dromedarius*). *Camel: An International Journal of Veterinary Sciences*, *1*, 13–27.

Deeth, H. C., & Datta, N. (2011). Heat Treatment of Milk; Ultra-High Temperature Treatment (UHT): Heating Systems. In Encyclopedia of Dairy Sciences (2nd ed.; pp. 699-707). San Diego, CA: Academic Press.

Deeth, H. C. (2002). Lipolysis in Milk and Dairy Products – A Research Journey. *Food Australia*, *54*, 433–436.

Dell'Orto, V., Cattaneo, D., Beretta, E., Baldi, A., & Savoini, G. (2000). Effect of trace element supplementation on milk yield and composition in camels. *International Dairy Journal*, *10*(12), 873–879. doi:10.1016/S0958-6946(01)00023-1

Delves-Broughton, J., Blackburn, P., Evans, R. J., & Hugenholtz, J. (1996). Applications of the bacteriocin, nisin. *Antonie van Leeuwenhoek*, *69*(2), 193–202. doi:10.1007/BF00399424

Dennis, E., Russell, L., & Edwards, G. (2010). Feral camels in the Australian rangelands (2010). In *Proceedings of the 16th Biennial Conference of the Australian Rangeland Society*. Australian Rangeland Society.

Deosarkar, S., Khedkar, C., Kalyankar, S., & Sarode, A. (2016). Ice cream: uses and method of manufacture. In B. Caballero, P. Finglas, & F. Toldrá (Eds.), *The Encyclopedia of food and health* (pp. 391–397). Oxford, UK: Academic Press. doi:10.1016/B978-0-12-384947-2.00384-6

Desert farms®. (2019). *Desert farms camel milk*. Retrieved in 22nd May, 2019 from: https://desertfarms.com/pages/our-practices

Desorby-Banon, S., Richard, F., & Hardy, J. (1994). Study of Acid and Rennet Coagulation of High Pressurized Milk. *Journal of Dairy Science*, *77*(11), 3267–3274. doi:10.3168/jds.S0022-0302(94)77267-2

Desouky, M., Shalaby, M., & Soryal, K. (2013). Compositional, rheological and organoleptic qualities of camel milk *Labneh* as affected by some milk heat treatments. *World Journal of Dairy & Food Sciences*, *8*(2), 118–130.

Desrosier, N. (2008). *Food Preservation Technology* (M. Mulyoharjo & D. Wijoyono, Trans.). Jakarta: University of Indonesia Press.

Devi, A. F., Buckow, R., Singh, T., Hemar, Y., & Kasapis, S. (2015). Colour Change and Proteolysis of Skim Milk during High Pressure Thermal–Processing. *Journal of Food Engineering*, *147*, 102–110. doi:10.1016/j.jfoodeng.2014.09.017

Diaz-Medina, E. (2017) *Studies on identification, lactation and rearing of dromedaries in the Island of Fuerteventura (Canary Islands)* (PhD thesis). University Autonomous of Barcelona, Spain. Available: http://camelides.cirad.fr/fr/science/these_diaz_medina.html

Dickson, H. R. (1951). *The Arab of the desert*. London: George Allen & Unwin Ltd.

Dikeman, M. E., Hunt, M. C., Addist, P. B., Schoenbeck, H. J., Pullen, M., Katsanidis, E., & Yancey, E. J. (2003). Effects of postexsanguination vascular infusion of cattle with a solution of saccharides, sodium chloride, and phosphates or with calcium chloride on quality and sensory traits of steaks and ground beef. *Journal of Animal Science*, *81*(1), 156–166. doi:10.2527/2003.811156x PMID:12597386

Dina, D., & Klintegerg, R. (1977). *Proposal for a rural development training project and study concerned with camel utilization in arid lands in Ethiopia*. Academic Press.

Dittmann, M.T., Runge, U., Lang, R.A., Moser, D., Galeffi, C., Kreuzer, M., & Clauss, M. (2014). Methane emission by camelids. *Plos One*, *9*(4).

Djadouni, F., & Kihal, M. (2012). Antimicrobial activity of lactic acid bacteria and the spectrum of their biopeptides against spoiling germs in foods. *Brazilian Archives of Biology and Technology*, *55*(3), 435–444. doi:10.1590/S1516-89132012000300015

Donkor, O. N., Henriksson, A., Singh, T. K., Vasiljevic, T., & Shah, N. P. (2007). ACE-inhibitory activity of probiotic yoghurt. *International Dairy Journal*, *17*(11), 1321–1331. doi:10.1016/j.idairyj.2007.02.009

Dowelmadina, M. M., El Zubeir, I. E. M., Salim, A. D. A., & Arabi, O. H. M. H. (2014). Influence of Some Factors on Composition of Dromedary Camel Milk in Sudan. *Global Journal of Animal Scientific Research*, *2*(2), 120–129.

Doyon, M., & Labrecque, J. A. (2008). Functional foods: A conceptual definition. *British Food Journal*, *110*(11), 1133–1149. doi:10.1108/00070700810918036

Draelos, Z. D. (1995). Photoaging, sunscreens and cosmeceuticals. In Z. D. Draelos (Ed.), *Cosmetics in dermatology* (pp. 233–244). New York, NY: Churchill Living Stone.

Draelos, Z. D. (2018). Cosmetics and cosmeceuticals. In J. L. Bolognia, J. V. Schaffer, & L. Cerroni (Eds.), *Dermatology* (pp. 2578–2580). New York, NY: Elsevier.

Dransfield, E. (1981). Eating quality of DFD beef. *Veterinary Medicine and Animal Science*, *10*, 344–361.

Dreiucker, J., & Vetter, W. (2011). Fatty acids patterns in camel, moose, cow and human milk as determined with GC/MS after silver ion solid phase extraction. *Food Chemistry*, *126*(2), 762–771. doi:10.1016/j.foodchem.2010.11.061

Driot, C., Kamili, A., Bengoumi, M., Faye, B., Delverdier, M., & Taleban, Y. (2011). Study on the epidemiology and of sarcoptic mange and ringworm in the one-humped camel in South of Morocco. *Journal of Camel Practice and Research*, *18*(1), 107–114.

Duance, V. C., Stephens, H. R., Dunn, M., Bailey, A. J., & Dubowitz, V. (1980). A role for collagen in the pathogenesis of muscular dystrophy. *Nature*, *284*(5755), 470–472. doi:10.1038/284470a0 PMID:7360283

Dubey, U., Lal, M., Mittal, A., & Kapur, S. (2015). *Therapeutic potential of Camel Milk*. doi:10.9755/ejfa.2015-04-122

Dubost, M. (2006). La nutrition. Chenelière.

Duconseille, A., Astruc, T., Quintana, N., Meersman, F., & Sante-Lhoutellier, V. (2015). Gelatin structure and composition linked to hard capsule dissolution: A review. *Food Hydrocolloids*, *43*, 360–376. doi:10.1016/j.foodhyd.2014.06.006

Dunne, C. P. (2005). *High Pressure Keeps Food Fresher*. Available At http://www.Natick.Army.Mil/About/Pao/05/05-22.Htm

Dunnett, M., & Harris, R. C. (1997). High-performance liquid chromatographic determination of imidazole dipeptides, histidine, 1 -methylhistidine and 3- methylhistidine in equine and camel muscle and individual muscle fibres. *Journal of Chromatography. B, Biomedical Sciences and Applications*, *688*(1), 47–55. doi:10.1016/S0378-4347(97)88054-1 PMID:9029312

Dunnett, M., Harris, R. C., Soliman, M. Z., & Suwar, A. A. S. (1997). Carnosine, anserine and taurine contents in individual fibres from the middle gluteal muscle of the camel. *Research in Veterinary Science*, *62*(3), 213–216. doi:10.1016/S0034-5288(97)90192-2 PMID:9300536

Dyer, W. J., & Dingle, J. R. (1967). *Fish as Food* (G. Borgstrom, Ed.). Academic.

Dziuba, B., & Dziuba, M. (2014). Milk proteins-derived bioactive peptides in dairy products: Molecular, biological and methodological aspects. *Acta Scientiarum Polonorum. Technologia Alimentaria*, *13*(1), 5–25. doi:10.17306/J.AFS.2014.1.1 PMID:24583380

Earnshaw, R. (1996). High Pressure Food Processing. *Nutrition & Food Science*, *2*(2), 8–11. doi:10.1108/00346659610108966

Ebaid, H. (2014). Promotion of immune and glycaemic functions in streptozotocin-induced diabetic rats treated with undenatured camel milk whey proteins. *Nutrition & metabolism*, *11*(1), 31. doi:10.1186/1743-7075-11-31 PMID:25009576

Ebaid, H., Abdel-salam, B., Hassan, I., Al-Tamimi, J., Metwalli, A., & Alhazza, I. (2015). Camel milk peptide improves wound healing in diabetic rats by orchestrating the redox status and immune response. *Lipids in Health and Disease*, *14*(1), 132–142. doi:10.118612944-015-0136-9 PMID:26498022

Ebaid, H., Abdel-Salam, B., Hassan, I., Al-Tamimi, J., Metwalli, A., & Alhazza, I. (2017). Erratum to: Camel milk peptide improves wound healing in diabetic rats by orchestrating the redox status and immune response. *Lipids in Health and Disease*, *16*(1), 43. doi:10.118612944-017-0421-x PMID:28219371

Ebaid, H., Salem, A., Sayed, A., & Metwalli, A. (2011). Whey protein enhances normal inflammatory responses during cutaneous wound healing in diabetic rats. *Lipids in Health and Disease*, *10*(1), 235. doi:10.1186/1476-511X-10-235 PMID:22168406

Eberhard, P., Strahm, W., & Eyer, H. (1999). High Pressure Treatment of Whipped Cream. *Agrarforschung*, *6*(9), 352–354.

Eckel, R. H., Grundy, S. M., & Zimmet, P. Z. (2005). The metabolic syndrome. *Lancet*, *365*(9468), 1415–1428. doi:10.1016/S0140-6736(05)66378-7 PMID:15836891

Edwards, G. P., Zeng, B., Saalfeld, W. K., Vaarzon-Morel, P., & McGregor, M. (Eds.). (2008). *Managing the impacts of feral camels in Australia: a new way of doing business. DKCRC Report 47*. Alice Springs: Desert Knowledge Cooperative Research Centre. Available at http://www.desertknowledgecrc.com.au/publications/contractresearch.html

Egbal, A. S., Marwa-Babiker, A. E., Mohamed, O. E., & Ismail, E. F. (2017). Morphology and Morphometry of Raw Camel Hair of Some Sudanese Camel types in Kordofan States. *Nova Journal of Medical and Biological Sciences*, *6*, 1–8.

Ehlayel, M., Hazeima, K., Al-Mesaifri, F., & Bener, A. (2011). Camel milk: An alternative for cow's milk allergy in children. *Allergy and Asthma Proceedings*, *32*(3), 255–258. doi:10.2500/aap.2011.32.3429 PMID:21703103

Eisa, M. O., & Hassabo, A. A. (2009). Variations in milk yield and composition between fore and rear udder-halves in she-camel (*Camelus dromedarius*). *Pakistan Journal of Nutrition*, *8*(12), 1868–1872. doi:10.3923/pjn.2009.1868.1872

Ejtahed, H. S., Naslaji, A. N., Mirmiran, P., Yeganeh, M. Z., Hedayati, M., Azizi, F., & Movahedi, A. M. (2015). Effect of camel milk on blood sugar and lipid profile of patients with type 2 diabetes: A pilot clinical trial. *International Journal of Endocrinology and Metabolism*, 13. PMID:25745496

Ejtahed, H., Niasari Naslaji, A., Mirmiran, P., Zraif Yeganeh, M., Hedayati, M., Azizi, F., & Moosavi Movahedi, A. (2014). Effect of Camel Milk on Blood Sugar and Lipid Profile of Patients with Type 2 Diabetes: A Pilot Clinical Trial. *International Journal of Endocrinology and Metabolism, 13*(1). doi:10.5812/ijem.21160 PMID:25745496

Eksterend, B., Larsson, M., & Perlmann, C. (1980). Casein micelle size and composition related to the enzymatic coagulation process. *Biochimica et Biophysica Acta, 660*(3), 361–366. doi:10.1016/0304-4165(80)90284-6 PMID:6772232

El Hatmi, H., Jrad, Z., Oussaief, O., Nasri, W., Sbissi, I., Khorchani, T., & Canabady-Rochelle, L. L. (2018). Fermentation of dromedary camel (*Camelus dromedarius*) milk by *Enterococcus faecium, Streptococcus macedonicus* as a potential alternative of fermented cow milk. *Lebensmittel-Wissenschaft + Technologie, 90*, 373–380. doi:10.1016/j.lwt.2017.12.040

El Khasmi, M., Riad, F., Safwate, A., El Abbadi, N., Farh, M., Faye, B., & Coxam, V. (2005). La chamelle allaitante face au stress calcique: une fonction endocrine adaptée aux conditions désertiques. *Science et changements planétaires/ Sécheresse, 16*(4), 261-267.

El Miniawy, H. M. F., Ahmed, K. A., Tony, M. A., Mansour, S. A., & Salah Khattab, M. M. (2014). *Camel milk inhibits murine hepatic carcinogenesis, initiated by diethylnitrosamine and promoted by phenobarbitone.* doi:10.1016/j.ijvsm.2014.10.004

El Owni, O., & Khater, Z. (2010). Effect of type of flavor on sensory characteristics of ice cream from Factories and Machines. *Australian Journal of Basic and Applied Sciences, 4*(8), 3257-3260.

El Wathig, M., Faye, B., Thevenon, S., Ravel, S., & Bossard, G. (2016). Epidemiological surveys of camel trypanosomosis in Al-jouf, Saudi Arabia based on PCR and ELISA. *Emirates Journal of Food and Agriculture, 28*(3), 212–216. doi:10.9755/ejfa.2015-09-759

El-Abd, M., Abdel-Hamid, M., Ahmed-Farid, O., El-demerdash, M., & Mohamed, Z. (2018). Protective effect of synbiotic fermented camel milk on non-alcoholic fatty liver disease in rats. *Current Science International, 7*(4), 466–480.

El-Agamy, E. I. (1989). *Biological activity of protective proteins of camel milk against pathogenic and nonpathogenic bacteria and viruses* (Ph.D. Thesis). Alexandria University, Alexandria, Egypt.

El-Agamy, E. I. (1994, October). Camel colostrum. II. Antimicrobial factors. In *Proceedings of the Workshop on Camels and Dromedaries as Dairy Animal* (pp. 24-26). Academic Press.

El-Agamy, E. I. (1998). Antimicrobial factors and nutritive value of human milk and other species. Journal of Agricultural Science. *Mansoura University., 23*, 245–254.

El-Agamy, E. I. (2009). Chapter 6: bioactive components in camel milk. In Y.W. Park (Ed.), Bioactive components in milk and dairy products (pp. 159-194). Wiley-Blackwell.

El-Agamy, E. (2007). The challenge of cow milk protein allergy. *Small Ruminant Research, 68*(1-2), 64–72. doi:10.1016/j.smallrumres.2006.09.016

Elagamy, E. I. (2000). Effect of heat treatment on camel milk proteins with respect to antimicrobial factors: A comparison with cows' and buffalo milk proteins. *Food Chemistry, 68*(2), 227–232. doi:10.1016/S0308-8146(99)00199-5

El-Agamy, E. I. (2009). Bioactive components in camel milk. In Y. W. Park (Ed.), *Bioactive components in milk and dairy products* (pp. 159–194). Ames, IA: Wiley-Blackwell Publ. doi:10.1002/9780813821504.ch6

El-Agamy, E. I., Ruppanner, R., Ismail, A., Champagne, C. P., & Assaf, R. (1992). Antibacterial and antiviral activity of camel milk protective proteins. *The Journal of Dairy Research, 59*(2), 169–175. doi:10.1017/S0022029900030417 PMID:1319434

El-Agamy, E., Nawar, M., Shamsia, S., Awad, S., & Haenlein, G. (2009). Are camel milk proteins convenient to the nutrition of cow milk allergic children. *Small Ruminant Research*, *82*(1), 1–6. doi:10.1016/j.smallrumres.2008.12.016

Elayan, A. A., Sulieman, A., & Saleh, F. (2008). The hypocholesterolemic effect of Gariss and Gariss containing bifidobacteria in rats fed on a cholesterol-enriched diet. *Asian J Biochem*, *3*, 43–47. doi:10.3923/ajb.2008.43.47

El-Bashir, O. M. (1997). *Physiological characters and Diseases of camel in the Sudan*. Omdurman Islamic University. (in Arabic)

El-Faer, M. Z., Rawdah, T. N., Attar, K. M., & Dawson, M. V. (1991). Mineral and proximate composition of the meat of the one-humped camel (*Camelus dromedaries*). *Food Chemistry*, *42*(2), 139–143. doi:10.1016/0308-8146(91)90029-N

El-Fakharany, E. N., Abedelbaky, B., Haroun, L., Sanchez, N., Redwan, E., & Redwan, E. M. (2012). Anti-infectivity of camel polyclonal antibodies against hepatitis C virus in Huh 7.5 hepatoma. *Virology Journal*, *16*(9), 201–211. doi:10.1186/1743-422X-9-201 PMID:22978304

El-Fattah, A. M. A., Rabo, F. H. A., El-Dieb, S. M., & El-Kashef, H. A. (2012). Changes in composition of colostrum of Egyptian buffaloes and Holstein cows. *BMC Veterinary Research*, *8*(1), 19. doi:10.1186/1746-6148-8-19 PMID:22390895

Elgasim, E. A., & Alkanhal, M. A. (1992). Proximate composition, amino acids and inorganic mineral content of Arabian Camel meat: Comparative study. *Food Chemistry*, *45*(1), 1–4. doi:10.1016/0308-8146(92)90002-J

El-Gawad, I. A., El-Sayed, E. M., Mahfouz, M. B., & Abd El-Salam, A. M. (1996). Changes of lactoferrin concentration in colostrum and milk from different species. *Egyptian Journal of Dairy Science*, *24*, 297–308.

Elhardallou, S. B., & El-Naggar, A. Y. (2016). Determination of Micro Minerals in Milk from Farm and Pasture-Reared Cow, Goat and Camel using Inductively Coupled Plasma-Optical Emission Spectrometry. *Oriental Journal of Chemistry*, *32*(1), 341–347. doi:10.13005/ojc/320138

Elhasan, S. M., Bushara, A. M., Abdelhakam, K. E., Elfaki, H. A., Eibaid, A. I., Farahat, F. H., ... Sukrab, A. M. (2017). Effect of heat treatments on physico-chemical properties of milk samples. *Journal of Academia and Industrial Research*, *6*, 40–46.

El-Hatmi, H., Girardet, J. M., Gaillard, J. L., Yahyaoui, M. H., & Attia, H. (2007). Characterization of whey proteins of camel (Camelus dromedarius) milk and colostrum. *Small Ruminant Research*, *70*(2-3), 267–271. doi:10.1016/j.smallrumres.2006.04.001

El-Hatmi, H., Levieux, A., & Levieux, D. (2006). Camel (*Camelus dromedarius*) immunoglobulin G, α-lactalbumin, serum albumin and lactoferrin in colostrum and milk during the early *post-partum* period. *The Journal of Dairy Research*, *73*(3), 288–293. doi:10.1017/S0022029906001713 PMID:16566855

Elobied, A. A., Osman, A. M., Abu Kashwa, S. M., Ali, A. S., Ibrahim, M. T., & Salih, M. M. (2015). Effect of parity and breed on some physico-chemical components of Sudanese camel milk. *Research Opinions in Animal & Veterinary Sciences*, *5*(1), 20–24.

El-Sayed, M. (2011). Effects of camels milk as a vehicle for insulin on glycaemic control and lipid profile in Type 1 diabetics. *American Journal of Biochemistry and Biotechnology*, *7*(4), 179–189. doi:10.3844/ajbbsp.2011.179.189

El-Sayed, M. A., El-Shafei, S. M. S., & Khalifa, S. A. (2018). Manufacture of processed cheese spread from camel cheese based: Evaluation of cheese characteristics. *American Journal of Food Science and Nutrition Research*, *5*(4), 76–86.

El-Zeini, H. M. (2006). Microstructure, rheological and geometrical properties of fat globules of milk from different animal species. *Polish Journal of Food and Nutrition Sciences*, *15*, 147–154.

Elzhrani, M. S. (2018). Camel milk improvement of antioxidant and lipid profile in hypercholesterolemic rabbits. *Journal of Cell and Animal Biology*, *12*(1), 1–4. doi:10.5897/JCAB2017.0455

El-Ziney, M., De Mayer, H., & Debeyera, J. (1997). Growth and survival kinetics of Yersinia enterocolitica IP 383 0:9 as affected by equimolar concentrations of undissociated short-chain organic acids. *International Journal of Food Microbiology*, *34*(3), 233–247. doi:10.1016/S0168-1605(96)01194-4

El-Zubeir, I. E. M., & Jabreel, S. O. (2008). Fresh cheese from camel milk coagulated with Camifloc. *International Journal of Dairy Technology*, *61*(1), 90–95. doi:10.1111/j.1471-0307.2008.00360.x

Enright, J. B., Sadler, W. W., & Thomas, R. C. (1957). Thermal Inactivation of *Coxiella Burnetii* and Its Relation to Pasteurization of Milk. *American Journal of Public Health*, *47*, 695–700. doi:10.2105/AJPH.47.6.695 PMID:13424814

Epstein, H. (1971). History and origin of the African camel. In *The origin of the domestic animals in Africa* (pp. 558–564). New York: African Publishing Corporation.

Epstein, H. (1971). *The origin of domestic animals of Africa*. New York: Africana Publ. Corp.

Ereifej, K. I., Alu'datt, M. H., Al-Khalidy, A., Alli, I., & Rabab, T. (2011). Comparison and characterization of fat and protein composition for camel milk from eight Jordanian locations. *Food Chemistry*, *127*(1), 282–289. doi:10.1016/j.foodchem.2010.12.112

Espinosa-Marrón, A., Quiñones-Capistrán, C. A., Rubio-Blancas, A., del Pilar Milke-García, M., & Castillejos-Molina, R. A. (2019). *Hyperglycemia: The Metabolic Syndrome Component That Aggravates Erectile Dysfunction in Mexican Patients*. Academic Press.

Essamadi, K., Bengoumi, M., Tressol, J. C., Chacornac, J. P., & Faye, B. (1998). Comparative relationship of plasma copper concentration and ceruloplasmin activity of camel and cow. *Trends in Comparative Biochemistry & Physiology*, *5*, 211–220.

Essen-Gustavsson, B. (1986). Activity and inactivity-related muscle adaptation in the animal kingdom. In B. Saltin (Ed.), *Biochemistry of Exercise VI* (pp. 435–444). Champaign, IL: Human Kinetics Publishers.

Etzion, Z., Alfassi, Z., Lavi, N., & Yagil, R. (1987). Halide concentration in camel plasma in various state of dehydration. *Biological Trace Element Research*, *12*(1), 411–418. doi:10.1007/BF02796697 PMID:24254620

European food. (2019). *Al Nassma Chocolate LLC*. Retrieved in 13th May, 2019 from: https://www.european-food.com/al-nassma-chocolate-llc/interview/camel-milk-chocolate-an-arab-superfood/

Fakhoury, M., Negrulj, R., Mooranian, A., & Al-Salami, H. (2014). Inflammatory bowel disease: Clinical aspects and treatments. *Journal of Inflammation Research*, *7*, 113–120. doi:10.2147/JIR.S65979 PMID:25075198

Fallah, Z., Feizi, A., Hashemipour, M., & Kelishadi, R. (2018). Positive Effect of Fermented Camel Milk on Liver Enzymes of Adolescents with Metabolic Syndrome: A Double Blind, Randomized, Cross-over Trial. *Materia Socio-Medica*, *30*(1), 20. doi:10.5455/msm.2018.30.20-25 PMID:29670474

Fallah, Z., Feizi, A., Hashemipour, M., Namazi, N., Azarbayejani, L., & Kelishadi, R. (2019). Effect of Fermented Camel Milk on Obesity Measures and Blood Pressure of Adolescents with Metabolic Syndrome. *Journal of Pediatrics Review*, *7*, 181–189. doi:10.32598/jpr.7.3.181

Fantuz, F., Salimei, E., & Papademas, P. (2016). Macro-and micronutrients in non-cow milk and products and their impact on human health. In *Non-Bovine Milk and Milk Products* (pp. 209–261). Cambridge, UK: Academic Press. doi:10.1016/B978-0-12-803361-6.00009-0

Fan, W., Chen, Y., Sun, J., & Zheng, Y. (2014). Effects of tea polyphenol on quality and shelf life of pork sausages. *Mboxemph Journal of Food Science and Technology*, *51*(1), 191–195. doi:10.100713197-013-1076-x PMID:24426069

FAO. (1982). *Camels and camel milk*. Retrieved from http://www.fao.org/3/X6528E/X6528E03.htm#chIII

FAO. (1990). *The technology of traditional milk products in developing countries*. Rome, Italy: FAO.

FAO. (2006). *Livestock's long shadow. Environmental issues and options*. FAO publ.

FAO. (2013). Milk and Dairy Products in Human Nutrition. Rome: Wiley-Blackwell. doi:10.1186/1471-2458-11-95

FAO. (2013). *Statistical Year Book*. Rome, Italy: Food and Agriculture Organization of the United Nations.

FAOSTAT. (2015). *Food and Agricultural Organization, United Nations statistics*. Retrieved from http://faostat.fao.org/site/339/default.aspx

FAOSTAT. (2019). *Food and Agricultural Organization of the United Nations/Statistics*. Retrieved from: http://www.fao.org/faostat/en/#data/QV/visualize

Farah, Z., Eberhard, P., Meyer, J., Rehberger, B., Thomet, A., & Gallmann, P. U. (2004). *UHT processing of camel milk*. Retrieved from http://www.agroscope.admin.ch/publikationen/einzelpublikation/index.html?lang=en&aid=11827&pid=19150

Farah, Z. (1986). Effect of Heat Treatment on Whey Proteins of Camel Milk. *Milchwissenschaft. Milk Science International*, *41*(12), 763–765.

Farah, Z. (1993). Composition and characteristics of camel milk. *The Journal of Dairy Research*, *60*(4), 603–626. doi:10.1017/S0022029900027953 PMID:8294611

Farah, Z. (1996). *Camel milk properties and products*. St. Gallen, Switzerland: SKAT, Swiss Centre for Developments Cooperation in Technology and Management.

Farah, Z., & Atkins, D. (1992). Heat coagulation of camel milk. *The Journal of Dairy Research*, *59*(2), 229–231. doi:10.1017/S002202990003048X

Farah, Z., & Bachmann, M. R. (1987). Rennet coagulation properties of camel milk. *Milchwissenschaft. Milk Science International*, *42*, 689–692.

Farah, Z., Rettenmaier, R., & Atkins, D. (1992). Vitamin content of camel milk. *International Journal for Vitamin and Nutrition Research*, *62*(1), 30–33. PMID:1587705

Farah, Z., Rettenmaier, R., & Atkins, D. (1992). Vitamin Content of Camel Milk. *International Journal for Vitamin and Nutrition Research*, *62*, 30–33. PMID:1587705

Farah, Z., & Rüegg, M. (1991). The Creaming Properties and Size Distribution of Fat Globules in Camel Milk. *Journal of Dairy Science*, *74*(9), 2901–2904. doi:10.3168/jds.S0022-0302(91)78472-5

Farah, Z., & Rüegg, M. W. (1989). The size distribution of casein micelles in camel milk. *Food Microstructure*, *8*, 211–216.

Farah, Z., Streiff, T., & Bachmann, M. (1990). Preparation and consumer acceptability tests of fermented camel milk in Kenya. *The Journal of Dairy Research*, *57*(2), 281–283. doi:10.1017/S002202990002690X

Fares, S., Sethom, M. M., Feki, M., Cheour, M., Sanhaji, H., Kacem, S., & Kaabachi, N. (2016). Fatty acids profile in preterm Colostrum of Tunisian women. Association with selected maternal characteristics. *Prostaglandins, Leukotrienes, and Essential Fatty Acids*, *112*, 32–36. doi:10.1016/j.plefa.2016.08.002 PMID:27637338

Farida, M., & Srikumar, T. (2001). Trace elements and their distribution in protein fractions of camel milk in comparison to other commonly milks. *The Journal of Dairy Research*, *68*(3), 463–469. doi:10.1017/S0022029901005003 PMID:11694048

Farkas, D. F., & Hoover, D. G. (2000). High Pressure Processing: Kinetics of Microbial Inactivation for Alternative Food Processing Technologies. *Journal of Food Science*, *65*, 47–64. doi:10.1111/j.1750-3841.2000.tb00618.x

Farouk, M. M., & Bekhit, A. E. (2012). Processed camel meats. CAB International publ.

Farouk, M. M., & Bakhit, A. E. (2013). Processed Camel Meats. In I. T. Kadim, O. Mahgoub, B. Faye, & M. M. Farouk (Eds.), *Camel Meat and Meat Products* (pp. 186–204). CAB International. doi:10.1079/9781780641010.0186

Faye, B. & Bengoumi, M. (2018). Camel clinical biochemistry and haematology. In *Trace-elements*. Springer Publ.

Faye, B. (2004). Dairy productivity potential of camels. *Proc. of the 34th meeting FAO/ICAR (International Committee for Animal Recording)*, 93-105.

Faye, B. (2018). What future for camel pastoralism in the world? In *Proceedings of the 5th Conference ISOCARD "Recent advances in camelids biology, health and Production"* (pp. 32-38). Laâyoune, Morocco: IAV Hassan II.

Faye, B., & Bonnet, P. (2012). Camel sciences and economy in the world: Current situation and perspectives. In *Proceedings of the 3rd ISOCARD Conference. Keynote presentations* (pp. 2-15). Muscat, Oman: Sultan Qaboos University.

Faye, B., & Konuspayeva, G. (2016). Innovations in camel milk processing: The new challenges for marketing camel dairy products and the consequences on genetic selection. In *Regional conf. for animal genetic resources conservation. Towards Sustainable Utilization*. Available on: https://oapgrc.gov.om/Documents/The new challenges for marketing camel dairy products and the consequences on genetic selection_Bernard Fye.pdf

Faye, B., & Konuspayeva, G. (2016). Innovations in camel milk processing: The new challenges for marketing camel dairy products and the consequences on genetic selection. In: *Regional conf. for animal genetic resources conservation. Towards Sustainable Utilization*. Available on: https://oapgrc.gov.om/Documents/The new challenges for marketing camel dairy products and the consequences on genetic selection_Bernard Fye.pdf

Faye, B., & Tisserand, J. L. (1989). Problèmes de la détermination de la valeur alimentaire des fourrages prélevés par le dromadaire. In Séminaire sur la nutrition et l'alimentation du dromadaire. Ouargla, Algérie: Options Méditerranéennes.

Faye, B., Abdallah, H., Almathen, F., Harzallah, B., & Al-Mutairi, S. (2011). Camel biodiversity. Camel phenotypes in the Kingdom of Saudi Arabia. In Camel Breeding, Protection and Improvement Center. project UTF/SAU/021/SAU. FAO publ.

Faye, B., Bengoumi, M., Al-Masaud, A. & Konuspayeva, G. (2015b). Comparative milk and serum cholesterol content in dairy cow and camel. *Journal of King Saud University-Science*, *27*, 168-175.

Faye, B., Bengoumi, M., Al-Masaud, A., & Konuspayeva, G. (2015a). Low milk cholesterol in camel milk: true or not? *Scientific and Practical Journal Veterinariya*, *2*(42), 189-191.

Faye, B. (2011). Combating desertification: The added value of the camel farming. *Annals of Arid Zone*, *50*(3&4), 1–11.

Faye, B. (2013). Camel Farming Sustainability: The Challenges of the Camel Farming System in the XXIth Century. *Journal of Sustainable Development*, *6*(12), 74–82. doi:10.5539/jsd.v6n12p74

Faye, B. (2013). Camel meat in the world. CAB International.

Faye, B. (2013). Classification, history and distribution of the camel. In I. Kadim, O. Maghoub, B. Faye, & M. Farouk (Eds.), *Camel meat and meat products* (pp. 1–7). Oxfordshire, UK: CAB International. doi:10.1079/9781780641010.0001

Faye, B. (2015). *Activity report UTF/SAU/044/SAU Improvement of research for sustainable development of camel production in the Kingdom of Saudi Arabia*. FAO.

Faye, B. (2016). The camel, new challenges for a sustainable development. *Tropical Animal Health and Production*, *48*(4), 689–692. doi:10.100711250-016-0995-8 PMID:26922737

Faye, B. (2018). The enthusiasm for camel production [Editorial]. *Emirates Journal of Food and Agriculture*, *30*(4), 249–250.

Faye, B., Abdelhadi, O., Raiymbek, G., Kadim, I., & Hocquette, J. F. (2013). La production de viande de chameau: État des connaissances, situation actuelle et perspectives. *Productions Animales*, *26*(3), 247–258.

Faye, B., Althamma, O. M., Musaad, A., Konuspayeva, G., & Bengoumi, M. (2014). Effect of selenium injection in pregnant camels on selenium status of their new-born and milk. *Emirates Journal of Food and Agriculture*, *26*(4), 342–348. doi:10.9755/ejfa.v26i4.17272

Faye, B., & Bengoumi, M. (2018). *Camel clinical biochemistry and hematology*. Springer Publ. doi:10.1007/978-3-319-95562-9

Faye, B., Bengoumi, M., Al-Masaud, A., & Konuspayeva, G. (2015). Comparative milk and serum cholesterol content in dairy cow and camel. *Journal of King Saud University-Science*, *27*(2), 168–175. doi:10.1016/j.jksus.2014.11.003

Faye, B., & Bonnet, P. (2012). Camel sciences and economy in the world: Current situation and perspectives. In *Proceedings of the 3rd ISOCARD Conference. Keynote presentations* (pp. 2-15). Muscat, Oman: Sultan Qaboos University.

Faye, B., & Bonnet, P. (2012). Camel sciences and economy in the world: current situation and perspectives. *Proc. 3rd ISOCARD conference*, 2-15.

Faye, B., Chaibou, M., & Vias, G. F. (2012). Integrated impact of climate change and socioeconomic development on the evolution of camel farming systems. *British Journal of Environment & Climate Change*, *2*(3), 227–244. doi:10.9734/BJECC/2012/1548

Faye, B., Jaouad, J., Bhrawi, K., Senoussi, A., & Bengoumi, M. (2014). Elevage camelin en Afrique du Nord: État des lieux et perspectives. *Revue d'Élevage et de Médecine Vétérinaire des Pays Tropicaux*, *67*(4), 213–221. doi:10.19182/remvt.20563

Faye, B., & Konuspayeva, G. (2012). The Encounter between Bactrian and Dromedary Camels in Central Asia. In E.-M. Knoll & P. A. Burger (Eds.), *Camels in Asia and North-Africa- Interdisciplinary perspectives on their past and present significance* (pp. 27–33). Wien: Austrian Academy of Sciences Press.

Faye, B., & Konuspayeva, G. (2012). The sustainability challenge of the dairy sector- The growing importance of the non-cattle milk production worldwide. *International Dairy Journal*, *24*(2), 50–56. doi:10.1016/j.idairyj.2011.12.011

Faye, B., & Konuspayeva, G. (2015). *Camel cheese making workshop: short report. Rapport FAO, projet UTF/SAU/044/SAU*. Riyadh: FAO Publ.

Faye, B., Konuspayeva, G. S., Almasaud, A., Alafaliq, A., & Ben Abdallah, A. (2018). The effect of date-urea blocks as supplementary feeding on growth of young camels. *Emirates Journal of Food and Agriculture*, *30*(4), 320–325. doi:10.9755/ejfa.2018.v30.i4.1668

Faye, B., Konuspayeva, G., Messad, S., & Loiseau, G. (2008a). Discriminant milk components of Bactrian camel (*Camelus bactrianus*), dromedary (*Camelus dromedarius*) and hybrids. *Dairy Science & Technology*, *88*(6), 607–617. doi:10.1051/dst:2008008

Faye, B., Konuspayeva, G., Narmuratova, M., & Loiseau, G. (2008b). The comparative fatty acid composition of milk in Bactrian camel, dromedary, mare, cow and goat. *Journal of Camelid Science*, *1*, 49–54.

Faye, B., Konuspayeva, G., Narmuratova, M., Serikbaeva, A., Musaad, A. M., & Mehri, H. (2013a). Effect of crude olive cake supplementation on camel milk production and fatty acid composition. *Dairy Science & Technology*, *93*(3), 225–239. doi:10.100713594-013-0117-6

Faye, B., Madani, H., & El-Rouili, A. H. (2014). Camel milk value chain in Northern Saudi Arabia. *Emirates Journal of Food and Agriculture*, *26*(4), 359–365. doi:10.9755/ejfa.v26i4.17278

Faye, B., Saleh, S., Konuspayeva, G., Musaad, A., Bengoumi, M., & Seboussi, R. (2013b). Comparative effect of organic and inorganic selenium supplementation on selenium status in camel. *Journal of King Saud University-Science*, *26*(2), 149–158. doi:10.1016/j.jksus.2013.10.003

Faye, B., Seboussi, R., & Alhadrami, G. (2011). Maternal transfer of selenium by blood and milk in camels. *Journal of Camelid Science*, *4*, 30–39.

Faye, B., Senoussi, H., & Jaouad, M. (2017). Le dromadaire et l'oasis: Du caravansérail à l'élevage périurbain. *Cahiers Agricultures*, *26*(1), 14001. doi:10.1051/cagri/2017005

Faye, B., & Vias, G. (2004). Scientific support of the camel sub-sector development project in Niger. *Proceedings of International Conference. On « Saving the camel and peoples' livelihood »*, 64-70.

Feldstein, A. E., Papouchado, B. G., Angulo, P., Sanderson, S., Adams, L., & Gores, G. J. (2005). Hepatic stellate cells and fibrosis progression in patients with nonalcoholic fatty liver disease. *Clinical Gastroenterology and Hepatology*, *3*(4), 384–389. doi:10.1016/S1542-3565(04)00616-0 PMID:15822044

Felfoul, I., Jardin, J., Gaucheron, F., Attia, H., & Ayadi, M. A. (2017). Proteomic profiling of camel and cow milk proteins under heat treatment. *Food Chemistry*, *216*, 161–169. doi:10.1016/j.foodchem.2016.08.007 PMID:27596405

Feligini, M., Bonizzi, I., Buffoni, J. N., Consenza, G., & Ramunno, L. (2009). Identification and quantification of α-s1, α-s2, β, and κ-caseins in water buffalo milk by reverse phase-high performance liquid chromatography and mass spectrometry. *Journal of Agricultural and Food Chemistry*, *57*(7), 2988–2992. doi:10.1021/jf803653v PMID:19256489

Feng, D. Z. (2007). Study on Growth and Development and Production Model of Alashan Bactrian Camel. China Agricultural University.

Fernández, M., Hudson, J. A., Korpela, R., & de los Reyes-Gavilán, C. G. (2015). Impact on human health of microorganisms present in fermented dairy products: An overview. *BioMed Research International*, *2015*, 412714–412714. doi:10.1155/2015/412714

Ferragut, V., Martinez, V. M., Trujillo, A. J., & Guamis, B. (2000). Properties of Yogurts Made from Whole Ewe's Milk Treated by High Hydrostatic Pressure. *Milchwissenschaft. Milk Science International*, *55*(5), 267–269.

Ferraro, V., Anton, M., & Santé-lhoutellier, V. (2016). The "sisters" α-helices of collagen, elastin and keratin recovered from animal by-products: Functionality, bioactivity and trends of application. *Trends in Food Science & Technology*, *51*, 65–75. doi:10.1016/j.tifs.2016.03.006

Fguiri, I., Ziadi, M., Sboui, A., Ayeb, N., Atigui, M., Arroum, S., & Khorchani, T. (2018). Effect of the production system and stage of lactation on the microbiological and biochemical characteristics of camel milk. *Journal of Camelid Science*, *11*, 57–63.

Figueiredo, M. M., Gamelas, J. A. F., & Martins, A. G. (2012). Characterization of bone and bone-based graft materials using FTIR spectroscopy. *Infrared Spectroscopy: Life and Biomedical Sciences*. Retrieved from www.intechopen.com

Figueiredoa, M. S. C., Martinsa, G., Freitasb, J., Judasb, F., & Figueiredo, H. (2011). Influence of hydrochloric acid concentration on the demineralization of cortical bone. *Chemical Engineering Research*, *89*(1), 116–124. doi:10.1016/j.cherd.2010.04.013

Finke, B. (2000). *Isolierung und charakterisierung von oligosaccharide naushumanen und tierischenmilchen* (Ph.D. thesis). University of Giessen, Shaker Verlag, Aachen, Germany.

Fitak, R. R., Mohandesan, E., Corander, J., & Burger, P. A. (2016). The de novo genome assembly and annotation of a female domestic dromedary of north african origin. *Molecular Ecology Resources*, *16*(1), 314–324. doi:10.1111/1755-0998.12443 PMID:26178449

Fitzpatrick, J., Barry, K., Cerqueira, P., Iqbal, T., O'Neill, J., & Roos, Y. (2007). Effect of composition and storage conditions on the flowability of dairy powders. *International Dairy Journal*, *17*(4), 383–392. doi:10.1016/j.idairyj.2006.04.010

Fonseca, F., Passot, S., Cunin, O., & Marin, M. (2004). Collapse temperature of freeze-dried *Lactobacillus bulgaricus* suspensions and protective media. *Biotechnology Progress*, *20*(1), 229–238. doi:10.1021/bp034136n PMID:14763847

Food and Agricultural Organization. (1982). *Camel and camel milk.* Rome: Author.

Food and Agriculture Organization. FAOSTAT. (2019). *Food and Agricultural Organization of the United Nations/ Statistics*. Retrieved May 4, 2019 from: http://www.fao.org/faostat/en/#data/QV/visualize

Fowler, M. E. (1998). *Medicine and surgery of south American camelids*. Iowa State Press Blackwell.

Fox, P. F. (1993). *Cheese: Chemistry, physics and microbiology*. London, UK: Chapman & Hall.

Fox, P. F. (2003). The major constituents of milk. In G. Smit (Ed.), *Dairy Processing, Improving Quality* (pp. 5–38). Cambridge, UK: Woodhead Publishing Limited. doi:10.1533/9781855737075.1.5

Fox, P., & McSweeney, P. (1998). Lactose chapter. In *Dairy Chemistry and Biochemistry* (1st ed.; pp. 21–66). Thomson Science.

Fraga Cotelo, M., Perelmuter Schein, K., Salvo, G., Solange, S., Abirad, Z., Miguel, P., ... Beatriz, S. (2013). Antimicrobial properties of lactic acid bacteria isolated from uruguayan artisan cheese. *Food Science and Technology (Campinas)*, *33*(4), 801–804. doi:10.1590/S0101-20612013000400029

Frenken, L. G., Howell, S., Ledeboer, A. M., & van der Logt, C. P. (2003). *U.S. Patent No. 6,670,453*. Washington, DC: U.S. Patent and Trademark Office.

Frost, M., Heymann, H., Bredie, W., Djksterhuis, G., & Martens, M. (2005). Sensory Measurement of Dynamic Flavor Intensity in Ice Cream with Different Fat Levels and Flavorings. *Food Quality and Preference*, *16*(4), 305–314. doi:10.1016/j.foodqual.2004.05.009

Fuente, M. A., Olano, A., Casal, V., & Juárez, M. (1999). Effects of high pressure and heat treatment on the mineral balance of goats' milk. *The Journal of Dairy Research*, *66*(1), 65–72. doi:10.1017/S0022029998003264 PMID:10191474

Fujita, K.-i., Matsuda, E., Sekine, K., Iigo, M., & Tsuda, H. (2004). Lactoferrin enhances Fas expression and apoptosis in the colon mucosa of azoxymethane-treated rats. *Carcinogenesis*, *25*(10), 1961–1966. doi:10.1093/carcin/bgh205 PMID:15192017

Fukuda, K., Yamamoto, A., Ganzorig, K., Khuukhenbaatar, J., Senda, A., Saito, T., & Urashima, T. (2010). Chemical characterization of the oligosaccharides in Bactrian camel (*Camelus bactrianus)* milk and colostrum. *Journal of Dairy Science*, *93*(12), 5572–5587. doi:10.3168/jds.2010-3151 PMID:21094729

Funk, A., Goutard, F., Miguel, E., Bourgarel, M., Chevalier, V., Faye, B., ... Roger, F. (2016). Mers-coV at the animal–human interface: Inputs on exposure Pathways from an expert-Opinion elicitation. *Frontiers in Veterinary Science*, *3*, 88. doi:10.3389/fvets.2016.00088 PMID:27761437

Gadaga, T. H., Nyanga, L. K., & Mutukumira, A. N. (2004). The occurrence, growth and control of pathogens in African fermented foods. *African Journal of Food, Agriculture, Nutrition and Development*, *4*(1). doi:10.4314/ajfand.v4i1.19155

Gaili, E. S. E., Al-Eknah, M. M., & Sadek, M. H. (2000). Comparative milking performance of three types of Saudi camels (*Camelus dromedarius*). *Journal of Camel Practice and Research*, *7*(1), 73–76.

Galali, Y., & Al-Dmoor, H. M. (2019). Miraculous properties of camel milk and perspective of modern science. *Journal of Family Medicine and Disease Prevention*, *5*(1), 1–7.

Galeboe, O., Seifu, E., & Sekwati-Monang, B. (2018). Production of camel milk yoghurt: Physicochemical and microbiological quality and consumer acceptability. *International Journal of Food Studies*, *7*(2), 51–63. doi:10.7455/ijfs/7.2.2018.a5

Galindar & Chagan. (2012). *Gobi Bactrian camel*. Inner Mongolia Peoples Publishing House.

Gangwar, L., Singh, R., & Deepak, D. (2018). Structure elucidation of a novel oligosaccharide (Medalose) from camel milk. *Journal of Molecular Structure*, *1153*, 157–161. doi:10.1016/j.molstruc.2017.10.006

Garcella, H. G., Garciab, E. G., Pueyob, P. V., Martínb, I. R., Arias, A. V., & Serranoa, R. N. A. (2016). Outbreaks of brucellosis related to the consumption of unpasteurized camel milk. *Journal of Infection and Public Health*, *9*(4), 523–527. doi:10.1016/j.jiph.2015.12.006 PMID:26796768

Garcia, C., Lutz, N. W., Confort-Gouny, S., Cozzone, P., Armand, M., & Bernard, M. (2012). Phospholipid fingerprints of milk from different mammalians determined by 31P NMR: Towards specific interest in human health. *Food Chemistry*, *135*(3), 1777–1783. doi:10.1016/j.foodchem.2012.05.111 PMID:22953921

García, P., Rodríguez, L., Rodríguez, A., & Martínez, B. (2010). Food biopreservation: Promising strategies using bacteriocins, bacteriophages and endolysins. *Trends in Food Science & Technology*, *21*(8), 373–382. doi:10.1016/j.tifs.2010.04.010

Gardner, G. E., Kennedy, L., Milton, J. T. B., & Pethick, D. W. (1999). Glycogen metabolism and ultimate pH of muscle merino, first-cross, and second-cross whether lambs as affected by stress before slaughter. *Australian Journal of Agricultural Research*, *50*(2), 175–181. doi:10.1071/A98093

Gaucheron, F. (2011). Diversité des laits et des produits laitiers dans le monde. In *Culture des laits du monde*. Paris, France: Les cahiers de l'OCHA.

Gaucheron, F., Famelart, M. H., Mariette, F., Raulot, K., & Michel, F. (1997). Combined Effects of Temperature and High-Pressure Treatments on Physicochemical Characteristics of Skim Milk. *Food Chemistry*, *59*(3), 439–447. doi:10.1016/S0308-8146(96)00301-9

Gauthier-Pilters, H. (1961). Observations sur l'écologie du dromadaire dans le Sahara nord-occidental. *Mammalia*, *25*(2), 195–280. doi:10.1515/mamm.1961.25.2.195

Gebreyohanes, M. G., & Assen, A. M. (2017). Adaptation mechanisms of camels (Camelus dromedarius) for desert environment: a review. Journal of Veterinary Science & Technology, 8(6).

Gedam, K., Prasad, R., & Vijay, V. K. (2007). The Study on UHT Processing of Milk: A Versatile Option for Rural Sector. *World Journal of Dairy & Food Sciences*, *2*(2), 49–53.

Gee, P. (1996). The camel in Australia. *Journal of Camel Practice and Research*, *3*(2), 139–140.

Gehan, T., & El-Bassyouni, O. W. G. (2013). Morphological and macrostructural studies of dog cranial bone demineralized with different acids. *Current Applied Physics*, *13*(5), 864–874. doi:10.1016/j.cap.2012.12.026

Gemechu, A. T., & Tola, Y. B. (2017). Traditional butter and ghee production, processing and handling in Ethiopia: A review. *African Journal of Food, Agriculture, Nutrition and Development*, *11*(4), 95–105.

Genene, A., Hansen, E., Eshetu, M., Hailu, Y., & Ipsen, R. (2019). Effect of heat treatment on denaturation of whey protein and resultant rennetability of camel milk. *LWT*, *101*, 404–409. doi:10.1016/j.lwt.2018.11.047

Gensler, H. L., & Magdaleno, M. (1991). Topical vitamin E inhibition of immunosuppression and tumorigenesis induced by ultraviolet irradiation. *Nutrition and Cancer*, *15*(2), 97–106. doi:10.1080/01635589109514117 PMID:2038569

Gervilla, R., Capellas, M., Ferragut, V., & Guamis, B. (1997). Effect of High Hydrostatic Pressure on Listeria Innocua 910 CECT. *Journal of Food Protection*, *60*(1), 33–37. doi:10.4315/0362-028X-60.1.33 PMID:10465037

Gervilla, R., Ferragut, V., & Guamis, B. (2001). High Hydrostatic Pressure Effects on Color and Milk-Fat Globule of Ewe's Milk. *Journal of Food Science*, *66*(6), 880–885. doi:10.1111/j.1365-2621.2001.tb15190.x

Gheisari, H. R., Aminlari, M., & Shekarforoush, S. S. (2009). A comparative study of the biochemical and functional properties of camel and cattle meat during frozen storage. *Veterinarski Arhiv*, *79*, 51–68.

Gill, C., & Rowland, I. (2003). Cancer. In Functional Dairy Products (pp. 19-53). Cambridge, UK: Woodhead Publishers.

Gioacchini, A. M., De Santi, M., Guescini, M., Brandi, G., & Stocchi, V. (2010). Characterization of the volatile organic compounds of Italian 'Fossa' cheese by solid-phase microextraction gas chromatography/mass spectrometry. *Rapid Communications in Mass Spectrometry*, *24*(23), 3405–3412. doi:10.1002/rcm.4782 PMID:21072795

Gizachew, A., Teha, J., & Birhanu, T. (2014). Review on Medicinal and Nutritional Values of Camel Milk. *Nature and Science*, *12*(120), 35–40.

Gizachew, A., Teha, J., Birhanu, T., & Nekemte, E. (2014). Review on medicinal and nutritional values of camel milk. *Nature and Science*, *12*(12), 35–41.

GMIA. (2012). Gelatin handbook. New York: Gelatin Manufacturers Institute of America, GMIA.

Gnädig, S., Xue, Y., Berdeaux, O., Chardigny, J. M., & Sebedio, J. L. (2003). Conjugated linoleic acid (CLA) as a functional ingredient. In Functional Dairy Products (pp. 263-298). CRC Press.

Gobbetti, M., Minervini, F., & Rizzello, C. G. (2004). Angiotensin I-converting enzyme-inhibitory and antimicrobial bioactive peptides. *International Journal of Dairy Society*, *57*(2-3), 173–188. doi:10.1111/j.1471-0307.2004.00139.x

Goff, H. (1997). Colloidal Aspects of Ice Cream—A Review. *International Dairy Journal*, *7*(6-7), 363–373. doi:10.1016/S0958-6946(97)00040-X

Goff, H., Freslon, B., Sahagian, M. E., Hauber, T. D., Stone, A. P., & Stanley, D. W. (1995). Structural Development in Ice Cream—Dynamic Rheological Measurements. *Journal of Texture Studies*, *26*(5), 517–536. doi:10.1111/j.1745-4603.1995.tb00801.x

Golik, F. (2014). Case study: The effects of excess fructose in a patient with autism spectrum disorder infections. *Journal of the Australasian College of Nutritional and Environmental Medicine*, *33*(3), 13.

Gomez-Guillen, M. C., Gimenez, B., Lopez-Caballero, M. E., & Montero, M. P. (2011). Functional and bioactive properties of collagen and gelatin from alternative sources: A review. *Food Hydrocolloids*, *25*(8), 1813–1827. doi:10.1016/j.foodhyd.2011.02.007

Gómez-Guillén, M., Pérez-Mateos, M., Gómez-Estaca, J., López-Caballero, E., Giménez, B., & Montero, P. (2009). Fish gelatin: A renewable material for developing active biodegradable films. *Trends in Food Science & Technology*, *20*(1), 3–16. doi:10.1016/j.tifs.2008.10.002

Gómez-Guillén, M., Turnay, J., Fernández-Dıaz, M., Ulmo, N., Lizarbe, M., & Montero, P. (2002). Structural and physical properties of gelatin extracted from different marine species: A comparative study. *Food Hydrocolloids*, *16*(1), 25–34. doi:10.1016/S0268-005X(01)00035-2

Gonzalez, F., Smulders, F. J. M., Paulsen, P., Skewes, O., & Konig, H. E. (2004). Anatomical investigations on meat cuts of guanacos (Lama guanicoe, Muller, 1776) and chemical composition of selected muscles. *Wiener Tierärztliche Monatsschrift*, *91*, 77–84.

Gopal, P. K., & Gill, H. S. (2000). Oligosaccharides and glycoconjugates in bovine milk and colostrum. *British Journal of Nutrition*, *84*(S1), 69–74. doi:10.1017/S0007114500002270 PMID:11242449

Gorban, A. M. S., & Izzeldin, O. M. (1997). Mineral Content of Camel Milk and Colostrums. *The Journal of Dairy Research*, *64*(3), 471–474. doi:10.1017/S0022029997002264

Gorban, A. M., & Izzeldin, O. M. (1999). Study on cholesteryl ester fatty acids in camel and cow milk lipid. *International Journal of Food Science & Technology*, *34*(3), 229–234. doi:10.1046/j.1365-2621.1999.00254.x

Gorelik, O., Shatskikh, Y., Rebezov, M., Kanareikina, S., Kanareikin, V., Lihodeyevskaya, O., ... Okuskhanova, E. (2017). Study of Chemical and Mineral Composition of New Sour Milk Bio-product with Sapropel Powder. *Annual Research & Review in Biology*, *18*(4), 1–5. doi:10.9734/ARRB/2017/36937

Gorini, F., Muratori, F., & Morales, M. A. (2014). The Role of Heavy Metal Pollution in Neurobehavioral Disorders: A Focus on Autism. *Review Journal of Autism and Developmental Disorders*, *1*(4), 354–372. doi:10.100740489-014-0028-3

Gossner, C., Danielson, N., Gervelmeyer, A., Berthe, F., Faye, B., Kaasik-Aaslav, K., ... Coulombier, D. (2015). Human–Dromedary Camel Interactions and the Risk of Acquiring Zoonotic Middle East Respiratory Syndrome Coronavirus Infection. *Zoonoses and Public Health*, *12171*. doi:10.1111/zph PMID:25545147

Goyal, A., Sharma, V., Upadhyay, N., Sihag, M., & Kaushik, R. (2013). High Pressure Processing and Its Impact on Milk Proteins: A Review. *Journal of Dairy Science and Technology*, *2*, 1–9.

Grandval, F. (2012). Tiviski: une entreprise de valorisation du lait local en Mauritanie. *Inter-réseaux, développement rural*, 5. Retrieved from http://www.inter-reseaux.org/IMG/pdf/Note_Tiviski_final.pdf

Griffiths, M. W. (2010). Improving the safety and quality of milk. In *Milk production and processing* (Vol. 1). Guelph, Canada: Woodhead Publishing Limited, University of Guelph.

Groenen, M. A. M., Dijkhof, R. J. M., & Van der Poel, J. J. (1995). Characterization of a GlyCAM1-like gene (glycosylation dependent cell adhesion molecule 1) which is 19 highly and specifically expressed in the lactating bovine mammary gland. *Gene*, *158*(2), 189–195. doi:10.1016/0378-1119(95)00138-V PMID:7607540

Guilloteau, P., Huërou-Luron, I. L., Chayvialle, J. A., Toullec, R., Zabielski, R., & Blum, J. W. (1997). Gut regulatory peptides in young cattle and sheep. *Journal of Veterinary Medicine Series A*, *44*(1-10), 1-23.

Gul, W., Farooq, N., Anees, D., Khan, U., & Rehan, F. (2015). Camel milk: A boon to mankind. *Int J Res Stud Biosci*, *3*, 23–29.

Gul, W., Farooq, N., Anees, D., Khan, U., & Rehan, F. (2015). Camel Milk: A Boon to Mankind. *International Journal of Research Studies in Biosciences*, *3*, 23–29.

Gumus, P., & Hayaloglu, A. A. (2019). Effects of blends of camel and calf chymosin on proteolysis, residual coagulant activity, microstructure, and sensory characteristics of Beyaz peynir. *Journal of Dairy Science*, *102*(7), 5945–5956. doi:10.3168/jds.2018-15671 PMID:31079909

Guzel-Seydim, Z., Kök-Tas, T., & Greene, A. K. (2010). Kefir and koumiss: microbiology and technology. In F. Yildiz (Ed.), *Development and Manufacture of Yogurt and Functional Dairy Products* (pp. 143–163). Boca Raton, FL: CRC Press.

Guzel-Seydim, Z., Seydim, A., Grenee, A., & Bodine, A. (2000). Determination of organic acids and volatile flavour substances in kefir during fermentation. *Journal of Food Composition and Analysis*, *13*(1), 35–43. doi:10.1006/jfca.1999.0842

Habib, H. M., Ibrahim, W. H., Schneider-Stock, R., & Hassan, H. M. (2013). *Camel milk lactoferrin reduces the proliferation of colorectal cancer cells and exerts antioxidant and DNA damage inhibitory activities*. doi:10.1016/j.foodchem.2013.03.039

Habtegebriel, H., Edwardb, D., Wawire, M., Silaa, D., & Seifu, E. (2018). Effect of operating parameters on the surface and physico-chemical properties of spray-dried camel milk powders. *Food and Bioproducts Processing*, *1*(12), 137–149.

Habtegebriel, H., Edward, D., Wawire, M., Sila, D., & Seifu, E. (2018). Effect of operating parameters on the surface and physico-chemical properties of spray-dried camel milk powders. *Food and Bioproducts Processing*, *112*, 137–149. doi:10.1016/j.fbp.2018.09.010

Habtegebriel, H., Wawire, M., & Sila, D. (2018). The effect of pretreatment (spray drying) on the yield and selected nutritional components of whole camel milk powder. *Food Science*, *83*(12), 2983–2991. doi:10.1111/1750-3841.14361 PMID:30440084

Haddadin, M. S. Y., Gammoh, S. I., & Robinson, R. K. (2008). Seasonal variations in the chemical composition of camel milk in Jordan. *The Journal of Dairy Research*, *75*(1), 8–12. doi:10.1017/S0022029907002750 PMID:17971263

Haeusler, R. A., McGraw, T. E., & Accili, D. (2018). Biochemical and cellular properties of insulin receptor signalling. *Nature Reviews. Molecular Cell Biology*, *19*(1), 31–44. doi:10.1038/nrm.2017.89

Hailu, Y., Hansen, E. B., Seifu, E., Eshetu, M., & Ipsena, R. (2016). Factors influencing the gelation and rennetability of camel milk using camel chymosin. *International Dairy Journal*, *60*, 62–69. doi:10.1016/j.idairyj.2016.01.013

Hailu, Y., Hansen, E. B., Seifu, E., Eshetu, M., Ipsen, R., & Kappeler, S. (2016a). Functional and Technological Properties of Camel Milk Proteins: A Review. *The Journal of Dairy Research*, *83*(4), 422–429. doi:10.1017/S0022029916000686 PMID:27845026

Hailu, Y., Hansen, E., Seifu, Y., Eshetu, M., Agerlin, M., Petersen, M. A., ... Ipsen, R. (2018). Rheological and sensory properties and aroma compounds formed during ripening of soft brined cheese made from camel milk. *International Dairy Journal*, *81*, 122–130. doi:10.1016/j.idairyj.2018.01.007

Hailu, Y., Seifu, E., & Yilma, Z. (2014). Physicochemical properties and consumer acceptability of soft unripened cheese made from camel milk using crude extract of ginger (*Zingiber officinale*) as coagulant. *African Journal of Food Science*, *8*(2), 87–91. doi:10.5897/AJFS2013.1102

Hal, J., & Hedrick, T. (1975). *Drying of milk and milk products*. Westport, CT: AVI Publ. Co. Ltd.

Hamad, S. H., Al Eid, S. M., Al Jassas, F. M., & Abu Tarboush, H. (2013). *Use of High Hydrostatic Pressure for The Preservation of Camel's Milk*. International Conference Animal & Dairy Sciences, Las Vegas, NV.

Hamad, S.H., Al Eid, S.M., Al Jassas, F.M., & Abu Tarboush, H. (2013). Use of high hydrostatic pressure for the preservation of camel's milk. *Journal of Veterinary Science and Technology, 4*.

Hamad, E., Abdel-Rahim, E., & Romeih, E. (2011). Beneficial effect of camel milk on liver and kidneys function in diabetic Sprague-Dawley rats. *Int J Dairy Sci*, *6*(3), 190–197. doi:10.3923/ijds.2011.190.197

Hamed, H., Chaari, F., Ghannoudi, Z., ElFeki, A., Ellouz, S. C., & Gargouri, A. (2018). Beneficial effects of fermented camel milk by lactococcus lactis subsp cremoris on cardiotoxicity induced by carbon tetrachloride in mice. *Biomedicine & Pharmacotherapy = Biomedecine & Pharmacotherapie, 97*, 107–114. doi:10.1016/j.biopha.2017.10.057

Hamed, H., El Feki, A., & Gargouri, A. (2019). Evaluation of the hepatoprotective effect of combination between fermented camel milk and Rosmarinus officinalis leaves extract against CCl 4 induced liver toxicity in mice. *Journal of Food Science and Technology*, *56*(2), 824–834. doi:10.100713197-018-3542-y PMID:30906040

Hamed, H., El-Feki, A., & Gargouri, A. (2016). Influence of Wet and Dry Season on Milk Composition of Dromedary Camels (*Camelus dromedarius*) from Tunisia. *Iranian Journal of Applied Animal Science*, *7*(1), 163–167.

Hamed, H., Gargouri, M., Boulila, S., Chaari, F., Ghrab, F., Kallel, R., ... El Feki, A. (2018). Fermented camel milk prevents carbon tetrachloride induced acute injury in kidney of mice. *The Journal of Dairy Research*, *85*(2), 251–256. doi:10.1017/S0022029918000250 PMID:29785914

Hamers-Casterman, C., Atahouch, T., Muyldermans, S., Robinson, G., Hamers, C., Songa, E. B., ... Hamers, R. (1993). Naturally-occuring antibodies devoid of light chains. *Nature*, *363*(6428), 446–448. doi:10.1038/363446a0 PMID:8502296

Hamidi, M., Choukri, A., & Hachi, M. (2017). Influence de la race cameline sur la production fromagère avec un extrait de kaolin du gésier de poulet en Algérie; étude préliminaire. *Livestock Research for Development, 29*(5). Retrieved from http://www.lrrd.org/lrrd29/5/med29085.html

Ham, J. S., Shin, J. H., Noh, Y. B., Jeong, S. G., Han, G. S., Chae, H. S., ... Jo, C. (2008). Chemical and microbiological quality, capillary electrophoresis pattern, and rennet coagulation of UHT-treated and irradiated milk. *Food Science and Biotechnology*, *17*, 58–65.

Ham, J. S., Shin, J. H., Noh, Y. B., Jeong, S. G., Han, G. S., Chae, H. S., ... Jo, C. (2008). Chemical and Microbiological Quality, Capillary Electrophoresis Pattern, and Rennet Coagulation of UHT-Treated and Irradiated Milk. *Food Science and Biotechnology*, *17*, 58–65.

Hammadi, M., Atigui, M., Ayadi, M., Barmat, A., Belgacem, A., Khaldi, G., & Khorchani, T. (2010). Training period and short time effects of machine milking on milk yield and milk composition in Tunisian Maghrebi camels (*Camelus dromedarius*). *Journal of Camel Research and Practice*, *17*(1), 1–7.

Hammam, A. R. (2019). Compositional and therapeutic properties of camel milk: A review. *Emirates Journal of Food and Agriculture*, *31*(3), 148–152. doi:10.9755/ejfa.2019.v31.i3.1919

Hamoud, A. M. (2015). *Characterisation of proteins in camel milk, the effect of heat treatment on physicochemical and functional properties related to yogurt* (PhD thesis). School of Life Sciences, Heriot-Watt University.

Hamzawy, M. A., El-Ghandour, Y. B., Abdel-Aziem, S. H., & Ali, Z. H. (2018). Leptin and camel milk abate oxidative stress status, genotoxicity induced in valproic acid rat model of autism. *International Journal of Immunopathology and Pharmacology*, *32*. doi:10.1177/2058738418785514 PMID:30004275

Harahap, Y., Jaswir, I., & Anwar, E. (2016). Physicochemical and functional properties of gelatin extracted from goat (*Capra hircus*) skin using the partial acid hydrolysis method. *Proceedings of the 3rd International Halal Conference (INHAC 2016)*, 565-576.

Harrison, J. A. (1985). Giant Camels from the Cenozoic of North America. *Smithsonian Contributions to Paleobiology*, *57*(57), 1–29. doi:10.5479i.00810266.57.1

Harrison, R. (2006). Milk xanthine oxidase: Properties and physiological roles. *International Dairy Journal, 16*(6), 546–554. doi:10.1016/j.idairyj.2005.08.016

Hartley, J. B. (1979). *Camels in the Horn of Africa.* Paper presented in IFS Symposium Camels.

Hashim, I. B., Khalil, A. H., & Habib, H. (2009). Quality and acceptability of a set-type yogurt made from camel milk. *Journal of Dairy Science, 92*(3), 857–862. doi:10.3168/jds.2008-1408 PMID:19233778

Hassaïne, O., & Zadi-Karam, H., & Karam. (2007). Technologically important properties of lactic acid bacteria isolated from raw milk of three breeds of Algerian dromedary (Camelus dromedarius). *African Journal of Biotechnology, 6*(14), 1720–1727.

Hassan, R. A., El Zubei, I. E. M., & Babiker, S. A. (2007). Effect of Pasteurization of Raw Camel Milk and StorageTemperature on the Chemical Composition of Fermented Camel Milk. *International Journal of Dairy Science, 2*(2), 166–171. doi:10.3923/ijds.2007.166.171

Hassan, R., El Zubeir, I., & Babiker, S. (2006). Microbiology of camel fermented milk (Gariss) in Sudan. *Research Journal of Microbiology, 1*(2), 160–165. doi:10.3923/jm.2006.160.165

Hassl, M., Jorgensen, B. D., & Janhoj, T. (2011). Rennet gelation properties of ultrafiltration retentates from camel milk. *Milchwissenschaft. Milk Science International, 66*, 80–84.

Hasson, S., Al-Busaidi, J. Z., Al-Qarni, Z. A., Rajapakse, S., Al-Bahlani, S., Idris, M. A., & Sallam, T. A. (2015). In vitro apoptosis triggering in the BT-474 human breast cancer cell line by lyophilised camel's milk. *Asian Pacific Journal of Cancer Prevention, 16*(15), 6651–6661. doi:10.7314/APJCP.2015.16.15.6651 PMID:26434890

Haug, I. J., & Draget, K. I. (2009). Gelatin. In G. O. Phillips & P. A. Williams (Eds.), *Handbook of hydrocolloids* (2nd ed.; pp. 142–163). Cambridge, UK: Woodhead Publishing Limited. doi:10.1533/9781845695873.142

Haug, I. J., & Draget, K. I. (2011). Gelatin. In G. O. Phillips & P. A. Williams (Eds.), *Handbook of food proteins* (pp. 92–115). Cambridge, UK: Woodhead Publishing Limited. doi:10.1533/9780857093639.92

Hayakawa, I., Kanno, T., Yoshiyama, K., & Fujio, Y. (1994). Oscillatory Compared with Continuous High-Pressure Sterilization on *Bacillus Stearothermophilus* Spores. *Journal of Food Science, 59*(1), 164–167. doi:10.1111/j.1365-2621.1994.tb06924.x

Hayes, J. E., Stepanyan, V., Allen, P., O'Grady, M. N., & Kerry, J. P. (2011). Evaluation of the effects of selected plant-derived nutraceuticals on the quality and shelf-life stability of raw and cooked pork sausages. *Lebensmittel-Wissenschaft + Technologie, 44*, 164–172.

Hazra, T., & Parmar, P. (2014). Natural Antioxidant Use in Ghee-A Mini Review. *Journal of Food Research and Technology, 2*(3), 101–105.

Heba, H. S., Hussein, A.-H., & Mohamed, M. H. (2016). Improving the physico-chemical and sensory characteristics of camel meat burger patties using ginger extract and papain. *Meat Science, 118*, 52–60.

Heller, K. J. (2001). Probiotic bacteria in fermented foods: Product characteristics and starter organisms. *The American Journal of Clinical Nutrition, 73*(2), 374s–379s. doi:10.1093/ajcn/73.2.374s

Helliwell, T. R. (1999). Muscle: Part 1- Normal structure and function. *Current Orthopaedics, 13*(1), 33–41. doi:10.1016/S0268-0890(99)90083-X

Hemida, M. G., Elmoslemany, A., Al-Hizab, F., Alnaeem, A., Almathen, F., Faye, B., ... Peiris, M. (2015). Dromedary Camels and the Transmission of Middle East Respiratory Syndrome Coronavirus (MERS-CoV). *Transboundary and Emerging Diseases*, 1–10. PMID:26256102

Hendrickx, M. L., Van Den, B. I., & Weemaes, C. (1998). Effects of High Pressure on Enzymes Related to Food Quality. *Trends in Food Science & Technology*, *9*(5), 197–203. doi:10.1016/S0924-2244(98)00039-9

Heneiksen-larsen, K. B., Lexell, J., & Sjostrom, M. (1983). Distribution of different fibre types in human skeletal muscles. I. Method for the preparation and analysis of cross-sections of whole tibialis anterior. *The Histochemical Journal*, *15*, 167–178. doi:10.1007/BF01042285 PMID:6343306

Hernández, D., Cardell, E., & Zárate, V. (2005). Antimicrobial activity of lactic acid bacteria isolated from Tenerife cheese: Initial characterization of plantaricin TF711, a bacteriocin-like substance produced by Lactobacillus plantarum TF711. *Journal of Applied Microbiology*, *99*(1), 77–84. doi:10.1111/j.1365-2672.2005.02576.x

Herrman, K., & Fischer, A. (2004). Method for hygienic slaughter of camels. In Z. Farah, & A. Fisher (Eds.), Milk and meat from the camel. Handbook on products and processing. Zuric: vdf Hochschulverlag AG an der ETH Zurich.

Hertzler, S., & Clancy, S. (2003). Kefir improves lactose digestion and tolerance in adults with lactose mal-digestion. *Journal of the American Dietetic Association*, *103*(5), 582–587. doi:10.1053/jada.2003.50111 PMID:12728216

Hite, B. H. (1899). The Effect of Pressure in the Preservation of Milk. *West Virginia Agricultural Experimental Station Bulletin*, *58*, 15–35.

Hjort af Ornäs, A. (1993). *The Multi-Purpose Camel: Interdisciplinary Studies on Pastoral Production in Somalia*. Uppsala, Sweden: EPOS, MO Print.

Hjört af Ornäs, A., & Ali Hussein, M. (1993). Camel herd dynamics in southern Somalia: Long term development and milk production implications. In A. Hjort af Ornäs (Ed.), The Multi-Purpose Camel: Interdisciplinary Studies on Pastoral Production in Somalia (pp. 31-42). Uppsala University.

Ho, T., Chan, S., Yago, A., & Shravya, R. (2019). Changes in physiochemical properties of spray-dried camel milk powder over accelerated storage. Food Chemistry. (Accepted for publication)

Hocquette, J. F., Malek, I. C., Jailler, R., & Picard, B. (2005). Recent advances in research on bovine muscle and meat sensory quality. II. Influence of rearing factors on muscle characteristics. *Cahiers Agricultures*, *14*, 365–372.

Holt, L. J., Herring, C., Jespers, L. S., Woolven, B. P., & Tomlinson, I. M. (2003). Domain antibodies: Proteins for therapy. *Trends in Biotechnology*, *21*(11), 484–490. doi:10.1016/j.tibtech.2003.08.007 PMID:14573361

Holzapfel, W. (1997). Use of starter cultures in fermentation on a household scale. *Food Control*, *8*(5), 241–258. doi:10.1016/S0956-7135(97)00017-0

Holzapfel, W. H. (2002). Appropriate starter culture technologies for small-scale fermentation in developing countries. *International Journal of Food Microbiology*, *75*(3), 197–212. doi:10.1016/S0168-1605(01)00707-3

Horbanczuk, O. K., & Wierzbicka, A. (2016). Technological and nutritional properties of ostrich, emu and rhea meat quality. *Journal of Veterinary Research (Pulawy)*, *60*, 279–286.

Horneman, D. A., Ottens, M., Hoorneman, M., van der Wielen, L. A., & Tesson, M. (2004). Reaction and diffusion during demineralization of animal bone. *AIChE Journal. American Institute of Chemical Engineers*, *50*(11), 2682–2690. doi:10.1002/aic.10264

Hosseini, S. M. a.-R., Zibaee, S., Yousefi, M., Taghipour, A., & Noras, M. (2015). Camels Milk: Nutrition and Health Perspectives Iranian Traditional Medicine. *International Journal of Pediatrics, 3*(5.1), 915-920.

Hosseini, S. M. A., Anushiravani, M., Mojahedi, M. J., Hami, M., Zibaee, S., Rakhshandeh, H., ... Tavassoli, A. P. (2019). The efficacy of camel milk and Tarangabin (manna of Alhagi maurorum (combination therapy on glomerular filtration rate in patients with chronic kidney disease: A randomized controlled trial. *Avicenna Journal of Phytomedicine*.

Ho, T. M., Chan, S., Yago, A. J., Shravya, R., Bhandari, B. R., & Bansal, N. (2019). Changes in physicochemical properties of spray-dried camel milk powder over accelerated storage. *Food Chemistry, 295*, 224–233. doi:10.1016/j.foodchem.2019.05.122 PMID:31174753

Huang, T., Tu, Z., Wang, H., & Zhang, L. (2017). Rheological and structural properties of fish scales gelatin: Effects of conventional and ultrasound- assisted extraction. *International Journal of Food Properties, 2912*.

Huppertz, T., Fox, P. F., & Kelly, A. L. (2004). High Pressure Treatment of Bovine Milk: Effects on Casein Micelles and Whey Proteins. *The Journal of Dairy Research, 71*(1), 97–106. doi:10.1017/S002202990300640X PMID:15068072

Huppertz, T., Hinza, K., Zobrista, M. R., Uniacke, T., Kellya, A. L., & Fox, P. F. (2005). Effects of High-Pressure Treatment on The Rennet Coagulation and Cheesemaking Properties of Heated Milk. *Innovative Food Science & Emerging Technologies, 6*(3), 279–285. doi:10.1016/j.ifset.2005.03.005

Huppertz, T., Smiddy, M. A., Upadhyay, V., & Kelly, A. L. (2006). High-Pressure-Induced Changes in Bovine Milk: A Review. *International Journal of Dairy Technology, 59*(2), 58–66. doi:10.1111/j.1471-0307.2006.00246.x PMID:16410058

Hussen, M., Selamawit, H., Ashenafi, G., Fikre, Z., & Ashenafi, F. (2016). Assessment on Safety Status of Camel Raw Milk Marketed in Samara-Logia Town of Afar National Regional State, Northeast Ethiopia. *Food Science and Quality Management, 49*, 88–88.

Hwang, I. H., Devine, C. E., & Hopkins, D. L. (2003). The biochemical and physical effects of electrical stimulation on beef and sheep meat tenderness. *Meat Science, 65*(2), 677–691. doi:10.1016/S0309-1740(02)00271-1 PMID:22063428

Hynd, J. (1980). Drying of whey. *International Journal of Dairy Technology, 33*(2), 52–54. doi:10.1111/j.1471-0307.1980.tb01471.x

Ibn-e-Sina, A. (2005). *Al-Qanun fit-tib, volume three* [The Canon of Medicine]. Beirut: Alaalami Beirut library Press (research of ebrahim shamsedine).

Ibrahem, S. A., & El Zubeir, I. E. M. (2016). Processing, composition and sensory characteristic of yoghurt made from camel milk and camel–sheep milk mixtures. *Small Ruminant Research, 136*, 109–112. doi:10.1016/j.smallrumres.2016.01.014

Ibrahim, A. (2015). *Effects of exopolysaccharide-producing starter cultures on physicochemical, rheological and sensory properties of fermented camel's milk* (Vol. 27). doi:10.9755/ejfa.v27i4.19911

Ibrahim, A., & Khalifa, S. (2015). *The effects of various stabilizers on physiochemical properties of camel milk yoghurt* (Vol. 11).

Ibrahim, A. H., & Khalifa, S. A. (2015). The effects of various stabilizers on physiochemical properties of camel milk yoghurt. *The Journal of American Science, 11*(1).

Ibrahim, A., & Khalifa, S. (2015). Effect of freeze-drying on camel's milk nutritional properties. *International Food Research Journal, 22*(4), 1438–1445.

Ibrahim, G. A., Nour, I. A., & Al-Maqbali, R. (2018). Determination of pesticide and antibiotic residues in musclkes of Sudanese camel (Camelus dromedaries). *Journal of Camel Practice and Research*, *25*(2), 163–169. doi:10.5958/2277-8934.2018.00023.1

Ibrahim, G. A., Nour, I. A., Al-Maqbali, R., & Kadim, I. T. (2017). Effect of age on concentrations of nutrients in four muscles of Sudanese dromedary (Camelus dromedaries) camel. *Journal of Applied Animal Research*, *45*(1), 577–584. doi:10.1080/09712119.2016.1232266

Ibrahim, G. A., Nour, I. A., & Kadim, I. T. (2015). Effect of age on quality characteristics and composition of muscles of Sudanese camel (Camelus dromedaries). *Journal of Camel Practice and Research*, *22*(2), 209–216. doi:10.5958/2277-8934.2015.00033.8

Ibrahim, H. R., Isono, H., & Miyata, T. (2018). Potential antioxidant bioactive peptides from camel milk proteins. *Animal Nutrition*, *4*(3), 273–280. doi:10.1016/j.aninu.2018.05.004 PMID:30175255

IDF. (1984). *The Thermization Of Milk, Document No. 182*. Brussels: International Dairy Federation.

IFIC. (2019). *Functional foods, International Food Information Council Foundation*; Retrieved January 12, 2019, from http://www.foodinsight.org

Ikechukwu, P., Okafor, D., Kabuo, N., Ibeabuchi, J., Odimegwu, O., Alagbaoso, E., ... Mbah, N. (2017). Production and evaluation of cookies from whole wheat and date palm fruit pulp as sugar substitute. *International Journal of Advancement in Engineering Technology Management and Applied Science*, *4*(4), 1–31.

Indra, R., Magash, A., & Biichee, N. (1998). *Studies of Bactrian camel*. Washington, DC: Institution Press.

International livestock Institute. (2013). *Camel milk, a practical guid to hygenic production and handling for improved market access*. Author.

Ip, C., Singh, M., Thompson, H. J., & Scimeca, J. A. (1994). Conjugated linoleic acid suppresses mammary carcinogenesis and proliferative activity of the mammary gland in the rat. *Cancer Research*, *54*(5), 1212–1215. PMID:8118808

Irigoyen, A., Arana, I., Castiella, M., Torre, P., & Ibànez, F. (2005). Microbiological, physicochemical, and sensory characteristics of kefir during storage. *Food Chemistry*, *90*(4), 613–620. doi:10.1016/j.foodchem.2004.04.021

Ishag, I. A., Eisa, M. O., & Ahmed, M.-K. A. (2011). Phenotypic characteristics of Sudanese camels (*Camelus dromedarius). Livestock Research for Rural Development*. Retrieved from http://www.lrrd.org/lrrd23/4/isha23099.htm

Ismael, A. B., El Hafez, S. M. A., Mahmoud, M. B., Elaraby, A. K. A., & Hassan, H. M. (2013). Development of new strategy for non-antibiotic therapy: Dromedary camel lactoferrin has a potent antimicrobial and immunomodulator effects. *Advances in Infectious Diseases*, *3*(04), 231–237. doi:10.4236/aid.2013.34034

Izadi, A., Khedmat, L., & Mojtahedi, S. Y. (2019). Nutritional and therapeutic perspectives of camel milk and its protein hydrolysates: A review on versatile biofunctional properties. *Journal of Functional Foods*, *60*, 103441. doi:10.1016/j.jff.2019.103441

Jafarpour, A. (2017). Feasibility of manufacture and investigation of physicochemical properties of camel milk – based ice cream. *Journal of Scientific Agriculture*, *1*, 300–302. doi:10.25081/jsa.2017.v1.838

Jagtiani, H. C., Jr., & Sakai, W. (1998). Tropical Fruit Processing (Food Science and Technology). London: Academic Press Inc.

Jakhar, J. K., Reddy, A. D., Maharia, S., Devi, M., Reddy, G. V. S., & Venkateshwarlu, G. (2012). Characterization of fish gelatin from blackspotted croaker (Protonibea diacanthus). *Archives of Applied Science Research*, *4*(3), 1353–1358.

Jang, A., & Lee, M. (2005). Purification and identification of angiotensin converting enzyme inhibitory peptides from beef hydrolysates. *Meat Science*, *69*(4), 653–661. doi:10.1016/j.meatsci.2004.10.014 PMID:22063143

Jans, C. (2011). *Biodiversity of lactic acid bacteria in raw camel milk products of East Africa including genomic and functional characterization of predominant lactose-adapted Streptococcus infantarius subsp. Infantarius.* (PhD Thesis No. 19835). ETH Zurich, Zurich, Switzerland.

Jans, C., Bugnard, J., Njage, P., Lacroix, C., & Meile, L. (2012). Lactic acid bacteria diversity of African raw and fermented camel milk products reveals a highly competitive, potentially health-threatening predominant. *Lebensmittel-Wissenschaft + Technologie*, *47*(2), 371–379. doi:10.1016/j.lwt.2012.01.034

Jans, C., Follador, R., Hochstrasser, M., Lacroix, C., Meile, L., & Stevens, M. J. A. (2013). Comparative genome analysis of Streptococcus infantarius subsp. InfantariusCJ18, an African fermented camel milk isolate with adaptations to dairy environment. *BMC Genomics*, *14*(1), 200. doi:10.1186/1471-2164-14-200

Jans, C., Follador, R., Lacroix, C., Meile, L., & Stevens, M. J. A. (2012). Complete Genome Sequence of the African Dairy Isolate Streptococcus infantarius subsp. Infantarius Strain CJ18. *Journal of Bacteriology*, *194*(8), 2105–2106. doi:10.1128/JB.00160-12

Jans, C., Gerber, A., Bugnard, J., Njage, P. M. K., Lacroix, C., & Meile, L. (2012). Novel Streptococcus infantarius subsp. Infantarius variants harboring lactose metabolism genes homologous to Streptococcus thermophilus. *Food Microbiology*, *31*(1), 33–42. doi:10.1016/j.fm.2012.02.001

Jans, C., Kaindi, D. W. M., Böck, D., Njage, P. M. K., Kouamé-Sina, S. M., Bonfoh, B., ... Meile, L. (2013). Prevalence and comparison of Streptococcus infantarius subsp. Infantarius and Streptococcus gallolyticus subsp. Macedonicus in raw and fermented dairy products from East and West Africa. *International Journal of Food Microbiology*, *167*(2), 186–195. doi:10.1016/j.ijfoodmicro.2013.09.008

Jans, C., Meile, L., Kaindi, D. W. M., Kogi-Makau, W., Lamuka, P., Renault, P., ... Bonfoh, B. (2017). African fermented dairy products – Overview of predominant technologically important microorganisms focusing on African Streptococcus infantarius variants and potential future applications for enhanced food safety and security. *International Journal of Food Microbiology*, *250*, 27–36. doi:10.1016/j.ijfoodmicro.2017.03.012

Jans, C., Meile, L., Lacroix, C., & Stevens, M. J. A. (2015). Genomics, evolution, and molecular epidemiology of the Streptococcus bovis/Streptococcus equinus complex (SBSEC). *Infection, Genetics and Evolution*, *33*, 419–436. doi:10.1016/j.meegid.2014.09.017

Jassim, S. A., & Naji, M. A. (2002). The desert ship: Heritage and science - unique camel antibodies. *Middle East Laboratory*, *5*, 6–11.

Jaturasitha, S., Thirawong, P., Leangwunta, V., & Kreuzer, M. (2004). Reducing toughness of beef from BosIndicus draught steers by injection of calcium chloride: Effect of concentration and time postmortem. *Meat Science*, *68*(1), 61–69. doi:10.1016/j.meatsci.2004.02.004 PMID:22062008

Jazieh, A. R., Al Sudairy, R., Abulkhair, O., Alaskar, A., Al Safi, F., Sheblaq, N., ... Tamim, H. (2012). Use of complementary and alternative medicine by patients with cancer in Saudi Arabia. *Journal of Alternative and Complementary Medicine (New York, N.Y.)*, *18*(11), 1045–1049. doi:10.1089/acm.2011.0266 PMID:22906212

Jelliffe, D. B., & Jelliffe, E. F. (1978). *Human milk in the modern world: Psychosocial, nutritional and economic significance.* Oxford, UK: Oxford University Press. doi:10.1136/bmj.2.6151.1573

Ji, R. M. T. (2006). *Studies on molecular evolution of domestic and wild bac-trian and the physical–chemical properties of camel milk.* Diss. ETHNo. 219208.

Jiang, P. E. (2005). An analysis on the factors influencing the spinning ability of camel hair. *Journal of Wenzhou Vocational and Technical College*, *5*, 39–40.

Jilo, K. (2016). Medicinal Values of Camel Milk. *International Journal of Veterinary Science and Research*, *2*(1), 18-25.

Ji, R. M. T., Zhang, H. P., & So, Y. L. M. (2007). Chemical compositions and dynamic changes of Mongolian Gobi Red Bactrian camel milk. *Chinese Journal of Food Science*, *28*(8), 399–403.

Ji, R., Cui, P., Ding, F., Geng, J., Gao, H., Zhang, H., ... Meng, H. (2009). Monophyletic origin of domestic bactrian camel (*Camelus bactrianus*) and its evolutionary relationship with the extant wild camel (*Camelus bactrianus ferus*). *Animal Genetics*, *40*(4), 377–382. doi:10.1111/j.1365-2052.2008.01848.x PMID:19292708

Jirimutu, B., Li, J., Alam, M. S., Li, H., Guo, M., & Zhang, H. (2010). Fatty acid and protein profiles, and mineral content of milk from the wild Bactrian camel (*Camelus bactrianus ferus*) in Mongolia. *Milchwissenschaft. Milk Science International*, *65*, 21–25.

Jirimutu, W. Z. (2012). Genome sequences of wild and domestic Bactrian camels. *Nature Communications*, *3*(1), 1202. doi:10.1038/ncomms2192 PMID:23149746

Johnston, D. E., Austin, B. A., & Murphy, P. M. (1992). Effects of High Hydrostatic Pressure on Milk. *Milchwissenchaft*, *47*, 760–763.

Johnston, D. E., Austin, B. A., & Murphy, R. J. (1992). Effects of High Hydrostatic Pressure on Milk. *Milchwissenschaft. Milk Science International*, *47*(12), 760–763.

Johnston, D. E., Murphy, R. J., & Birks, A. W. (1994). Stirred-Style Yogurt-Type Product Prepared from Pressure Treated Skim-Milk. *High Pressure Research*, *12*(4-6), 215–219. doi:10.1080/08957959408201660

Jones-Abeiderrhamane, N. (2013). *Camel cheese: seemed like a good idea*. Nouakchott, Mauritania: Nancy Jones-Abeiderrahmane.

Jones, P., & Kenny, A. (2010). *Australia's Muslim Cameleers: Pioneers of the Inland, 1860s-1930s*. Wakefield press Publishers.

Jouany, J. P. (2000). La digestion chez les camélidés; comparaison avec les ruminants. *Productions Animales*, *13*(3), 165–176.

Jouppila, K., & Roos, Y. (1994). Water sorption and time-dependent phenomena of milk powders. *Journal of Dairy Science*, *77*(7), 1798–1808. doi:10.3168/jds.S0022-0302(94)77121-6

Jrad, Z., El Hatmi, H., Adt, I., Girardet, J. M., Cakir-Kiefer, C., Jardin, J., ... Oulahal, N. (2014). Effect of digestive enzymes on antimicrobial, radical scavenging and angiotensin I converting enzyme inhibitory activities of camel colostrum and milk proteins. *Dairy Science & Technology*, *94*(3), 205–224. doi:10.100713594-013-0154-1

Jrad, Z., El-Hatmi, H., Adt, I., Gouin, S., Jardin, J., Oussaief, O., ... Oulahal, N. (2019). Antilisterial activity of dromedary lactoferrin peptic hydrolysates. *Journal of Dairy Science*, *102*(6), 4844–4856. doi:10.3168/jds.2018-15548 PMID:31005319

Jrad, Z., Girardet, J.-M., Adt, I., Oulahal, I., Degraeve, N., Khorchani, P., & El Hatmi, H. (2014). Antioxidant activity of camel milk casein. *Mljekarstvo*, *64*, 287–294. doi:10.15567/mljekarstvo.2014.0408

Jrad, Z., Oulahal, N., Adt, I., Khorchani, T., Degraeve, P., & El-Hatmi, H. (2015). Camel colostrum: Nutritional composition and improvement of the antimicrobial activity after enzymatic hydrolysis. *Emirates Journal of Food and Agriculture*, *27*(4), 384–389. doi:10.9755/ejfa.v27i4.19912

Jrad, Z., Oussaief, O., Bouhemda, T., Khorchani, T., & EL-Hatmi, H. (2019). Potential effects of ultrafiltration process and date powder on textural, sensory, bacterial viability, antioxidant properties and phenolic profile of dromedary Greek yogurt. *International Journal of Food Science & Technology*, *54*(3), 854–861. doi:10.1111/ijfs.14005

Juffs, H., & Deeth, H. C. (2007). *Scientific Evaluation of Pasteurisation For Pathogen Reduction in Milk and Milk Products*. Canberra: Food Standards Australia and New Zealand.

Jumah, R., Shaker, R., & Abu-Jadayil, B. (2001). Effect of milk source on therheological properties of yoghurt during the gelation process. *International Journal of Dairy Technology*, *54*(3), 89–93. doi:10.1046/j.1364-727x.2001.00012.x

Jurjanz, S., Nurseitova, M., Toregozhina, Z., Konuspayeva, G., & Faye, B. (2018). Kinetics of polychlorinated biphenyls in Bactrian camels. *Emirates Journal of Food and Agriculture*, *30*(4), 312–319. doi:10.9755/ejfa.2018.v30.i4.1667

Kadim, I. (2013). A Review of the Nutritive Value and Meat Quality Characteristics of the Dromedary (*Camelus dromedaries*) Camel Meats. *CAMEL: International Journal of Veterinary Science*, *1*(2), 129–156.

Kadim, I. T., Al-Ani, M. R., Al-Maqbaly, R. S., Mansour, M. H., Mahgoub, O., & Johnson, E. H. (2011). Proximate, amino acid, fatty acid and mineral composition of raw and cooked camel (Camelus dromedarius) meat. *British Food Journal*, *113*(4), 482–493. doi:10.1108/00070701111123961

Kadim, I. T., Al-Karousi, A., Mahgoub, O., Al-Marzooqi, W., Al-Maqbaly, R., Khalaf, S. K., & Raiymbek, G. (2013a). Physical, chemical, quality and histochemical characteristics of infraspinatus, triceps brachii, longissimus thoraces, biceps femoris, semitendinosus, and semimembranosus of dromedary camel (Camelus dromedaries) muscles. *Meat Science*, *93*, 564–571. doi:10.1016/j.meatsci.2012.11.028 PMID:23273465

Kadim, I. T., & Mahgoub, O. (2008). Effect of age on quality and composition of one-humped camel Longissimus thoracis muscle. *International Journal of Postharvest Technology and Innovation*, *1*(3), 327–336. doi:10.1504/IJPTI.2008.021467

Kadim, I. T., Mahgoub, O., Al-Marzooqi, W., Al-Zadgali, S., Annamali, K., & Mansour, M. H. (2006). Effects of age on composition and quality of muscle Longissimus thoracic of the Omani Arabian Camel (*Camelus dromedarius*). *Meat Science*, *73*(4), 619–625. doi:10.1016/j.meatsci.2006.03.002 PMID:22062561

Kadim, I. T., Mahgoub, O., Al-Marzooqi, W., & Khalaf, S. K. (2009a). Effect of low voltage electrical stimulation and splitting carcass on histochemical and meat quality characteristics of the one-humped camel (Camelus dromedaries) Longissimus thoracic muscle. *Journal of Camelid Science*, *2*, 30–40.

Kadim, I. T., Mahgoub, O., Al-Marzooqi, W., & Khalaf, S. K. (2009a). Effect of low voltage electrical stimulation and splitting carcass on histochemical and meat quality characteristics of the one-humped camel (Camelus dromedaries) Longissimus thoracis muscle. *Journal of Camelid Science*, *2*, 30–40.

Kadim, I. T., Mahgoub, O., Al-Marzooqi, W., Khalaf, S. K., Mansour, M. H., Al-Sinani, S. S. H., & Al-Amri, I. S. (2009b). Effects of electrical stimulation on histochemical muscle fibre staining, quality, and composition of camel and cattle Longissimus thoracic muscles. *Journal of Food Science*, *74*(1), S44–S52. doi:10.1111/j.1750-3841.2008.00992.x PMID:19200120

Kadim, I. T., Mahgoub, O., Al-Marzooqi, W., Khalaf, S. K., & Raiymbek, G. (2013b). Nutritive Value, Quality and Health Aspects of the Dromedary (Camelus dromedaries) and Bactrian (Camelus bacterianus) Camel Meats: A Review. *Agricultural and Marine Sciences*, *18*, 7–24.

Kadim, I. T., & Sahi, A. B. A. (2018). Health aspects of camel meat: A review of literature. *Advances in Animal and Veterinary Sciences*, *6*(7), 271–272. doi:10.17582/journal.aavs/2018/6.7.271.272

Kaindi, D.W.M., Schelling, E., Wangoh, J., Imungi, J.K., Farah, Z. & Meile, L. (2011). Microbiological quality of raw camel milk across the Kenya market chain. *Food, 5*(1), 79-83.

Kajimoto, O., Kurosaki, T., Mizutani, J., Ikeda, N., Kaneko, K., Aihara, K., ... Nakamura, Y. (2002). Antihypertensive effects of liquid yogurts containing "lactotripeptides (VPP, IPP)" in mild hypertensive subjects. *Journal of Nutrition and Food, 5*, 55–66.

Kalejman, H., & Sheva, B. (2011). *United State Patent.* US Patent No. US7, 883, 691, B2.

Kalla, K., Manthani, V., & Keerthi, S. (2017). Camel Milk An White Gold Of Dessert-A Review. *International Archive of Applied Sciences and Technology, 8*(3), 74–83.

Kalyankar, S., Deshmukh, M., Chopde, S., Khedkar, C., Lule, V., & Deosarkar, S. (2016). Milk Powder. In B. Caballero, P. Finglas, & F. Toldrá (Eds.), *The Encyclopedia of Food and Health*. Oxford, UK: Academic Press. doi:10.1016/B978-0-12-384947-2.00465-7

Kamal, A. M., Omar, A., & El-Saied, K. M. (2007). Changes in amino acids profile of camel milk protein during the early lactation. *International Journal of Dairy Science, 2*(3), 226–234. doi:10.3923/ijds.2007.226.234

Kamal, A. M., & Salama, O. A. (2009). Lipid fractions and fatty acid composition of colostrums, transitional and mature she-camel milk during the first month of lactation. *Asian Journal of Clinical Nutrition, 1*, 23–30. doi:10.3923/ajcn.2009.23.30

Kamal, M., Foukani, M., & Karoui, R. (2017a). Rheological and physical properties of camel and cow milk gels enriched with phosphate and calcium during acid-induced gelation. *Journal of Food Science and Technology, 54*(2), 439–446. doi:10.100713197-016-2480-9 PMID:28242943

Kamal, M., Foukani, M., & Karoui, R. (2017b). Effects of heating and calcium and phosphate mineral supplementation on the physical properties of rennet-induced coagulation of camel and cow milk gels. *The Journal of Dairy Research, 84*(2), 220–228. doi:10.1017/S0022029917000152 PMID:28524011

Kamal, M., & Karoui, R. (2017). Monitoring of mild heat treatment of camel milk by front-face fluorescence spectroscopy. *Lebensmittel-Wissenschaft + Technologie, 79*, 586–593. doi:10.1016/j.lwt.2016.11.013

Kamoun, M. (1995a). Dromedary meat: production, qualitative aspects and acpability for transformation. *Option Mediterraneennes.Serie B, Etudes Recherches,* (13), 105-130.

Kamoun, M. (1995b). *Evolution de la qualite de la carcasse et de la viande des dromadaires En function de la conduit zootechnique des animaux.* Rapport final relative a la bourse de recherché FIS no. 1372-2.

Kappeler, S. R., Van den Brink, H. J., Rahbek-Nielsen, H., Farah, Z., Puhan, Z., Hansen, E. B., & Johansen, E. (2006). Characterizations of recombinant camel chymosin reveals superior properties for the coagulation of bovine and camel milk. *Biochemical and Biophysical Research Communications, 342*(2), 647–654. doi:10.1016/j.bbrc.2006.02.014 PMID:16488399

Kappeler, S., Farah, Z., & Puhan, Z. (1998). Sequence analysis of *Camelus dromedarius* milk caseins. *The Journal of Dairy Research, 65*(2), 209–222. doi:10.1017/S0022029997002847 PMID:9627840

Kappeler, S., Farah, Z., & Puhan, Z. (1999). Alternative splitting of lactophorin mRNA from lactating mammary gland of the camel (*Camelus dromedarius*). *Journal of Dairy Science, 82*(10), 2084–2093. doi:10.3168/jds.S0022-0302(99)75450-0 PMID:10531593

Kappeler, S., Farah, Z., & Puhan, Z. (2003). 5′-Flanking regions of camel milk genes are highly similar to homologue regions of other species and can be divided into two distinct groups. *Journal of Dairy Science*, *86*(2), 498–508. doi:10.3168/jds.S0022-0302(03)73628-5 PMID:12647956

Kappeler, S., Heuberger, C., Farah, Z., & Puhan, Z. (1998). *Compositional and structural analysis of camel milk proteins with emphasis on protective proteins*. ETH Zurich.

Kappeler, S., Heuberger, C., Farah, Z., & Puhan, Z. (2004). Expression of the Peptidoglycan Recognition Protein, PGRP, in the Lactating Mammary Gland. *Journal of Dairy Science*, *87*(8), 2660–2668. doi:10.3168/jds.S0022-0302(04)73392-5 PMID:15328291

Kappeler, S., Heuberger, C., Farah, Z., & Puhan, Z. (2004). Expression of the peptidoglycan recognition protein, PGRP, in the lactating mammary gland. *Journal of Dairy Science*, *87*(8), 2660–2668. doi:10.3168/jds.S0022-0302(04)73392-5 PubMed

Kappeler, S., Manfred, A., Farah, Z., & Puhan, Z. (1999). Sequence analysis of camel milk (*Camelus dromedarius*) lactoferrin. *International Dairy Journal*, *9*(7), 481–486. doi:10.1016/S0958-6946(99)00117-X

Karaca, O., Guven, M., Kaya, S., & Kahyaoglu, A. (2009). The Functional, Rheological and Sensory Characteristics of Ice Creams with Various Fat Replacers. *International Journal of Dairy Technology*, *62*(1), 93–99. doi:10.1111/j.1471-0307.2008.00456.x

Karaman, S., Toker, Ö., Yüksel, F., Çam, M., Kayacier, A., & Dogan, M. (2014). Physicochemical, bioactive, and sensory properties of persimmon-based ice cream: Technique for order preference by similarity to ideal solution to determine optimum concentration. *Journal of Dairy Science*, *97*(1), 97–110. doi:10.3168/jds.2013-7111 PMID:24268400

Kargozari, M., Moini, S., Basti, A. A., Emam-Djomeh, Z., Ghasemlou, M., Martin, I. R., ... Szumny, A. (2014). Development of Turkish dry-fermented sausage (sucuk) reformulated with camel meat and hump fat and evaluation of physicochemical, textural, fatty acid and volatile compound profiles during ripening. *Food Science and Technology (Campinas)*, *59*, 849–858.

Karim, A. A., & Bhat, R. (2009). Fish gelatin: Properties, challenges, and prospects as an alternative to mammalian gelatins. *Food Hydrocolloids*, *23*(3), 563–576. doi:10.1016/j.foodhyd.2008.07.002

Karthikeyan, S., Yadav, S., Paramasivam, M., Srinivasan, A., & Singh, T. P. (2000). Structure of buffalo lactoferrin at 3.3 Å resolution at 277 K. *Acta Crystallographica. Section D, Biological Crystallography*, *56*(6), 684–689. doi:10.1107/S0907444900005151 PMID:10818344

Kashyap, D.R, Rompca, A., & Gaballa, A. (2014). Peptidoglycan recognition proteins kill bacteria by inducing oxidative, thiol, and metal stress. *PLoS Pathog, 10*(7), 1-17.

Kaskous, S. (2016). Importance of camel milk for human health. *Emirates Journal of Food and Agriculture*, *28*(3), 158–163. doi:10.9755/ejfa.2015-05-296

Kassem, A., ElSayed, M. T., & Ahmed, A. (2004). Microstructural characteristics of Arabian camel meat. *Journal of Camelid Science*, *1*, 86–95.

Kaushik, R., Sachdeva, B., Arora, S., & Gupta, C. (2015). Effect of content on sensory and physico-chemical properties of laboratory-pasteurized calcium and vitamin D-fortified mixture of cow and buffalo milk. *International Journal of Dairy Technology*, *68*(1), 135–143. doi:10.1111/1471-0307.12166

Kavas, G. (2015). Kefirs manufactured from camel (*Camelus dramedarius*) milk and cow milk: Comparison of some chemical and microbial properties. *Italian Journal of Food Science*, *27*, 357–365.

Kavas, N., & Kavas, G. (2016). Probiotic frozen yoghurt production using camel milk (*Camelus dromedarius*) with improved functions by strawberry guava (*Psidium littorale* var. *cattleianum*) fortification. *British Journal of Applied Science and Technology*, *14*(5), 1–12. doi:10.9734/BJAST/2016/23683

Kawabata, S., & Niwa, M. (1989). Fabric Performance in Clothing Manufacture. *Journal of the Textile Institute*, *80*(1), 19–50. doi:10.1080/00405008908659184

Kaya, G., Tran, C., Sorg, O., Hotz, R., Grand, D., Carraux, P., & Saurat, J. H. (2006). Hyaluronate fragments reverse skin atrophy by a CD44- dependent mechanism. *PLoS Medicine*, *3*(12), 493. doi:10.1371/journal.pmed.0030493 PMID:17177600

Kebir, N., Aichouni, A., & Zahzeh, T. (2017). Raw camel milk properties on alloxan-induced diabetic Wistar rats. *Romanian Journal of Diabetes, Nutrition, and Metabplic Disorders*, *24*(1), 41-47. doi:10.1515/rjdnmd-2017-0005

Keeney, P., & Kroger, M. (1974). *Fundamentals of dairy chemistry* (2nd ed.). Westport, CT: AVI Publishing Co.

Kehoe, T. J., & Prescott, E. C. (2007). *Great depressions of the twentieth century*. Research Department, Federal Reserve Bank of Minneapolis.

Kessler, E. C., Bruckmaier, R. M., & Gross, J. J. (2019). Immunoglobulin G content and colostrum composition of different goat and sheep breeds in Switzerland and Germany. *Journal of Dairy Science*, *102*(6), 5542–5549. doi:10.3168/jds.2018-16235 PMID:30904298

Keykanlu, H., Zibaei, S., Ardjmand, M., & Safekordi, A. (2016). Fluorocarbon nanostructures (PFOB-NEP) as camel milk lactoferrin and its anti-cancer effects on human breast cancer cell line MCF7. *Izvestiia po Himiia*, *48*(2), 323–331.

Khalafalla, A. I., Saeed, I. K., Ali, Y. H., Abdurrahman, M. B., Kwiatek, O., Libeau, G., ... Abbas, Z. (2010). An outbreak of peste des petits ruminants (PPR) in camels in the Sudan. *Acta Tropica*, *116*(2), 161–165. doi:10.1016/j.actatropica.2010.08.002 PMID:20707980

Khalesi, M., Salami, M., Moslehishad, M., Winterburn, J., & Moosavi-Movahedi, A. A. (2017). Biomolecular content of camel milk: A traditional superfood t owards future healthcare industry. *Trends in Food Science & Technology*, *62*, 49–58. doi:10.1016/j.tifs.2017.02.004

Khalil, M. S., Beheri, H. H., & Fattah, W. I. A. (2002). Structural and electrical properties of zirconia/hydroxyapatite porous composites. *Ceramics International*, *28*(4), 451–458. doi:10.1016/S0272-8842(01)00118-3

Khalil, R., & Blassy, K. (2011). The Use Modified Date Pulp Fibers in Functional Low Fat Ice Cream. *Egyptian Journal of Dairy Science*, *39*, 275–283.

Khan, A. A., Alzohairy, M. A., & Mohieldein, A. H. (2013). Antidiabetic Effects of Camel Milk in Streptozotocin-induced Diabetic Rats. *American Journal of Biochemistry and Molecular Biology*, *3*(1), 151–158. doi:10.3923/ajbmb.2013.151.158

Khan, A., & Alzohairy, M. (2011). Hepatoprotective effects of camel milk against CCl4-induced hepatotoxicity in Rats. *Asian Journal of Biochemistry*, *6*(2), 171–180. doi:10.3923/ajb.2011.171.180

Khan, H., Athar, I. H., & Aslam, M. (2004). Evaluation of Cheese Prepared by Processing Camel Milk. *Pakistan Journal of Zoology*, *36*, 323–326.

Khan, J. A., Kumar, P., Paramasivam, M., Yadav, R. S., Sahani, M. S., Sharma, S., ... Singh, T. P. (2001). Camel lactoferrin, a transferrin-cum-lactoferrin: Crystal structure of camel apo-lactoferrin at 2.6 Å resolution and structural basis of its dual role. *Journal of Molecular Biology*, *309*(3), 751–761. doi:10.1006/jmbi.2001.4692 PMID:11397094

Khaskheli, M., Arain, M. A., Chaudhry, S., Soomro, A. H., & Qureshi, T. A. (2005). Physico-chemical quality of camel milk. *Journal of Agriculture and Social Sciences*, *2*, 164–166.

Khatoon, H., & Najam, R. (2017). Bioactive Components in Camel Milk: Their Nutritive Value and Therapeutic Application. In Nutrients in Dairy and their Implications on Health and Disease (pp. 377-387). Elsevier.

Khatoon, H., & Najam, R. (2017). Bioactive Components in Camel Milk: Their Nutritive Value and Therapeutic Application. In R. R. Watson, R. J. Collier, & V. R. Preedy (Eds.), Nutrients in Dairy and their Implications on Health and Disease (pp. 377–387). Academic Press. doi:10.1016/B978-0-12-809762-5.00029-2

Khedid, K., Faid, M., Mokhtari, A., Soulaymani, A., & Zinedine, A. (2009). Characterization of lactic acid bacteria isolated from the one humped camel milk produced in Morocco. *Microbiological Research*, *164*(1), 81–91. doi:10.1016/j.micres.2006.10.008

Khezrian, A., & Shahbazi, Y. (2018). Application of nanocompostie chitosan and carboxymethyl cellulose films containing natural preservative compounds in minced camel's meat. *International Journal of Biological Macromolecules*, *106*, 1146–1158. doi:10.1016/j.ijbiomac.2017.08.117 PMID:28847602

Khorchani, T., Hammadi, M., & Moslah, M. (2005). Artificial nursing of camel calves: an effective technique for calves' safeguard and improving herd productivity. In *Proceedings of the International Workshop Desertification Combat and Food Safety: The Added Value of Camel Producers, Ashkabad (Turkmenistan)*, (Vol. 362, pp. 177-182). Amsterdam, The Netherlands: IOS press Publishers.

Khunger, N., & Gupta, J. (2017). Approach to management of aging skin. In M. Venktaram (Ed.), *ACS(I) Textbook of cutaneous & aesthetic surgery* (pp. 711–715). New Delhi, India: Jaypee Brothers Medical Publisher.

Kieselev, N. (1956). Bacteriological examination of chal (Ru). *Mol. Prom*, *17*, 31–34.

Kimaryo, V. M., Massawe, G. A., Olasupo, N. A., & Holzapfel, W. H. (2000). The use of a starter culture in the fermentation of cassava for the production of "kivunde", a traditional Tanzanian food product. *International Journal of Food Microbiology*, *56*(2–3), 179–190. doi:10.1016/S0168-1605(00)00159-8

Kimassoum, D., Bawe, N. M., Nadjilem, D., Nji, A. M., Tidjani, A., Bughe, R. N., & Mbacham, W. F. (2016). Evaluation of some nutritional and physicochemical properties of camel meat originating from Chad. *African Journal of Food Science*, *10*(12), 368–373.

Kim, H. Y., Kim, S. H., Choi, M. J., Min, S. G., & Kwak, H. S. (2008). The Effect of High Pressure–Low Temperature Treatment on Physicochemical Properties in Milk. *Journal of Dairy Science*, *91*(11), 4176–4282. doi:10.3168/jds.2007-0883 PMID:18946121

Kim, S. J., Cho, A. R., & Han, J. (2013). Antioxidant and antimicrobial activities of leafy green vegetable extracts and their applications to meat product preservation. *Food Control*, *29*(1), 112–120. doi:10.1016/j.foodcont.2012.05.060

Kinoti, M. F. (1996). *The potential of condensed camel milk in contributing to food security in greater Baragoi, Samburu district* (Doctoral dissertation). University of Nairobi.

Kitts, D., & Weiler, K. (2003). Bioactive proteins and peptides from food sources. Applications of bioprocesses used in isolation and recovery. *Current Pharmaceutical Design*, *9*(16), 1309–1323. doi:10.2174/1381612033454883 PMID:12769739

Kligman, A. M., & Grave, G. L. (1986). Topical tretinoin for photoaged skin. *Journal of the American Academy of Dermatology*, *15*(4), 836–838. doi:10.1016/S0190-9622(86)70242-9 PMID:3771853

Kniazeva, M., Crawford, Q. T., Seiber, M., Wang, C. Y., & Han, M. (2004). Monomethyl branched-chain fatty acids play an essential role in *Caenorhabditis elegans* development. *PLoS Biology*, *2*(9), e257. doi:10.1371/journal.pbio.0020257 PMID:15340492

Knoess, K. H., Makhudum, A. J., Rafiq, M., & Hafeez, M. (1986). Milk production potential of the dromedary with special reference to the province of Punjab, *Pakistan World Anim. Rev. FAO Rome*, *57*, 11–21.

Koç, A., & Atasever, S. (2016). *Production and characteristics of camel milk.* Paper presented in International Selçuk-Ephesus Symposium on Culture of Camel-Dealing and Camel Wrestling, Turkey.

Köhler-Rollefson, I., & Rathore, H. S. (2004). The camel in Rajasthan: Agrobiodiversity under threat. *Annals of Arid Zone*, *43*(3&4), 401–412.

Kojda, G., & Harrison, D. (1999). Interactions between NO and reactive oxygen species: Pathophysiological importance in atherosclerosis, hypertension, diabetes and heart failure. *Cardiovascular Research*, *43*(3), 652–671. doi:10.1016/S0008-6363(99)00169-8 PMID:10690328

Kolakowski, P., Reps, A., Dajnowiec, F., Szczepek, J., & Porowski, S. (1997). Effect of High Pressures on The Microflora of Raw Cow's Milk. In Proceedings of Process Optimization and Minimal Processing of Foods. Leuven, Belgium: Leuven University Press.

Koletzko, B. (2016). Human Milk Lipids. *Annals of Nutrition & Metabolism*, *69*(suppl 2), 28–40. doi:10.1159/000452819 PMID:28103608

Konuspayeva, G. (2007). *Variabilité physico-chimique et biochimique du lait des grands camélidés (Camelus bactrianus, Camelus dromedarius et hybrides) au Kazakhstan* (Doctoral dissertation). Université Montpellier II, France.

Konuspayeva, G., & Faye, B. (2004, November). A better knowledge of milk quality parameters: A preliminary step for improving the camel milk market opportunity in a transition economy–The case of Kazakhstan. In *Saving the Camel and Peoples' Livelihoods Building a Multi-Stakeholder Platform for the Conservation of the Camel in Rajasthan. International Conference* (pp. 28-36). Academic Press.

Konuspayeva, G., Al-Hammad, K., Algruin, K., Alshammari, F., Al-Rasheedi, F. S., & Faye, B. (2015). Manufacturing camel cheese: the experience of Saudi Arabia. *Scientific and Practical Journal Veterinariya,* 2(42), 203-205.

Konuspayeva, G., Faye, B., & Serikbaeva, A. (2003). Les produits laitiers traditionnels à base de lait de chamelle en Asie Centrale. In Atelier Intl. sur le lait de chamelle en Afrique. FAO-CIRAD-KARKARA. FAO Publ.

Konuspayeva, G., Faye, B., Loiseau, G., & Levieux, D. (2007). *Lactoferrin and Immunoglobulin Contents in Camel's Milk (Camelus bactrianus, Camelus dromedarius, and Hybrids) from Kazakhstan.* doi:10.3168/jds.s0022-0302(07)72606-1

Konuspayeva, G., Shomamrey, M., Aleliwi, N., Camier, B. & Faye, B. (2014b). New trials to make camel mozzarella. *Bulletin of Al-Farabi University, Série biologie*, *1/2*(60), 138-140.

Konuspayeva, G., Baubekova, A., Akhmetsadykova, Sh., Akhmetsadykov, N., & Faye, B. (2019). Concentrations in D- and L-lactate in rawx cow and camel milk. *Journal of Camel Practice and Research*, *26*(1), 111–113. doi:10.5958/2277-8934.2019.00016.X

Konuspayeva, G., Camier, B., Aleilawi, N., Al-Shumeimyri, M., Al-Hammad, K., Algruin, K., & Faye, B. (2017). Manufacture of dry-and brine-salted soft camel cheeses for the camel dairy industry. *International Journal of Dairy Technology*, *70*(1), 92–101. doi:10.1111/1471-0307.12319

Konuspayeva, G., Camier, B., Gaucheron, F., & Faye, B. (2014a). Some parameters to process camel milk into cheese. *Emirates Journal of Food and Agriculture*, *26*(4), 354–358. doi:10.9755/ejfa.v26i4.17277

Konuspayeva, G., Faye, B., Baubekova, A., & Loiseau, G. (2012). Camel gruyere cheese making. *Proceedings of the 3rd ISOCARD conference*, 218-219.

Konuspayeva, G., Faye, B., & Loiseau, G. (2009a). The composition of camel milk: A meta-analysis of the literature data. *Journal of Food Composition and Analysis*, *22*(2), 95–101. doi:10.1016/j.jfca.2008.09.008

Konuspayeva, G., Faye, B., & Loiseau, G. (2011b). Variability of vitamin C content in camel milk from Kazakhstan. *Journal of Camelid Science*, *4*, 63–69.

Konuspayeva, G., Faye, B., Loiseau, G., Ivashchenko, A., Meldebekova, A., & Davletov, S. (2009b). Physiological change in camel milk composition 1- Effect of lactation stage. *Tropical Animal Health and Production*, *42*, 495–499. doi:10.100711250-009-9449-x PMID:19757134

Konuspayeva, G., Faye, B., Loiseau, G., & Levieux, D. (2007). Lactoferrin and Immunoglobin content in camel milk from Kazakhstan. *Journal of Dairy Science*, *90*, 38–46. doi:10.3168/jds.S0022-0302(07)72606-1 PMID:17183073

Konuspayeva, G., Faye, B., Loiseau, G., Narmuratova, M., Ivashchenko, A., Meldebekova, A., & Davletov, S. (2010). Physiological change in camel milk composition (*Camelus dromedarius*) 2: Physico-chemical composition of colostrum. *Tropical Animal Health and Production*, *42*(3), 501–505. doi:10.100711250-009-9450-4 PMID:19763867

Konuspayeva, G., Jurjanz, S., Loiseau, G., Barci, V., Akhmetsadykova, Sh., Meldebekova, A., & Faye, B. (2011a). Contamination of Camel milk (heavy metals, organic pollutants and radionuclides) in Kazakhstan. *Journal of Environmental Protection*, *2*(01), 90–96. doi:10.4236/jep.2011.21010

Konuspayeva, G., Lemarie, E., Faye, B., Loiseau, G., & Montet, D. (2008). Fatty acid and cholesterol composition of camel's (*Camelus bactrianus, Camelus dromedarius* and hybrids) milk in Kazakhstan. *Dairy Science & Technology*, *88*(3), 327–340. doi:10.1051/dst:2008005

Konuspayeva, G., Loiseau, G., & Faye, B. (2004). La plus-value « santé » du lait de chamelle cru et fermenté: L'expérience du Kazakhstan. *Rencontre Recherches Ruminants*, *11*, 47–50.

Koohmaraie, M. (1988). The role of endogenous proteases in meat tenderness. *Reciprocal Meat Conference Proceedings*, *41*, 89-100.

Korashy, H. M., El Gendy, M. A., Alhaider, A. A., & El-Kadi, A. O. (2012). Camel milk modulates the expression of aryl hydrocarbon receptor-regulated genes, Cyp1a1, Nqo1, and Gsta1, in murine hepatoma Hepa 1c1c7 cells. *BioMed Research International*. PMID:22570534

Korashy, H. M., Maayah, Z. H., Abd-Allah, A. R., El-Kadi, A. O., & Alhaider, A. A. (2012). Camel milk triggers apoptotic signaling pathways in human hepatoma HepG2 and breast cancer MCF7 cell lines through transcriptional mechanism. *BioMed Research International*. PMID:22654482

Korashy, H., Maayah, Z., Abd-Allah, A., El-Kadi, A., & Alhaider, A. (2012). Camel Milk Triggers Apoptotic Signaling Pathways in Human Hepatoma HepG2 and Breast CancerMCF7 Cell Lines through Transcriptional Mechanism. *Journal of Biomedicine & Biotechnology*, 1–9. doi:10.1155/2012/593195

Korhonen, H. J. (2009). Bioactive Components in Bovine Milk. In Bioactive Components in Milk and Dairy Products (pp. 15-42). Wiley-Blackwell. doi:10.1002/9780813821504.ch2

Korish, A. (2014). The antidiabetic action of camel milk in experimental type 2 diabetes mellitus: An overview on the changes in incretin hormones, insulin resistance, and inflammatory cytokines. *Hormone and Metabolic Research. Hormon- und Stoffwechselforschung. Hormones et Metabolisme*, *46*(06), 404–411. doi:10.1055-0034-1368711 PMID:24627103

Korish, A. A., & Arafah, M. M. (2013). Camel milk ameliorates steatohepatitis, insulin resistance and lipid peroxidation in experimental non-alcoholic fatty liver disease. *BMC Complementary and Alternative Medicine*, *13*(1), 264. doi:10.1186/1472-6882-13-264 PMID:24119413

Korlepara, R. G., Kalla, A. M., Manthani, V., & Keerthi, S. (2017). Camel milk a white gold of desert: A review. *International Archive of Applied Sciences and Technology*, *8*(3), 74–83.

Korlepara, R., Kalla, A., Manthani, V., & Keerthi, S. (2017). Camel milk a white gold of dessert- a review. *International Archive of Applied Sciences and Technology*, *8*(3), 74–83.

Koroleva, N. S. (1991). Starters for fermented milks. Section 4, Kefir and kumis starters. *IDF Bulletin*, *227*, 35–40.

Kozhamkulova, B. S. (1986). The Late Cenozoic two-humped (Bactrian) camels of Asia. *Quartärpläontolgie*, *6*, 93–97.

Krebbers, B., Matser, A., Hoogerwerf, S., Moezelaar, R., Tomassen, M., & Berg, R. (2003). Combined High-Pressure and Thermal Treatments for Processing of Tomato Puree: Evaluation of Microbial Inactivation and Quality Parameters. *Innovative Food Science & Emerging Technologies*, *4*(4), 377–385. doi:10.1016/S1466-8564(03)00045-6

Krishnankutty, R., Iskandarani, A., Therachiyil, L., Uddin, S., Azizi, F., Kulinski, M., ... Mohammad, R. M. (2018). Anticancer Activity of Camel Milk via Induction of Autophagic Death in Human Colorectal and Breast Cancer Cells. *Asian Pacific journal of cancer prevention. APJCP*, *19*(12), 3501. PMID:30583676

Król, J., Brodziak, A., Litwińczuk, Z., & Barłowska, J. (2012). Selected Factors Determining the Content of Lactoferrin, Lysozyme and Immunoglobulins G in Bovine Milk. In *A Search for Antibacterial Agents*. IntechOpen. Available from: https://www.intechopen.com/books/a-search-for-antibacterial-agents/selected-factors-determining-the-content-of-lactoferrin-lysozyme-and-immunoglobulins-g-in-bovine-milk

Kula, J. (2016). Medicinal Values of Camel Milk. *International Journal of Veterinary Scientific Research*, *2*(1), 18-25. Doi:10.17352/ijvsr.000009

Kula, J. (2016). Camel milk and its therapeutic effects: A review. *Global Veterinaria*, *16*(4), 378–388.

Kula, J. T., & Tegegne, D. (2016). Chemical composition and medicinal values of camel milk. *Int J Res Stud Biosci*, *4*(4), 13–25.

Kula, J. T., & Tegegne, G. (2016). Chemical composition and medicinal values of camel milk. [IJRSB]. *International Journal of Research Studies in Biosciences*, *4*(4), 13–25.

Kula, J., & Tegegne, D. (2016). Chemical composition and medicinal value of camel milk. *International Journal of Research Studies in Bioscience*, *4*(4), 13–25.

Kumar, D., Chatli, M. K., Singh, R., Mehta, N., & Kumar, P. (2016). Enzymatic hydrolysis of camel milk casein and its antioxidant properties. *Dairy Science & Technology*, *96*(3), 391–404. doi:10.100713594-015-0275-9

Kumar, D., Chatli, M. K., Singh, R., Mehta, N., & Kumar, P. (2016). Enzymatic hydrolysis of camel milk proteins and its antioxidant properties. *Journal of Camel Practice and Research*, *23*(1), 33–40. doi:10.5958/2277-8934.2016.00005.9

Kumar, D., Chatli, M. K., Singh, R., Mehta, N., & Kumar, P. (2016b). Antioxidant and antimicrobial activity of camel milk casein hydrolysates and its fractions. *Small Ruminant Research*, *139*, 20–25. doi:10.1016/j.smallrumres.2016.05.002

Kumar, K., Venu, L., & Manchala, R. (2016). Anti-hyperglycemic activity of camel milk in rat models of diabetes / insulin resistance. *International Journal of Research Studies in Medical and Health Sciences*, *1*(1), 7–14.

Kumar, M., Pandya, H. B., Dodiya, K. K., Bhatt, R., & Mangukiya, M. (2017). Advancement in industrial method of ghee making process at sarvottam dairy, Bhavnagar, Gujarat (India). *International Journal of Science. Environment ISSN*, *6*(3), 1727–1736.

Kumar, P., & Mishra, H. (2004). Yoghurt powder- a review of process technology storage and utilization. *Food and Bioproducts Processing*, *82*(2C2), 133–142. doi:10.1205/0960308041614918

Kunz, C., Niesem, M., Lilienfeld Toal, H., & Burmeister, W. (1984). Vitamin D, 25-hydroxyvitamin D and 1,25-dihydroxyvitamin D in cow milk, infant formulas and breast milk during different stages of lactation. *International Journal for Vitamin and Nutrition Research*, *54*, 141–148. PMID:6548730

Kunz, C., & Rudloff, S. (2002). Health benefits of milk derived carbohydrates. *Bulletin of the International Dairy Federation*, *375*, 72–79.

Kunz, C., & Rudloff, S. (2006). Health promoting aspects of milk oligosaccharides. *International Dairy Journal*, *16*(11), 1341–1346. doi:10.1016/j.idairyj.2006.06.020

Kurtu, M. Y. (2004). An assessment of the productivity for meat and carcass yield of camel (Camelus dromedaries) and the consumption of camel meat in the Eastern region of Ethiopia. *Tropical Animal Health and Production*, *36*(1), 65–76. doi:10.1023/B:TROP.0000009520.34657.35 PMID:14979560

Kuwabara, Y., Nagai, S., Yoshimitsu, N., Nakagawa, I., Watanabe, Y., & Tamai, Y. (1995). Antihypertensive effect of the milk fermented by culturing with various lactic acid bacteria and yeast. *Journal of Fermentation and Bioengineering*, *80*(3), 294–295. doi:10.1016/0922-338X(95)90834-M

Laack, R. V., Kauffman, R., & Greaser, M. (2001). Determinants of ultimate pH of meat. *Proceedings of 47th International Congress of Meat Science and Technology*, *1*, 22-26.

Lacotte, P., Gomez, F., Bardeau, F., Muller, S., Acharid, A., Quervel, X., ... Birlouez-Aragon, I. (2015). A fluorescence-based analyzer to assess cheese milk denatured whey proteins. *Journal of Dairy Science*, *98*(10), 1–10. doi:10.3168/jds.2015-9412 PMID:26210276

Lakosa, I., & Shokin, V. (1964). Milk production. In Camels (pp. 113–120). Science. Technical Agricultural Publ.

Laleye, L. C., Jobe, B., & Wasesa, A. A. (2008). Comparative study on heat stability and functionality of camel and bovine whey proteins. *Journal of Dairy Science*, *91*(12), 4527–4534. doi:10.3168/jds.2008-1446 PMID:19038927

Larson, J. A. (2009). *Information Resources on the South American Camelids: Llamas, Alpacas, Guanacos, and Vicunas 2004-2008*. AWIC Resource Series No. 12. Retrieved from: https://pubs.nal.usda.gov/sites/pubs.nal.usda.gov/files/Camelids2009.pdf

Laurent, T. C., & Fraser, J. R. (1992). Hyaluronan. *The FASEB Journal*, *6*(7), 2397–2404. doi:10.1096/fasebj.6.7.1563592 PMID:1563592

Law, A. J. R., Leaver, J., Felipe, X., Ferragut, V., Pla, R., & Guamis, B. (1998). Comparison of The Effects of High Pressure and Thermal Treatments on The Casein Micelles in Goat's Milk. *Journal of Agricultural and Food Chemistry*, *46*(7), 2523–2530. doi:10.1021/jf970904c

Lawrie, R. A. (2006). *Lawrie's Meat Science* (7th ed.). Cambridge, UK: Woodhead Publishing Limited. doi:10.1533/9781845691615

Lee, S. K., Kim, Y. S., Liang, C. Y., & Song, Y. H. (2003). Effects of dietary vitamin E supplementation on color stability, lipid oxidation and reducing ability of Hanwoo (Korean cattle) beef during retail display. *Asian-Australasian Journal of Animal Sciences*, *10*(10), 1529–1534. doi:10.5713/ajas.2003.1529

Leeson, C. R., Lesson, T. S., & Paparo, A. A. (1985). Textbook of Histology (5th ed.). W. B. Saunders Company.

Lee, Y. P., & Lardy, H. A. (1965). Influence of thyroid hormones on 1-α-glycerophosphate dehydrogenases and other dehydrogenases in various organs of the rat. *The Journal of Biological Chemistry*, *240*, 1427–1436. PMID:14284758

Legarreta, I. G. (2010). Canned products and Pâté. In F. Toldra (Ed.), *Handbook of Meat Processing* (pp. 337–349). Ames, IA: Wiley-Blackwell. doi:10.1002/9780813820897.ch19

Legesse, Y. W., Dunn, C. D., Mauldin, M. R., Ordonez-Garza, N., Rowden, G. R., Gebre, Y. M., ... Bradley, R. D. (2018). Morphometric and genetic variation in 8 breeds of Ethiopian camels (*Camelus dromedarius*). *Journal of Animal Science*, *96*(12), 4925–4934. PMID:30189034

Legrand, D., Elass, E., Carpentier, M., & Mazurier, J. (2005). Lactoferrin. *Cellular and Molecular Life Sciences*, *62*(22), 2549–2559. doi:10.100700018-005-5370-2 PMID:16261255

Lemhadri, A., Zeggwagh, N.-A., Maghrani, M., Jouad, H., & Eddouks, M. (2004). Anti-hyperglycaemic activity of the aqueous extract of Origanum vulgare growing wild in Tafilalet region. *Journal of Ethnopharmacology*, *92*(2-3), 251–256. doi:10.1016/j.jep.2004.02.026

Leprovost, F., Nocart, M., Guerin, G., & Martin, P. (1994). Characterization of the goat lactoferrin cDNA: Assignment of the relevant locus to bovine U12 synteny group. *Biochemical and Biophysical Research Communications*, *203*(2), 1324–1332. doi:10.1006/bbrc.1994.2327 PMID:8093048

Leroy, F., & De Vuyst, L. (2004). Lactic acid bacteria as functional starter cultures for the food fermentation industry. *Trends in Food Science & Technology*, *15*(2), 67–78. doi:10.1016/j.tifs.2003.09.004

Lev, E. (2006). Healing with animals in the Levant from the 10th to the 18th century. *Journal of Ethnopharmacology and Ethnomedicine*, *2*. doi:10.1186/1746-4269-2-11 PMID:16504024

Levieux, D., Morgan, F., Geneix, N., Masle, I., & Bouvier, F. (2002). Caprine immunoglobulin G, β-lactoglobulin, α-lactalbumin and serum albumin in colostrum and milk during the early *post-partum* period. *The Journal of Dairy Research*, *69*(3), 391–399. doi:10.1017/S0022029902005575 PMID:12369410

Levieux, D., & Ollier, A. (1999). Bovine immunoglobulin G, beta-lactoglobulin, alpha-lactalbumin and serum albumin in colostrum and milk during the early post-partum period. *The Journal of Dairy Research*, *66*(3), 421–430. doi:10.1017/S0022029999003581 PMID:10480080

Levy, A., Steiner, L., & Yagil, R. (2013). Camel milk: Disease control and dietary laws. *Journal of Health Science*, *1*, 48–53.

Lewis, M. J., & Heppell, N. (2000). *Continuous Thermal Processing of Foods: Pasteurization and UHT Sterilization*. Gaithersburg, MD: Aspen Publishers.

Lianou, A., Kakouri, A., Pappa, E. C., & Samelis, J. (2017). Growth interactions and antilisterial effects of the bacteriocinogenic Lactococcus lactis subsp. Cremoris M104 and Enterococcus faecium KE82 strains in thermized milk in the presence or absence of a commercial starter culture. *Food Microbiology*, *64*, 145–154. doi:10.1016/j.fm.2016.12.019

Liepa, M., Zagorska, J., & Galoburda, R. (2017). Effect of High Pressure Processing on Milk Coagulation Properties. *Research for Rural Development*, *1*, 223–229. doi:10.22616/rrd.23.2017.033

Liepa, M., Zagorska, J., Galoburda, R., & Kostascuka, S. (2018). Effect of High-Pressure Processing on Microbial Quality of Skimmed Milk. Proc. Latvian Acad. *Sci., Section B*, *72*, 118–122.

Li, G., Le, G., Shi, Y., & Shrestha, S. (2004). Angiotensin I-converting enzyme inhibitory peptides derived from food proteins and their physiological and pharmacological effects. *Nutrition Research (New York, N.Y.)*, *24*(7), 469–486. doi:10.1016/S0271-5317(04)00058-2

Li, H., & Papadopoulos, V. (1998). Peripheral-type benzodiazepine receptor function in cholesterol transport. Identification of a putative cholesterol recognition/interaction amino acid sequence and consensus pattern. *Endocrinology*, *139*(12), 4991–4997. doi:10.1210/endo.139.12.6390 PMID:9832438

Liu, C., Xie, C. P., & Liu, X. J. (2017). Properties of Yak Wool in Comparison to Cashmere and Camel Hairs. *Journal of Natural Fibers*, *6*, 1–12.

Liu, D., Nikoo, M., Boran, G., Zhou, P., & Regenstein, J. M. (2015). Collagen and gelatin. *Annual Review of Food Science and Technology*, *6*(1), 527–557. doi:10.1146/annurev-food-031414-111800 PMID:25884286

Liu, H., Han, J., & Guo, S. (2009). Characteristics of the gelatin extracted from Channel Catfish (Ictalurus Punctatus) head bones. *Lebensmittel-Wissenschaft + Technologie*, *42*(2), 540–544. doi:10.1016/j.lwt.2008.07.013

Li, Y.-J., Ou, J.-J., Li, Y.-M., & Xiang, D.-X. (2017). Dietary supplement for core symptoms of autism spectrum disorder: Where are we now and where should we go? *Frontiers in Psychiatry*, *8*, 155. doi:10.3389/fpsyt.2017.00155 PMID:28878697

Locker, R. H. (1989). Muscle in to meat. In Meat Production and Processing. New Zealand Society of Animal Production.

Loden, M. (2003). Role of topical emollients and moisturizers in the treatment of dry skin barrier disorders. *American Journal of Clinical Dermatology*, *4*, 771–788. doi:10.2165/00128071-200304110-00005 PMID:14572299

Loiseau, G., Faye, B., Serikbaeva, A., & Montet, D. (2001). Enzymes ability to serve as markers of pasteurized camel milk. *Int. Conf. On new horizons in biotechnology.*

Lomholt, S. B., & Qvist, K. B. (1997). Relationship between Rheological Properties and Degree of K-Casein Proteolysis During Renneting Of Milk. *The Journal of Dairy Research*, *64*(4), 541–549. doi:10.1017/S002202999700246X

Longo, N., Frigeni, M., & Pasquali, M. (2016). Carnitine transport and fatty acid oxidation. *Biochimica et Biophysica Acta (BBA)-. Molecular Cell Research*, *1863*(10), 2422–2435.

Lonnecker, S., Boyle, E. A., Getty, K. J. K., Buege, D. R., Ingham, S. C., Searls, G., & Harper, N. M. (2010). Production methods and product characteristics of jerky produced by small and very small meat processing businesses. *Journal of Muscle Foods*, *21*(4), 826–833. doi:10.1111/j.1745-4573.2010.00222.x

López Aranguren, D. J. (1930). Camélidos fósiles argentinos. *Anales de la Sociedad Científica Argentina (Buenos Aires)*, *109*, 97–126.

Lopez Fandino, R., Carrascosa, A. V., & Olano, A. (1996). The Effects of High Pressure on Whey Protein Denaturation and Cheese-Making Properties of Raw Milk. *Journal of Dairy Science*, *79*(6), 929–1126. doi:10.3168/jds.S0022-0302(96)76443-3

Lopez Fandino, R., De La Fuente, M. A., Ramos, M., & Olano, A. (1998). Distribution of Minerals and Proteins between the Soluble and Colloidal Phases of Pressurized Milks from Different Species. *The Journal of Dairy Research*, *65*(1), 69–78. doi:10.1017/S0022029997002653

López-Fandiño, R. (2006). High pressure-induced changes in milk proteins and possible applications in dairy technology. *International Dairy Journal*, *16*(10), 1119–1131. doi:10.1016/j.idairyj.2005.11.007

López-Fandiño, R., Otte, J., & Van Camp, J. (2006). Review: Physiological, chemicaland technological aspects of milk-protein-derived peptides with antihypertensiveand ACE-inhibitory activity. *International Dairy Journal*, *16*(11), 1277–1293. doi:10.1016/j.idairyj.2006.06.004

Lorenzen, P. C., Wernery, R., Johnson, B., Jose, S., & Wernery, U. (2011). Evaluation of indigenous enzyme activities in raw and pasteurised camel milk. *Small Ruminant Research*, *97*(1-3), 79–82. doi:10.1016/j.smallrumres.2011.01.014

Lore, T. A., Mbugua, S. K., & Wangoh, J. (2005). Enumeration and identification of microflora in suusac, a Kenyan traditional fermented camel milk product. *Lebensmittel-Wissenschaft + Technologie*, *38*(2), 125–130. doi:10.1016/j.lwt.2004.05.008

Lucey, J. A., Hauth, B., Gorry, C., & Fox, P. F. (1993). Acid–base buffering of milk. *Milchwissenschaft. Milk Science International*, *48*, 268–272.

Ludwig, W., Schleifer, K. H., & Whitman, W. B. (2009). Order II. Lactobacillales ord. Nov. In P. De Vos, G. M. Garrity, D. Jones, N. R. Krieg, W. Ludwig, F. A. Rainey, … W. B. Whitman (Eds.), Bergey's manual of systematic bacteriology. The firmicutes (2nd ed.; Vol. 3, pp. 464–735). New York, NY: Springer.

Lynch, M. F., Tauxe, R. V., & Hedberg, C. W. (2009). The growing burden of foodborne outbreaks due to contaminated fresh produce: Risks and opportunities. *Epidemiology and Infection*, *137*(03), 307–315. doi:10.1017/S0950268808001969

Maaroufi, S. H., Rezaei, K., Raftaniamiri, Z., & Mirzaei, F. (2015). Evaluating the effects of herbal essences from spearmint and wild thyme on the quality of camel's milk. *International Journal of Food Science & Technology*, *50*(10), 2168–2174. doi:10.1111/ijfs.12855

MacDonald, L. E., Brett, J., Kelton, D., Majowicz, S. E., Snedeker, K., & Sargeant, J. M. (2011). A systematic review and meta-analysis of the effects of pasteurization on milk vitamins, and evidence for raw milk consumption and other health related outcomes. *Journal of Food Protection*, *74*(11), 1814–1832. doi:10.4315/0362-028X.JFP-10-269 PMID:22054181

Mader, J., Salsman, D., Conrad, D., & Hoskin, D. (2005). Bovine lactoferricin selectively induces apoptosis in human leukemia and carcinoma cell lines. *Molecular Cancer Therapeutics*, *4*(4), 612–624. doi:10.1158/1535-7163.MCT-04-0077 PMID:15827335

Madsen, B. D., Rasmussen, M. D., Nielsen, M. O., Wiking, L., & Larsen, L. B. (2004). Physical properties of mammary secretions in relation to chemical changes during transition from colostrum to milk. *The Journal of Dairy Research*, *71*(3), 263–272. doi:10.1017/S0022029904000263 PMID:15354571

Mahmoud, M. H., Badr, G., & El Shinnawy, N. A. (2016). Camel whey protein improves lymphocyte function and protects against diabetes in the offspring of diabetic mouse dams. *International Journal of Immunopathology and Pharmacology*, *29*(4), 632–646. doi:10.1177/0394632016671729

Maiorano, G., Cavone, C., Mccormick, R. J., Ciarlariello, A., Gambacorta, M., & Manchisi, A. (2007). The effect of dietary energy and vitamin E administration on performance and intramuscular collagen properties of lambs. *Meat Science*, *76*(1), 182–188. doi:10.1016/j.meatsci.2006.11.001 PMID:22064205

Maitha, I. (2019). *Microbial safety of traditional milk products From North Eastern Kenya and functional characterization of selected Lactic Acid Bacteria* (Thesis). University of Nairobi, Nairobi, Kenya.

Maitha, I., Kaindi, D. W. M., Wangoh, J., & Mbugua, S. K. (2019). Microbial Quality and Safety of Traditional Fermented Camel Milk Product Suusac Sampled from Different Regions in North Eastern, Kenya. *Asian Food Science Journal*, *8*(2), 1–9. doi:10.9734/afsj/2019/v8i229986

Makhdoomi, D. M., Gazi, M. A., Nabi, S., & Ahmed, S. (2013). Morphometric studies on adult double humped camel of Ladakh, India. *Emirates Journal of Food and Agriculture*, *25*(7), 544–548. doi:10.9755/ejfa.v25i7.15999

Mal, G., & Pathak, K. M. L. (2009). *Camel Milk- properties and its products*. 2nd conference of ISOCARD-2009, Djerba, Tunisia.

Malacarne, M., Martuzzi, F., Summer, A., & Mariani, P. (2002). Protein and fat composition of mare's milk: Some nutritional remarks with reference to human and cow's milk. *International Dairy Journal*, *12*(11), 869–877. doi:10.1016/S0958-6946(02)00120-6

Malbe, M., Otstavel, T., Kodis, I. & Viitak, A. (2010). Content of selected micro and macro elements in dairy cows. *Agronomy Research, 8*(S2), 323-26.

Maldonado, J., Gil, A., Narbona, E., & Molina, J. A. (1998). Special formulas in infant nutrition: A review. *Early Human Development*, *53*, S23–S32. doi:10.1016/S0378-3782(98)00062-0 PMID:10102652

Mal, G. D., & Sena, S. (2007). Milk composition among different breeds of camel. *The Indian Veterinary Journal*, *84*(10), 1064–1065.

Mal, G., Bjakhat, C., Suchitra Sena, D., & Pathak, K. M. L. (2010). Effect of coagulants on preparation of camel milk paneer. *Journal of Camel Practice and Research*, *17*(2), 181–184.

Mal, G., & Pathak, K. (2010). *Camel milk and milk products.* National Research Center on Camel.

Mal, G., Suchitra, D. S., & Sahani, M. S. (2007). Changes in chemical and macro-minerals content of dromedary milk during lactation. *Journal of Camel Practice and Research*, *14*(2), 195–197.

Malik, A., Al-Senaidy, A., Jankun, E., & Jankun, J. (2012). A study of the anti-diabetic agents of camel milk. *International Journal of Molecular Medicine*, *30*(3), 585–592. doi:10.3892/ijmm.2012.1051 PMID:22751901

Malmgren, B. (2015). *Challenges in processing of goat, buffalo and camel milk for longer shelf life.* Presentation to 7th international symposium on Sheep, Goat and other non-cow milk, Limossol, Cyprus.

Mankor, A., & Koussou, M. O. (2015). *Etude du sous-secteur camelin du Tchad.* N'Djamena, Chad: Rapport FAO.

Maqsood, S., Al Haddad, N. A., & Mudgil, P. (2016). Vacuum packaging as an effective strategy to retard off-odour development, microbial spoilage, protein degradation and retain sensory quality of camel meat'. *Lebensmittel-Wissenschaft + Technologie*, *72*, 55–62.

Maqsood, S., Al-Dowaila, A., Mudgil, P., Kamal, H., Jobe, B., & Hassan, H. M. (2019). Comparative characterization of protein and lipid fractions from camel and cow milk, their functionality, antioxidant and antihypertensive properties upon simulated gastro-intestinal digestion. *Food Chemistry*, *279*, 328–338. doi:10.1016/j.foodchem.2018.12.011 PMID:30611498

Maqsood, S., Manheem, K., Abushelaibil, A., & Kadim, I. T. (2014). Characterization of the lipid and protein fraction of fresh camel meat and the associated changes during refrigerated storage. *Journal of Food Composition and Analysis*, *41*, 212–220. doi:10.1016/j.jfca.2014.12.027

Margarida Figueiredoa, Martinsa, Freitasb, Judasb, & Figueiredo. (2011). Influence of hydrochloric acid concentration on the demineralization of cortical bone. *Chemical Engineering Research and Design, 89*, 116–124.

Mariod, A. A., & Adam, H. F. (2013). Review: Gelatin, source, extraction and industrial applications. *Acta Scientiarum Polonorum. Technologia Alimentaria*, *12*(2), 135–147.

Markiewicz-Górka, I., Zawadzki, M., Januszewska, L., Hombek-Urban, K., & Pawlas, K. (2011). Influence of selenium and/or magnesium on alleviation alcohol induced oxidative stress in rats, normalization function of liver and changes in serum lipid parameters. *Human and Experimental Toxicology*, *30*(11), 1811–1827. doi:10.1177/0960327111401049 PMID:21474619

Markiewicz-kęszycka, M., Czyżak-runowska, G., Lipińska, P., & Wójtowski, J. (2013). Fatty acid profile of milk - a review. *Bulletin of the Veterinary Institute in Pulawy*, *57*(2), 135–139. doi:10.2478/bvip-2013-0026

Marnila, P., Korhonen, H., Roginski, H., Fuquay, J. W., & Fox, P. F. (2002). *Encyclopedia of Dairy Science*.

Marshall, E., & Mejia, D. (2011). *Traditional fermented food and beverage for improved livelihoods*. Rome, Italy: FAO.

Martini, P., Costeur, L., Le Tonsorer, J.-M., & Schmid, P. (2015). Pleistocene camelids from the Syrian Desert: The diversity in El Kowm. *L'Anthropologie*, *119*(5), 687–693. doi:10.1016/j.anthro.2015.10.005

Martin, M., Martin-Sosa, S., Garcia-Pardo, L., & Hueso, P. (2001). Distribution of bovine sialoglycoconjugates during lactation. *Journal of Dairy Science*, *84*(5), 995–1000. doi:10.3168/jds.S0022-0302(01)74558-4 PMID:11384055

Martín-Ortiz, A., Salcedo, J., Barile, D., Bunyatratchata, A., Moreno, F. J., Martin-García, I., & Ruiz-Matute, A. I. (2016). Characterization of goat colostrum oligosaccharides by nano-liquid chromatography on chip quadrupole time-of-flight mass spectrometry and hydrophilic interaction liquid chromatography-quadrupole mass spectrometry. *Journal of Chromatography. A*, *1428*, 143–153. doi:10.1016/j.chroma.2015.09.060 PMID:26427327

Marty, A., Eberschweiler, A., & Dangbet, Z. (2009). *Au Cœur De La Transhumance. Un Campement Chamelier Au Tchad Central*. Paris, France: Khartala.

Maryniak, N., Hansen, E., Ballegaard, A.S., Sancho, A., & Bøgh, K. (2018). Comparison of the Allergenicity and Immunogenicity of Camel and Cow's Milk—A Study in Brown Norway Rats. *Nutrients*, *10*(12), 1-18.

Marziali, S., Guerra, E., Cerdán-Garcia, C., Segura-Carretero, A., Caboni, M. F., & Verardo, V. (2018). Effect of early lactation stage on goat colostrum: Assessment of lipid and oligosaccharide compounds. *International Dairy Journal*, *77*, 65–72. doi:10.1016/j.idairyj.2017.09.004

Mason, J. (2012). Vitamins, trace minerals and other micronutrients. In L. Goldman & A. I. Schafer (Eds.), *Cecil textbook of medicine* (pp. 1–10). Philadelphia: Saunders.

Maswadeh, H. M., Aljarbou, A. N., Alorainy, M. S., Alsharidah, M. S., & Khan, M. A. (2015). *Etoposide Incorporated into Camel Milk Phospholipids Liposomes Shows Increased Activity against Fibrosarcoma in a Mouse Model*. doi:10.1155/2015/743051

Mati, A., Girardet, J.-M., Xenakis, D., & Linden, G. (1991). Isolation and characterization of proteose-peptone hydrophobic fractions of cow's, ewe's and goat's milk. *Le Lait*, *71*, 259–273. doi:10.1051/lait:1991320

Mati, A., Senoussi-Ghezali, C., Zennia, S., Almi-Sebbane, D., Elhatmi, H., & Giradet, J.-M. (2017). Dromedary camel milk proteins, a source of peptides having biological activities: A review. *International Dairy Journal*, *73*, 25–37. doi:10.1016/j.idairyj.2016.12.001

Maurad, K., & Meriem, K. (2008). Probiotic characteristics of *Lactobacillus plantarum* strains from traditional butter made from camel milk in arid regions (Sahara) of Algeria. *Grasas y Aceites*, *59*(3), 218–224. doi:10.3989/gya.2008.v59.i3.511

Ma, Y., & Barbano, D. M. (2003). Milk pH As A Function Of co2 Concentration, Temperature, And Pressure in A Heat Exchanger. *Journal of Dairy Science*, *86*(12), 3822–3830. doi:10.3168/jds.S0022-0302(03)73989-7 PMID:14740816

Mc Mahon, D. J., & Brown, R. J. (1984). Composition, structure and integrity of casein micelles: A review. *Journal of Dairy Science*, *67*(3), 499–512. doi:10.3168/jds.S0022-0302(84)81332-6

McClements, J. M. J., Patterson, M. F., & Linton, M. (2001). The effect of growth stage and growth temperature in high hydrostatic pressure inactivation of some psychotropic bacteria in milk. *Journal of Food Protection*, *64*(4), 514–522. doi:10.4315/0362-028X-64.4.514 PMID:11307889

McGinnis, W. R. (2004). Oxidative stress in autism. *Alternative Therapies in Health and Medicine, 10*(6), 22–36. PMID:15624347

Mcgrath, B. A., Fox, P. F., Mcsweeney, P. L. H., & Kelly, A. L. (2016). Composition and properties of bovine colostrum: A review. *Dairy Science & Technology, 96*(2), 133–158. doi:10.100713594-015-0258-x

McIntyre, R. T., Parrish, D. B., & Fountaine, F. C. (1952). Properties of the colostrum of the dairy cow. VII. pH, buffering capacity and osmotic pressure. *Journal of Dairy Science, 23*, 405–422.

McNees, A. L., Markesich, D., Zayyani, N. R., & Graham, D. Y. (2015). Mycobacterium paratuberculosis as a cause of Crohn's disease. *Expert Review of Gastroenterology & Hepatology, 9*(12), 1523–1534. doi:10.1586/17474124.2015.1093931 PMID:26474349

Medhammar, E., Wijesinha-Bettoni, R., Stadlmayr, B., Nilsson, E., Charrondiere, U. R., & Burlingame, B. (2012). Composition of milk from minor dairy animals and buffalo breeds: a biodiversity perspective. *Journal of the Science of Food and Agriculture, 92*, 445-474.

Meguid, N. A., Atta, H. M., Gouda, A. S., & Khalil, R. O. (2008). Role of polyunsaturated fatty acids in the management of Egyptian children with autism. *Clinical Biochemistry, 41*(13), 1044–1048. doi:10.1016/j.clinbiochem.2008.05.013 PMID:18582451

Mehaia, M. A. (1993). Fresh soft white cheese (Domiati-type) from camel milk: Composition yield and sensory evaluation. *Journal of Dairy Science, 76*(10), 2845–2855. doi:10.3168/jds.S0022-0302(93)77623-7

Mehaia, M. A. (2006). Manufacture of fresh soft white cheese (Domiati type) from dromedary camel's milk using ultrafiltration process. *Journal of Food Technology, 4*, 206–212.

Mehaia, M. A., Hablas, M. A., Abdel-Rahman, K. M., & El-Mougy, S. A. (1995). Milk composition of Majaheim, Wadah and Hamra camels in Saudi Arabia. *Food Chemistry, 52*(2), 115–122. doi:10.1016/0308-8146(94)P4189-M

Mehra, R., & Kelly, P. (2006). Milk oligosaccharides: Structural and technological aspects [Review]. *International Dairy Journal, 16*(11), 1334–1340. doi:10.1016/j.idairyj.2006.06.008

Mehrin, B., Saeid, Z., Maryam, I., Samane, L. A., Somaye, B., Mahbobe, M., & Ali, H. (2011). The extract of lactoperoxidase enzyme from camel milk using chromatography methods and its antibacterial effects on *Pseudomonas aeruginosa*. *Clinical Biochemistry, 44*(13), S92–S92. doi:10.1016/j.clinbiochem.2011.08.208

Mehta, B., Jain, A., Patel, D., & Aparnathi, K. (2019). Camel Milk: Opportunity and Challenges. National Seminar on "Indian Dairy Industry - Opportunities and Challenges". *National Seminar on "Indian Dairy Industry - Opportunities and Challenges"*. Retrieved from http://www.dairyknowledge.in/sites/default/files/ch9_0.pdf

Mehta, R. D., & Pathak, K. M. L. (2012). *Camel milk cream: The candidate cosmeceutical* (A Pilot Study, Unpublished).

Meisel, H. (2004). Multifunctional peptides encrypted in milk proteins. *BioFactors (Oxford, England), 21*(1-4), 55–61. doi:10.1002/biof.552210111 PMID:15630170

Meisel, H., Walsh, D., Murray, B., & FitzGerald, R. (2006). ACE inhibitory peptides. In Y. Mine & F. Shahidi (Eds.), *Nutraceutical Proteins and Peptides in Health and Disease* (Vol. 4, pp. 269–315). Taylor & Francis Group Publisher.

Menegaz, A. N., Goin, F. J., & Jaureguizar, E. O. (1989). Análisis morfológico y morfométrico multivariado de los representantes fósiles y vivientes del género *Lama (Artiodactyla, Camelidae). Sus implicancias sistemáticas biogeográficas, ecológicas y biocronológicas. Ameghiniana, 26*, 153–172.

Menzies, D. J., & Hopkins, D. L. (1996). Relationship between color and ph in lamb loins. *Proceedings of Australian Society of Animal Production*, *21*, 353.

Merin, U., Bernstein, S., Bloch-Damti, A., Yagil, R., van Creveld, C., Lindner, P., & Gollop, N. (2001). A comparative study of milk serum proteins in camel (*Camelus dromedarius*) and bovine colostrum. *Livestock Production Science*, *67*(3), 297–30. doi:10.1016/S0301-6226(00)00198-6

Metcalfe, D., & Bui, E. (2016). Land: Resources and capacity for management. In *Australia state of the environment*. Canberra: Australian Government Department of the Environment and Energy. Retrieved from https://soe.environment.gov.au/theme/land/topic/2016/resources-and-capacity-management

Metwalli, A. A. M. (1992). *Changes in casein micellar structure during heating in the presence and absence of whey proteins* (Thesis). Minia University, Egypt.

Metwalli, N. H., Shalabi, S. I., Bayoumi, S. E., & Metwalli, A. A. M. (1988a). Effect of Ultra-High Temperature and Subsequent Storage on the Constituent of Recombined Milk: 1- Selected Chemical Characteristics and Nitrogen Distribution. *Minia Journal of Agricultural. Research for Development*, *10*(3), 1225-1240.

Metwalli, A. A. M., Ismail, E. A., Alhaj, O. A., Saleh, K. A., & Ibrahim, F. S. (2013). The Effect of Urea and Formaldehyde on Heat Coagulation Time (HCT) Of Camel Milk. *Life Science Journal*, *10*(3), 2113–2119.

Metwalli, A., Mahmoud, A., Ebaid, H., Ahmed, O. M., & Ahmed, R. R. (2015). Up-regulation of Hsp72 and keratin16 mediates wound healing in streptozotocin diabetic rats. *Biological Research*, *48*(1), 54. doi:10.118640659-015-0044-5 PMID:26428860

Meyer, J., Butikofer, U., Walther, B., Wechsler, D., & Sieber, R. (2009). Hot topic: Changes in angiotensin-converting enzyme inhibition and concentration of the teripeptides Val-Pro-Pro and Ile-Pro-Pro during ripening of different Swiss cheese varieties. *Journal of Dairy Science*, *92*(3), 826–836. doi:10.3168/jds.2008-1531 PMID:19233775

Miezeliene, A., Alencikiene, G., Gruzauskas, R., & Barstys, T. (2011). The effect of dietary selenium supplementationon meat quality of broiler chickens. *Biotechnologie, Agronomie, Société et Environnement*, *15*, 61–69.

Migdal, W., & Žirković, B. (2007). Meat–from functional food to disease of modern civilization. *Biotechnology in Animal Husbandry*, *23*, 19–31.

Mihic, T., Rainkie, D., Wilby, K., & Pawluk, S. (2016). The Therapeutic Effects of Camel Milk: A Systematic Review of Animal and Human Trials. *Journal of Evidence-Based Complementary & Alternative Medicine*, *21*(4), NP110–NP126. doi:10.1177/2156587216658846 PMID:27432772

Mihretie, Y., Tadesse, N., Amakelew, S., & Fikru, S. (2018). Cheese production from camel milk using lemon juice as a coagulant. *Journal of Environmental and Agricultural Sciences*, *17*, 11–19.

Mikesell, M. W. (1955). Notes on the dispersal of the dromedary. *Southwestern Journal of Anthropology*, *11*(3), 231–245. doi:10.1086outjanth.11.3.3629022

Miller, W. O., Staffle, R. L., & Zirkle, S. B. (1968). Factors, which influence the water-holding capacity of various types of meat. *Food Technology*, *22*, 11390.

Mills, O. H., Berger, R. S., & Baker, M. D. (1993). A controlled comparison of skin cleansers in photoaged skin. *Journal of Geriatric Dermatology*, *1*, 173–179.

Ming, L., Yuan, L., Yi, L., Ding, G., Hasi, S., Chen, G., Jambl, T., … Jirimutu. (2019). *Whole-genome sequencing of 128 camels across Asia provides insights into origin and migration of domestic Bactrian camels*. Retrieved from https://www.biorxiv.org/content/biorxiv/early/2019/06/03/656231.full.pdf

Miniero, R., Mazza, G., Pasqua, A., Dolceamore, T., Zurlo, F., Mahdi, A., & Britti, D. (2014). Composition and therapeutic use of camel milk. *Large Animal Review*, *20*(3), 125–132.

Mirghani, A. (1994). *Microbial and biochemical properties of fermented camel's milk (gariss)* (Unpublished MSc thesis).

Mirmiran, P., Ejtahed, H. S., Angoorani, P., Eslami, F., & Azizi, F. (2017). Camel milk has beneficial effects on diabetes Mellitus: A systematic review. *International Journal of Endocrinology and Metabolism*, *15*(2), e42150.

Mirmiran, P., Ejtahed, H.-S., Angoorani, P., Eslami, F., & Azizi, F. (2017). Camel Milk Has Beneficial Effects on Diabetes Mellitus: A Systematic Review. *International Journal of Endocrinology and Metabolism*, *15*(2), e42150–e42150. doi:10.5812/ijem.42150 PMID:29026408

Mistry, V. (2004). Fermented liquid milk products. In Y. H. Hui, L. Meunier-Goddik, Ö. S. Hansen, J. Josephsen, W. Nip, P. S. Stanfield, & F. Toldra (Eds.), *Handbook of Food and beverage fermentation technology* (pp. 939–957). New York: Marcel Dekker. doi:10.1201/9780203913550.ch45

Moatsou, G., Samolada, M., Katsabeki, A., & Anifantakis, E. (2004). Casein fraction of ovine milk from indigenous Greek breeds. *Dairy Science & Technology*, *84*(3), 285–296. doi:10.1051/lait:2004006

Mohamad, R. H., Zekry, Z. K., Al-Mehdar, H. A., Salama, O., El-Shaieb, S. E., El-Basmy, A. A., ... Sharawy, S. M. (2009). Camel milk as an adjuvant therapy for the treatment of type 1 diabetes: Verification of a traditional ethnomedical practice. *Journal of Medicinal Food*, *12*(2), 561–465. doi:10.1089/jmf.2008.0009

Mohamed, I. M. A., & El Zubeir, E. M. I. (2012). Effect of pasteurization on the keeping quality of camel milk. In *ISO-CARD International Conference Sultanate of Oman 29thJanuary–1th February* (*Vol. 3*, pp. 232-233). Academic Press.

Mohamed, A. E., Babiker, I. A., & Mohamed, T. E. (2013). Preparation of fresh soft cheese from dromedary camel milk using acid and heat method. *Research Opinions in Animal & Veterinary Sciences*, *3*, 289–292.

Mohamed, E., & Mustafa, A. (2016). Fatty acids content in milk of dromedary camel (*Camelus dromedarius*) from farming and pastoral systems in Sudan. *International Journal of Science and Research*, *5*(6), 570–573.

Mohamed, H. E., Mousa, H. M., & Beynen, A. C. (2005). Ascorbic acid concentrations in milk from Sudanese camels. *Journal of Animal Physiology and Animal Nutrition*, *89*(1-2), 35–37. doi:10.1111/j.1439-0396.2004.00507.x PMID:19112713

Mohamed, M. A., Larsson-Raznikiewicz, M., & Mohamud, M. A. (1990). Hard cheese making from camel milk. *Milchwissenschaft. Milk Science International*, *45*, 716–718.

Mohamed, W. A., Schaalan, M. F., & El-Abhar, H. S. (2015). Camel Milk: Potential Utility as an Adjunctive Therapy to Peg-IFN/RBV in HCV-4 Infected Patients in Egypt. *Nutrition and Cancer*, *67*(8), 1307–1315. doi:10.1080/01635581.2015.1087041 PMID:26492130

Mohammad, D. (2009). Camel's milk protects against cadmium chloride-induced hypochromic microcytic anemia and oxidative stress in red blood cells of white albino rats. *American Journal of Pharmacology and Toxicology*, *4*(4), 136–143. doi:10.3844/ajptsp.2009.136.143

Mohammed, S., Eshetu, M., Tadesse, Y., & Hailu, Y. (2019). Rheological Properties and Shelf Life of Soft Cheese Made from Camel Milk Using Camel Chymosin. *Journal of Dairy & Veterinary Sciences, 10*.

Mohammed, S., Eshetu, M., Tadesse, Y., & Hailu, Y. (2019). Rheological properties and shelf life of soft cheese made from camel milk using camel chymosin. *Journal of Dairy & Veterinary Sciences*, *10*(4), 555794. doi:10.19080/JDVS.2019.10.555794

Mohandesan, E., Fitak, R., Corander, J., Yadamsuren, A., Chuluunbat, B., Abdelhadi, O., ... Burger, P. A. (2017). Mitogenome sequencing in the genus camelus reveals evidence for purifying selection and long-term divergence between wild and domestic Bactrian camels. *Scientific Reports*, *7*(1), 9970–9982. doi:10.103841598-017-08995-8 PMID:28855525

Mohsin, A. (2019). Qualitative Improvement of Camel Milk Date Yoghurt by Addition of Biosynthesized Xanthan from Orange Waste. *Food Science and Technology (Campinas)*, *108*, 61–68.

Mona, E. (2010). Biochemical effects of fermented camel milk on diarrhea in rats. *New York Science Journal*, *3*(5), 106–111.

Monchot, H. (2015). From paleontology to zooarchaeology, importance of camels through time and history. *Proceedings of 4th Conference of ISOCARD, "Silk Road Camel: The Camelids, main stakes for sustainable development"*.

Monod, T. (1992). Du désert. *Sécheresse*, *1*(3), 7–24.

Montgomery, J. L., King, M. B., Gentry, J. G., Barham, A. R., Barham, B. L., Hilton, G. G., ... Miller, M. F. (2004). Supplemental vitamin D3 concentration and biological type of steers. II. Tenderness, quality, and residues of beef. *Journal of Animal Science*, *82*(7), 2092–2104. doi:10.2527/2004.8272092x PMID:15309957

Moreira, F. B., de Souza, N. E., Matsushita, M., do Prado, I. N., & Nascimento, W. G. (2003). Evaluation of carcass characteristics and meat chemical composition of Bos indicus and Bos indicus x Bos taurus crossbred steers fi nished in pasture systems. *Brazilian Archives of Biology and Technology*, *46*(4), 609–616. doi:10.1590/S1516-89132003000400016

Moreno-Indias, I., Sánchez-Macías, D., Castro, N., Morales-delaNuez, A., Hernández-Castellano, L. E., Capote, J., & Argüello, A. (2012). Chemical composition and immune status of dairy goat colostrum fractions during the first 10 h after partum. *Small Ruminant Research*, *103*(2-3), 220–224. doi:10.1016/j.smallrumres.2011.09.015

Morr, C. V., & Ha, E. Y. W. (1993). Whey protein concentrates and isolates: Processing and functional properties. *Critical Reviews in Food Science and Nutrition*, *33*(6), 431–476. doi:10.1080/10408399309527643 PMID:8216810

Moslehishad, M., Ehsani, M. R., Salami, M., Mirdamadi, S., Ezzatpanah, H., Niasari, A., & Moosavi-Movahedi, A. (2013). The comparative assessment of ACE-inhibitory and antioxidant activities of peptide fractions obtained from fermented camel and bovine milk by *Lactobacillus rhamnosus* PTCC 1637. *International Dairy Journal*, *29*(2), 82–87. doi:10.1016/j.idairyj.2012.10.015

Mostafidi, M., Moslehishad, M., Piravivanak, Z., & Pouretedal, Z. (2016). Evaluation of mineral content and heavy metals of dromedary camel milk in Iran. *Food Science and Technology (Campinas)*, *36*(4), 717–723. doi:10.1590/1678-457x.16116

Motarjemi, Y., Käferstein, F., Moy, G., & Quevedo, F. (1993). Contaminated weaning food: A major risk factor for diarrhoea and associated malnutrition. *Bulletin of the World Health Organization*, *71*(1), 79–92.

Mounir, S. (2017). Foam Mat Drying. In *Drying technologies for foods-fundamentals and applications*. CRC Press.

Moura, F. A., De Andrade, K. Q., Dos Santos, J. C. F., Araújo, O. R. P., & Goulart, M. O. F. (2015). *Antioxidant therapy for treatment of inflammatory bowel disease: Does it work?* doi:10.1016/j.redox.2015.10.006

Mourad, K., & Nour-Eddine, K. (2006). Physicochemical and microbiological studies of 'Shmen' a traditional butter made from camel milk in the Sahara (Algeria); isolation and identification of lactic acid bacteria and yeast. *Journal of Animal Science*, *12*, 45–65.

Moure, A., Domínguez, H., & Parajó, J. (2006). Antioxidant properties of ultrafiltration-recovered soy protein fractions from industrial effluents and their hydrolysates. *Process Biochemistry*, *41*(2), 447–456. doi:10.1016/j.procbio.2005.07.014

Mousa, H. M., Ali, K. E., & Hume, I. D. (1983). Effects of water deprivation on urea metabolism in camels, desert sheep and desert goats fed dry desert grass. *Comparative Biochemistry and Physiology*, *74A*(3), 715–720. doi:10.1016/0300-9629(83)90574-1 PMID:6132716

Moustafa, M. G. F., Abdel-Mohsen, A. M., Ebaid, H., Hassan, I., & Al-Tamimi, J. (2016). Wound healing of different molecular weight of hyaluronan; in-vivo study. *International Journal of Biological Macromolecules*, *89*, 582–591. doi:10.1016/j.ijbiomac.2016.05.021 PMID:27174907

Mozaffarian, D., Micha, R., & Wallace, S. (2010). Effects on Coronary Heart Disease of Increasing Polyunsaturated Fat in Place of Saturated Fat: A Systematic view and Meta-Analysis of Randomized Controlled Trials. *PLoS Medicine*, *7*(3), e1000252. doi:10.1371/journal.pmed.1000252 PMID:20351774

Mudgil, P., & … . (2018). Rheological, Micro-Structural and Sensorial Properties of Camel Milk Yogurt as Influenced by Gelatin. *Food Science and Technology (Campinas)*, *98*, 646–653. Retrieved from https://linkinghub.elsevier.com/retrieve/pii/S0023643818307400

Mudgil, P., Kamal, H., Yuen, G. C., & Maqsood, S. (2018). Characterization and identification of novel antidiabetic and anti-obesity peptides from camel milk protein hydrolysates. *Food Chemistry*, *259*, 46–54. doi:10.1016/j.foodchem.2018.03.082

Muhialdina, B. J., & Algboory, H. L. (2018). Identification of low molecular weight antimicrobial peptides from Iraqi camel milk fermented with *Lactobacillus plantarum. PharmaNutrition*, *6*(2), 69–73. doi:10.1016/j.phanu.2018.02.002

Mukasa-Mugerwa, E. (1981). The camel (Camelus dromedaries): A biographical review. International Livestock Centre for Africa.

Mukherjee, S., Date, A., Patarvale, V., Korting, H. C., Roeder, A., & Weindl, G. (2006). Retinoids in the treatment of skin aging: An overview of clinical efficacy & clinical interventions in aging. *Clinical Interventions in Aging*, *1*, 327–348. doi:10.2147/ciia.2006.1.4.327 PMID:18046911

Mullaicharam, A. (2014). A review on medicinal properties of Camel milk. *World Journal of Pharmaceutical Sciences*. Available online at: http://www.wjpsonline.com/

Mullaicharam, A. (2014). A review on medicinal properties of camel milk. *World J Pharm Sci*, *2*(3), 237–242.

Mullaicharam, A. (2014). A review on medicinal properties of Camel milk. *World Journal of Pharmaceutical Science*, *2*(3), 237–242.

Mullaicharam, A. R. (2014). A review on medicinal properties of camel milk. *World Journal of pharmaceutic. Science*, *2*, 237–242.

Muloi, D., Alarcon, P., Ombui, J., Ngeiywa, K. J., Abdullahi, B., Muinde, P., ... Fèvre, E. M. (2018). Value chain analysis and sanitary risks of the camel milk system supplying Nairobi city, Kenya. *Preventive Veterinary Medicine*, *159*, 203–210. doi:10.1016/j.prevetmed.2018.09.010 PMID:30314783

Murray, J., Darr, D., & Reich, J. (1991). Topical vitamin C treatment reduces UV radiation-induced erythema in human skin. *The Journal of Investigative Dermatology*, *96*, 587.

Musaad, A., Faye, B., & Abu-Nikhela, A. (2013b). Lactation curves of dairy camels in an intensive system. *Tropical Animal Health and Production*, *4*(4), 1039–1046. doi:10.100711250-012-0331-x PMID:23212839

Musaad, A., Faye, B., & Al-Mutairi, S. (2013a). Seasonal and physiological variation of gross composition of camel milk in Saudi Arabia. *Emirates Journal of Food and Agriculture*, *25*(8), 618–624. doi:10.9755/ejfa.v25i8.16095

Mushref, F. (2006). In vitro anticancer agent I-Tissue culture study of human lung cancer cells A549 II-Tissue culture study of mice leukemia cells L1210. *Int J Cancer Res*, *2*(4), 330–344. doi:10.3923/ijcr.2006.330.344

Muslim, E. T. (2018). Effect of usage Iraqi camel colostrum extract on some blood parameters in albino rats. *Al-Qadisiyah Journal of Veterinary Medicine Sciences*, *17*(1), 138–141. doi:10.29079/vol17iss1art489

Mutlag, A., Al-Zoreky, N., & El-Dermerdash, H. (2013). Camel's milk as a natural source for probiotics. *Research Journal of Microbiology*, *8*, 70–80. doi:10.3923/jm.2013.70.80

Muyonga, J., Cole, C., & Duodu, K. (2004). Fourier transform infrared (FTIR) spectroscopic study of acid soluble collagen and gelatin from skins and bones of young and adult Nile perch (*Lates niloticus*). *Food Chemistry*, *86*(3), 325–332. doi:10.1016/j.foodchem.2003.09.038

Mwangi, L. W., Matofari, J. W., Muliro, P. S., & Bebe, B. O. (2016). Hygienic assessment of spontaneously fermented raw camel milk (suusa) along the informal value chain in Kenya. *International Journal of Food Contamination*, *3*(1), 18. doi:10.118640550-016-0040-8

Nadia, A. (2007). *Ice cream between health and disease* (1st ed.). Aleskandaria, Egypt: AlMaaref Alhaditha Library. (In Arabic)

Nagao, K., & Yanagita, T. (2008). Bioactive lipids in metabolic syndrome. *Progress in Lipid Research*, *47*(2), 127–146. doi:10.1016/j.plipres.2007.12.002 PMID:18177744

Nagasawa, T., Kiyosawa, I., & Takase, M. (1974). Lactoferrin and serum albumin of human casein in colostrum and milk. *Journal of Dairy Science*, *57*(10), 1159–1163. doi:10.3168/jds.S0022-0302(74)85030-7 PMID:4473469

Nagy, P., Fábri, Zs. N., Varga, L., Reiczigel, J., & Juhász, J. (2017). Effect of genetic and nongenetic factors on chemical composition of individual milk samples from dromedary camels (*Camelus dromedarius*) under intensive management. *Journal of Dairy Science*, *100*(11), 8680–8693. doi:10.3168/jds.2017-12814 PMID:28843681

Nagy, P., Faigl, V., Reiczigel, J., & Juhasz, J. (2015). Effect of pregnancy and embryonic mortality on milk production in dromedary camels (*Camelus dromedarius*). *Journal of Dairy Science*, *98*(2), 975–986. doi:10.3168/jds.2014-8546 PMID:25434338

Nahar, N., Khan, W., & Shoeb, M. (2016). Physico-Chemical analysis and composition of camel milk of Bangladesh. *Journal of Basic and Applied Sciences*, 231–235.

Nakamura, T., Kawase, H., Kimura, K., Watanabe, Y., Ohtani, M., Arai, I., & Urashima, T. (2003). Concentrations of sialyloligosaccharides in bovine colostrum and milk during the prepartum and early lactation. *Journal of Dairy Science*, *86*(4), 1315–1320. doi:10.3168/jds.S0022-0302(03)73715-1 PMID:12741556

Nakamura, Y., Yamamoto, N., Sakai, K., Okubo, A., Yamazaki, S., & Takano, T. (1995a). Purification and characterization of angiotensin I-converting enzyme inhibitors from sour milk. *Journal of Dairy Science*, *78*(4), 777–783. doi:10.3168/jds.S0022-0302(95)76689-9 PMID:7790570

Nakamura, Y., Yamamoto, N., Sakai, K., & Takano, T. (1995b). Antihypertensive effect of sour milk and peptides isolated from it that are inhibitors to angiotensin I-converting enzyme. *Journal of Dairy Science*, *78*(6), 1253–1257. doi:10.3168/jds.S0022-0302(95)76745-5 PMID:7673515

Narmuratova, M., Konuspayeva, G., Loiseau, G., Serikbaeva, A., Barouh, N., Montet, D., & Faye, B. (2006). Fatty acids composition of dromedary and Bactrian camel milk in Kazakhstan. *Journal of Camel Practice and Research*, *13*(1), 45–50.

Naser, S. A., Sagramsingh, S. R., Naser, A. S., & Thanigachalam, S. (2014). Mycobacterium avium subspecies paratuberculosis causes Crohn's disease in some inflammatory bowel disease patients. *World Journal of Gastroenterology*, *20*(23), 7403–7415. doi:10.3748/wjg.v20.i23.7403 PMID:24966610

Navarrete-Rodríguez, E. M., Ríos-Villalobosaet, L. A., Alcocer-Arreguína, C. R., Del-Rio-Navarro, B. E., & … . (2018). Cross-over clinical trial for evaluating the safety of camel's milk intake in patients who are allergic to cow's milk protein. *Allergologia et Immunopathologia*, *46*(2), 149–154. doi:10.1016/j.aller.2017.06.005 PMID:29223706

Navas-Carretero, S., Pérez-Granados, A. M., Sarriá, B., & Vaquero, P. M. (2009). Iron absorption from meat pate fortified with ferric pyrophosphate in iron-deficient women. *Nutrition (Burbank, Los Angeles County, Calif.)*, *25*(1), 20–24. doi:10.1016/j.nut.2008.07.002 PMID:18752926

Nduko, J. M., Matofari, J. W., Nandi, Z. O., & Sichangi, M. B. (2017). Spontaneously fermented kenyan milk products: A review of the current state and future perspectives. *African Journal of Food Science*, *11*(1), 1–11. doi:10.5897/AJFS2016.1516

Needs, E. C., Stenning, R. A., Gill, A., Ferragut, V., & Rich, G. T. (2000). High-Pressure Treatment of Milk: Effects on Casein Micelle Structure and On Enzymic Coagulation. *The Journal of Dairy Research*, *67*(1), 31–42. doi:10.1017/S0022029999004021 PMID:10717841

Newton, A. E., Fairbanks, A. J., Golding, M., Andrewes, P., & Gerrard, J. A. (2012). The role of the Maillard reaction in the formation of flavour compounds in dairy products – not only a deleterious reaction but also a rich source of flavour compounds. *Food & Function*, *3*(12), 1223–1326. doi:10.1039/c2fo30089c PMID:22948260

Niasari-Naslaji, A., Arabha, H., Atakpour, A., Salami, M., & Moosavi-Movahedi, A. (2012). Camel Milk and its Bioactive Molecules in Medical Treatments. *Science Cultivation*, *2*(1), 20–24.

Niaz, B., Zahoor, T., Randhawa, M. A., & Jamil, I. A. (2017). Solation of Lactoferrin from Camel Milk through Fast Protein Liquid Chromatography and its Antagonistic Activity against *Escherichia coli* and *Staphylococcus aureus*. *Pakistan Journal of Zoology*, *49*(4), 1307–1313. doi:10.17582/journal.pjz/2017.49.4.1307.1313

Nigussie, H., & Seifu, E. (2007). Effect of the lactoperoxidase system and container smoking on the microbial quality of cows' milk produced in Kombolcha woreda, eastern Ethiopia. *Livestock Research for Rural Development*, *19*, 157.

Nijdam, J., Ibach, A., & Kind, M. (2008). Fluidisation of whey powders above the glass-transition temperature. *Powder Technology*, *187*(1), 53–61. doi:10.1016/j.powtec.2008.01.013

Nikkhah, A. (2011). Science of Camel and Yak Milks: Human Nutrition and Health Perspectives. *Food and Nutrition Sciences*, *2*(06), 667–673. doi:10.4236/fns.2011.26092

Njage, P. (2010). *Microbial diversity, safety and role of predominant lactic acid bacteria in raw and spontaneously fermented camel milk from Kenya and Somalia* (PhD Thesis). University of Nairobi, Nairobi, Kenya.

Njage, P. M. K. (2011). *Microbial diversity, safety and role of predominant lactic acid bacteria in raw and spontaneously fermented camel milk in Kenya and Somalia* (PhD Thesis). University of Nairobi, Kenya.

Nongonierm, A. B., Paolella, S., Mudgil, P., Maqsood, S., & FitzGerald, R. J. (2018). Identification of novel dipeptidyl peptidase IV (DPP-IV) inhibitory peptides in camel milk protein hydrolysates. *Food Chemistry*, *244*, 340–348. doi:10.1016/j.foodchem.2017.10.033 PMID:29120791

Norbu, Z. (1988). Alasha Bactrian camel. Inner Mongolia Science and Technology Press.

Nova, C. L. (1970). Reproduction in *Camelidae*. *Journal of Reproduction and Fertility*, *22*(1), 3–20. doi:10.1530/jrf.0.0220003 PMID:4911974

Nuñez, M. (2016). Existing Technologies in Non-cow milk processing and traditional non-cow milk products. In E. Tsakalidou & K. Papadimitriou (Eds.), *Non-Bovine Milk and Milk Products*. Elsevier.

NUTTAB. (2010). *Nutrient data tables*. Food Standard Australia New Zealand (FSANZ). Accessed Aug. 2, 2012. http://www.foodstandards.gov.au/consumerinformation/nuttab2010/

Nyagoya, S. (2016). *Cow Milk Fermentation trials with Streptococcus infantarius subsp. Infantarius and its effect on the growth of selected pathogenic bacteria* (Thesis). University of Nairobi. Retrieved from https://foodtech.uonbi.ac.ke/sites/default/files/cavs/agriculture/foodtech/Final%20dissertation.pdf

Odamaki, T., Xiao, J. Z., Yonezawa, S., Yaeshima, T., & Iwatsuki, K. (2011). Improved viability of bifidobacteria in fermented milk by cocultivation with Lactococcus lactis subspecies lactis. *Journal of Dairy Science*, *94*(3), 1112–1121. doi:10.3168/jds.2010-3286

Odongo, N. O., Lamuka, P. O., Matofari, J. W., & Abong, G. O. (2016). Risk factors associated with the post-harvest loss of milk along camel milk value chain in Isiolo County, Kenya. *African Journal of Agricultural Research*, *11*(8), 674–682. doi:10.5897/AJAR2015.9988

Oftedal, O. T. (1995). Comparative analysis of nonhuman milks. In R. G. Jensen (Ed.), *Handbook of milk composition* (p. 749-788). San Diego, CA: Academic Press. doi:10.1016/B978-012384430-9/50035-4

Ogier, J., & Serror, P. (2008). Safety assessment of dairy microorganisms: The Enterococcus genus. *International Journal of Food Microbiology*, *126*(3), 291–301. doi:10.1016/j.ijfoodmicro.2007.08.017

Ogolla, J. A., Dede, C., Okoth, M. W., Hensel, O., & Sturm, B. (2017). Strategies and technologies for camel milk preservation and utilization of non-marketed milk in arid and semi-arid areas. *East African Agricultural and Forestry Journal*, *82*(2-4), 144–167. doi:10.1080/00128325.2017.1363686

Oldfield, D. J., Taylor, M. W., & Singh, H. (2005). Effect of preheating and other process parameters on whey protein reactions during skim milk powder manufacture. *International Dairy Journal*, *15*(5), 501–511. doi:10.1016/j.idairyj.2004.09.004

Olsvig-Whittaker, I., Frankenberg, E., Perevolotsky, A., & Ungar, E. D. (2006). Grazing, overgrazing and conservation. Changing concepts and practices in the Negev rangelands. *Sécheresse*, *17*, 195–199.

Omar, A., Harbourne, N., & Oruna-Concha, M. J. (2016). Quantification of major camel milk proteins by capillary electrophoresis. *International Dairy Journal*, *58*, 31–35. doi:10.1016/j.idairyj.2016.01.015

Omar, A., Harbourne, N., & Oruna-Concha, M. J. (2018). Effects of industrial processing methods on camel skimmed milk properties. *International Dairy Journal*, *84*, 15–22. doi:10.1016/j.idairyj.2018.03.011

Omer, R. H., & Eltinay, A. H. (2008). Chemical composition of camel's colostrum and milk in United Arab Emirates. *Arab University Journal of Agricultural Science*, *16*(1), 127–134. doi:10.21608/ajs.2008.14620

Omer, R. H., & Eltinay, A. H. (2009). Changes in chemical composition of camel's raw milk during storage. *Pakistan Journal of Nutrition*, *8*(5), 607–610. doi:10.3923/pjn.2009.607.610

Ono, K., Berry, B. W., & Douglass, L. W. (1986). Nutrient content of some fresh and retail cuts of veal. *Journal of Food Science*, *51*(5), 1352–1357. doi:10.1111/j.1365-2621.1986.tb13120.x

Ono, K., Berry, B., Johnson, H. K., Russek, E., Parker, C. F., Cahill, V., & Althouse, P. (1984). Nutrient composition of lamb of two age groups. *Journal of Food Science*, *49*(5), 1233–1239. doi:10.1111/j.1365-2621.1984.tb14961.x

Ontsouka, C. E., Bruckmaier, R. M., & Blum, J. W. (2003). Fractionized milk composition during removal of colostrum and mature milk. *Journal of Dairy Science*, *86*(6), 2005–2011. doi:10.3168/jds.S0022-0302(03)73789-8 PMID:12836936

Ortonne, J. P. (2006). Retinoid therapy for pigmentary disorders. *Dermatologic Therapy*, *19*(5), 280–288. doi:10.1111/j.1529-8019.2006.00085.x PMID:17014483

Otles, S., & Cadingi, O. (2003). Kefir: A probiotic dairy-composition, nutritional and therapeutic aspects. *Pakistan Journal of Nutrition*, *2*(2), 54–59. doi:10.3923/pjn.2003.54.59

Otte, J., Shalaby, S., Zakora, M., & Neilsen, M. (2007). Fractionation and identification of ACE-inhibitory peptides from α-lactalbumin and β-casein produced by thermolysin-catalysed hydrolysis. *International Dairy Journal*, *17*(12), 1460–1472. doi:10.1016/j.idairyj.2007.04.008

Oudah, L. (2016). The effect of camel milk in the tissue changes to the kidneys of laboratory male rats treated by cadmium. *International Journal of Animal Health and Livestock Production Research*, *1*(2), 8–14.

Oulad Belkhir, A., Chehma, A., & Faye, B. (2013). Phenotypic variability of two principal Algerian camel's populations (Targui and Sahraoui). *Emirates Journal of Food and Agriculture*, *25*(3), 231–237. doi:10.9755/ejfa.v25i3.15457

Pan, D., & Guo, Y. (2010). Optimization of sour milk fermentation for the production of ACE inhibitory peptides and purification of a novel peptide from whey protein hydrolysate. *International Dairy Journal*, *20*(7), 472–479. doi:10.1016/j.idairyj.2010.01.007

Pan, D., Luo, Y., & Tanokura, M. (2005). Antihypertensive peptides from skimmed milk hydrolysate digested by cell-free extract of Lactobacillus helveticus JCM1004. *Food Chemistry*, *91*(1), 123–129. doi:10.1016/j.foodchem.2004.05.055

Pandya, A. J., & Haenlein, G. F. W. (2009). Chapter 5: bioactive components in buffalo milk. In Y. W. Park (Ed.), Bioactive components in milk and dairy products (pp. 105-158). Wiley-Blackwell.

Panesar, P. S. (2011). Fermented Dairy Products: Starters Cultures and Potential Nutritional Benefits. *Food and Nutrition Sciences*, *02*(01), 47–51. doi:10.4236/fns.2011.21006

Pan, Y., Rowney, M., Guo, P., & Hobman, P. (2007). Biological properties of lactoferrin: An overview. *Australian Journal of Dairy Technology*, *62*, 31–42.

Pari, L., & Satheesh, M. A. (2004). Antidiabetic activity of Boerhaavia diffusa L.: Effect on hepatic key enzymes in experimental diabetes. *Journal of Ethnopharmacology*, *91*(1), 109–113. doi:10.1016/j.jep.2003.12.013

Pariza, M. (1999). *Conjugated linoleic acid and the control of cancer and obesity*. doi:10.1093/toxsci/52.suppl_1.107

Park, Y. (2009). Overview of bioactive components in milk and dairy products. In *Bioactive Components in Milk and Dairy Products* (p. 14). Ames, IA: Wiley-Blackwell Publishers. doi:10.1002/9780813821504.ch1

Park, Y. W., Juárez, M., Ramos, M., & Haenlein, G. F. W. (2007). Physico-chemical characteristics of goat and sheep milk. *Small Ruminant Research*, *68*(1–2), 88–113. doi:10.1016/j.smallrumres.2006.09.013

Parmar, N. B. (2013). *Characterization of ghee prepared from camel milk and evaluation of its shelf life during storage* (Master Thesis). SMC College of Dairy Science, Anand Agricultural University, Anand, Gujarat, India.

Parrish, D. B., Wise, G. H., Hughes, J. S., & Atkeson, F. W. (1948). Properties of the colostrum of the dairy cow. II. Effect of prepartal rations upon the nitrogenous constituents. *Journal of Dairy Science*, *31*(10), 889–895. doi:10.3168/jds.S0022-0302(48)92273-5

Patel, K., Wakhisi, J., Mining, S., Mwangi, A., & Patel, R. (2013). Esophageal cancer, the topmost cancer at MTRH in the Rift Valley, Kenya, and its potential risk factors. *ISRN Oncology*. PMID:24490085

Patterson, M. F. (2005). Microbiology of pressure-treated foods. *Journal of Applied Microbiology*, *98*(6), 1400–1409. doi:10.1111/j.1365-2672.2005.02564.x PMID:15916652

Pearce, K., & Jacob, R. (2004). Saltbush lifts sheep meat vitamin content. *Farming Ahead*, *153*, 63.

Pearson, A. M., & Greaser, M. L. (1999). Flesh food and their analogues. In A. J. Rosenthal (Ed.), *Food texture: Measurement and Perception* (Vol. 1, pp. 228–255). Aspen Publishers, Inc.

Pellegrini, A., Dettling, C., Thomas, U., & Hunziker, P. (2001). Isolation and characterization of four bactericidal domains in the bovine β-lactoglobulin. *Biochemicaet Biophysica Acta*, *1526*(2), 131–140. doi:10.1016/S0304-4165(01)00116-7 PMID:11325534

Perez, P., Maino, M., Guzman, R., Vaquero, A., Kobrich, C., & Pokniak, J. (2000). Carcass characteristics of liama (*Lama glama*) reared in central Chile. *Small Ruminant Research*, *37*(1-2), 93–97. doi:10.1016/S0921-4488(99)00127-3 PMID:10818308

Perkins, M. L., D'Arcy, B. R., Lisle, A. T., & Deeth, H. C. (2005). Solid phase microextraction of stale flavour volatiles from the headspace of UHT milk. *Journal of the Science of Food and Agriculture*, *85*(14), 2421–2428. doi:10.1002/jsfa.2243

Perkins, M. L., & Deeth, H. C. (2002). Ultra-High-Temperature (UHT) Treatment of Milk: Comparison of Direct and Indirect Modes of Heating. *Australian Journal of Dairy Technology*, *57*, 211–227.

Pessione, E., & Cirrincione, S. (2016). Bioactive Molecules Released in Food by Lactic Acid Bacteria: Encrypted Peptides and Biogenic Amines. *Frontiers in Microbiology*, *7*, 876. doi:10.3389/fmicb.2016.00876

Peters, J. (1998). *Camelus thomasi Pomel*, 1893, a possible ancestor of the one-humped camel? *Mammalian Biology*, *63*, 372–376.

Petrovic, L., Grujic, R., & Petrovic, M. (1993). Definition of the optimum freezing rate –2. Investigation of the physico-chemical properties of beef m. Longissimus dorsi frozen at different freezing rates. *Meat Science*, *33*(3), 319–331. doi:10.1016/0309-1740(93)90004-2 PMID:22060150

Pette, C., & Staron, S. (1990). Cellular and molecular diversities of mammalian skeletal muscle fibres. *Reviews of Physiology, Biochemistry and Pharmacology*, *116*, 1–76. PMID:2149884

Philanto, A., Virtanen, T., & Korhonen, H. (2010). Angiotensin I converting enzyme (ACE) inhibitory activity and antihypertensive effect of fermented milk. *International Dairy Journal*, *20*(1), 3–10. doi:10.1016/j.idairyj.2009.07.003

Pickford, M., Morales, J., & Soria, D. (1995). Fossil camels from the Upper Miocene of Europe: Implications for biogeography and faunal change. *Geobios-Lyon*, *28*(5), 641–650. doi:10.1016/S0016-6995(95)80217-7

Picot, L., Bordenave, S., Didelot, S., Fruitier-Arnaudin, I., Sannier, F., Thorkelsson, G., ... Piot, J. M. (2006). Antiproliferative activity of fish protein hydrolysates on human breast cancer cell lines. *Process Biochemistry*, *41*(5), 1217–1222. doi:10.1016/j.procbio.2005.11.024

Pierce, A., Colavizza, D., Benaissa, M., Maes, P., Tartar, A., Montreuil, J., & Spik, G. (1991). Molecular cloning and sequence analysis of bovine lactotransferrin. *European Journal of Biochemistry*, *196*(1), 177–184. doi:10.1111/j.1432-1033.1991.tb15801.x PMID:2001696

Pilkington, S. M., Watson, R. E., Nicolaou, A., & Rhodes, L. E. (2011). Omega-3 polyunsaturated fatty acids: Photoprotective macronutrients. *Experimental Dermatology*, *20*(7), 537–543. doi:10.1111/j.1600-0625.2011.01294.x PMID:21569104

Platteeuw, C., van Alen-Boerrigter, I., van Schalkwijk, S., & de Vos, W. M. (1996). Food-grade cloning and expression system for Lactococcus lactis. *Applied and Environmental Microbiology*, *62*(3), 1008–1013.

Pogorzelska-Nowicka, E., Atanasov, A. G., Horba ́nczuk, J., & Wierzbicka, A. (2018). Review: Bioactive compounds in functional meat products. *Molecules (Basel, Switzerland)*, *23*(2), 307. doi:10.3390/molecules23020307

Poławska, E., Zdanowska-Sa̜siadek, Z., Horbanczuk, J. O., Pomianowski, J., Józ˙wik, A., Tolik, D., ... De Smet, S. (2016). Effect of dietary organic and inorganic selenium supplementation on chemical, mineral and fatty acid composition of ostrich meat. *CYTA: Journal of Food*, *14*(1), 84–87. doi:10.1080/19476337.2015.1046940

Polidori, P., Renieri, C., Antonini, M., Passamonti, P., & Pucclarelli, F. (2007). Meat fatty acid composition of llama (lama glama) reared in the Andean highlands. *Meat Science*, *75*(2), 356–358. doi:10.1016/j.meatsci.2006.07.010 PMID:22063670

Pospiech, E., Grzes, B., Lyczynski, A., Borzuta, K., Szalata, M., & Micolajczak, B. (2003). Muscle proteins and their changes in the process of meat tenderization. In Effect of genetic and non-genetic factors on carcass and meat quality of pigs. Poland Institute of Genetics and Animal Breeding.

Power, R. C., Salazar-García, D. C., Wittig, R. M., & Henry, A. G. (2014). Assessing use and suitability of scanning electron microscopy in the analysis of micro remains in dental calculus. *Journal of Archaeological Science*, *49*, 160–169. doi:10.1016/j.jas.2014.04.016

Purchas, R. W., & Busboom, J. R. (2005). The effect of production system and age on levels of iron, taurine, carnosine, coenzyme Q10, and creatine in beef muscles and liver. *Meat Science*, *70*(4), 589–596. doi:10.1016/j.meatsci.2005.02.008 PMID:22063884

Purchas, R. W., Rutherfurd, S. M., Pearce, P. D., Vather, R., & Wilkinson, B. H. P. (2004). Concentrations in beef and lamb of taurine, carnosine, coenzyme Q10, and creatine. *Meat Science*, *66*(3), 629–637. doi:10.1016/S0309-1740(03)00181-5 PMID:22060873

Purchas, R. W., Triumf, E. C., & Egelandsdal, B. (2010). Quality characteristics and composition of the Longissimus muscle in the short-loin from male and female farmed red deer in New Zealand. *Meat Science*, *86*(2), 505–510. doi:10.1016/j.meatsci.2010.05.043 PMID:20584574

Purchas, R. W., Wilkinson, B. H. P., Carruthers, F., & Jackson, F. (2014). A comparison of the nutrient content of uncooked and cooked lean from New Zealand beef and lamb. *Journal of Food Composition and Analysis*, *35*(2), 75–82. doi:10.1016/j.jfca.2014.04.008

Qadeer, Z., Huma, N., Sameen, A., & Iqbal, T. (2015). Camel milk cheese: Optimization of processing conditions. *Journal of Camelid Science*, *8*, 18–25.

Quan, S., Burentegusi, Y., & Miyamoto, T. (2006). Microflora in traditional starter cultures for fermented milk, Hurunge, from inner Mongolia. *China Journal of Animal Science Journal*, *77*(2), 235–241. doi:10.1111/j.1740-0929.2006.00343.x

Quan, S., Tsuda, H., & Miyamoto, T. (2008). Angiotensin I-converting enzyme inhibitory peptides in skim milk fermented with *Lactobacillus helveticus* 130B4 from camel milk in Inner Mongolia, China. *Journal of the Science of Food and Agriculture*, *88*(15), 2688–2692. doi:10.1002/jsfa.3394

Quigley, L., McCarthy, R., O'Sullivan, O., Beresford, T. P., Fitzgerald, G. F., Ross, R. P., ... Cotter, P. D. (2013). The microbial content of raw and pasteurized cow milk as determined by molecular approaches. *Journal of Dairy Science*, *96*(8), 4928–4937. doi:10.3168/jds.2013-6688

Quigley, L., O'Sullivan, O., Beresford, T. P., Ross, R. P., Fitzgerald, G. F., & Cotter, P. D. (2011). Molecular approaches to analysing the microbial composition of raw milk and raw milk cheese. *International Journal of Food Microbiology*, *150*(2–3), 81–94. doi:10.1016/j.ijfoodmicro.2011.08.001

Quita, S., & Kurdi, A. (2010). Antigenotoxic and anticytotoxic effect of camel milk in mice treated with cisplatin. *Saudi Journal of Biological Sciences*, *17*(2), 159–166. doi:10.1016/j.sjbs.2010.02.010 PMID:23961073

Rachman, A. B., Maheswari, R. R. A., & Bachroem, M. S. (2015). Composition and isolation of lactoferrin from colostrum and milk of various goat breeds. *Procedia Food Science*, *3*, 200–210. doi:10.1016/j.profoo.2015.01.022

Radlowski, E. C., & Johnson, R. W. (2013). Perinatal iron deficiency and neurocognitive development. *Frontiers in Human Neuroscience*, *7*, 34–43. doi:10.3389/fnhum.2013.00585 PMID:24065908

Radwan, A. I., Bekair1, S. I., Mukayel, A. A., AL-Bokmy, A. M., Prasad, P.V.S., Azar, F.N., & Coloyan, E. R. (1995). Control of *Brucella melitensis* infection in a large camel herd in Saudi Arabia using antibiotherapy and vaccination with Rev. 1 vaccine. *Revue Scientifique et Technique de.l'Office International des Epizooties, 14*, 719-732.

Rafiq, S., Huma, N., Pasha, I., Sameen, A., Mukhtar, O., & Khan, M. (2016). Chemical composition, nitrogen fractions and amino acids profile of milk from different animal species. *Asian-Australasian Journal of Animal Sciences*, *29*(7), 1022–1028. doi:10.5713/ajas.15.0452 PMID:26954163

Rahelic, S., & Puac, S. (1981). Fibre types in longissimus dorsi from wild and highly selected pig breeds. *Meat Science*, *5*(6), 451–455. doi:10.1016/0309-1740(81)90042-5 PMID:22054604

Rahmeh, R., Alomirah, H., Akbar, A., & Sidhu, J. (2019). Composition and properties of camel milk. In Milk Production, Processing and Marketing. IntechOpen. doi:10.5772/intechopen.82592

Raiymbek, G., Faye, B., Kadim, I. T., Serikbaeva, A., & Konuspayeva, G. (2019). Comparative fatty acids composition and cholesterol content in Bactrian (*Camelus bactrianus*) and dromedary camel (*Camelus dromedaries*) meat. *Tropical Animal Health and Production*, *51*(7), 2025–2035. doi:10.100711250-019-01894-2 PMID:31011922

Raiymbek, G., Kadim, I. T., Al-Amri, I. S., Abdulaziz, Y. A., & Faye, B. (2018). Concentration of nutrients in six muscles of Bactrian (Camelus bacterianus) camel. *Journal of Camel Practice and Research*, *25*(1), 109–121. doi:10.5958/2277-8934.2018.00016.4

Ramadan, S., & Inoue-Murayama, M. (2017). Advances in camel genomics and their applications: A review. *The Journal of Animal Genetics*, *45*(2), 49–58. doi:10.5924/abgri.45.49

Ramet, J. P. (1984). Les enzymes coagulantes en fromagerie. In *Le fromage*. Paris: Ed. Sepaic.

Ramet, J. P. (1989). L'aptitude fromagère du lait de dromadaire. *Revue d'Élevage et de Médecine Vétérinaire des Pays Tropicaux*, *42*(1), 105–111.

Ramet, J. P. (1993). *La technologie des fromages au lait de dromadaire (Camelus dromedarius)* (Vol. 113). Food & Agriculture Org.

Ramet, J. P. (2001). The Technology of Making Cheese from Camel Milk (*Camelus Dromedarius*). *FAO Animal Production and Health Paper*, *113*, 31–33.

Ramet, J. P. (2001). The technology of making cheese from camel milk (Camelus dromedarius). In *Animal production and health paper n°113*. Rome, Italy: FAO.

Rao, D. R., Chawan, C., & Pulusani, S. (1981). Influence of milk and thermophilus milk on plasma cholesterol levels and hepatic cholesterogenesis in rats. *Journal of Food Science*, *46*(5), 1339–1341. doi:10.1111/j.1365-2621.1981.tb04168.x

Rasheed, Z. (2017). Medicinal values of bioactive constituents of camel milk: A concise report. *International Journal of Health Sciences*, *11*(5), 1–2. PMID:29114185

Rathore, G. S. (1986). *Camels and their Management. ICAR publ.*

Ratnasari, I., Sudarminto, S. Y., Nusyam, H., & Widjanarko, S. B. (2014). Extraction process modification to enhance properties of skin gelatin of pangas catfish (Pangasius pangasius). *Food and Public Heath*, *4*(3), 140–150.

Ratnasari, I., Yuwono, S. S., Nusyam, H., & Widjanarko, S. B. (2013). Extraction and characterization of gelatin from different fresh water fishes as alternative sources of gelatin. *International Food Research Journal*, *20*(6), 3085–3091.

Rawdah, T. N., El-Faer, M. Z., & Koreish, S. A. (1994). Fatty acid composition of the meat and fat of the one-humped camel (*Camelus dromedarius*). *Meat Science*, *37*(1), 149–155. doi:10.1016/0309-1740(94)90151-1 PMID:22059419

Ray, R., & Mishra, S. (2017). Technological Innovations in Processing of Fermented Foods An Overview. In *Fermented Foods, Part II Technological Interventions* (1st ed.; pp. 21–45). Boca Raton, FL: CRC Press.

Raziq, A., Tareen, A. M., & de Verdier, K. (2011). Characterization and significance of Raigi camel, a livestock breed of the Pashtoon pastoral people in Afghanistan and Pakistan. *Journal of Livestock Science*, *2*, 11–19.

Raziq, K., Younas, M., & Kakar, M. A. (2008). Camel – a potential dairy animal in difficult environments. *Pakistan Journal of Agricultural Sciences*, *45*(2), 263–267.

Rea, H. (1983). *Studies on the Manufacture of Frozen Yogurt* (Unpublished MSc thesis). Ein Shams University, Egypt.

Redwan, E. M., El-Baky, N. A., Al-Hejin, A. M., Baeshen, M. N., Almehdar, H. A., Elsaway, A., & Uversky, V. N. (2016). Significant antibacterial activity and synergistic effects of camel lactoferrin with antibiotics against methicillin-resistant *Staphylococcus aureus* (MRSA). *Research in Microbiology*, *167*(6), 480–491. doi:10.1016/j.resmic.2016.04.006 PMID:27130281

Redwan, E., & Tabll, A. (2007). Camel lactoferrin markedly inhibits hepatitis C virus genotype 4 infection of human peripheral blood leukocytes. *Journal of Immunoassay & Immunochemistry*, *28*(3), 267–277. doi:10.1080/15321810701454839 PMID:17613672

Refaey, A. T. A.-J. S. E. (2013). *Nutritional and medicinal value of camel (Camelus dromedarius) milk*. Food and Environment. doi:10.2495/fenv130201

Renand, G., Picard, B., Touraille, C., Berge, P., & Lepetit, J. (2001). Relationships between muscle characteristics and meat quality traits of young Charolais bulls. *Meat Science*, *59*(1), 49–60. doi:10.1016/S0309-1740(01)00051-1 PMID:22062505

Reps, A., Warminska Radyko, I., & Dajnowiec, F. (1999). Effect of High Pressure on Yoghurt. In H. Ludwig (Ed.), *Advances in High Pressure Bioscience and Biotechnology* (pp. 453–456). Heidelberg, Germany: Springer. doi:10.1007/978-3-642-60196-5_102

Reps, A., Warminska Radyko, I., Krzyzewska, A., & Tomasik, J. (2001). Effect of High Pressures on *Streptococcus Salivarius* Subsp. *Thermophilus. Milchwissenschaft. Milk Science International*, *56*(3), 131–133.

Rey, M. W., Woloshuk, S. L., deBoer, H. A., & Pieper, F. R. (1990). Complete nucleotide sequence of human mammary gland lactoferrin. *Nucleic Acids Research*, *18*(17), 5288. doi:10.1093/nar/18.17.5288 PMID:2402455

Rhee, S. J., Lee, J.-E., & Lee, C.-H. (2011). Importance of lactic acid bacteria in Asian fermented foods. *Microbial Cell Factories*, *10*(1Suppl 1), S5. doi:10.1186/1475-2859-10-S1-S5

Richard, D. (1985). *Le dromadaire et son élevage. In IEMVT, Coll. « études et synthèses*. Montpellier, France: CIRAD.

Ridzoulis, C. (2013). *Introduction to the physical chemistry of foods* (J. Rhoades, Ed.). CRC Press, Taylor & Francis Group. doi:10.1201/b14705

Robinson, R. K. (1990). Dairy microbiology: Volume 1-The microbiology of milk. Elsevier Applied Science Publishers Ltd.

Rodríguez-Figueroa, J. C., Reyes-Díaz, R., González-Córdova, A. F., Troncoso-Rojas, R., Vargas-Arispuro, I., & Vallejo-Cordoba, B. (2010). Angiotensin-converting enzyme inhibitory activity of milk fermented by wild and industrial Lactococcus lactis strains. *Journal of Dairy Science*, *93*(11), 5032–5038. doi:10.3168/jds.2010-3103

Rodr, L. M., Gomez, M. P.-G., Pimentel, L. L., & Fontecha, J. (2017). Milk fat components with potential anticancer activity—a review. *Bioscience Reports*, *37*. doi:10.1042/BSR20170705 PMID:29026007

Roger, F., Diallo, A., Yigezu, L. M., Hurard, C., Libeau, G., Mebratu, G. Y., & Faye, B. (2000). Investigations of a new pathological condition of camels in Ethiopia. *Journal of Camel Practice and Research*, *7*(2), 163–166.

Rolfes, S., Pinna, K., & Whitney, E. (2015). Understanding Normal and Clinical Nutrition (10th ed.). Cengage learning.

Ronald de Almeida, C. (2011). Camel milk: Characteristics and perspectives for use in clinical practice. *Revista Chilena de Nutrición*, *38*(2), 211–218.

Roohani, N., Hurrell, R., Kelishadi, R., & Schulin, R. (2013). Zinc and its importance for human health: An integrative review. *Journal of Research in Medical Sciences*, *18*, 144–157. PMID:23914218

Ross, P. R., Morgan, S., & Hill, C. (2002). Preservation and fermentation: Past, present and future. *International Journal of Food Microbiology*, *79*(1–2), 3–16. doi:10.1016/S0168-1605(02)00174-5

Ross, R., Desmond, C., Fitzgerald, G., & Stanton, C. (2005). Overcoming the technological hurdles in the development of probiotic foods. *Journal of Applied Microbiology*, *98*(6), 1410–1417. doi:10.1111/j.1365-2672.2005.02654.x

Rostan, E. F., DeBuys, H. V., Madey, D. L., & Pinnell, S. R. (2002). Evidence supporting zinc as an important antioxidant for skin. *International Journal of Dermatology*, *41*(9), 606–611. doi:10.1046/j.1365-4362.2002.01567.x PMID:12358835

Roy, T., & Deepak, D. (2014). Antioxidant properties of milk oligosaccharides from various ruminants. *International Journal of Pharma and Bio Sciences*, *5*(2), 400–408.

Ruas-Madiedo, P., Hugenholtz, J., & Zoon, P. (2002). An overview of the functionality of exopolysaccharides produced by lactic acid bacteria. *NIZO Dairy Conference on Food Microbes 2001*, *12*(2), 163–171. 10.1016/S0958-6946(01)00160-1

Rufian-Henares, J. A., Guerra-Hernandez, E., & Garcıa-Villanova, B. (2006). Colour measurement as indicator for controlling the manufacture and storage of enteral formulas. *Food Control*, *17*(6), 489–493. doi:10.1016/j.foodcont.2005.02.011

Rusniok, C., Couvé, E., Cunha, V. D., Gana, R. E., Zidane, N., Bouchier, C., ... Glaser, P. (2010). Genome Sequence of Streptococcus gallolyticus: Insights into Its Adaptation to the Bovine Rumen and Its Ability To Cause Endocarditis. *Journal of Bacteriology*, *192*(8), 2266–2276. doi:10.1128/JB.01659-09

Russo, C. (2019). *Meet the Camels behind the Celebrated Camel Milk Chocolate*. Retrieved in 13th May, 2019 from: https://millerchocolate.com/blogs/news/the-story-of-the-camel-milk-chocolate-bar

Rutagwenda, T., Lechner-Doll, M., Schwartz, H. J., Schultka, W., & Von Engelhardt, W. (1990). Dietary preference and degrability of forage on a semi-arid thornbush savannah indigenous ruminants, camels and donkeys. *Animal Feed Science and Technology*, *35*(3-4), 179–192. doi:10.1016/0377-8401(90)90123-P

Rybczynski, N., Gosse, J. C., Harington, R., Wogelius, R. A., Hidy, A. J., & Buckley, M. (2013). Mid-Pliocene warm-period deposits in the High Arctic yield insight into camel evolution. *Nature Communications*, *4*(1550), 1–9. PMID:23462993

Rybicka, I., & Gliszczyńska-Świgło, A. (2017). Minerals in grain gluten-free products. The content of calcium, potassium, magnesium, sodium, copper, iron, manganese, and zinc. *Journal of Food Composition and Analysis*, *59*, 61–67. doi:10.1016/j.jfca.2017.02.006

Ryskaliyeva, A., Henry, C., Miranda, G., Faye, B., Konuspayeva, G., & Martin, P. (2018). Complex milk protein fractions' in Bactrian camel milk. In *The 5th Conference ISOCARD "Recent advances in camelids biology, health and Production"*, 275-277.

Ryskaliyeva, A., Henry, C., Miranda, G., Faye, B., Konuspayeva, G., & Martin, P. (2019b). The main WAP isoform usually found in camel milk arises from the usage of an improbable intron cryptic splice site in the precursor to mRNA in which a GC-AG intron occurs. BMC Genetics, 20, 14. doi:10.118612863-018-0704-x

Ryskaliyeva, A., Henry, C., Miranda, G., Faye, B., Konuspayeva, G., & Martin, P. (2018). Combining different proteomic approaches to resolve complexity of the milk protein fraction of dromedary, Bactrian camels and hybrids, from different regions of Kazakhstan. *PLoS One*, *13*(5), e0197026. doi:10.1371/journal.pone.0197026 PMID:29746547

Ryskaliyeva, A., Henry, C., Miranda, G., Faye, B., Konuspayeva, G., & Martin, P. (2019a). Alternative splicing events expand molecular diversity of camel CSN1S2 increasing its ability to generate potentially bioactive peptides. *Scientific Reports*, *9*(1), 5243. doi:10.103841598-019-41649-5 PMID:30918277

Saad, B. (2015). Greco-Arab and Islamic diet therapy: Tradition, research and practice. *Surge, 1*(1).

Saadaoui, B., Henry, C., Khorchani, T., Mars, M., Martin, P., & Cebo, C. (2013). Proteomics of the milk fat globule membrane from *Camelus dromedarius. Proteomics*, *13*(7), 1180–1184. doi:10.1002/pmic.201200113 PMID:23349047

Saadoun, A., & Cabrera, M. C. (2008). A review of the nutritional content and technological parameters of indigenous sources of meat in South America. *Meat Science*, *80*(3), 570–581. doi:10.1016/j.meatsci.2008.03.027 PMID:22063568

Saalfeld, W. K., & Edwards, G. P. (2010). Distribution and abundance of the feral camel (*Camelus dromedarius*) in Australia. *The Rangeland Journal*, *32*(1), 1–9. doi:10.1071/RJ09058

Sabahelkheir, M. K., Faten, M. M., & Hassan, A. A. (2012). Amino acid composition of human and animal's milk (camel, cow, sheep and goat). *Journal of Science and Technology*, *2*(2), 32–34.

Sabahelkhier, M. K., Faten, M. M., & Omer, F. I. (2012). Comparative determination of biochemical constituents between animals (goat, sheep, cow and camel) milk with human milk. *Research Journal of Recent Sciences*, *1*(5), 69–71.

Sachdeva, M. (2010). Cosmeceuticals. In N. Khunger & M. Sachdeva (Eds.), *Practical manual of cosmetic dermatology and surgery* (pp. 213–223). New Delhi, India: Mehta Publishers.

Sachdeva, M., & Khunger, N. (2010). Principles of normal skin care. In N. Khunger & M. Sachdeva (Eds.), *Practical manual of cosmetic dermatology and surgery* (pp. 1–15). New Delhi, India: Mehta Publishers.

Sadick, N. S. (2018). The pathophysiology of the male aging face and body. In N. S. Sadick & B. H. Thiers (Eds.), *Dermatologic clinics cosmetic dermatology for men* (pp. 1–4). New York, NY: Elsevier. doi:10.1016/j.det.2017.08.002

Sagar, S., Mehta, B., Wadhwani, K., Darji, V., & Aparnathi, K. (2017). Evaluation of camel milk for selected processing related parameters and comparisons with cow and buffalo milk. *International Journal of Health, Animal Science and Food Safety, 3*, 27 – 37.

Sagar, S. P., Mehta, B. M., Wadwani, K. N., Dargi, V. B., & Aparnthi, K. D. (2016). Evaluation of Camel Milk for Selected Processing Related Parameters and Composition with Cow and Buffalo Milk. *Int. J. Of Health. Animal Science and Food Safety*, *3*, 27–37.

Sahani, M., Agrawal, R., Tuteja, F., Ghouri, S., Aminudeen, R., & Sena, D. (2005). Hypoglycemic activity of camel milk in straptozotocin induced hyperglycemia in rats. *The Indian Journal of Animal Sciences*, *75*, 1436–1437.

Sah, B., Vasiljevic, T., McKechnie, S., & Donkor, O. (2014). Effect of probiotics on antioxidant and antimutagenic activities of crude peptide extract from yogurt. *Food Chemistry*, *156*, 264–270. doi:10.1016/j.foodchem.2014.01.105 PMID:24629967

Saikia, R. (2008). *Microbial Biotechnology*. New India Publishing.

Saini, N., Bhati, A., Singh, N., & Tuteja, F. (2007). Trace mineral and vitamin C content of camel milk: A comparative study. *Veterinary Practitioner*, *8*(1), 20–21.

Saipolda, T. (2005). Mongolian camels: current status of genetic resources, recording and production system in African, Asian and American Camelids. *Proceedings of the 34th meeting FAO/ICAR (International Committee for Animal Recording)* (pp. 73-80). Academic Press.

Saito, Z. (1985). Particle structure in spray-dried whole milk and in instant skim milk powder as related to lactose crystallization. *Food Microstructure*, *4*, 333–340.

Salami, M., Moosavi-Movahedi, A., Ehsani, M., Yousefi, R., Haertlé, T., Chobert, J., ... Niasari-Naslaji, A. (2010). Improvement of the antimicrobial and antioxidant activities of camel and bovine whey proteins by limited proteolysis. *Journal of Agricultural and Food Chemistry*, *58*(6), 3297–3302. doi:10.1021/jf9033283 PMID:20175528

Salami, M., Moosavi-Movahedi, A., Moosavi-Movahedi, F., Ehsani, M. R., Yousefi, R., Farhadi, M., ... Haertlé, T. (2011). Biological activity of camel milk casein following enzymatic digestion. *The Journal of Dairy Research*, *78*(4), 471–478. doi:10.1017/S0022029911000628 PMID:21910944

Saldo, J., Mcsweeney, P. L. H., Sendra, E., Kelly, A. L., & Guamis, B. (2002). Proteolysis in Caprine Milk Cheese Treated by High Pressure to Accelerate Cheese Ripening. *International Dairy Journal*, *12*(1), 35–44. doi:10.1016/S0958-6946(01)00169-8

Salem, S., Fardous, M., Meead, G., & El-Rashody, H. (2017). Effect of Camel Milk Fortified with Dates in Ice Cream Manufacture on Viscosity, Overrun, and Rheological Properties during Storage Period. *Food and Nutrition Sciences*, *8*(05), 551–564. doi:10.4236/fns.2017.85038

Saljooghi, S., Mansouri-Najand, L., Ebrahimnejad, H., Doostan, F., & Askari, N. (2017). Microbiological, biochemical and organoleptic properties of fermented probiotic drink produced from camel milk. *Veterinary Research Forum: An International Quarterly Journal*, *8*(4), 313–317. PMID:29326790

Sallam, K. I., & Morshedy, A. E. M. A. (2008). Organochlorine pesticides residues in camel, cattle and sheep carcasses slaughtered in Sharkia province, Egypt. *Food Chemistry*, *18*(1), 154–164. doi:10.1016/j.foodchem.2007.10.066

Salmen, S. H., Abu-Tarboush, H. M., Al-Saleh, A. A., & Metwalli, A. A. (2012). Amino acids content and electrophoretic profile of camel milk casein from different camel breeds in Saudi Arabia. *Saudi Journal of Biological Sciences*, *19*(2), 177–183. doi:10.1016/j.sjbs.2011.12.002 PMID:23961177

Saltanat, H., Li, H., Xu, Y., Wang, J., Liu, F., & Geng, X. H. (2009). The influences of camel milk on the immune response of chronic hepatitis B. *Chinese Journal of Cellular and Molecular Immunology*, *25*(5), 431-433.

Saltin, B., Rose, R. J., & Henckel, P. (1994). Skeletal muscle morphology and metabolic potential. *Acta Physiologica Scandinavica*, *150*(617), 24–32. PMID:8010123

Samet-Bali, O., Bellila, A., Ayadi, M.-A., Marzouk, B., & Attia, H. (2010). A comparison of the physicochemical, microbiological and aromatic composition of Traditional and Industrial Leben in Tunisia. *International Journal of Dairy Technology*, *63*(1), 98–104. doi:10.1111/j.1471-0307.2009.00546.x

Sarmadi, B., & Ismail, A. (2010). Antioxidative peptides from food proteins: A review. *Peptides*, *31*(10), 1949–1956. doi:10.1016/j.peptides.2010.06.020 PMID:20600423

Savadogo, A., Ouattara, C. A., Savadogo, P. W., Barro, N., Ouattara, A. S., & Traoré, A. S. (2004). Identification of exopolysaccharides-producing lactic acid bacteria from Burkina Faso fermented milk samples. *African Journal of Biotechnology*, *3*(3), 189–194. doi:10.5897/AJB2004.000-2034

Savadogo, A., Ouattara, A. C., Bassole, H. I., & Traore, S. A. (2006). Bacteriocins and lactic acid bacteria—A minireview. *African Journal of Biotechnology*, *5*(9). Retrieved from https://www.ajol.info/index.php/ajb/article/view/42771

Sawaya, W. N., Khalil, J. K., Al-Shalahat, A., & Al-Mohammed, H. (1984). Chemical composition and nutritional quality of camel milk. *Journal of Food Science*, *49*(3), 744–747. doi:10.1111/j.1365-2621.1984.tb13200.x

Sboui, A., Djegham, M., Belhadj, O. & Khorchani, T. (2016). Le lait de chamelle: qualités nutritives et effet sur les variations de la glycémie. *Options Méditerranéennes, A, 115*, 487-492.

Sboui, A., Djegham, M., Belhadj, O. & Khorchani, T. (2016). Le lait de chamelle: qualités nutritives et effet sur les variations de la glycémie. *Options Méditerranéennes, A*, 487-492.

Sboui, A., Khorchani, T., Djegham, M., & Belhadj, O. (2009). Comparaison de la composition physicochimique du lait camelin et bovin du Sud tunisien; variation du pH et de l'acidité à différentes températures. *Afrique Science: revue internationale des sciences et technologie, 5*.

Sboui, A., Djegham, M., Khorchani, T., Hammadi, M., Barhoumi, K., & Belhadj, O. (2010). Effect of camel milk on blood glucose, cholesterol and total proteins variations in alloxan-induced diabetic dogs. *International Journal of Diabetes and Metabolism*, *18*(1), 5–11. doi:10.1159/000497686

Sboui, A., Khorchani, T., Djegham, M., Agrebi, A., Dalleli, A., & Belhadj, O. (2012). Camel Milk as Adjuvant to Treat Alloxan Diabetes: Effect of Heat Treatment on this Property. *Journal of Diabetes & Metabolism*, *3*(04), 190. doi:10.4172/2155-6156.1000190

Sboui, A., Khorchani, T., Djegham, M., Agrebi, A., Elhatmi, H., & Belhadj, O. (2009). Anti-diabetic effect of camel milk in alloxan-induced diabetic dogs: A dose response experiment. *Journal of Animal Physiology and Animal Nutrition*. PMID:19906135

Sboui, A., Khorchani, T., Djegham, M., Agrebi, A., Elhatmi, H., & Belhadj, O. (2010). Anti-diabetic effect of camel milk in alloxan-induced diabetic dogs: A dose–response experiment. *Journal of Animal Physiology and Animal Nutrition*, *94*(4), 540–546. doi:10.1111/j.1439-0396.2009.00941.x PMID:19906135

Schönfeldt, H., & Gibson, N. (2008). Changes in the nutrient quality of meat in an obesity context. *Meat Science*, *80*(1), 20–27. doi:10.1016/j.meatsci.2008.05.025 PMID:22063166

Schreiber, R., & Hinrichs, J. (2000). Rennet coagulation of heated milk concentrates. *Le Lait*, *80*(1), 33–42. doi:10.1051/lait:2000105

Schrieber, R., & Gareis, H. (2007). *Gelatine handbook: Theory and industrial practice*. Weinheim: Wiley-VCH Verlag GmbH & Co. doi:10.1002/9783527610969

Seboussi, R., Faye, B., Askar, M., Hassan, K., & Alhadrami, G. (2009). Effect of selenium supplementation on blood status and milk, urine and fecal excretion in pregnant and lactating camel. *Biological Trace Element Research*, *128*(1), 45–57. doi:10.100712011-008-8251-3 PMID:18972072

See, S. F., Hong, P. K., Ng, K. L., Wan Aida, W. M., & Babji, A. S. (2010). Physicochemical properties of gelatins extracted from skins of different freshwater fish species. *International Food Research Journal*, *17*(3), 809–816.

Seifried, H. E., Anderson, D. E., Fisher, E. I., & Milner, J. A. (2007). A review of the interaction among dietary antioxidants and reactive oxygen species. *The Journal of Nutritional Biochemistry*, *18*(9), 567–579. doi:10.1016/j.jnutbio.2006.10.007 PMID:17360173

Seifu, E. (2007). Handling, preservation and utilization of camel milk and camel milk products in Shinile and Jijiga Zones, eastern Ethiopia. *Marketing, 10.*

Serri, R., & Lorrizo, M. (2008). Cosmeceuticals: Focus on topical in photoaging. *Clinics in Dermatology*, *26*(6), 633–638. doi:10.1016/j.clindermatol.2007.09.016 PMID:18940544

Shabo, Y., Barzel, & Yagil, R. (2008). Etiology of Crohn's Disease and Camel Milk Treatment. *Journal of Camel Practice and Research*, *15*, 55–59.

Shabo, Y., Barzel, R., Margoulis, M., & Yagil, R. (2005). Camel milk for food allergies in children. *Immunology and Allergies*, *7*, 796–798. PMID:16382703

Shabo, Y., Barzel, R., Margoulis, M., & Yagil, R. (2005). Camel Milk for Food Allergies in Children. *Immunology and Allergies*, *7*, 796–798. PMID:16382703

Shabo, Y., Barzel, R., & Yagil, R. (2008). Etiology of Crohn's disease and camel milk treatment. *Journal of Camel Practice and Research*, *15*(1), 55–59.

Shabo, Y., & Yagil, R. (2005). Etiology of autism and camel milk as therapy. *International Journal on Disability and Human Development: IJDHD*, *4*(2), 67–70. doi:10.1515/IJDHD.2005.4.2.67

Shafi, F., Reshi, M., Bashir, A., & Bashir, I. (2018). Chocolate processing. *International Journal of Advanced Biological Research*, *8*(3), 408–419.

Shahaj, A., Monguidi, M., & Stoicescu, A-V. (2019). Guidelines for reporting surveillance data on Transmissible Spongiform Encephalopathies (TSE) in the EU within the framework of Regulation (EC) No 999/2001. EFSA Supporting Publications.

Shahein, M. R., Hassanein, A. M., & Zayan, A. F. (2014). Evaluation of soft cheese manufactured from camel and buffalo milk. *World Journal of Dairy Food Science*, *9*(2), 213–219.

Shah, M. G., Qureshi, A. S., & Reissmann, M. (2014). *Phenotypic and genetic differentiation of Pakistani camel breeds.* Lambert Academic Publishing.

Shah, R. A. (2005). Cosmeceuticals. In S. Savant, D. Gore, R. A. Shah, & K. Sarangi (Eds.), *Textbook of dermato-surgery & cosmetology* (pp. 519–524). Mumbai, India: ASCAD.

Shalash, M. R. (1984). The production and utilization of camel milk. In W. R. Cockrill (Ed.), *The Camelid: An all-purpose animal* (pp. 196–208). Uppsala, Sweden: Scandinavian Institute of African Studies.

Shamsia, S. M. (2009). Nutritional and therapeutic properties of camel and human milks. *International Journal of Genetics and Molecular Biology*, *1*(2), 52–58.

Shariatikia, M., Behbahani, M., & Mohabatkar, H. (2017). Anticancer activity of cow, sheep, goat, mare, donkey and camel milks and their caseins and whey proteins and in silico comparison of the caseins. *Molecular Biology Research Communications*, *6*(2), 57. PMID:28775991

Sharma, A. K., & Singh, T. P. (1999). Lactoferrin–metal interactions: First crystal structure of a complex of lactoferrin with a lanthanide ion (Sm3+) at 3.4 Å resolution. *Acta Crystallographica. Section D, Biological Crystallography*, *55*(11), 1799–1804. doi:10.1107/S0907444999009865 PMID:10531475

Sharma, A., Jana, A., & Chavan, R. (2012). Functionality of milk powders and milk-based powders for end use applications—A review. *Comprehensive Reviews in Food Science and Food Safety*, *11*(5), 518–528. doi:10.1111/j.1541-4337.2012.00199.x

Sharma, A., & Pant, S. (2013). Studies on camel hair merino-wool blended knitted fabrics. *Indian Journal of Fibre and Textile Research*, *38*, 317–319.

Sharma, C., & Singh, C. (2014). Therapeutic value of camel milk–a review. *Advanced Journal of Pharmacie and Life Science Research*, *2*(3), 7–13.

Sharma, P., Dube, D., Singh, A., Mishra, B., Singh, N., Sinha, M., ... Singh, T. P. (2011). *Structural Basis of Recognition of Pathogen-associated Molecular Patterns and Inhibition of Proinflammatory Cytokines by Camel Peptidoglycan Recognition Protein*. doi:10.1074/jbc.m111.228163

Sharma, P., Dube, D., Singh, A., Mishra, B., Singh, N., Sinha, M., ... Singh, T. P. (2011). Structural basis of recognition of pathogen-associated molecular patterns and inhibition of proinflammatory cytokines by camel peptidoglycan recognition protein. *The Journal of Biological Chemistry*, *286*(18), 16208–16217. doi:10.1074/jbc.M111.228163 PMID:21454594

Sharma, P., Dube, D., Sinha, M., Dey, S., Kaur, P., Sharma, S., & Singh, T. P. (2012). Structural basis of heparin binding to camel peptidoglycan recognition protein-S. *International Journal of Biochemistry and Molecular Biology*, *3*(1), 86. PMID:22509483

Sharma, S., Sinha, M., Kaushik, S., Kaur, P., & Singh, T. (2013). C-lobe of lactoferrin: The whole story of the half-molecule. *Biochemistry Research International*, *ID271641*, 1–8. doi:10.1155/2013/271641 PMID:23762557

Shehadeh, N., Gelertner, L., Blazer, S., Perlman, R., Solovachik, L., & Etzioni, A. (2001). Importance of insulin content in infant diet: Suggestion for a new infant formula. *Acta Paediatrica (Oslo, Norway)*, *90*(1), 93–95. doi:10.1111/j.1651-2227.2001.tb00262.x

Shehata, M. F. (2005). Carcass traits and meat quality of one-humped camels fed different halophytic forages: 2-Physical, chemical, and sensory characteristics of camel meat. *Journal of Agriculture Science*, *30*, 1943–1952.

Sheng, Q., & Fang, X. (2009). Bioactive components in mare milk. In Y. W. Park (Ed.), Bioactive components in milk and dairy products (pp. 195-213). Wiley-Blackwell.

Shewangizaw, A. (2016). Review on the dual functions of camel milk processing and marketing for unmet demand. *Middle East Journal of Scientific Research*, *24*(10), 3058–3066.

Shimada, K., Sakuma, Y., Wakamatsu, J., Fukushima, M., Sekikawa, M., Kuchida, K., & Mikami, M. (2004). Species and muscle differences in L-carnitine levels in skeletal muscles based on a new simple assay. *Meat Science*, *68*(3), 357–362. doi:10.1016/j.meatsci.2004.04.003 PMID:22062403

Shohami, E., Beit-Yannai, E., Horowitz, M., & Kohen, R. (1997). Oxidative stress in closed-head injury: Brain antioxidant capacity as an indicator of functional outcome. *Journal of Cerebral Blood Flow and Metabolism*, *17*(10), 1007–1019. doi:10.1097/00004647-199710000-00002 PMID:9346425

Shori, A. (2012). Comparative study of chemical composition, isolation and identification of micro-flora in traditional fermented camel milk products: Gariss, Suusac, and Shubat. *Journal of the Saudi Society of Agricultural Sciences*, *11*(2), 79–88. doi:10.1016/j.jssas.2011.12.001

Shori, A. (2013). Antioxidant activity and viability of lactic acid bacteria in soybean-yogurt made from cow and camel milk. *Journal of Taibah University for Science*, *7*(4), 202–208. doi:10.1016/j.jtusci.2013.06.003

Shori, A. B. (2015). Camel milk as a potential therapy for controlling diabetes and its complications: A review of in vivo studies. *Journal of Food and Drug Analysis*, *23*(4), 609–618. doi:10.1016/j.jfda.2015.02.007 PMID:28911476

Shori, A. B., & Baba, A. S. (2012). Viability of lactic acid bacteria and sensory evaluation in Cinnamomum verum and Allium sativum-bio-yogurts made from camel and cow milk. *Journal of the Association of Arab Universities for Basic and Applied Sciences*, *11*(1), 50–55. doi:10.1016/j.jaubas.2011.11.001

Shori, A., & Baba, A. (2014). Comparative antioxidant activity, proteolysis and in vitro-amylase and glucosidase inhibition of Allium sativum yogurts made from cow and camel milk. *Journal of Saudi Chemical Society*, *18*(5), 456–463. doi:10.1016/j.jscs.2011.09.014

Shuiep, E. S., Zubeir, I. E. M., El Owni, O. A. O., & Musa, H. H. (2008). Raw camel (*Camelus dromedarius*) milk in Khartoum state, Sudan. *Tropical and Subtropical Agroecosystems*, *8*, 101–106.

Siboukeur, A. (2013). Effect of cameline nisin isolated from Lactococcus lactis sub sp. lactis on Staphylococcus aureus sp. *Emirates Journal of Food and Agriculture*, *25*(5), 398–402. doi:10.9755/ejfa.v25i5.15511

Siboukeur, O., Mati, A., & Hessas, B. (2005). Amélioration de l'aptitude à la coagulation du lait cameline (Camelus dromedarius): Utilisation d'extraits enzymatiques coagulants gastriques de dromadaires. *Cahiers Agricultures*, *14*(5), 473–478.

Silbermayr, K., Orozco-terWengel, P., Charruau, P., Enkhbileg, D., Walzer, C., Vogl, C., ... Burger, P. A. (2010). High mitochondrial differentiation levels between wild and domestic Bactrian camels: A basis for rapid detection of maternal hybridization. *Animal Genetics*, *41*(3), 315–318. doi:10.1111/j.1365-2052.2009.01993.x PMID:19968638

Silva, R. S. G., Bandeira, S. F., & Pinto, L. A. A. (2014). Characteristics and chemical composition of skins gelatin from cobia (*Rachycentron canadum*). *Lebensmittel-Wissenschaft + Technologie*, *57*(2), 580–585. doi:10.1016/j.lwt.2014.02.026

Simek, J., Vorlova, L., Malota, L., Steinhauserova, I., & Steinhauser, L. (2003). Post-mortal changes of pH value and lactic acid content in the muscles of pigs and bulls. *Journal of Animal Science*, *7*, 295–299.

Simmons, N. J., Daley, C. C., Cummings, T. L., Morgan, S. K., Johnson, N. V., & Lombard, A. (2008). Reassessing the principles of electrical stimulation [Review]. *Meat Science*, *80*(1), 110–122. doi:10.1016/j.meatsci.2008.05.006 PMID:22063176

Sinclair, A. J., Slattery, W. J., & O'Dea, K. (1982). The analysis of polyunsaturated fatty acids in meat by capillary gas-liquid chromatography. *Journal of the Science of Food and Agriculture*, *33*(8), 771–776. doi:10.1002/jsfa.2740330814

Singh, H., Shalabi, S. I., Fox, P. F., Flynn, A., & Berry, A. (1988). Rennet coagulation of heated milk-influnce of pH adjustment before or after heating. *The Journal of Dairy Research*, *55*(2), 205–215. doi:10.1017/S0022029900026030

Singh, R., Mal, G., Kumar, D., Patil, D., & Pathak, K. (2017). Camel Milk: An Important Natural Adjuvant. *Agricultural Research*, *6*(4), 327–340. doi:10.100740003-017-0284-4

Sing, R. R. B., & Patil, G. R. (1989). Storage stability of UHT buffalo milk. 1. Change in physico-chemical properties. *Indian Journal of Dairy Science*, *42*, 150–154.

Şireli, U., & Orhan, C. (2015). Frozen yogurt. *Turkish Food Journal*, *40*(3), 179–185.

Sisay, F., & Awoke, K. (2015). Review on production quality and use of camel milk in Ethiopia. *Journal of Fisheries & Livestock Production*, *3*(3), 155–162.

Sisay, F., & Awoke, K. (2015). Review on production, quality and use of camel milk in Ethiopia. *Journal of Fisheries & Livestock Production*, *3*(3), 1–4.

Sliwinski, S., Croonenberghs, J., Christophe, A., Deboutte, D., & Maes, M. (2006). Polyunsaturated fatty acids: Do they have a role in the pathophysiology of autism? *Neuroendocrinology Letters*, *27*(4), 465–472. PMID:16891996

Smelt, J. M. (1998). Recent Advances in the Microbiology of High-Pressure Processing. *Trends in Food Science & Technology*, *9*(4), 152–158. doi:10.1016/S0924-2244(98)00030-2

Smith, D., Bakshi, A., & Lomauro, C. (1984). Changes in Function of Sweetener System and Whey Substitution. *Milchwissenschaft. Milk Science International*, *39*, 455.

Smits, M. G., Huppertz, T., Alting, A. C., & Kiers, J. (2011). Composition, constituents and properties of Dutch camel milk. *Journal of Camel Practice and Research*, *18*, 1–6.

Smits, M. G., & Montety, G. J. (2009). Ammonia emission from camel dairy in the Netherlands. *Journal of Camel Practice and Research*, *16*(2), 139–142.

Snow, D. H., & Harris, R. C. (1985). Thoroughbreds and greyhounds: biochemical adaptations in creatures of nature and of man. In Circulation, respiration and metabolism. Springer-Verlag. doi:10.1007/978-3-642-70610-3_17

Snow, D. H., & Guy, P. S. (1981). Fibre type and enzyme activities of the gluteus medius in different breeds of horse. In J. Poortmans & G. Niset (Eds.), *Biochemistry of Exercise IV-B* (pp. 275–282). Baltimore, MD: University of Park Press.

Sobczuk-Szul, M., Wielgosz-Groth, Z., Wronski, M., & Rzemieniewski, A. (2013). Changes in the bioactive protein concentrations in the bovine colostrum of Jersey and Polish Holstein–Friesian cows. *Turkish Journal of Veterinary and Animal Sciences*, *37*(1), 43–49.

Soboleva, S. E., Sedykh, S. E., Alinovskaya, L. I., Buneva, V. N., & Nevinsky, G. A. (2019). Cow Milk Lactoferrin Possesses Several Catalytic Activities. *Biomolecules*, *9*(6), 208. doi:10.3390/biom9060208 PMID:31146486

Sockalingam, K., Nelson, H., Idris, M. I., & Abdullah, H. Z. (2016). Effects of pre-treatment durations on properties of black tilapia (*Oreochromis Mossambicus*) skin gelatin. *Materials Science Forum*, *840*, 146–150. doi:10.4028/www.scientific.net/MSF.840.146

Soetikno, V., Watanabe, K., Sari, F. R., Harima, M., Thandavarayan, R. A., Veeraveedu, P. T., ... Suzuki, K. (2011). Curcumin attenuates diabetic nephropathy by inhibiting PKC-a and PKC-b1 activity in streptozotocin-induced type I diabetic rats. *Molecular Nutrition & Food Research*, *55*(11), 1655–1665. doi:10.1002/mnfr.201100080 PMID:22045654

Sofjan, R., & Hartel, R. (2004). Effects of overrun on structural and physical characteristics of ice cream. *International Dairy Journal*, *14*(3), 255–262. doi:10.1016/j.idairyj.2003.08.005

Solanki, D., & Hati, S. (2018). Fermented camel milk: A Review on its bio-functional properties. *Emirates Journal of Food and Agriculture*, *30*(4), 268–274. doi:10.9755/ejfa.2018.v30.i4.1661

Solanki, D., Hati, S., & Sakure, A. (2017). In silico and in vitro analysis of novel angiotensin I-converting enzyme (ACE) inhibitory bioactive peptides derived from fermented camel milk (Camelus dromedarius). *International Journal of Peptide Research and Therapeutics*, *23*(4), 441–459. doi:10.100710989-017-9577-5

Soleymanzadeh, N., Mirdamadi, S., & Kianirad, M. (2016). Antioxidant activity of camel and bovine milk fermented by lactic acid bacteria isolated from traditional fermented camel milk (Chal). *Dairy Science Technology*, *96*(4), 443-457. ff.ffhal01532393 doi:10.100713594-016-0278-1ff

Soleymanzadeh, N., Mirdamadi, S., Mirzaei, M., & Kianirad, M. (2019). Novel β-casein derived antioxidant and ACE-inhibitory active peptide from camel milk fermented by Leuconostoc lactis PTCC1899: Identification and molecular docking. *International Dairy Journal*.

Soliman, G. Z. A. (2005). Comparison of chemical and mineral content of milk from human, cow, buffalo, camel and goat in Egypt. *Egyptian Journal of Hospital Medicine*, *21*, 116–130.

Soltani, M., Boran, O. S., & Hayaloglu, A. A. (2016). Effect of various blends of camel chymosin and microbial rennet (*Rhizomucor miehei*) on microstructure and rheological properties of Iranian UF White cheese. *Lebensmittel-Wissenschaft + Technologie*, *68*, 724–728. doi:10.1016/j.lwt.2016.01.028

Sorensen, J., Palmer, D. S., Qvist, K. B., & Schiott, B. (2011). Initial stage of cheese production: A molecular modeling study of bovine and camel chymosin complexed with peptides from the chymosin-sensitive region of κ-casein. *Journal of Agricultural and Food Chemistry*, *59*(10), 5636–5647. doi:10.1021/jf104898w PMID:21476511

Soukoulis, C., Lebesi, D., & Tzia, C. (2009). Enrichment of Ice Cream with Dietary Fiber: Effects on Rheological Properties, Ice Crystallization and Glass Transition Phenomena. *Food Chemistry*, *115*(2), 665–671. doi:10.1016/j.foodchem.2008.12.070

Soukoulis, C., Lyroni, E., & Tzia, C. (2010). Sensory Profiling and Hedonic Judgment of Probiotic Ice Cream as a Function of Hydrocolloids, Yogurt and Milk Fat Content. *Lebensmittel-Wissenschaft + Technologie*, *43*(9), 1351–1358. doi:10.1016/j.lwt.2010.05.006

Sow, L. C., & Yang, H. (2015). Effects of salt and sugar addition on the physicochemical properties and nanostructure of fish gelatin. *Food Hydrocolloids*, *45*, 72–82. doi:10.1016/j.foodhyd.2014.10.021

Spencer, T. S. (1988). Dry skin and skin moisturizers. *Clinics in Dermatology*, *6*(3), 24–28. doi:10.1016/0738-081X(88)90028-4 PMID:3071400

Stahl, T., Sallmann, H. P., Duehlmeier, R., & Wernery, U. (2006). Selected vitamins and fatty acid patterns in dromedary milk and colostrum. *Journal of Camel Practice and Research*, *13*(1), 53–57.

Stahl, T., Sallmann, H. P., Duehlmeier, R., & Wernery, U. (2006). Selected vitamins and fatty acid patterns in dromedary milk and colostrums. *Journal of Camel Practice and Research*, *13*(1), 53–57.

Starodubtseva, N. L., Sobolev, V. V., Soboleva, A. G., Nikolaev, A. A., & Bruskin, S. A. (2011). Genes expression of metalloproteinases (MMP-1, MMP-2, MMP-9, and MMP-12) associated with psoriasis. *Russian Journal of Genetics*, *47*(9), 1117–1123. doi:10.1134/S102279541109016X PMID:22117411

Stave, C., & Törner, M. (2007). Exploring the organisational preconditions for occupational accidents in food industry: A qualitative approach. *Safety Science*, *45*(3), 355–371. doi:10.1016/j.ssci.2006.07.001

Steinfeld, H., De Haan, C., & Blackburn, H. (2003). Livestock - Environment Interactions: issues and options. FAO publ.

Stelwagen, K., Carpenter, E., Haigh, B., Hodgkinson, A., & Wheeler, T. T. (2009). Immune components of bovine colostrum and milk. *Journal of Animal Science*, *87*(suppl. 13), 3–9. doi:10.2527/jas.2008-1377 PMID:18952725

Stenberg, M., Marko-Varga, G., & Oste, R. (2002). Enantio separation of D- and L-amino acids by a coupled system consisting of an ion-exchange column and a chiral column and determination of D-aspartic acid and d-glutamic acid in soy products. *Food Chemistry*, *79*(4), 507–512. doi:10.1016/S0308-8146(02)00215-7

Stewart, B. W., & Kleihues, P. (2003). *World cancer report*. Academic Press.

Stiles, N. (1988). Le dromadaire contre l'avancée du désert. *La Recherche*, *201*, 948–952.

Su, X. B. (1988). Camel Raising Science. Agricultural Publishing House.

Su, X.B. (1989). Hair Characters and Ecological Environment of Bactrian Camels in China. *Livestock Ecology*, *4*, 11-13.

Sulieman, A. E., Elamin, O. M., Elkhalifa, E. A., & Laleye, L. (2018). A comparative study of physicochemical properties of freeze-dried camel's milk and cow's milk powder. *Discourse Journal of Agriculture & Food Science*, *6*, 11–16.

Sulieman, A. M. E., Elamin, O. M., Elkhalifa, E. A., & Laleye, L. (2014). Comparison of physicochemical properties of spray-dried camel's milk and cow's milk powder. *International Journal of Food Science and Nutrition Engineering*, *4*(1), 15–19.

Sulieman, A. M., Ilayan, A. A., & Faki, A. E. (2006). Chemical and microbiological quality of *Garris*, Sudanese fermented camel's milk product. *International Journal of Food Science & Technology*, *41*(3), 321–328. doi:10.1111/j.1365-2621.2005.01070.x

Sulieman, A., Elamin, O., Elkhalifa, E., & Laleye, L. (2018). A comparative study of physicochemical properties of freeze-dried camel's milk and cow's milk powder. *Discourse Journal of Agriculture and Food Sciences*, *6*(2), 11–16.

Suliman, G., Sami, A., Alowaimer, A., & Koohmaraie, M. (2011). Effect of breed on the quality attributes of camel meat. *The Indian Journal of Animal Sciences*, *81*, 407–411.

Suliman, S. O., Abdelrahman, S. H., & Khojali, S. M. E. (2013). Effect of Heat Treatment on Some Mineral Status of Camel Milk. *Journal of Animal Science*, *2*, 4–5.

Sulzer, G., & Busse, M. (1991). Growth inhibition of Listeria spp. On Camembert cheese by bacteria producing inhibitory substances. *International Journal of Food Microbiology*, *14*(3), 287–296. doi:10.1016/0168-1605(91)90120-E

Su, X. B. (1987). The histological structure of camel coarse hair and its character analysis. *Acta Veterinaria et Zootechnica Sinica*, *S1*, 52–58.

Swai, E. S., Moshy, W., Mshanga, D., Lutatina, J., & Bwanga, S. (2011). Intestinal parasitic infections of camels in the agro and pastoral areas of northern Tanzania. *Veterinary Research*, *4*, 4–38.

Swatland, H. J. (1984). The structure and properties of meat. In *Structure and Development of Meat Animals* (pp. 153–200). Englewood Cliffs, NJ: INC.

Tagliazucchi, D., Shamsia, S., & Conte, A. (2016). Release of angiotensin converting enzyme-inhibitory peptides during in vitro gastro-intestinal digestion of camel milk. *International Dairy Journal*, *56*, 119–128. doi:10.1016/j.idairyj.2016.01.009

Taheri, A., Abedian Kenari, A. M., Gildberg, A., & Behnam, S. (2009). Extraction and physicochemical characterization of greater lizardfish (*Saurida tumbil*) skin and bone gelatin. *Journal of Food Science*, *74*(3), E160–E165. doi:10.1111/j.1750-3841.2009.01106.x PMID:19397722

Takayama, Y., Mizumachi, K., & Takezawa, T. (2002). The bovine lactoferrin region responsible for promoting the collagen gel contractile activity of human fibroblasts. *Biochemical and Biophysical Research Communications*, *299*(5), 813–817. doi:10.1016/S0006-291X(02)02748-1 PMID:12470651

Tak, L., Bais, B., Singh, R., Singh, S., & Nayak, T. (2018). Assessment of Probiotic and Neutraceutical Properties of Camel Milk Yoghurt. *International Journal of Current Microbiology and Applied Sciences*, *7*(10), 3351–3357. doi:10.20546/ijcmas.2018.710.388

Tamime, A. Y., & McNulty, D. (1999). Kishk—A dried fermented milk / cereal mixture. 4. Microbiological quality. *Le Lait*, *79*(4), 449–456. doi:10.1051/lait:1999437

Tang, S. C., & Yang, J. H. (2018). Dual effects of alpha hydroxy acids on the skin. Molecules, 23(4), 863. doi:10.3390/molecules23040863

Tantawy, E., El-Sayed, G. R., & El-Said, E. S. (2010). Effect of Camel Milk on Oxidative Stresses in Experimentally Induced Diabetic Rabbits. *Veterinary Research Forum: An International Quarterly Journal*, *1*(1), 30–43.

Tas, A. A. (2018). Dietary strategies in autism spectrum disorder (ASD). *Progress in Nutrition*, *20*(4), 554–562.

Tayeb, M. A. F. (1950). La cavité buccale du chameau. *Revue d'Élevage et de Médecine Vétérinaire des Pays Tropicaux*, *4*(3), 157–160. doi:10.19182/remvt.6884

Taylor, S. (1986). Immunological and allergic properties of cows' milk proteins in humans. *Journal of Food Protection*, *49*(3), 239–250. doi:10.4315/0362-028X-49.3.239 PMID:30959730

Tay, T., & Chua, Y. (2015). High temperature short time (HTST) camel milk pasteurization pilot plant. *Journal of Engineering and Applied Sciences (Asian Research Publishing Network)*, *10*(15), 6241–6245.

Temerbayeva, M., Rebezov, M., Okuskhanova, E., Zinina, O., Gorelik, O., Vagapova, O., ... Yessimbekov, Z. (2018). Development of Yogurt from Combination of Goat and Cow Milk. *Annual Research & Review in Biology*, *23*(6), 1–7. doi:10.9734/ARRB/2018/38800

Terefe, M. A., Kebede, A., & Kebede, M. (2017). Clotting Activities of Partially Purified Extracts of *Moringa oleifera L.* on Dromedary Camel Milk. *East African Journal of Sciences*, *11*(2), 117–128.

Tettelin, H., Masignani, V., Cieslewicz, M. J., Eisen, J. A., Peterson, S., & Wessels, M. R., … Fraser, C. M. (2002). Complete genome sequence and comparative genomic analysis of an emerging human pathogen, serotype V Streptococcus agalactiae. *Proceedings of the National Academy of Sciences of the United States of America*, *99*(19), 12391–12396. 10.1073/pnas.182380799

Teuber, M. (2009). Genus II. Lactococcus. In P. De Vos, G. M. Garrity, D. Jones, N. R. Krieg, W. Ludwig, F. A. Rainey, … W. B. Whitman (Eds.), Bergey's manual of systematic bacteriology. The firmicutes (2nd ed.; Vol. 3, pp. 711–722). New York, NY: Springer.

Tewari, D., Stankiewicz, A., Mocan, A., Sah, A., Huminiecki, L., Horba ́nczuk, J. O., & Atanasov, A. G. (2018). Ethnopharmacological approaches for management of dementia and the therapeutic significance of natural products and herbal drugs. *Frontiers in Aging Neuroscience*, *10*, 3. doi:10.3389/fnagi.2018.00003

Thimson, W. J., & Short, A. J. (1965). Resistance of Microorganisms to Hydrostatic Pressure. *Biotechnology and Bioengineering*, *7*(1), 139–159. doi:10.1002/bit.260070124

Thompson, L., Reniers, D., Baker, L., & Siu, M. (1982). Succinylated whey protein concentrates in ice cream and instant puddings. *Journal of Dairy Science*, *66*(8), 1630–1637. doi:10.3168/jds.S0022-0302(83)81985-7

Thum, C., Cookson, A., McNabb, W. C., Roy, N. C., & Otter, D. (2015). Composition and enrichment of caprine milk oligosaccharides from New Zealand Saanen goat cheese whey. *Journal of Food Composition and Analysis*, *42*, 30–37. doi:10.1016/j.jfca.2015.01.022

Tierney, E., Bukelis, I., Thompson, R. E., Ahmed, K., Aneja, A., Kratz, L., & Kelley, R. I. (2006). Abnormalities of cholesterol metabolism in autism spectrum disorders. *American Journal of Medical Genetics. Part B, Neuropsychiatric Genetics*, *141*(6), 666–668. doi:10.1002/ajmg.b.30368 PMID:16874769

Toba, T., Arihara, K., & Adachi, S. (1987). Comparative study of polyssacharide from kefir grains, an encapsuled homofermentative Lactobacillus species and Lactobacillus kefir. *Milchwissenschaf*, *42*, 565–568.

Tomczyk, W. (2016). Camels on the Northeastern Frontier of the Roman Empire. *Papers from the Institute of Archaeology*, *26*(1), 1–13. doi:10.5334/pia-485

Tomonaga, S., Kaneko, K., Kaji, Y., Kido, Y., Denbow, D. M., & Furuse, M. (2006). Dietary β-alanine enhances brain, but not muscle, carnosine and anserine concentrations in broilers. *Animal Science Journal*, *77*(1), 79–86. doi:10.1111/j.1740-0929.2006.00323.x

Topo, E., Soricelli, A., D'Aniello, A., Ronsini, S., & D'Aniello, G. (2009). The role and molecular mechanism of D-aspartic acid in the release and synthesis of LH and testosterone in humans and rats. *Reproductive Biology and Endocrinology*, *7*(1), 120–131. doi:10.1186/1477-7827-7-120 PMID:19860889

Tourette, I., Messad, S., & Faye, B. (2002). Impact des pratiques de traite des éleveurs sur la qualité sanitaire du lait de chamelle en Mauritanie. *Revue d'Élevage et de Médecine Vétérinaire des Pays Tropicaux*, *55*(3), 229–233. doi:10.19182/remvt.9827

Towfik, A. I. (2018). Histological evaluation of camel colostrum extracts effects as a new biological therapy on auricular cartilage defect healing. *Al-Qadisiyah Journal of Veterinary Medicine Sciences*, *17*(2), 17–22. doi:10.29079/vol17iss2art497

Trabelsi, H., Chehma, A., Senoussi, A., & Faye, B. (2012). The Contribution of the dromedary in the spontaneous plant seeds transfer in the northern Algerian Sahara. *Journal of Life Science*, *6*(3), 300–303.

Trujillo, A. J., Capellas, M., Saldo, J., Gervilla, R., & Guamis, B. (2002). Applications of High-Hydrostatic Pressure on Milk and Dairy Products: A Review. *Innovative Food Science & Emerging Technologies*, *4*(4), 295–307. doi:10.1016/S1466-8564(02)00049-8

Trujillo, A. J., Royo, C., Guamis, B., & Ferragut, V. (1999). Influence of Pressurisation on Goat Milk and Cheese Composition and Yield. *Milchwissenschaft. Milk Science International*, *54*, 197–199.

Tsioulpas, A., Grandison, A. S., & Lewis, M. J. (2007). Changes in physical properties of bovine milk from the colostrum period to early lactation. *Journal of Dairy Science*, *90*(11), 5012–5017. doi:10.3168/jds.2007-0192 PMID:17954740

Tsuda, H., Sekine, K., Ushida, Y., Kuhara, T., Takasuka, N., Iigo, M., . . . Moore, M. A. (2000). *Milk and dairy products in cancer prevention: focus on bovine lactoferrin*. doi:10.10161383-5742(00)00040-5

Tsuda, H., & Sekine, K. (2000). Milk components as cancer chemopreventive agents. *Asian Pacific Journal of Cancer Prevention*, *1*(4), 277–282. PMID:12716300

Tumenbayar, E. S. (2015). Mongolian Bactrian camel. Menghe Text Publishing Company.

Tung, Y.-T., Chen, H.-L., Yen, C.-C., Lee, P.-Y., Tsai, H.-C., Lin, M.-F., & Chen, C.-M. (2013). Bovine lactoferrin inhibits lung cancer growth through suppression of both inflammation and expression of vascular endothelial growth factor. *Journal of Dairy Science*, *96*(4), 2095–2106. doi:10.3168/jds.2012-6153 PMID:23462173

Uerpmann, H., & Uerpmann, M. (2002). The appearance of the domestic camel in south-east Arabia. *Journal of Oman Studies*, *12*, 235–260.

Uniacke-Lowea, T., Huppertz, T., & Fox, P. F. (2010). Equine milk proteins: Chemistry, structure and nutritional significance. *International Dairy Journal*, *20*(9), 609–629. doi:10.1016/j.idairyj.2010.02.007

Urashima, T., Fukuda, K., & Messer, M. (2012). Evolution of milk oligosaccharides and lactose: A hypothesis. *Animal*, *6*(3), 369–374. doi:10.1017/S1751731111001248 PMID:22436215

Urashima, T., Kitaoka, M., Asakuma, S., & Messer, M. (2009). Milk oligosaccharides. In P. L. H. McSweeney & P. F. Fox (Eds.), *Advanced Dairy Chemistry. Lactose, Water, Salts and Minor Constituents* (Vol. 3, pp. 295–349). New York, NY: Springer Science Business Media.

Urashima, T., Murata, S., & Nakamura, T. (1997). Structural determination of monosialyltrisaccharides obtained from caprine colostrum. *Comparative Biochemistry and Physiology, 116B*(4), 431–435. doi:10.1016/S0305-0491(96)00269-6 PMID:9149396

Urashima, T., Saito, T., Nakamura, T., & Messer, M. (2001). Oligosaccharides of milk and colostrum in non-human mammals [review]. *Glycoconjugate Journal, 18*(5), 357–371. doi:10.1023/A:1014881913541 PMID:11925504

Uversky, V. N., El-Fakharany, E. M., Abu-Serie, M. M., Almehdar, H. A., & Redwan, E. M. (2017). Divergent anticancer activity of free and formulated camel milk α-lactalbumin. *Cancer Investigation, 35*(9), 610–623. doi:10.1080/07357907.2017.1373783 PMID:28949782

Valko, M., Rhodes, C., Moncol, J., Izakovic, M., & Mazur, M. (2006). Free radicals, metals and antioxidants in oxidative stress-induced cancer. *Chemico-Biological Interactions, 160*(1), 1–40. doi:10.1016/j.cbi.2005.12.009 PMID:16430879

Vandenplas, Y. (2002). Oligosaccharides in infant formula. *British Journal of Nutrition, 87*(S2), S293–S296. doi:10.1079/BJN/2002551 PMID:12088532

Varnam, A. H., & Sutherland, J. P. (1995). *Meat and meat products: technology, chemistry and microbiology*. London: Chapman and Hall.

Vasbinder, A. J., Rollema, H. S., & Kruif, C. G. (2003). Impaired rennetability of heated milk; study of enzymatic hydrolysis and gelation kinetics. *Journal of Dairy Science, 86*(5), 1548–1555. doi:10.3168/jds.S0022-0302(03)73740-0 PMID:12778565

Vazquez-Landaverde, P. A., Qian, M. C., & Torres, J. A. (2007). Kinetic Analysis of Volatile Formation in Milk Subjected to Pressure-Assisted Thermal Treatments. *Journal of Food Science, 72*(7), 389–398. doi:10.1111/j.1750-3841.2007.00469.x PMID:17995641

Vazquez-Landaverde, P. A., Torres, J. A., & Qian, M. C. (2006). Effect of high-pressuremoderate-temperature processing on the volatile profile of milk. *Journal of Agricultural and Food Chemistry, 54*(24), 9184–9192. doi:10.1021/jf061497k PMID:17117808

Vazquez-Landaverde, P. A., Torres, J. A., & Qian, M. C. (2006). Quantification of trace volatile sulfur compounds in milk by solid-phase microextraction and gas chromatography-pulsed flame photometric detection. *Journal of Dairy Science, 89*(8), 2919–2927. doi:10.3168/jds.S0022-0302(06)72564-4 PMID:16840607

Vazquez-Landaverde, P. A., Velazquez, G., Torres, J. A., & Qian, M. C. (2005). Quantitative determination of thermally derived off-flavor compounds in milk using solid-phase microextraction and gas chromatography. *Journal of Dairy Science, 88*(11), 3764–3772. doi:10.3168/jds.S0022-0302(05)73062-9 PMID:16230682

Velioglu Ogunc¸, A., Manukyan, M., Cingi, A., Eksioglu-Demiralp, M., Özdemir Aktan, A. O., & Yalçın, A. S. (2008). Dietary whey supplementation in experimental models of wound healing. *International Journal for Vitamin and Nutrition Research, 78*(2), 70–73. doi:10.1024/0300-9831.78.2.70

Verschoore, M., & Jerajani, H. (2015). Skin aging and antiaging cosmetics. In S. Chakaravarthi & M. Verschoore (Eds.), Basic sciences for modern cosmetic dermatology (pp. 148-161). New Delhi, India: Jaypee Brothers Medical Publishers.

Vessby, B. (2003). Dietary fat, fatty acid composition in plasma and the metabolic syndrome. *Current Opinion in Lipidology, 14*(1), 15–19. doi:10.1097/00041433-200302000-00004 PMID:12544656

Vias, G., Bonfoh, B., Garba, M., Ilou, I., Kamil, H., & Faye, B. (2003). Valorisation du lait de chamelle au Sahel: opération " fromages camélins " dans le Tadsit (Niger) et à Tombouctou (Mali). Séminaire sous-régional " lait sain pour le Sahel ", 24 fev.-3 mars 2003, Bamako. *Etudes et recherches sahéliennes, 8-9*, 39-46.

Vias, G., Faye, B., Kane, Y., Diarra, A., Laouali, G., & Daouda, H. (2006). Performances de reproduction de la femelle dromadaire (*Camelus dromedarius*) dans la zone pastorale de Zinder (Niger). *Revue Africaine de Santé et Productions Animales*, *4*, 111–116.

Vias, G., Ibrahim, Y., Vall, E., & Faye, B. (2004). La traction caméline, un apport important dans l'évolution des pratiques de traction animale au Niger. *Revue d'Élevage et de Médecine Vétérinaire des Pays Tropicaux*, *57*(3-4), 177–179. doi:10.19182/remvt.9888

Vici, G., Belli, L., Biondi, M., & Polzonetti, V. (2016). Gluten free diet and nutrient deficiencies: A review. *Clinical Nutrition (Edinburgh, Lothian)*, *35*(6), 1236–1241. doi:10.1016/j.clnu.2016.05.002 PMID:27211234

Vikas, M., & Farah, Z. (1991). *Manufacture of cheese from camel milk. Report on field studies in Kenya*. ETH Zürich.

Virtanen, T., Pihlanto, A., Akkanen, S., & Korhonen, H. (2007). Development of antioxidant activity in milk whey during fermentation with lactic acid bacteria. *Journal of Applied Microbiology*, *102*(1), 106–115. doi:10.1111/j.1365-2672.2006.03072.x PMID:17184325

Von den Driesch, A., & Obermaier, H. (2007). The hunt for wild dromedaries during the 3rd and 2nd millennia BC on the United Arab Emirates coast. Camel bone finds from the excavations at Al Sufouh 2 Dubai, UAE. In Documenta Archaeobiologiae Bd. 5 – Skeletal series and their socio-economic context (pp. 133-167). Rahden, Germany: Verlag Marie Leidorf GmbH.

Vuyst, L. D., & Leroy, F. (2007). Bacteriocins from Lactic Acid Bacteria: Production, Purification, and Food Applications. *Journal of Molecular Microbiology and Biotechnology*, *13*(4), 194–199. doi:10.1159/000104752

Wakabayashi, H., Yamauchi, K., & Takase, M. (2006). Lactoferrin research, technology and applications. *International Dairy Journal*, *16*(11), 1241–1251. doi:10.1016/j.idairyj.2006.06.013

Wali, A., Yanhua, G., Ishimov, U., Yili, A., Aisa, H. A., & Salikhov, S. (2019). Isolation and Identification of Three Novel Antioxidant Peptides from the Bactrian Camel Milk Hydrolysates. *International Journal of Peptide Research and Therapeutics*, 1–10.

Walstra, P., Wouters, J., & Geurts, T. (2008). Milk for liquid consumption. In Dairy Science and Technology (pp. 421-444). CRC, Taylor & Francis.

Wambui, J. M., Lamuka, P. O., & Njage, P. M. K. (2017). Lactic acid bacteria isolates from fermented camel milk (suusac) are potential protective cultures of raw camel meat. *International Journal of Agriculture and Environmental Research*, *3*, 2960–2975.

Wang, F., Garza, L. A., Kang, S., Varani, J., Orringer, J. S., Fisher, G. J., & Voorhees, J. J. (2007). In Vivo Stimulation of De Novo Collagen Production Caused by Cross-linked Hyaluronic Acid Dermal Filler Injections in Photodamaged Human Skin. *Archives of Dermatology*, *143*(2), 155–163. doi:10.1001/archderm.143.2.155 PMID:17309996

Wang, L., An, X., Yang, F., Xin, Z., Zhao, L., & Hu, Q. (2008). Isolation and characterisation of collagens from the skin, scale and bone of deep-sea redfish (*Sebastes mentella*). *Food Chemistry*, *108*(2), 616–623. doi:10.1016/j.foodchem.2007.11.017 PMID:26059140

Wangoh, J., Farah, Z., & Puhan, Z. (1993). Extraction of camel rennet and its comparison with calf rennet extract. *Milchwissenschaft. Milk Science International*, *48*, 322–325.

Wangoh, J., Farah, Z., & Puhan, Z. (1998). Composition of milk from three camel (camelus dromedarius) breeds in Kenya during lactation. *Milchwissenschaft. Milk Science International*, *53*(3), 136–139.

Wangoh, J., Farah, Z., & Puhan, Z. (1998). Composition of milk from three camel (*Camelus dromedarius*) breeds in Kenya during lactation. *Milchwissenschaft. Milk Science International*, *53*(3), 136–139.

Wang, S. Y., Liang, J. P., Shao, W. J., & Wen, H. (2011). Mineral, vitamin and fatty acid contents in the camel milk of dromedaries in the Anxi Gansu China. *Journal of Camel Practice and Research*, *18*(2), 273–276.

Wanjala, N. W., Matofari, J. W., & Nduko, J. M. (2016). Antimicrobial effect of smoking milk handling containers' inner surfaces as a preservation method in pastoral systems in Kenya. *Pastoralism*, *6*(1), 17. doi:10.118613570-016-0064-y

Warris, P. (1990). The handling of cattle pre-slaughter and its effects on carcass and meat quality. *Applied Animal Behaviour Science*, *28*(1-2), 171–186. doi:10.1016/0168-1591(90)90052-F

Wayua, F. O., Okoth, M. W., & Wangoh, J. (2012). Survey of postharvest handling, preservation and processing practices along the camel milk chain in Isiolo district, Kenya. *African Journal of Food, Agriculture, Nutrition and Development*, 12.

Webb, S. D. (Ed.). (1974). *Pleistocene mammals of Florida*. The University Press of Florida.

Weerathilake, W. A. D. V., Rasika, D. M. D., Ruwanmali, J. K. U., & Munasinghe, M. A. D. D. (2014). The evolution, processing, varieties and health benefits of yogurt. *International Journal of Scientific and Research Publications, 4*(4), 1–10. Retrieved from http://www.ijsrp.org/research-paper-0414/ijsrp-p2855.pdf

Wegmann, M., Santonnat, B., & Lersch, P. (2008). Low molecular weight hyaluronic acid: Its effect on epidermal gene expression and skin aging. *SOFW-Journal*, *134*, 17–22.

Wei, H. F., Yin, Z. C., & Wang, M. Q. (1985). Hair Characteristics and Fiber Types of Bactrian Camels. *Gansu Animal and Veterinary Sciences*, *1*, 10–12.

Wei, S. R., & Wu, J. G. (1983). Analysis of wool Quality of Sunid Bactrian Camel. *Zhongguo Xumu Zazhi*, *3*, 15–17.

Wernery, U. (2003). Novel observations on camel milk. *Proc. 9th Kenya camel forum.*

Wernery, U. (2008). Camel milk-new observations. In *Conference proceedings: International Camel conference. Recent trends in camel research and future strategies for saving camels* (pp. 200-204). Bikaner.

Wernery, R., Joseph, S., Johnson, B., Jose, S., Tesfamariam, M., Ridao-Alonso, M., & Wernery, U. (2012). Camel milk against Autism–A preliminary report. *Journal of Camel Practice and Research*, *19*(2), 143–147.

Wernery, R., & Yagil, R. (2012). Medicinal properties in camel milk for treatment of Epidemic Diseases. *Proceedings of the 3rd ISOCARD International Conference*, 225-227.

Wernery, U. (2006). Camel milk, the white gold of the desert. *Journal of Camel Practice and Research*, *13*(1), 15.

Wernery, U. (2007). Camel milk–new observations. In T.K. Gahlot (Eds.). *Proceedings of the International Camel Conference* (pp: 200-204). CVAS.

Wernery, U., Fischbach, S., Johnson, B., & Jose, S. (2008). Evaluation of alkaline phosphatase (ALP), γ-glutamyl transferase (GGT) and lactoperoxidase (LPO) activities for their suitability as markers of camel milk heat inactivation. *Milchwissenschaft. Milk Science International*, *63*(3), 265–267.

Wernery, U., Hanke, B., Braun, F., & Johnson, B. (2003). The effect of heat treatment on som constituents. Preliminary report. *Milchwissenschaft. Milk Science International*, *58*, 277–279.

Wernery, U., Johnson, B., & Tawfig Ishmail, W. (2006). Insulin content in raw dromedary milk and serum measured over one lactation period. *Journal of Camel Practice and Research*, *13*(2), 89–90.

Wernery, U., Nagy, P., Bhai, I., Schiele, W., & Johnson, B. (2006). The effect of heat treatment, pasteurization and different storage temperatures on insulin concentrations in camel milk. *Milchwissenschaft. Milk Science International, 61*(1), 25–28.

Wheeler, J. C. (2012). South American camelids - past, present and future. *Wheeler. Journal of Camelid Science, 5*, 1–24.

WHO. (2006). *Definition and diagnosis of diabetes mellitus and intermediate hyperglycaemia: report of a WHO/IDF consultation*. WHO.

WHO. (2019). *Estimated incidence, mortality and prevalence worldwide in 2019*. Retrieved January 19, 2019, from http://globocan.iarc.fr/Pages/fact_sheets_cancer.aspx

Wiecek, S., Wos, H., Radziewicz-Winnicki, I., Komraus, M., & Grzybowska-Chlebowczyk, U. (2014). Disaccharidase activity in children with inflammatory bowel. *The Turkish Journal of Gastroenterology, 25*(2), 185–191. doi:10.5152/tjg.2014.3994 PMID:25003680

Wiegand, B. R., Sparks, J. C., Beitz, D. C., Parrish, F. C. Jr, Horst, R. L., Trenkle, A. H., & Ewan, R. C. (2002). Short-term feeding of vitamin D3 improves color but does not change tenderness of pork-loin chops. *Journal of Animal Science, 80*, 2116–2121. PMID:12211380

Wiklund, E., Finstad, G., Johansson, L., Aguiar, G., & Bechtel, P. J. (2008). Carcass composition and yield of Alaskan reindeer (Rangifer tarandus tarandus) steers and effects of electrical stimulation applied during field slaughter on meat quality. *Meat Science, 78*(3), 185–193. doi:10.1016/j.meatsci.2007.06.004 PMID:22062269

Wild, S., Roglic, G., Green, A., Sicree, R., & King, H. (2004). Global prevalence of diabetes—estimates for the year 2000 and projections for 2030. *Diabetes Care, 27*(5), 1047–1053. doi:10.2337/diacare.27.5.1047

Wilhelm, K. P., Cua, A. B., & Maibach, H. I. (1991). Skin aging: Effect on trans-epidermal water loss, stratum corneum hydration, skin surface pH, and casual sebum content. *Archives of Dermatology, 127*(12), 1806–1809. doi:10.1001/archderm.1991.04520010052006 PMID:1845280

Williams, P. (2007). Nutritional composition of red meat. *Nutrition & Dietetics: the Journal of the Dietitians Association of Australia, 64*(s4), S113–S119. doi:10.1111/j.1747-0080.2007.00197.x

Wilson, D. E., & Reeder, D. M. (2005). *Mammal species of the world*. Smithsonian.

Wilson, R. T. (1989). *Ecophysiology of the Camelidae and desert ruminants*. Berlin, Germany: Springer-Verlag. doi:10.1007/978-3-642-74483-9

Wilson, R. T. (2019). The one-humped camel in Bangladesh. *Journal of Camel Practice and Research, 26*(1), 11–13. doi:10.5958/2277-8934.2019.00002.X

Wilson, R. T., & Gutierrez, C. (2015). The one-humped camel in the Canary Islands: History and present status. *Tropicultura, 33*(4), 288–298.

Witzler, J. J. P., Pinto, R. A., Font de Valdez, G., de Castro, A. D., & Cavallini, D. C. U. (2017). Development of a potential probiotic lozenge containing Enterococcus faecium CRL 183. *LWT, 77*, 193–199. doi:10.1016/j.lwt.2016.11.011

Wolf, J. S., Li, D., Taylor, R. J., & O'Malley, B. W. Jr. (2003). Lactoferrin inhibits growth of malignant tumors of the head and neck. *ORL, 65*(5), 245–249. doi:10.1159/000075220 PMID:14730178

Wolfschoon, A. (1997). Influence of calcium chloride addition to milk on the cheese yield. *International Dairy Journal, 7*(4), 249–254. doi:10.1016/S0958-6946(97)00005-8

Wood, J. D., Enser, M., Fisher, A. V., Nute, G. R., Sheard, P. R., Richardson, R. I., ... Whittington, F. M. (2008). Fat deposition, fatty acid composition and meat quality: A review. *Meat Science*, *78*(4), 343–358. doi:10.1016/j.meatsci.2007.07.019 PMID:22062452

Wu, H., Guang, X., Al-Fageeh, M., Cao, J., Pan, S., Zhou, H., . . . Alshanqeeti, A. (2014). Camelid genomes reveal evolution and adaptation to desert environments. *Nature Communications, 5*. Retrieved from https://www.nature.com/articles/ncomms6188

Wullschleger, S., Lacroix, C., Bonfoh, B., Sissoko-Thiam, A., Hugenschmidt, S., & Romanens, E. … Meile, L. (2012). Analysis of lactic acid bacteria communities and their seasonal variations in a spontaneously fermented dairy product (Malian fènè) by applying a cultivation/genotype-based binary model. *International Dairy Journal*. doi:10.1016/j.idairyj.2012.08.001

Wu, Y., Huang, P., Li, Y., Zhang, X. Y., Xu, Z. Z., Wang, B. F., & Shi, J. (2011). Molecular biological identification of lactic acid bacteria in fermented camel milk as a Kazakh traditional food in Xinjiang. *Food Science*, *32*(1), 173–176.

Xu, R., Xiu, L., Zhang, Y., Du, R., & Wang, X. (2019). Probiotic and hepatoprotective activity of lactobacillus isolated from Mongolian camel milk products. *Beneficial Microbes*, 1–12. PMID:31122041

Yadav, A. K., Kumar, R., Priyadarshini, L., & Singh, J. (2015). Composition and medicinal properties of camel milk: A Review. *Asian Journal of Dairy & Food Research*, *34*(2), 83–91. doi:10.5958/0976-0563.2015.00018.4

Yagil, R., Saran, A., & Etzion, Z. (1984). *Camels milk: for drinking only?* Academic Press.

Yagil, R., Zagorski, O., Van Creveld, C., & Saran, A. (1994, October). Science and camel's milk production. In *Actes du Colloque: Dromadaires et chameaux animaux laitier*. Academic Press.

Yagil, R. (1985). *The desert camel: comparative physiological adaptation. In Comparative animal nutrition*. Basel, Germany: Karger.

Yagil, R. (1987). Camel milk - A review. *Farm Animals*, *2*, 81–99.

Yagil, R., & Etzion, Z. (1979). Antidiuretic hormone and aldosterone in the dehydrated and rehydrated camel. *Comparative Biochemistry and Physiology*, *63A*(2), 275–278. doi:10.1016/0300-9629(79)90159-2

Yagil, R., & Etzion, Z. (1980). Effect of drought condition on the quality of camel milk. *The Journal of Dairy Research*, *47*(02), 159–166. doi:10.1017/S0022029900021026

Yagil, R., & Etzion, Z. (1980a). Milk yield of camels (Camelus dromedarius) in drought areas. *Comparative Biochemistry and Physiology. Part A, Physiology*, *67*(1), 207–209. doi:10.1016/0300-9629(80)90433-8

Yahya, M., Alhaj, O. & Al-Khalifah, A. (2017). Antihypertensive effect of fermented skim camel (*Camelus dromedarius*) milk on spontaneously hypertensive rats. *Nutricion hospitalaria: organo oficial de la Sociedad Espanola de Nutricion Parenteral y Enteral*, *34*, 416-421.

Yahya, M. A., Alhaj, O. A., AL-Khalifah, A. S., & Almnaizel, A. T. (2018). Hypocholesterolemic effect of camel milk on rats fed a high-cholesterol diet. *Emirates Journal of Food and Agriculture*, *30*(4), 288–294. doi:10.9755/ejfa.2018.v30.i4.1664

Yamamoto, N., Akino, A., & Takano, T. (1994). Antihypertensive effect of the peptides derived from casein by an extracellular proteinase from Lactobacillus helveticus CP790. *Journal of Dairy Science*, *77*(4), 917–922. doi:10.3168/jds.S0022-0302(94)77026-0 PMID:8201050

Yam, B. A. Z., Khomeiri, M., Mahounak, A. S., & Jafari, S. M. (2014). Hygienic Quality of Camel Milk and Fermented Camel Milk (Chal) in Golestan Province, Iran. *Journal of Microbiology Research (Rosemead, Calif.)*, *4*(2), 98–103.

Yam, B. A., & Khomeiri, M. (2015). Introduction to Camel origin, history, raising, characteristics, and wool, hair and skin: A review. *Research Journal of Agriculture and Environmental Management*, *4*, 496–508.

Yam, B., Khomeiri, M., Mahounak, A., & Jafari, S. (2014). Hygienic quality of camel milk and fermented camel milk (Chal) in Golestan Province, Iran. *Journal of Microbiology Research (Rosemead, Calif.)*, *4*(2), 98–103.

Yang, J., Dou, Z., Peng, X., Wang, H., Shen, T., Liu, J., & Lia, G. Y. G. (2018). Transcriptomics and proteomics analyses of anti-cancer mechanismsof TR35eAn active fraction from Xinjiang Bactrian camel milk inesophageal carcinoma cell. *Clinical Nutrition (Edinburgh, Lothian)*. doi:10.1016/j.clnu.2018.10.013

Yang, W. L., Chen, Y. P., Cheng, Y. F., Li, X. H., Zhang, R. Q., Wen, C., & Zhou, Y. M. (2016). An evaluation of zinc bearing palygorskite inclusion on the growth performance, mineral content, meat quality, and antioxidant status of broilers. *Poultry Science*, *95*(4), 878–885. doi:10.3382/ps/pev445 PMID:26787924

Yang, X.-Y., Chen, J.-P., & Zhang, F.-X. (2009). Research on the chemical composition of Saanen goat colostrum. *International Journal of Dairy Technology*, *62*(4), 500–504. doi:10.1111/j.1471-0307.2009.00515.x

Yassin, M. H., Soliman, M. M., Mostafa, S. A., & Ali, H. A. (2015). Antimicrobial effects of camel milk against some bacterial pathogens. *Journal of Food and Nutrition Research*, *3*(3), 162–168. doi:10.12691/jfnr-3-3-6

Yateem, A., Balba, M. T., Al-Surrayai, T., Al-Mutairi, B., & Al-Daher, R. (2008). Isolation of Lactic Acid Bacteria with Probiotic Potential from Camel Milk. *International Journal of Dairy Science*, *3*(4), 194–199. doi:10.3923/ijds.2008.194.199

Yazdanpanah, N., & Langrish, T. (2011). Fast crystallization of lactose and milk powder in fluidized bed dryer-crystallizer. *Dairy Science & Technology*, *91*(3), 323–340. doi:10.100713594-011-0015-8

Ye, A., Anema, S. G., & Singh, H. (2004). High-Pressure–Induced Interactions between Milk Fat Globule Membrane Proteins and Skim Milk Proteins in Whole Milk. *Journal of Dairy Science*, *7*(12), 4013–4022. doi:10.3168/jds.S0022-0302(04)73542-0 PMID:15545361

Yoganandi, J., Mehta, M. B., Wadhwani, K. N., Darji, V. B., & Aparnathi, K. D. (2014). Comparison of physico-chemical properties of camel milk with cow milk and buffalo milk. *Journal of Camel Practice and Research*, *21*(2), 253–258. doi:10.5958/2277-8934.2014.00045.9

Yokoyama, H., Sawamura, N., & Motobayashi, N. (1992). *Method for accelerating cheese ripening*. European Patent application EP 469 857 (0) A1.

Yorbik, O., Sayal, A., Akay, C., Akbiyik, D., & Sohmen, T. (2002). Investigation of antioxidant enzymes in children with autistic disorder. *Prostaglandins, Leukotrienes, and Essential Fatty Acids*, *67*(5), 341–343. doi:10.1054/plef.2002.0439 PMID:12445495

Younan, M., Bornstein, S., & Gluecks, I. V. (2016). MERS and the dromedary camel trade between Africa and the Middle East. *Tropical Animal Health and Production*, *48*(6), 1277–1282. doi:10.100711250-016-1089-3 PMID:27324244

Yuksekdag, Z. N., Beyatli, Y., & Aslim, B. (2004). Determination of some characteristics coccoid forms of lactic acid bacteria isolated from Turkish kefirs with natural probiotic. *Lebensmittel-Wissenschaft + Technologie*, *37*(6), 663–667. doi:10.1016/j.lwt.2004.02.004

Zafra, O., Fraile, S., Gutiérrez, C., Haro, A., Páez-Espino, A. D., Jiménez, J. I., & De Lorenzo, V. (2011). Monitoring biodegradative enzymes with nanobodies raised in Camelus dromedarius with mixtures of catabolic proteins. *Environmental Microbiology*, *13*(4), 960–974. doi:10.1111/j.1462-2920.2010.02401.x PMID:21219561

Zagorska, J., & Ciprovica, I. (2012). The influence of heat treatment on antimicrobial proteins in milk. *World Academy of Science, Engineering and Technology*, *64*, 832–836.

Zagorski, O., Maman, A., Yafee, A., Meisles, A., Van Creveld, C., & Yagil, R. (1998). Insulin in milk – a comparative study. *International Journal of Animal Science*, *13*, 241–244.

Zagorski, O., Maman, A., Yaffe, A., & Meisler, A., Van creveld, C., & Yagil, R. (1998). Insulin in milk-a comparative study. *International Journal of Animal Sciences*, *13*, 241–244.

Zaharia, N., Salamon, R., Pascal, C., Salamon, S., & Zaharia, R. (2011). Changes in fatty acid composition and cholesterol content of goat colostrum. *Biotechnology in Animal Husbandry*, *27*(3), 1201–1208. doi:10.2298/BAH1103201Z

Zahedi, M., Salami, M., & Moslehishad, M. (2016). Fermented camel milk (Chal): Chemical, microbial and functional properties. *Journal of Pharmaceutical and Health Sciences*, *4*(3), 193–204.

Zahedi, M., Salami, M., & Moslehishad, M. (2016). Fermented Camel Milk (Chal): Chemical, Microbial and Functional Properties. *Journal of Pharmaceutical and Health Sciences*, *4*(3), 193–204.

Zayas, J. F. (1997). Foaming properties of proteins. In J.F. Zayas (Ed.), Functionality of proteins in food (pp. 260-309). Springer - Verlag. doi:10.1007/978-3-642-59116-7_6

Zeina, R. M., Al-Ayadhi, L., & Bashir, S. (2014). Autism spectrum disorder: Main problem waiting for solution in Kingdom of Saudi Arabia. *Autism*, *8*(8), 487–490.

Zeleke, Z. M. (2007). Non-genetic factors affecting milk yield and milk composition of traditionally managed camels (*Camelus dromedarius*) in Eastern Ethiopia. *Livestock Research for Rural Development*, *19*(6), 85. Retrieved from http://www.lrrd.org/lrrd19/6/zele19085.htm

Zhang, B. T. (1984). The property of camel hair. *Journal of China Textile Engineering Association*, *5*, 649–653.

Zhang, H., Yao, J., Zhao, D., Liu, H., Li, M., & Guo, M. (2005). Change in chemical composition of Alxa Bactrian camel milk during lactation. *Journal of Dairy Science*, *88*(10), 3402–3410. doi:10.3168/jds.S0022-0302(05)73024-1 PMID:16162513

Zhang, J. L., Han, X., Shan, Y. J., Zhang, L. W., Du, M., Liu, M., ... Ma, Y. (2018). Effect of bovine lactoferrin and human lactoferrin on the proliferative activity of the osteoblast cell line MC3T3–E1 in vitro. *Journal of Dairy Science*, *101*(3), 1827–1833. doi:10.3168/jds.2017-13161 PMID:29290425

Zhang, L. Y., Wang, J. Q., Yang, Y. X., Bu, D. P., Li, S. S., & Zhou, L. Y. (2011). Comparative proteomic analysis of changes in the bovine whey proteome during the transition from colostrum to milk. *Asian-A Australian Journal Animal Science*, *24*(2), 272–278. doi:10.5713/ajas.2011.10122

Zhang, P. Y., Liu, G. L., & Bai, G. H. (1982). Physical Properties of Bactrian Camel coarse hair. *Zhongguo Xumu Zazhi*, *5*, 23–26.

Zhang, Y., Lima, C. F., & Rodrigues, L. R. (2014). Anticancer effects of lactoferrin: Underlying mechanisms and future trends in cancer therapy. *Nutrition Reviews*, *72*(12), 763–773. doi:10.1111/nure.12155 PMID:25406879

Zhao, D. B., Bai, Y. H., & Niu, Y. B. (2015). Composition and characteristics of Chinese Bactrian camel milk. *Small Ruminant Research*, *127*, 58–67. doi:10.1016/j.smallrumres.2015.04.008

Zhao, J., Unelius, L., Bengtsson, T., Cannon, B., & Nedergaard, J. (1994). Coexisting beta-adrenoceptor subtypes: Significance for thermogenic process in brown fat cells. *American Journal of Physiology. Cell Physiology*, *267*(4), C969–C979. doi:10.1152/ajpcell.1994.267.4.C969 PMID:7943293

Zhao, R. G. T., Bao, H. J., & Ha, S. S. R. (2007). Study on antibacterial activity and its influential factor of lactoferrin in Bactrian camel milk *in vitro. Progress of Veterinary. Medecine in China*, *28*(10), 22–26.

Zhao, S., Zhang, C., Wang, J., Liu, G., Bu, D., Cheng, J., & Zhou, L. (2010). Variations of immunoglobulins in colostrum and immune milk as affected by antigen releasing devices. *Asian-Australasian Journal of Animal Sciences*, *23*(9), 1184–1189. doi:10.5713/ajas.2010.90521

Zibaee, S., Hosseini, S. M. A.-R., Yousefi, M., Taghipour, A., Kiani, M. A., & Noras, M. R. (2015). Nutritional and Therapeutic Characteristics of Camel Milk in Children: A Systematic Review. *Electronic Physician*, *7*(7), 1523–1528. doi:10.19082/1523

Zilhadia, Y., Harahap, Y., Jaswir, I., & Effionora, A. (2018). Characterization and functional properties of gelatin extracted from goatskin. *International Food Research Journal*, *25*(1), 275–281.

Zomborszky, Z., Szentmihalyi, G., Sarudi, I., Horn, P., & Szabo, C. S. (1996). Nutrient composition of muscles in deer and boar. *Journal of Food Science*, *61*(3), 625–627. doi:10.1111/j.1365-2621.1996.tb13172.x

Zottola, E. A., Yezzi, T. L., Ajao, D. B., & Roberts, R. F. (1994). Utilization of cheddar cheese containing nisin as an antimicrobial agent in other foods. *International Journal of Food Microbiology*, *24*(1), 227–238. doi:10.1016/0168-1605(94)90121-X

Zouari, A., Perrone, T., Dolivet, A., Schuck, P., Gaucheron, F., Attia, H., & Ayadi, M. (2018). Physicochemical properties of spray dried camel milk powder: comparative study with cow milk powder. In *EuroDrying'2017 – In 6th European Drying Conference* (p. 19-21). Liège: Belgium: Academic Press.

Zou, X.-Q., Guo, Z., Huang, J.-H., Jin, Q.-Z., Cheong, L.-Z., Wang, X.-G., & Xu, X.-B. (2012). Human milk fat globules from different stages of lactation: A lipid composition analysis and microstructure characterization. *Journal of Agricultural and Food Chemistry*, *60*(29), 7158–7167. doi:10.1021/jf3013597 PMID:22747344

Zubeir, I. (2015). Fluid milk processing and marketing for sustainable development of the camels' herders communities. *SUST Journal of Agricultural and Veterinary Sciences*, *16*(1), 1–13.

Zussman, J., Ahdout, J., & Kim, J. (2010). Vitamin and photoaging: Do scientific data support their use. *Journal of the American Academy of Dermatology*, *63*(3), 507–525. doi:10.1016/j.jaad.2009.07.037 PMID:20189681

About the Contributors

Omar Alhaj has an excellent expertise in Dairy Biotechnology and currently working at University of Petra, Jordan. His Ph.D. and MSc. were awarded from Wales University, United Kingdom. He served as teaching professor and industry consultant at a number of institutions. He has been granted a number of research project funds in his field. He authored over 30 manuscripts and book chapters in reputable journals and publishers, and he served as reviewer for several peer reviewed reputable journals and has a number of international research collaborations worldwide.

Bernard Faye is a veterinarian, specialized in animal husbandry and veterinary medicine in tropical countries, PhD University of Paris XII and HDR (state doctorate) Montpellier University. From 1975 to 1983, work in Africa (Ethiopia, Niger) in research and development before joining the National Institute of Agronomic Research (INRA) as head of the Animal ecopathology Lab. In 1996, in CIRAD (Centre for International Cooperation in agronomic research for development) as head of the animal Productions program. Many research missions in nearly 80 countries. Researches focused on the large camelids (mineral metabolism). Founder and chairman t of the International Society for Research and Development on Camelids (ISOCARD) which organizes triennial conferences. More than 600 scientific papers and reports.

Rajendra Prasad Agrawal did his MBBS in 1983 with University position and top in Medial College and MD in Internal Medicine in 1987 from SP Medical College, Bikaner. He had procured special training in diabetes from UK for a year (1997-1998). He is now Principal & Controller of S.P.Medical College, Bikaner, Sr. Professor & Head, Department of Medicine and also Incharge of Diabetes Care & Research Centre, S P Medical College, Bikaner. At different National and International level his research work has been presented and has been honored by "Juvenile Diabetes Research Foundation (JDRF), European Association for the study of diabetes (EASD) and International Physician Association". Every body knows him by his research on "Role of Camel Milk in Diabetes". He is having more than 120 publications in National and International Journals.

* * *

Issa Al-Amri is currently holding the positions of Director of DARIS Research Center, Associate Professor of Biology, and Assistant Dean at the University of Nizwa, Oman. Previously worked at Sultan Qaboos University as the Director of Electron Microscopy Unit, Department of Pathology, College of Medicine & Health Sciences. Received BSc from Glasgow Caledonian University (UK), MSc from

University of Wales (UK) and PhD from University of Portsmouth (UK). More than 30 years of experience and over 90 publications. Research interests focused on life sciences, reproductive biology, cancer biology, and electron microscopy.

Hiba F. Al-Sayyed is an assistant professor at the Department of Nutrition /Faculty of Pharmacy and Medical Sciences/University of Petra/Amman/Jordan since 2014. She gained her PhD (since 2012), MSc (since 2003), and BSc (since 2000) from the Department of Nutrition and Food Technology/Faculty of Agriculture/The University of Jordan/Amman/Jordan. She aims to spread the science and awareness of nutrition using various tools such as performing related research, nutrition education, counseling, and conducting food analysis. Dr. Hiba is keen in helping people managing their health by having better food choices. She has experience in food analysis (as she was a laboratory technician in the food chemistry laboratories/Jordan Food and Drug Administration for 7 years) and scientific research (as she worked as a research assistant during her PhD studying period). Till date, she has published 13 articles; most of them are related to her PhD thesis on the effect of date palm fruit (Phoenix dactylifera L.) on 7,12-dimethylbenz(α)anthracene-induced mammary cancer in Sprague-Dawley rats. Dr. Hiba is dedicated to scientific research; her research interests are: antioxidants, cancer and especially mammary cancer, and community nutrition issues.

Nour El Sahory, a high energy and results- orientated person, had Doctor of Philosophy in clinical nutrition from Queen's university Belfast (QUB, UK), in 2018 and MSc in nutrition and food technology and the functional food from Jordan University of Science & Technology in 2013. She published her MSc research (effect of lupine flour on baking characteristics of gluten free cookies) and many researches during her PhD such as (association between overall fruit and vegetable intake, and sub-types and blood pressure).

Halima El-Hatmi is an Associate Professor at the High Institute of Applied Biology of Medenine (ISBAM) (University of Gabes, Gabes Tunisia) since 2007. She got a Ph.D. (2007) and Advanced Studies Diploma (2000) from the Faculty of Sciences of Sfax (University of Sfax, Tunisia) and an Engineering diploma (1995) in Food Technology from the National School of Engineers of Sfax (University of Sfax, Tunisia). She was the head of Food Technology Department from 2008 to 2011 at the ISBAM. Since 2011, her main achievements in the field of teaching activities are related to the PAQ (Plan d'amélioration de la Qualité dans l'Enseignement Supérieur, Improvement of the Quality of Higher Education in Tunisia Prject. She was the leader of this project for ISBAM entitled "Improvement of the Quality of Practical Teaching in agri-food". This project allowed the implementation of a Foods Technology platform with equipments adapted for practical courses. Within the framework of this project, a congress in 2014 (April 25-27 "AgroInnov: Technologies innovantes pour la production alimentaire (Innovative technologies for food manufacturing") was organized with continuing education courses regarding quality management in the food sector in order to get complementary ressources. Shis research topics and skills are mainly bioactive peptides derived from milk proteins, biochemistry and physico-chemistry of dairy products (mainly camel milk) and valorization of traditional ressources. She supervised 02 PhD (Supervisor or co-supervisor); 05 Students preparing Fundamental master, 03 engineers, more than 40 students preparing applied master and applied Licenses. She participated to research projects as coordinator or as a member (PROCAMED Cod. I-B/1.1/493: Promotion of innovative camel systems and local sectors for sustainable management of Saharan territories (2013-2015) and ARIMNET (AROMATIC: Natural Bioactive Molecules for Safe and Sustainable dairy Products (2018-2020)). She participated to 01 Erasmus+KA2 Project (SPAAT4FOOD). She published 16 Scientific articles in international journals with Impact Factor.

MoezAlIslam Faris got his three higher university degrees from the University of Jordan in the field of human nutrition. Recently, Dr. Faris has been completed Harvard Medical School/Global Clinical Scholar Research Training (GCSRT) Program. Dr. Faris works now as an associate professor the Department of Clinical Nutrition and Dietetics/the University of Sharjah, with seventeen years' experience in the academic field in four Arabian universities. Dr. Faris published more than 50 original research and review articles in scientific peer-reviewed journals and conference proceedings and abstracts, with dozens of public articles in popular magazines in different Arab countries. Dr. Faris is a an author and co-author in a list of scientific and academic refereed books and participated in editing and reviewing a number of important Arabic books in nutrition. Dr. Faris is a member and a founder of a number of associations and professional societies and specialized committees and editorial member of a number of journals.

Yonas Hailu has an MSc and PhD in dairy foods. He is an expert in dairy food chemistry and processing technologies and have been working in these areas for many years. He has worked on milk gelation, cheese maturation, proteolysis, peptide analysis, membrane filtration, drying and concentration of milk proteins, protein analysis, HPLC, milk powder analysis, sensory evaluation, aroma analysis. Currently, working on developing next generation Infant formula. His main area focus are dairy ingredient processing and new product development. Yonas has authored and co-authored more than seventeen articles in reputable journals and presented his findings in international conferences.

Surong Hasi is specialized in the research field of veterinary pharmacology and toxicology at the College of Veterinary Medicine, Inner Mongolia Agricultural University (IMAU). In 2004, he was awarded PhD degree on veterinary parasitology from China Agricultural University (CAU). He worked as post-doc at Leuven University, Belgium (2007.10-2008.10). Professor Hasi also worked as a visiting scholar at Paris LCH laboratory (2012.12-2013.3) and at Texas A & M University (2016.2-2016.8). He is the director of the Camel Protection Association of Inner Mongolia (2013-present). His research interests focus on parasitic diseases of domestic ruminants, drug-drug interactions and pharmacokinetics of drugs, bioinformatics.

Irwandi Jaswir has been known as a "Halal" Scientist. He contributes to the Muslim Ummah and serves to Islam through his tireless and never-ending studies on the scientific halal-related issues and return the findings back to the Community through research publications, books, book chapters, halal-related training, education, community services, etc. He believes "Halal Science", which includes halal materials as alternative for non halal materials and ingredients, halal authentications, development of rapid method for non-halal contamination, halal food and cosmetics, development of halal standard, etc., will not only the key element to protect the Muslims from consuming modern consumer products which are much more complex and very prone to non-halal contamination, but also the important component required to build the halal industry that can contribute to economy of Muslim Ummah. The market of halal industry nowadays is expected to be USD 2.5 trillion, unfortunately Muslims do not play their important roles and do not enjoy the huge market yet. He is the 2018 King Faisal International Prize

Laureate in Service to Islam. His commitment in conducting quality researches, coupled with a strong determination to publish quality research papers have a strong encouragement by his University, IIUM. Prof. Irwandi has completed more than 30 research studies, mostly in the area halal food science. Among the topics he researches are: Determination of non-halal substances in food using FTIR; Development of Halal Gelatin from various alternative sources; Development of Halal Nano-Particles from Camel Gelatin (Funded by Saudi Arabia); Portable Electronic Nose f or Rapid Detection of Lard and Alcohol in Food and Beverages; Anti-Cancer Compounds from Local Sources, etc. These research projects are funded from various funding agency such as the Ministry of Education (MOE), Ministry of Science, Technology and Innovation (MOSTI), Malaysia and National Plans for Science and Technology (NPST), Kingdom of Saudi Arabia. He also received research grants from Republic of Korea and Japan. To date, Irwandi's has chalked up a remarkable achievement in research which include: more than 180 scientific papers published in reputable international journals; contributed to 40 book-chapters; presented more than 250 research papers in international conferences – including keynote address and invited lectures; written more than 30 non-refereed and mass-media scientific articles. His dedication to research has enabled him to file 5 patents under his name, and his outstanding achievement is recognised both locally and internationally bagging more 60 scientific awards. Most importantly, his outstanding dedication and commitment in research has placed him in the same rank of other renowned scientist with the inclusion of his name in the annual publication of the "Who's Who in the World 2008." His name is also included in the book "25 Great Indonesian Scientist Abroad" to be published by the Indonesian Government. His current H-index is 24 with 1882 citations (Google Scholar), showing his high credibility as a renown scholars.

Zeineb Jrad (F) received his Ph.D. in Biological Sciences and Biotechnology from the Higher Institute of Biotechnology at Monastir in 2015. She is a Postdoctoral Fellow in the MOBIDOC Program (Device funded by the European Union under the Support Program for Education, Mobility, Research and Innovation). She works in collaboration between a social-economic organization specializing in the dairy industry "General Creamery", a research center "Laboratory of wildlife and livestock of the Institute of arid regions of Medenine "and" the technology hall of the Higher Institute of Applied Biology of Medenine, University of Gabes". Shis research interests include: (i) - Development of an innovative product based on camel milk on an industrial scale and approve its health value as a partial substitution for fresh milk currently marketed. (ii) Development of selected simple and effecient methods using natural and safe antimicrobials and antioxidants, notably some traditionnaly used for ancestarl dairy products, to better protect dromedary and goat raw milk from microbial contamination. She co-supervised 04 students preparing fundamental master, 01 engineer and supervised 10 students preparing applied master and liscences. She participated as a member of research project (i) PROCAMED: Promotion of innovative camel systems and local sectors for sustainable management of Saharan territories (2013-2015) (ii) ARIMNET: AROMATIC- Natural bioactive molecules for safe and substainable dairy products (2018-2020) AND (iii) PRIMA 2018-2020 (ArtiSaneFood: Innovative Bio-interventions and Risk Modelling Approaches for Ensuring Microbial Safety and Quality of Mediterranean Artisanal Fermented Foods) . She published 10 scientific articles in international journals with Impact Factor, 02 scientific articles in indexed journals and 03 publication in national journal. She participated in 10 national and international congress and 15 workshops and training courses.

Isam Kadim (Meat Scientists) Department of Biology Sciences and Chemistry College of Arts and Sciences University of Nizwa Nizwa, Sultanate of Oman BSC and MSC from Mosul University- Iraq PhD Massey University – New Zealand (1988) He has more than 33 years teaching experience at four different international institutes. He supervised many Master and PhD students. He published more than 120 refereed papers, 3 books and 17 book chapters and presented 95 papers at both national and international conferences. He obtained funding grants for 16 research projects (1,300,000 USD). He published many articles regarding health aspects of meat and safety and quality of various meat and meat products. He published two books on camel meat.

Dasel Wambua Mulwa Kaindi is a Lecturer at the Department of Food Science, Nutrition and Technology, University of Nairobi.

Touhami Khorchani is a Professor at Livestock and Wildlife Laboratory, Arid Lands Institute of Medenine (Tunisia).

Gaukhar Konuspayeva is a Professor at biological faculty of Al Farabi Kazakh National University (KazNU, Almaty, Kazakhstan). She graduated university at 2002 at KazNU (Kazakhstan), She achieved her doctorate at Montpellier-II University (France) in 2007 on Food Sciences. Title of dissertation is "Physico-chemical and biochemical variability of milk of large Camelidae (Camelus bactrianus, Camelus dromedaries and hybrids) in Kazakhstan". She participated to many camel conferences and workshops (Turkmenistan, India, Niger, Emirates, Senegal, Bolivia, Morocco, Oman…). From 2010 to 2015, she was camel expert at FAO camel project at Al-Jouf and Al-Kharj (Saudi Arabia). She is author of 175 scientific papers and achieved expertises for FAO (Morocco, Mauritania, Kazakhstan) or private companies (Tunisia, Algeria) in camel dairy sector.

Widya Lestari is an Assistant Professor at Oral Biology, Fundamental Dental and Medical Science Department, Kulliyyah of Dentistry, International Islamic University Malaysia. She received her Bachelor's degree in Dentistry in 2002. She conferred a Master in Oral Traumatology in 2011 at University of Malaya and a PhD in 2012 in Molecular Biology at Tokyo Medical and Dental University, Japan. She is currently the Head of Research at her faculty and her research of interests include molecular craniofacial and genetic, halal dental materials, biomaterials and clinical dentistry. She is currently leading a research project entitled " Physicochemical Characterization, In Vitro and In Vivo Evaluations of Chitosan Enriched with Sea Cucumber Extract Hydrogel as Dental Haemostatic Agent where her team is working to provide an halal dental material.

Msafiri Mbaga is an Associate Professor in the Department of Natural Resource Economics at Sultan Qaboos University. He received his B.Sc. degree from Tanzania and obtained both his M.Sc. and Ph.D. from the University of Manitoba, Canada. He worked as a postdoctoral research fellow at Laval University in Quebec Canada, thereafter at the World Bank Headquarters in Washington DC. In 2005 Dr. Mbaga joined the Agriculture and Agri-Food Canada in Ottawa as a Senior Economist. Dr. Mbaga has 25 years of experience in teaching and research and has published extensively in reputable academic journals. Over the years, he has supervised a number of M.Sc. and PhD students and garnered more than US$195,000 in research funding.

(Rajesh Mehta - Contributing Author) Senior Professor & Head, Deaprtment of Skin & VD, S. P. Medical College, Bikaner, Rajasthan.

Ali Ahmed Mohamed Metwalli is a Professor in Dairy chemistry and Microbiology Department of Dairy Science; College of Agriculture, Minia University, Egypt.

Ikhlas Nour is an Associate professor, Director of Institute for Studies and Promotion of Animal Exports University of Khartoum Sudan, Ph. D: Animal Production, University of Khartoum, M.VSc University of Khartoum, Sudan, BVSc Faculty of Veterinary Science, University of Khartoum. Staff member of the Department of Meat Production, Faculty of Animal Production University of Khartoum, Supervising post graduate students, conducting research in meat science and technology and meat production, teaching courses for under and post graduate students, member of Scientific Committees, Member of Board of Directors, Institute for Studies and Promotion of Animal Exports, Member of the Faculty of Animal Production Faculty Board and Research Council, Member of the Senate.

Fitri Octavianti completed her Bachelor of Dental Surgery from North Sumatera University, Indonesia and Master in Clinical Dentistry (Orthodontics) from Padjadjaran University, Indonesia. She has served as Senior Lecturer in the Faculty of Dentistry from Universiti Sains Islam Malaysia (USIM) several years before opting to focus on her clinical practices in orthodontics. She is an active active researcher in the area of dentistry, dental materials, and orthodontics, and lately conducting research in shari'a compliant dentistry. She published a number of article in dentistry in various international journals.

Olfa Oussaief is a PhD Student at Livestock and Wildlife Laboratory, Arid Lands Institute of Medenine (Tunisia).

Wenbin Zhang worked as researcher in Bactrian Camel Institute of Alxa, Inner Mongolia.

Index

A

B

C

D

E

F

G

H

I

L

M

N

O

P

www.ingramcontent.com/pod-product-compliance
Lightning Source LLC
LaVergne TN
LVHW080531300926
849162LV00007B/1583